Risk Management Handbook for Healthcare Organizations

Risk Management Handbook for Healthcare Organizations

Sixth Edition

VOLUME 2

Clinical Risk Management

Roberta Carroll, Series Editor
Sylvia M. Brown, Volume Editor

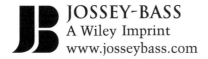

JOSSEY-BASS
A Wiley Imprint
www.josseybass.com

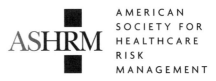

ASHRM

AMERICAN
SOCIETY FOR
HEALTHCARE
RISK
MANAGEMENT

Library of Congress Cataloging-in-Publication Data

Risk management handbook for healthcare organizations / Roberta Carroll, series editor. – 6th ed.
    p. ; cm.
    Includes bibliographical references and indexes.
    ISBN 978-0-470-62080-9 (set) – ISBN 978-0-470-62081-6 (v. 1 : cloth) – ISBN 978-0-470-62082-3 (v. 2 : cloth) – ISBN 978-0-470-62083-0 (v. 3 : cloth)
    1. Health facilities—Risk management.   I. Carroll, Roberta.
    [DNLM: 1. Health Facilities—organization & administration.   2. Risk Management.   3. Health Facilities—economics. WX 157 R59532 2010]
    RA971.38.R58 2010
    362.11068—dc22

2010017899

Printed in the United States of America

SIXTH EDITION
HB Printing   10 9 8 7 6 5 4 3 2 1

Contents

List of Boxes, Exhibits, Figures, Tables, and Appendices

EXHIBITS

FIGURES

TABLES

BOXES

APPENDICES

The Contributors

Joyce H. Benton, RN, MSA, ARM, CPHRM, DFASHRM, LHRM, is Risk control director for CNA HealthPro. Previously, Benton served as the director of quality management and safety at Henry General Hospital, an acute care hospital in the suburbs of Atlanta. In that role, she developed the risk management and infection control programs and assisted in restructuring the safety, workers' compensation, and quality improvement programs at the facility. Benton began her career as a registered nurse in surgical pediatrics at Grady Memorial Hospital in Atlanta and newborn nursery and childbirth education at Henry General Hospital. Benton is an active member of the American Society for Healthcare Risk Management (ASHRM), served on ASHRM's 2003–2004 board of directors, and is also an active member of the Georgia Society for Healthcare Risk Management and North Carolina ASHRM. She was awarded the Fellow designation (FASHRM) from ASHRM in 1992, and the Distinguished Fellow designation (DFASHRM) in 1998. Benton completed ASHRM's Healthcare Risk Management Certificate Program in 1996. She also received the certified professional in healthcare risk management (CPHRM) designation from ASHRM in 2000. Benton was the recipient of ASHRM's Excellence in Writing Award in 1999. In 2005, Benton was awarded ASHRM's highest honor, the Distinguished Service Award (DSA). In addition. Benton received the 1995–1996 Georgia Healthcare Risk Manager of the Year Award, the 2002 Distinguished Service Award for outstanding contributions in the advancement of the profession of risk management and service to the Georgia Society for Healthcare Risk Management (GSHRM), and the 2004 GSHRM Lifetime Achievement Award. Benton is a frequent speaker on healthcare risk management topics at the local, state, and national level, and she has written several articles. She was a contributing author to the fourth edition of the *Risk Management Handbook*. She has served as faculty for ASHRM's Healthcare Risk Management Certificate Program, CPHRM study course, and Insurance 101 program.

Sylvia M. Brown, RN, JD, is vice president, risk management Premier Insurance Management Services. Brown received her baccalaureate degree in English and nursing from Stanford University and a juris doctorate degree from The Washington College of Law at the American University. She has more than twenty-five years of experience in healthcare risk management. Her accomplishments include development of a total quality management program for a one hundred-hospital system, presentation of numerous education programs to clients, implementation of an international newsletter, and numerous ASHRM publications. She also worked with the Virginia Hospital Association to develop and implement risk management education seminars for hospital boards of directors. As the vice president of risk management for Premier Insurance Management Services, Brown provides a variety of risk management services to Premier members, including seminars, newsletters, and Web site resources.

Robert F. Bunting, Jr., MT (ASCP), MSA, DFASHRM, CPHRM, CPHQ, is clinical research manager for WellPoint, the nation's leading health benefits company. Bunting received clinical training as a laboratory scientist. His bachelor of science in medical technology and master of science in administration in healthcare degrees were awarded by Columbus State University in Columbus, Georgia. He has more than twenty years of healthcare experience, including ten years as the director of quality and risk management for a comprehensive healthcare system. He was the instructor of a graduate school risk management course for more than ten years. He has written several healthcare books and articles, and since 2002 he has served on the editorial board of the *Journal of Nursing Risk Management*, published by the Armed Forces Institute of Pathology. He is a frequent speaker on the state and national levels. He is a past president (1994–1995) of the Georgia Society for Healthcare Risk Management (GSHRM), and he received GSHRM's 1996–1997 Risk Manager of the Year Award. He served as chair of ASHRM's Certification Education Task Force in 1999–2001 and 2002–2003. He has been the editor of ASHRM's *A Study Guide for the Certified Professional in Healthcare Risk Management (CPHRM) Examination* since its inception. Bunting earned the Distinguished Fellow of the American Society for Healthcare Risk Management (DFASHRM) designation in 1998, won ASHRM's Excellence in Writing Award in 1999, earned his CPHRM designation in 2000, and received GSHRM's first Distinguished Service Award in 2001. He was awarded ASHRM's Distinguished Service Award in 2003.

Robin Burroughs, RN, CHRM, CPHRM, is risk control consulting director with CNA HealthPro, based in their New York City regional offices. She has been with CNA since 1995. Burroughs is responsible for providing risk management consulting services to the healthcare industry. While at CNA HealthPro, in addition to providing direct client consulting services, Burroughs has participated in the analysis of claims, including the long-term care claims studies and nurse practitioner claims study published by CNA HealthPro. In addition to coauthoring the chapter in the American Society of Healthcare Risk Management's *Risk Management Handbook, Risk Management for Behavioral Health*, along with a self-assessment checklist for facilities, she published an article on fall prevention that appeared in the May 2, 2005, edition of AAHSA's *Weekly Perspective*. Before joining CNA HealthPro, Burroughs was acting assistant vice president, quality management, and corporate risk manager for New York City's public healthcare system, Health and Hospitals Corporation (HHC). Before joining the New York City HHC, she was assistant vice president, risk management, for Interfaith Medical Center, another multihospital integrated healthcare delivery system in New York City. Burroughs is a registered nurse and a graduate of the Buffalo General Hospital School of Nursing, Her clinical and administrative nursing experience includes medical, oncology research, geriatric, and psychiatric specialties. She has also consulted to several New York City law firms in the assessment and investigation of medical malpractice and negligence cases. Burroughs also attended the State University of New York at Buffalo and D'Youville College. She is a graduate of the Institute of Medical Law, where she earned certification as a HealthCare Risk Manager (CHRM). She has achieved ASHRM designation as a Certified Professional HealthCare Risk Manager (CPHRM), and is licensed in Texas as a Field Safety Representative with a Specialty in Hospitals, and a Loss Control Representative for General Liability, Professional Liability, Commercial, and Auto. Burroughs is a member of the adjunct faculty of New York University's School of Professional and Continuing Education.

Christine L. Clark, MT (ASCP), JD, CPHRM, is director of risk management at Resurrection West Suburban Medical Center in Oak Park, Illinois. She has held several positions in claims and risk management and has quality- and performance-improvement experience in various healthcare settings, including academic hospitals, community hospitals, insurance companies, and the College of American Pathologists. She is a medical technologist with thirteen years of clinical experience in hospital and reference laboratories and was formerly a paramedic on a municipal fire department. She has published several articles on healthcare regulation, home healthcare, claims management, and patient safety–related topics. She serves on the ASHRM Journal Task Force and Pearls Task Force. Clark has also served as chair of the ASHRM Nominating Committee and the On-Line Education Task Force and as a member of the Safety/Security Special Interest Group, Video Education Task Force, and the Bloodborne Pathogens Task Force. She is currently treasurer of the Chicagoland Healthcare Risk Management Society and has served on the Executive Board, the Bylaws Committee, and as chair of the Program Committee. She has also chaired the Health Law Committee for the Women's Bar Association of Illinois, served on various Chicago Bar Association committees and the Chicago Area Nurse Attorneys' Association. She holds a bachelor of science degree in medical technology from Eastern Illinois University and a juris doctor degree from Loyola University Chicago School of Law. Clark is an Illinois licensed attorney. She also holds a Healthcare Leadership Certificate through Loyola University's School of Business Administration.

Hedy Cohen, RN, BSN, MS, is vice president for the institute for safe medication practices (ISMP) She received an associate of arts in nursing from Bucks County Community College in Newtown, Pennsylvania, a BSN from LaSalle University in Philadelphia, a master's degree in health systems administration from Rochester Institute for Technology in Rochester, New York, and is presently is a PhD candidate in health policy at the University of the Sciences in Philadelphia. Her clinical nursing background of more than eighteen years was focused in critical care and nursing management. She is a frequent speaker for healthcare organizations on current issues in medication safety and has written numerous articles on improving the medication-use process. She also edits ISMPs monthly newsletter *Nurse Advise-ERR*, cowrote a handbook on high-alert drugs, and is on the National Advisory Board for the *Nursing Advance Journal* and *Davis's Drug Guide for Nurses*. Cohen has been appointed adjunct associate professor at Temple School of Pharmacy and Faculty Fellow in the Executive Patient Safety Fellowship, which is offered through Virginia Commonwealth University in Richmond. She also serves as a medication error clinical analyst for the Pennsylvania Safety Authority's reporting program.

Roslyn M. Corcoran, RN MSN, is director of patient safety and clinical performance improvement at Barnes-Jewish Hospital. She directs and manages the hospital Patient Safety / Risk Management Program, medical staff office, GME Program, and the quality and compliance programs at Barnes-Jewish Hospital. She is providing interim coverage for the vice president of safety and quality and is accountable for administrative oversight for the Patient Safety and Quality Department and programs. She is accountable for organizational strategic goals and initiatives related to the Exceptional Patient Care experience. In addition to staff and budget responsibilities, she assumed interim oversight of Infection Prevention Department and Performance Measurement Department. Corcoran has oversight for data review, education, and monitoring of safety strategies, including risk identification and exposure, and coordinates investigation and defense with BJC System Risk Management. She also has oversight for the medical staff and allied health professional credentialing and peer reviews. The Quality and Compliance Department has oversight of state/CMS/The Joint Commission compliance for the organization as well as clinical quality support for the organization. She has worked at BJH for twenty-three years and has a background in critical care nursing. Previous positions include critical care manager, house supervisor, and manager of quality and compliance. She is a graduate of the Barnes School of Nursing in St. Louis, Missouri and received her BSN and MSN from the Barnes-Jewish College of Nursing in St. Louis.

Mary Lynn Curran, RN, MS, CPHRM, FASHRM, is the vice president of clinical risk management for Willis North America, Chicago, Illinois. Curran was with Thilman Filippini (TF) when Willis purchased the firm in 2008. Curran has been working in the healthcare risk management field as a consultant to healthcare organizations and insurance companies for many years. Her background includes nursing practice in acute, postacute, and clinical settings. Currently, Curran works with Willis's clients in the seniors housing and long-term care industry on risk and safety programs. Curran served on the executive board of Chicagoland Healthcare Risk Management Society (CHRMS) in 2002–2004 and 2006–2008 and on various committees, including bylaws, program, publications, and membership committees. Curran is a contributing author to *Assisted Living Executive* as well as publications of CHRMS and ASHRM. Curran contributed to the fourth and fifth editions of ASHRM's *Risk Management Handbook for Health Care Organizations*. Curran earned her nursing degree from St. Francis Hospital School of Nursing, Evanston, Illinois, and her bachelor's degree in science and master's degree in healthcare administration from the University of St. Francis, Joliet, Illinois. She earned the designation of Certification in Professional Healthcare Risk Management (CPHRM) in 2002, 2005, and 2008. She was awarded the designation of Fellow from the American Society of Healthcare

Risk Management (FASHRM) in 2005 and Chicagoland Healthcare Risk Management Society's Lifetime Achievement Award in 2008. Curran was also with AIG Consulting Inc.–Healthcare Management Division, Chicago, Illinois, where she worked as risk consultant to hospitals, long-term care organizations, and miscellaneous healthcare facilities. She also worked with Premier, Inc., Chicago, Illinois, in the insurance division and hospital relations division.

Bruce Dmytrow, BS, MBA, CPHRM, is vice president, CNA HealthPro, for Chicago-based CNA. He has been with CNA since 1995. Dmytrow is responsible for leading the risk management business unit of CNA HealthPro. The business unit comprises a group of consultants with diverse backgrounds who provide risk management consulting services to healthcare clients. Clients include hospitals, medical group practices, long-term care facilities, advanced medical technology companies, allied healthcare facilities, risk retention groups, and captive insurance companies. Before joining CNA, Dmytrow was a manager and healthcare consultant at MMI Companies, Inc. and Bio-Med Associates. Before his career in the insurance industry, Dmytrow served as a clinician at the University of Chicago Hospitals and Northwestern Memorial Hospital. Within the profession, Dmytrow provides education programs to healthcare professionals and participates in panel discussions for major insurance and healthcare-related associations. He is widely published and often quoted in industry journals. Dmytrow serves as an active member on several healthcare organization boards of directors and advisory boards. Dmytrow graduated cum laude from Boston College with a bachelor of science degree. He received a postgraduate degree in medical dosimetry from Yale University Medical School/Yale–New Haven Hospital and a master of business administration degree in entrepreneurship, with highest distinction, from DePaul University in Chicago.

Alice Epstein, LHRM, CPHQ, CPHRM, is risk control consulting director with CNA HealthPro. She holds a master's degree in hospital and healthcare administration from the University of Alabama in Birmingham. She holds the following honorary designations: Fellow of the National Association of HealthCare Quality and Distinguished Fellow of the American Society of Healthcare Risk Management. Epstein has received the following professional certifications and licenses: Certified Professional in Healthcare Risk Management from the American Society for Healthcare Risk Management, Certified Professional in Healthcare Quality from the Healthcare Quality Professional Board, Certified Professional Environmental Auditor from the Health & Safety, Board of Environmental Auditing, Field Safety Representative with Specialty in Hospitals for the State of Texas, Loss Control Representative for Commercial Auto, General Liability and Professional Liability for the State of Texas, Licensed Health Care Risk Manager for the State of Florida, and continuing education insurance instructor for the South Carolina Department of Insurance.

Asheesh Gupta, MBA, vice president Audax Management Company, LLC, a $4 billion middle-market private equity firm helping management teams add value in Boston, Massachusettes, has over twelve years of business strategy and management consulting experience focused on operations management. He has led projects to reduce costs through improved operations, grow revenue through marketing spend optimization, and focused management efforts through performance scorecards. He has worked in the high-tech manufacturing, food processing, ink manufacturing, consumer packaged goods, and healthcare services industries. Previously he served as the director of supply chain management as well as the director of the internal performance improvement consulting team at Dartmouth-Hitchcock Medical Center. Prior to entering the healthcare industry Gupta worked for Computer Sciences Corporation as a senior consultant in the SAP practice and with Andersen Consulting (now Accenture) prior to that. He has been involved with numerous SAP implementations with a focus on materials management and production planning. He has taught graduate school courses in healthcare service operations management. Gupta served as a Malcolm Baldrige National Quality Award (MBNQA) auditor in 2006, 2007, and 2009 and is an ASQ–certified quality engineer. He received an MBA from the Tuck School of Business at Dartmouth College and a BS in mechanical engineering from Carnegie Mellon University with University Honors.

Gary Harding, BS, is director of technical services for Greener Pastures, LLC and a career professional biomedical engineer. He received a magna cum laude biomedical engineering technology degree from Temple University College of Engineering and has postgraduate experience in law and social policy. He has direct experience in medical device and healthcare worker safety while a senior consultant and senior project engineer at ECRI, the manager of the National Clinical Risk Management program for Johnson & Higgins, and a national practice manager in the Health Care Risk Advisory Services of Laventhol & Horwath. Harding has reviewed, discussed, and published articles on such subjects as back injury, accidental needlesticks, exposure to hazardous materials, emergency medical systems, risk management, laser technology, and the evaluation of medical devices. He is experienced in reviewing and analyzing healthcare policies and procedures for a wide range of medical clients, including medical device manufacturers, acute and chronic care facilities, insurers, and psychiatric services. He is well experienced in OSHA requirements related to bloodborne pathogens. He has provided accident investigation and expert witness services throughout the country related to medical device–acquired infections and injuries for healthcare workers and others such as sanitation workers, police, and firefighters, and for several high technology and other devices. He has discussed methods to perform such investigations and methods to use to procure safer products.

Susan W. Harris, RN, MBA, is the director of perioperative, bariatric, and endoscopy services at Dekalb Medical in Decatur, Georgia, a suburb of Atlanta. Susan has worked in the operating room for over thirty years and has been director of perioperative services for the past twenty years. She is a member of the Association of Operating Room Nurses and has served as a board member of the Georgia Organization of Nurse Executives. She is currently a board member of the Dekalb Surgical Associates, a local physician joint venture. Susan has served as the chair of the Safety Committee at Dekalb Medical and has participated in many safety and risk initiatives. Ms. Harris has served as a member of the Information Technology Steering Committee and currently sits on the Infection Control Committee. She has designed and opened two surgery centers and developed a surgical weight loss center that received a Center of Excellence status from the Surgical Review Corporation. Susan has been the hospital's team leader for The Joint Commission's Operative and Invasive Standards for the past ten years. In addition to her position at Dekalb Medical, Susan also provides consulting services for Operations Solutions for Healthcare, Inc. She attended nursing school at Polk College School of Nursing in Winter Haven, Florida, and she received her MBA from Kennestone State University in Marietta, Georgia.

Kathryn Hyer, PhD, MPP, is associate professor in the School of Aging Studies at the University of South Florida and director of the Training Academy on Aging, a program sponsored by the university to promote geriatric and gerontological training for health-care professionals. Hyer is a nationally recognized leader in geriatric and gerontological education and holds joint faculty appointments in The College of Public Health's Health Policy and Management Department and the Division of Geriatric Medicine in the College of Medicine. Hyer played a key role in Florida's Nursing Home Reform Bill of 2001, the legislation that mandates all Florida nursing homes to report adverse incidents and create risk management programs. She is the course director for a state-approved licensed healthcare risk management program that emphasizes risk management in long-term care. Hyer holds a masters degree in public policy from the Kennedy School of Government at Harvard University and doctorate in public administration from Arizona State University. She is a member of ASHRM, Gerontological Society of America, American Geriatrics Society, a Fellow in the Association for Gerontology in Higher Education, has testified before the Federal Physician Payment Review Commission, and has contributed more than forty publications to the literature in the fields of geriatrics care, the education of healthcare professionals, and policy issues relating to the quality of long-term care.

Leilani Kicklighter, RN, ARM, MBA, CPHRM, DFASHRM, principle, The Kicklighter Group, is an independent consultant offering healthcare risk management, patient safety consulting, and stress management education. She serves as a risk management consultant to ambulatory surgery centers and is the course coordinator and instructor for the healthcare risk management online certificate course offered by the University of South Florida. This is a preparatory course laying the foundation for licensure in Florida as a healthcare risk manager. Most recently, she served as the corporate director of risk management services and patient safety officer for a large long-term care/skilled nursing facility. Previously, she was a healthcare risk management consultant with a large global insurance broker and consulted throughout the United States and internationally. Kicklighter began her career as a registered nurse. Her experience in healthcare risk management spans more than thirty years and has afforded her experience in a variety of healthcare organizational settings including a large teaching hospital, university medical school, large multispecialty clinic, for-profit community hospital, not-for-profit integrated healthcare multifacility system, and a large HMO. She has been a member of the American Society for Healthcare Risk Management (ASHRM) since its inception, serving on numerous committees, the board of directors, and as president in 1997–1998. Kicklighter has been awarded the DFASHRM designation from ASHRM. She is the past-president and board member of the Florida Society for Healthcare Risk Management and Patient Safety. She has a master's in business administration from Nova Southeastern University and has earned designations as an Associate in Risk Management (ARM), and Certified Professional in Healthcare Risk Management (CPHRM). Kicklighter is a licensed healthcare risk manager in the state of Florida. She is a well-known author and lecturer in the fields of infection control and risk management on the local, state, national, and international levels.

G. Eric Knox, MD, is the former director of patient safety and risk management, Children's Hospitals and Clinics, Minneapolis and St. Paul. Under his leadership, Children's Hospitals and Clinics was a finalist for the AHA McKesson Award for building a culture of safety and implementing a story-based knowledge network in 2002. Prior to joining Children's Hospitals and Clinics, Knox was president and chief medical officer of Obstetrix Medical Group, Inc., a for-profit publicly traded national group practice of maternal-fetal medicine specialists. Before Obstetrix, he founded Minnesota Perinatal Specialists and actively practiced maternal-fetal medicine for twenty-two years. In 2009, Knox joined PeriGen, a technology-enabled solutions firm providing a full suite of consulting and professional services to improve outcomes and increase patient safety in OB. As a senior physician consultant in PeriGen's Consulting Solutions Group, Knox works with experts in discreet areas of clinical risk management and obstetrics to evaluate client hospitals against current patient safety standards and best practices of care and to design solutions to help them meet their individual clinical and financial goals. Knox is a former professor of OB-GYN at the University of Minnesota, Minneapolis, Minnesota. His research and consulting has focused on high reliability and teamwork in preventing perinatal injury and malpractice claims. He has published over 115 articles concerning clinical practice and management of clinical risk. Currently, he is doing multidisciplinary qualitative research on patterns of nurse–physician communication and their effect on patient injury in obstetrics. From 1985 to 1997, Knox served as the medical director of MMI Companies, Inc., a medical malpractice insurer and clinical risk management group that served hospital, physician, and health plan clients throughout the United States, the UK, Germany, and Australia. He has given over two hundred lectures and seminars to nurses, physicians, and governing boards on all aspects of managing clinical risk and creating patient safety. He was a founding board member of the National Patient Safety Foundation. He currently consults and advises leadership and governance of healthcare organizations throughout the United States.

David Lickerman, MD, FACEP, ABIM, CHQM, is an emergency physician at St. Luke's Hospital in Chesterfield, Missouri. Previously, he was associate director of Emergency Medical Services at Christian Hospitals NE-NW in St. Louis for twenty-three years. He is a graduate of Indiana University School of Medicine. His residency training was in primary care internal medicine at St. Luke's Hospital–Washington University in St. Louis. His board certifications include internal medicine, emergency medicine, and quality improvement.

In 1993, he founded MeduLogic, LLC, to produce and distribute computer-based continuing medical education materials. Software written by Lickerman and published by MeduLogic include Clinical Communication and Risk Management Strategies for Emergency Medicine, The Many Faces of Family Violence, and Risk Management & the Art of Primary Care. He has also published CME courses on the Internet at the Virtual Lecture Hall (www.vlh.com). Current course offerings include EMTALA: An ER Law that Affects All Physicians and Risk Management and the Art of Medicine. While at Christian Hospital, he was chair of the Emergency Department's Quality Improvement Committee for twenty-one years and developed and edited the QI Notes and QI FlashNotes newsletters. He has served as an ED risk management consultant for the Medical Protective Company and Farmers Insurance Company Professional Liability Division. Lickerman is a well-known legal expert in ED medical-legal and risk management issues. He has written and lectured nationally on the subjects of ED quality improvement, risk management, ED redesign, family violence, and physician–patient communication.

Stephanie Lickerman, EMT, RN, BSN, is director of community education for the Melanoma Hope Network, St. Louis. A graduate of St. Luke's School of Nursing and St. Louis University, she has been editor of the Christian Hospital QI Notes newsletter since 1989. Additionally, she has edited three medical education software packages: Clinical Communication and Risk Management Strategies for Emergency Medicine, The Many Faces of Family Violence, and Risk Management and The Art of Primary Care. Previously, Lickerman served as Chair of the Planning Commission, Wildwood, Missouri (1995–1997); coauthored the master plan, ordinances, and natural resource matrix; was one of the original founders of the city; and served as City Science Coordinator (1997–2003). Her medical background is in cardiothoracic, cardiac medicine, neuro and surgical intensive care, and in-service, ACLS, and CPR instructing (both hospital and corporate). She has received the following awards: Recognition of Outstanding Service, Southern Illinois University, Edwardsville, 1996; Resolution 97–13, Stephanie Lickerman Month, December 1997, for public service and city development; Melanoma Hope Network service Award, 2004; Rose Award, Rockwood School District's highest honor, 2005, for outstanding service in education. Lickerman has spoken on the national level regarding her city science work and is well known in her community for educational outreach in the environmental and medical sciences.

Denise Murphy, RN, BSN, MPH, CIC, is chief patient safety and quality officer at Barnes-Jewish Hospital at Washington University Medical Center in St. Louis. Before taking that position, she spent seven years as director of healthcare epidemiology and patient safety for BJC HealthCare. Murphy went to nursing school in Philadelphia, received her BSN in Portland, Maine, and a master's degree in public health degree from St. Louis University, School of Public Health. Murphy's early nursing experience was in pediatric ICUs, surgical nursing, and nursing management. She entered the field of infection control in 1981, sitting for the first certification in infection control (CIC) exam in 1983. She has been an infection control practitioner in hospitals ranging from 100 to 1200 beds in rural and urban settings. Her presentations and publications are numerous on prevention of surgical site infections, bloodstream infections and ventilator-associated pneumonia; on redesigning infection control services; the business of infection control; and establishment of patient safety programs. Murphy is an active member of The Association for Professionals in Infection Control and Epidemiology (APIC), the Society for Healthcare Epidemiology of America (SHEA), and the American Society for Healthcare Risk Managers (ASHRM). She is a past president of the APIC Greater St. Louis chapter, and currently serves as a director on the APIC national board and chair of strategic planning. Murphy was a four-year member of the APIC Annual Conference Task Force, and is currently the ICP representative on the SHEA Educational Conference Planning Committee. She graduated from the first AHA/National Patient Safety Foundation-sponsored Leadership Fellowship training program in August, 2003.

Sara Ratner, BA, JD, is chief compliance officer, Prime Therapeutics, Minneapolis, MN. Previously Sara was senior legal counsel MinuteClinic, a division of CVS Caremark. She joined MinuteClinic in 2006 as senior legal counsel, where she leads the legal, government affairs, and regulatory strategy in support of the business's growth objectives. During her tenure, MinuteClinic has become the largest retail clinic in the country, currently operating over 560 clinics in twenty-five states. In 2008, she received added responsibilities as vice president of human resources, as well as leader of the strategy related to business-to-business partnerships with other integrated healthcare delivery systems. Previously, she served as vice president, deputy general counsel and chief compliance officer at Fiserv Health, where she also chaired the company's political action committee. Prior to Fiserv Health, Ratner was an associate in the health law practice at Minneapolis-based law firm, Leonard Street and Deinard, where she worked with multistate health plans and provider organizations. Ratner is frequently invited to speak about the retail clinic business model, including appearances on XM Radio's Oprah & Friends with Dr. Mehmet Oz. She has published a number of healthcare articles in various journals, including the *Journal of Health Law* and the *American Health Lawyers Association*. In 2007, Ratner was appointed to serve on the National Governors Association Health Care Task Force, as well as participate in the Women Business Leaders of the U.S. Health Care Industry Foundation and the Healthcare Leadership Trust. She also participates as an appointed member of the Minnesota State Bar Association Health Law Section Governing Council. Ratner received her BA, cum laude, from Washington University in St. Louis and her JD, magna cum laude, with a concentration in health law from St. Louis University.

Fay A. Rozovsky, JD, MPH, DFASHRM, has more than twenty years of experience as a healthcare risk management consultant and attorney. She has lectured extensively and has written or coauthored numerous articles and books, including *Consent to Treatment: A Practical Guide, Clinical Trials and Human Research* (with Rodney Adams), and *What Do I Say? Communicating Intended or Unanticipated Outcomes in Obstetrics* (with Dr. James R. Woods). She coedited with Woods *The Patient Safety Compliance Handbook: A Practical Guide for Healthcare Organizations*, published in March 2005. Rozovsky's expertise in consent law has been recognized by several courts, including the U.S. Supreme Court and appellate courts in Hawaii, Kentucky, West Virginia, and several other states. Rozovsky received a JD from Boston College Law School and an MPH from the Harvard School of Public Health. She is an affiliate associate professor in the Department of Legal Medicine at Virginia Commonwealth University School of Medicine. Rozovsky is admitted to the practice of law in Florida and Massachusetts. Rozovsky is a distinguished fellow and past president of the American Society for Healthcare Risk Management and a recipient of the Distinguished Service Award, the highest honor bestowed on a member of ASHRM. Currently, she is the chair of the Professional Technical Advisory Committee for Hospitals of The Joint Commission on Accreditation of Healthcare Organizations.

Jeffrey M. Sconyers, JD, vice president and general counsel of Children's Hospital and Regional Medical Center, Seattle, the regional pediatric referral and teaching center for Washington, Alaska, Idaho, Montana, and Wyoming. Sconyers received his law degree from Yale Law School and has practiced health law for more than twenty years. He is a past president of the Washington State Society of Healthcare Attorneys and its program czar in perpetuity. He was a founding coeditor of the *Washington Health Law Manual*, published by WSSHA and the Washington State Hospital Association. He is a member of the Executive Committee of the Board of Directors of the American Health Lawyers Association and chair of its Professional Resources Committee. At Children's Hospital, he chairs the Compliance Committee, staffs the Governance and the Audit and Corporate Responsibility Committees, and oversees the departments of safety, security, risk management, compliance, and legal affairs.

Laurence A. Sherman, BA, BS, MD, JD, FACP, FCAP, is professor emeritus of pathology at Northwestern Medical School, Chicago, and is board certified in internal medicine, clinical pathology, and blood banking. Sherman consults part-time in medical legal, compliance, and billing areas, including for the Northwestern faculty, and is part of the Northwestern Transplantation Ethics group. He also intermittently surveys for JCAHO. Previously at Northwestern, he was director of clinical laboratories and blood bank at Northwestern Memorial and director of the blood bank at Children's Memorial. His earliest clinical laboratory experience was as a medical technologist in the army. Previous academic positions include professor of pathology and medicine at Washington University in St. Louis and director of its (NHLBI) National Heart, Lung, and Blood Institute Institutional Training Program in Blood Banking; associate director of its NHLBI Specialized Center of Research in Thrombosis; and director of the Blood Bank at Barnes Hospital. Nationally, he held many offices in the American Association of Blood Banks, including president, and received its Quinn Jordan Award for contributions in transfusion medicine and government affairs. Sherman received his bachelor of science degree from the University of Chicago, his doctor of medicine from Albany Medical College, and juris doctor from Loyola (Chicago). He has served on committees of the American Society of Hematology, American Society of Clinical Pathology, American Heart Association, College of American Pathologists, and National Veterans Administration, and also served in local and regional groups. He has written or edited books in clinical pathology and coagulation research and has published more than one hundred journal articles and book chapters on blood transfusion, coagulation and thrombosis, clinical pathology, medical legal matters, and medical ethics and has given many presentations around the country.

Cynthia S. Siders, RN, MSN, DFASHRM, CPHRM, is vice president of Insured Services Risk Management & Patient Safety Institute. Siders has more than twenty-five years of healthcare, administrative, and insurance experience, twenty of those focused on risk management and patient safety. Responsibilities as vice president of insured services include providing leadership, education, information, and consultative support for clients in eleven states. These services include local, regional, and national educational programs; comprehensive risk management, patient safety, and quality improvement evaluations; and consultative services for healthcare systems, hospitals, physician office practices, community health centers, and long-term care facilities. She is also responsible for the development of proactive risk management and patient safety products and services, clinical risk management guideline development, and staff development and mentoring. Siders has bachelor's and master's of science degrees in nursing from the University of North Dakota and is a graduate of the Healthcare Risk Management Certificate Program cosponsored by MMI Companies, Inc. and the University of Health Sciences/The Chicago Medical School. She is a Distinguished Fellow with the American Society for Healthcare Risk Management and a Certified Professional in Healthcare Risk Management from the American Hospital Association. Siders is past president of the North Dakota Society for Healthcare Risk Management and serves as faculty for the ASHRM Barton Certificate Program. She was awarded the ASHRM Research Incentive Award in 1994.

Kathleen Rice Simpson, PhD, RNC, FAAN, is a perinatal clinical nurse specialist at St. John's Mercy Medical Center in St. Louis. Simpson is responsible for perinatal nursing practice and research and consultation on clinical issues for the antepartum, intrapartum, and obstetric triage units. She coordinates the perinatal nursing fellowship program and orientation, continuing education, and competence validation for the professional nursing staff. Simpson is a fellow in the American Academy of Nursing and a member of the Association of Women's Health, Obstetric, and Neonatal Nurses, the Association of Critical Care Nurses, Sigma Theta Tau, and Alpha Sigma Nu, the Jesuit Honor Society. She is the chair of the National Certification Corporation (NCC) Obstetric Content Team for the In-Patient OB and Electronic Fetal Monitoring Certification Examinations. Simpson is the editor of AWHONN's Perinatal Nursing and Competence Validation for Perinatal Care Providers and the author of AWHONN's *Practice Monograph Cervical Ripening and Induction and Augmentation of Labor*. She is a member of the National Nurse Advisory Council of the March of Dimes and a member of the editorial boards of the *Journal of Perinatal Neonatal Nursing* and *MCN, The American Journal of Maternal-Child Nursing*. She is the author of many articles and text chapters on perinatal patient safety and has been principal investigator on numerous research studies about safe care during labor and birth. She has provided perinatal risk management consultation to many hospitals and healthcare systems across the country and has been a labor and delivery nurse for more than twenty years.

David M. Sine, MA, ARM, CSP, CPHRM, is president and founder of SafetyLogic Systems in Austin, Texas. Sine serves as a member of the NFPA 101 Life Safety Code

Subcommittee on Health Care Occupancies, the JCAHO Committee on Healthcare Safety, and acts as a risk management and clinical ethics advisor to the National Association of Psychiatric Health Systems. Previously, he has been state safety director for two eastern states, the senior staff engineer for The Joint Commission (TJC), a senior consultant for the AHA and vice chair of the board of Brackenridge Hospital in Austin, Texas. He is a founding partner and one-time contributing editor for Briefings on Hospital Safety, coauthor of Quality Improvement Techniques for Hospital Safety, and the Design Guide for Behavior Heath Facilities. Mr. Sine is a Certified Safety Professional, a Certified Professional in Healthcare Risk Management, and currently serves as chair of the ASHRM Ethics Committee. A healthcare risk management consultant since 1980, he has conducted over 1,300 JCAHO compliance assessment surveys.

David M. Stallings, MHA, CPHQ, FASHRM, is director of risk management of Children's Hospital and Regional Medical Center, Seattle, the regional pediatric referral and teaching center for Washington, Alaska, Idaho, Montana, and Wyoming. Stallings received his bachelor of science degree from San Jose State University and a master of health administration degree from the University of Southern California. He is the former director of risk management and quality assessment at UCLA Medical Center/UCLA Health Network and has more than sixteen years of experience managing risk in community, tertiary, and academic medical centers. Stallings is an active member, and former board member, of the Washington Health Care Risk Management Society. He has served in various member and leadership capacities with ASHRM and is a current member of the ASHRM Board of Directors. He has been a Certified Professional in Healthcare Quality since 1994 and was awarded the Fellow of ASHRM designation in 2003.

Marshall K. Steele, MD, is an orthopedic surgeon, author, lecturer, and consultant. Until 2006 he was a practicing orthopedic surgeon and founder and president of a sixteen-surgeon subspecialty musculoskeletal center in Annapolis, Maryland. At Anne Arundel Medical Center in Annapolis, Maryland, he served for over ten years as medical director of surgical business development and the operating room. In 1995, he created a system of care in joint surgery that was named "Joint Camp" by one of his patients. This patient care system addressed every aspect of the experience from the patient and family perspective as well as creating a structure and tools that would ensure long-term success and promote safety. This model was reproduced in other surgical programs in multiple subspecialties. He has taught these concepts to hundreds of physicians and hospitals in the United States and abroad. In 2005, Steele founded Marshall Steele & Associates. Since then, his team has implemented over one hundred Destination Centers of Superior Performance in surgical subspecialties. Their model has become known as the gold standard for service lines in orthopedics and spine. He has received numerous awards for his work in improving the patient experience, safety, and outcomes. Steele was a physician to the 1994 Olympic Games, and his sports medicine book *Sideline Help* (Human Kinetics 1995) is used by youth coaches. His latest book, *Orthopedics and Spine, Strategies for Superior Service Line Performance*, was published in September 2009 by Healthleaders.

Sally T. Trombly, RN, MPH, JD, DFASHRM, is executive director of the Dartmouth-Hitchcock Risk Management Program, based at Dartmouth-Hitchcock Medical Center in Lebanon, New Hampshire, and an adjunct instructor in community and family medicine at Dartmouth Medical School. Dartmouth-Hitchcock's risk management and self-insured liability insurance program covers tertiary care services and graduate medical education at Mary Hitchcock Memorial Hospital, a network of more than nine hundred Dartmouth-Hitchcock Clinic specialty and primary care physicians practicing throughout New Hampshire and Vermont, and an affiliated group of regional hospitals and related health-care organizations. Her background includes extensive risk management experience in several healthcare delivery sites, including fourteen years at the Risk Management Foundation working with the institutions participating in Harvard's self-insured liability insurance program. Trombly has served on ASHRM's board of directors, its legislative committees, various ASHRM task forces, and has participated at the state chapter level. Since 1995, she has been on the board of directors of the Anesthesia Patient Safety Foundation (APSF) and participates in review of research grant proposals as a member of the APSF's Scientific Evaluation Committee. She also serves on the editorial advisory review board for ECRI Institute. She has written and lectured on several risk management and health law topics.

Nancy Tuohy, RN, MSN, is a medication safety specialist at the Institute of Safe Medication Practices (ISMP). Tuohy is also the assistant editor for ISMP *Nurse Advise-ERR* and a contributor to the other ISMP *Medication Safety Alert!* publications. Tuohy's interests include patient safety and healthcare systems analysis, including the evolution of health-care informatics. Her previous work experiences cover a broad range of healthcare settings, including pediatrics, critical care, outpatient clinic, elementary school settings, pharmaceutical research, and prehospital care as an emergency medical technician. Tuohy obtained her BSN at the University of North Carolina at Chapel Hill and her MSN at University of Pennsylvania. She also holds a bachelor's degree in psychology from Wake Forest University.

Cynthia Wallace, CPHRM, is senior risk management analyst with ECRI Institute, an independent nonprofit that researches best approaches to improving patient care. Wallace researches and writes risk management and patient safety guidance materials and educational programs for use in acute care, aging services, and ambulatory and physician office settings. She has written on numerous topics ranging from the integration of risk management and quality improvement to falls reduction initiatives. Additionally, Wallace provides consultation and advisory services to members of ECRI Institute's various print and online risk management services. These include ECRI Institute's Healthcare Risk Control System, Continuing Care Risk Management System, and Operating Room Risk Management, as well as various online newsletter services. She also serves as one of the course developers and instructors for ECRI Institute's risk management certification program provided to professional staff within aging services communities. In addition, Wallace has overseen special reports and projects developed by ECRI Institute's risk management publications group and assisted in developing educational conferences on topics related to risk management for ECRI Institute customers. Special projects include ECRI Institute's Physician Office Fundamentals in Risk Management and Patient Safety, Critical Care Safety: Essentials for ICU Patient Care and Technology, and Falls Prevention Strategies in Healthcare Settings. She is a member of the American Society for Healthcare Risk Management and the Philadelphia Area Society for Healthcare Risk Managers. Before joining ECRI Institute, she was the Los Angeles and Washington, DC, bureau chief for *Modern Healthcare*, a weekly magazine for the healthcare industry. Wallace received her of bachelor of arts degree from Colgate University, Hamilton, New York and is a certified professional in healthcare risk management (CPHRM).

Linda Wallace, MSN, BSN, RN, CPHRM, is program director at ECRI Institute. Wallace has more than twenty years of experience as a healthcare risk manager and ten years of experience in the area of patient safety and medical error prevention. Wallace has a clinical background in critical care nursing and nursing administration and risk management experience with the medical malpractice insurance industry and community-based and national healthcare systems. As well, Wallace has a background in the engineering approach to predictive and reactive systems. Wallace was the codeveloper, with a division of ABS, of a healthcare medical error prevention, identification, and analysis program for managers and directors. This program offers tools for use by managers in event investigation and analysis, in predictive analysis, and in change analysis. Currently, Wallace is responsible for the risk management and culture of safety programs for continuing care and senior services clients. Wallace revised the Web-based Continuing Care Risk Assessment and developed the reporting mechanism to track implementation of three best practice toolkits. She is currently involved in the development and implementation of a series of educational programs for continuing care and senior services risk managers. Wallace facilitated two groups of eastern Pennsylvania hospitals in the identification and implementation of best practice strategies in the areas of preoperative antibiotic administration and medication reconciliation. She has spoken at state and national conferences on the topics of culture of safety and disclosure. Wallace holds a bachelor of science in nursing from the Medical College of Virginia and a master of science in nursing from the University of Virginia. She has been associated with the American Society of Healthcare Risk Management since 1987 and received a certificate for completion of the Barton Module Series. Wallace is also a certified professional in healthcare risk management (CPHRM).

Craig Westling, MS, MPH, is currently vice president of operations and client services at Marshall Steele & Associates, where he is responsible for leading the musculoskeletal, OR, and vascular consulting practices. He has over twenty years of healthcare and corporate operations experience. In his previous position at Dartmouth-Hitchcock Medical Center, Westling led a broad range of operational improvement initiatives in areas such as orthopedics, central sterile, air rescue, and more. Before Dartmouth, Westling improved work processes as the director of quality assurance at PeopleSoft and as a client relations manager at Oracle. He holds a BA from Middlebury College, an MS in health administration from New England College, and an MPH from the Dartmouth Medical School.

Kelley Woodfin RN, BS, DFASHRM, CPHRM, is president and CEO of CORE Risk Services, Inc., providing healthcare risk management consulting services in the western United States. Woodfin has extensive experience in the development and implementation of clinical and enterprise risk management programs for acute care, managed care, and long-term care systems. She coauthored the textbook *Emergency Preparedness: Disaster Planning for Health Care Facilities*, Aspen Publishers, 1986, is published in four emergency nursing textbooks, and has produced numerous articles for professional clinical journals.

Sheila Cohen Zimmet, BSN, JD, is senior associate vice president for regulatory affairs at Georgetown University (GU). She previously served as associate dean for research integrity for Weill Cornell Medical College, until returning to GU in her current role. At GU, Zimmet has oversight responsibility for research integrity, protection of human and animal subjects of research, medical center conflict of interest management, environmental health and safety, and the clinical trials office. She is a former neonatal intensive care nurse, senior associate counsel to the GU Medical Center, and GU's first director of research assurance and compliance. Zimmet also is a former two-term member of the NCRR Advisory Council (1996–2000 and 2004–2008) and a current member of the NCRR Chimpanzee Management Plan Working Group. She frequently speaks on issues related to research compliance matters at local, national and international professional meetings.

Preface

As I prepared the sixth edition of the *Risk Management Handbook* for publication, an initial, but critical task was to identify what changes have occurred since publication of the last edition that could significantly impact the practice of healthcare risk management. In essence, it was necessary to determine what new developments have added risks to the organization and therefore added responsibilities to the risk management professional's daily tasks and how we can address these new developments; what tasks can be eliminated, if any; and what remains the same and needs to be continued. While this task sounds relatively easy, it was by no means simple.

Responsibilities of the healthcare risk management professional continue to evolve. What used to be a role focused primarily on education to clinical staff and reacting to and managing incidents reported through the facility's incident reporting system has changed. The risk management professional is now focusing efforts on identifying and managing risks to the enterprise through what is commonly called enterprise risk management (ERM). The risk management professional's role in managing ERM risks necessitates a set of skills that have not previously been appreciated by those in the healthcare professions. Those skills focus on coordination, facilitation, and the ability to manage and lead teams of people to identify, analyze, manage, and monitor risks across organizational settings. *Risk management professionals cannot manage risk on an enterprisewide basis by themselves.*

Focusing on risks to the enterprise requires a different set of skills for the risk management professional, skills not required in the past but now in demand, such as the ability to see the big picture, and the ability to "connect the dots" among and between identified risks so that strategies and solutions can take them into account and become less focused on tactics. The following table represents the transition of the traditional risk manager to the risk management professional managing ERM programs today. This sixth edition was written to support the new ERM risk management professional.

Transitioning from Risk Management to Enterprise Risk Management Requires a Set of New Skills

FROM	>	TO
Following	>	Leading
Educated	>	Experienced
Information	>	Knowledge
Single Topic	>	Big Picture
Tactician	>	Strategist
Clinical Risk	>	All Risks
Team Member	>	Team Builder
Task Manager	>	Change Agent
Closed	>	Open
Risk / Loss	>	Risk / Opportunity
Doer	>	Facilitator
Individual Autonomy	>	Standardized
Personal Opinion	>	Consensus

The adage that "nothing ever goes away in healthcare risk management; we just keep adding to the responsibilities" continues to be supported by the changes that are necessary in each edition of the *Handbook*. What was a soft-back, single-volume first edition published in the mid-1990s has become what is now considered the premier reference text in healthcare risk management—the 2010, sixth edition is a series of separate hardback textbooks including the works of over ninety authors in fifty-six chapters of three volumes.

Many who use the *Risk Management Handbook* as a reference text are not aware that all the editors and contributing authors are volunteers, meaning that they have graciously donated their time and expertise to advance our profession and the discipline of healthcare risk management to this *Handbook* project. We thank them for their time and appreciate the efforts made in making this *Handbook* series a success. Authors writing material new to the sixth edition include Ronni Solomon on the role of patient safety organizations; Ann Gaffey and Sharon Groves writing on the clinical record; David Sine writing an appendix on design for safety in the behavioral health environment to support the chapter on risk management and behavioral health and Leilani Kicklighter writing an appendix on complementary and alternative medicine for the chapter on managing primary care risks in the ambulatory care environment; Sylvia Brown writing on risk management and patient safety in oncology; Sara Ratner lending her expertise on risk management and retail clinics; Cindy Siders writing on the care of the obese patient; W. Patrick Downes, David Elliott Jose, and Leigh Ann Lauth O'Neill authoring the new chapter on Medicare RAC Audits; and returning author Shelia Hagg-Rickert with Nancy Poblenz writing on medical tourism.

Most authors from the previous edition agreed to revise their current work; however, as expected, several were unable to continue as a contributing author, so new authors were solicited to take their place. They include Rachel Remaley, Krishna Lynch, Michelle Hoppes, Jeanie Taylor, Keith Higdon, Craig L. Allen, Mary Lynn Curran, Marshall Steele,

Susan Harris, Craig Westling, Asheesh Gupta, Cindy Wallace, Linda Wallace, Roslyn Corcoran, Melissa (Lisa) Thompson, Leeanne R. Coons, Kurt Davis, Karen M. Buesing, Michelle Boyd, Tim Gorman, Susan E. Ziel, and Neil Austin.

Returning authors who graciously consented to update their previously published works include Gisele Norris, Roberta L. Carroll, Michael Zuckerman, Peter Hoffman, John C. West, John Horty, Jane McCaffrey, Sheila Hagg-Rickert, Kimberly Willis, Dominic A. Colaizzo, Ellen L. Barton, Geri Amori, Sheila Cohen Zimmet, Peggy Berry Martin, Frank Federico, Fay A. Rozovsky, Mark A. Kadzielski, Ronni Solomon, Madelyn Quattrone, Harlan Hammond, Peggy L. B. Nakamura, Denise Murphy, Hedy Cohen and Nancy Tuohy, Sally T. Trombly, G. Eric Knox, Kathleen Rice Simpson, David Stallings, Jeff Sconyers, Christine Clark, Lawrence Sherman, Sylvia Brown, David Lickerman and Stephanie Lickerman, Alice L. Epstein and Gary H. Harding, Robin Burroughs and Bruce W. Dmytrow, Robert F. Bunting, Jr. and Joyce H. Benton, Kelley Woodfin, Kathryn Hyer, Mark Cohen, Frederick Robinson, and Melissa (Lisa) Thompson, Berni Bussell, Glenn Troyer, William M. Klimon, Rebecca Havlisch, Lorrie J. Neiburg, Brad R. Norrick, Thomas M. Jones, Thomas M. Hermes, Pamela J. Para, and Phyllis Ruez.

Authors writing two or more chapters include John C. West, Ellen L. Barton, Roberta L. Carroll, Dominic A. Colaizzo, Ronni Solomon, Sheila Hagg-Rickert, Sheila Cohen Zimmet, Peggy L. B. Nakamura, and Sylvia Brown.

Projects of this magnitude are never done alone. I would like to thank all the contributing authors, because without their collective efforts this *Handbook* series could never have been published. I also wish to thank and acknowledge the hard work and dedication of the editors for the three volumes: Peggy Nakamura, Sylvia Brown, and Glenn Troyer. They are extraordinarily dedicated professionals who graciously gave of their time and expertise to review content and make editorial changes to the chapters within the individual volumes. Simultaneously editing and preparing three books for publication is a time-consuming task occurring around the end-of-the-year holidays every few years. As with past editions, I thank my family for allowing me to disappear on occasion to devote my time to this project with little complaint, and a special "thank you" to my brother Terrance (Red) Carroll for his continued patience and support.

We have enjoyed bringing the sixth edition to you and hope you find this series an invaluable resource and addition to your risk management library. Share it with others within your organization, so that they can better understand and support the evolving role of the healthcare risk management professional.

Submitted by
Roberta Carroll
Series Editor
Risk Management Handbook for Healthcare Organizations, sixth edition

About This Book

Carrying forward the theme of previous editions, this volume on clinical risk management in the sixth edition of the *Risk Management Handbook for Healthcare Organizations* series had three goals.

The first was to update information previously published in the handbook concerning clinical environments such as perinatal, emergency, and surgical services, and long-term care, as well as key clinical risk management topics such as informed consent and medication safety. This could not have been done without the support of returning authors (Joyce Benton, Robert Bunting, Robin Burroughs, Bruce Dmytrow, Alice Epstein, Gary Harding, Kathryn Hyer, Mary Lynn Curran, Fay Rozovsky, Jeff Sconyers, David Stallings, Sally Trombly, Sheila Zimmet, Denise Murphy, Hedy Cohen, Nancy Tuohy, Eric Knox, Kathleen Rice Simpson, Kelley Woodfin, David Lickerman, Stephanie Lickerman, Christine Clark, and Laurence Sherman). Contributing new ideas to the chapter on patient safety was Roslyn Corcoran.

The second goal was to add new clinical area-specific chapters. New authors contributed the following: Marshall Steele, Susan Harris, Craig Westling, and Asheesh Gupta shared their perspective on surgical patient safety; Sara Ratner provided insight on risk management in the retail clinic environment; Cindy Wallace and Linda Wallace shared comprehensive risk management strategies for the intensive care unit; Cindy Siders gave a thorough overview of bariatric risk management issues and solutions, David Sine contributed his expertise in a new appendix to the behavioral health chapter on latent risk in the built environment, and Leilani Kicklighter shared innovative risk management issues and solutions pertaining to complementary and alternative medicine.

The third goal was to help the reader internalize key clinical risk management and patient safety principles, such as SBAR, and apply such principles in the various clinical settings. To achieve this goal, the chapters have been organized in a way that transitions the information from generic risk management resources and issues first, followed by chapters on risk management related to specific clinical environments. These chapters are intended to be primers that address complex risks in terms that can be quickly absorbed by anyone unfamiliar with the particular clinical area.

The dedication of contributing authors to this volume is gratefully acknowledged. We hope readers will appreciate the energy, expertise, and time spent in bringing to the reader these topics in clinical risk management.

Sylvia M. Brown
Editor, Volume 2

Risk Management Handbook for Healthcare Organizations

1

Patient Safety and the Risk Management Professional: New Challenges and Opportunities

Denise Murphy
Roslyn Corcoran

The field of healthcare risk management grew out of the insurance crisis of the 1970s, when professional liability premiums skyrocketed due, in part, to the dissolution of the doctrine of charitable immunity, which once shielded a hospital's assets from malpractice lawsuits.[2] The Joint Commission (TJC), formerly known as the Joint Commission on Accreditation of Healthcare Organizations, or JCAHO, defines risk management as "clinical and administrative activities undertaken to identify, evaluate, and reduce the risk of injury to patients, staff, and visitors, and the risk of loss to the organization itself."[3] In other words, healthcare risk management is committed to reducing loss associated with patient safety-related events in healthcare settings.

Like the malpractice crisis of the 1970s, the patient safety movement today is forcing great changes in healthcare risk management. One of the greatest catalysts has been the Institute of Medicine's 1999 report, *To Err Is Human: Building a Safer Health System.* Also known as the IOM report, this extensive document attempted to shed light on the growing problem of medical errors.[4] The problems exposed by the IOM report have since

Note: The authors gratefully acknowledge the significant contribution made by Gina Pugliese and Katrina Shannon, coauthors of this chapter in the fifth edition of book. Risk management has been practiced in the world of business for more than a century, beginning in the fields of engineering and economics. In the 1960s, risk management became associated with insurance strategies aimed at minimizing or financing predictable business losses.[1] Philosophically, risk management aims to bring order from chaos and to facilitate certainty in an environment of uncertainty.

given rise to mounting regulations and government scrutiny, and the healthcare industry has responded in many innovative ways.

Most importantly, risk managers today must assist healthcare professionals meet an unprecedented standard of care because the evidence used to determine whether they acted as reasonably prudent providers now potentially includes highly prescriptive standards, such as The Joint Commission's requirement that every procedure be preceded by a *time-out* to verify parameters such as right patient and correct procedural site. Even more challenging, to help providers implement new approaches the risk management professional must work with other managers to transform a traditionally hierarchical healthcare environment into a culture of patient safety. Risk management professionals today are also increasingly responsible for helping their employers satisfy patient safety reporting requirements. To do this, they must stay abreast of state-specific reporting requirements as well as new federal patient safety-related legislation, such as the Patient Safety and Quality Improvement Act of 2005 (the patient safety act).[5] The act authorized the creation of patient safety organizations (PSOs) to improve the quality and safety of U.S. healthcare delivery by encouraging clinicians and healthcare organizations to voluntarily report and share quality and patient safety information without fear of legal discovery. (Please see Volume 1, Chapter 10 in this series for more information on patient safety organizations.)

Even though the patient safety movement has created challenges, it has also provided opportunities for risk management professionals to expand their knowledge. Not only are these professionals gaining a broader understanding of the dynamics of error from the patient safety theory perspective, they are also learning from new tools such as electronic incident reporting, which is designed to capture relevant information, help providers learn from errors, and implement processes to prevent errors in the future. Armed with additional information on the frequency and nature of errors, risk management professionals are better able to negotiate resources and support from organizational leaders to enhance safety programs. The patient safety movement has provided a fresh context for the risk management professional's discussion with healthcare executives because keeping patients safe from harm is now more clearly tied to protection of market share, reimbursement levels, organizational reputation, and accreditation status. Today, safety has become a top priority in every healthcare organization, and the risk management professional is now engaged in efforts to restore trust in a healthcare system whose safety track record is being closely scrutinized by decision makers, legislators, payers, and consumers.

This chapter will discuss the scope of medical errors in healthcare, provide an overview of patient safety theory and related safety guidelines, and highlight strategies to leverage patient safety concepts to reduce loss and improve care.

· · · · · · · · ·
THE SCOPE OF MEDICAL ERRORS

In the IOM report, an adverse event is defined as an injury caused by medical management rather than by the underlying disease or condition of the patient. Some, but not all, adverse events are the result of medical errors. The IOM report defines medical error as the failure of a planned action to be completed as intended or the use of a wrong plan to achieve an aim. Two studies of large patient populations, one an analysis of New York data known as the Harvard Medical Practice Study[6] and another based on data from Colorado and Utah,[7] found that adverse events occurred in 2.9 and 3.7 percent of hospitalizations, respectively. Data from these two studies were extrapolated in the IOM report to the more than 33.6 million admissions to U.S. hospitals in 1997. It is possible to conclude from these studies that at least 44,000 to 98,000 patients in U.S. hospitals die each year as a result of medical errors.

The accuracy of the IOM's nearly 100,000 patient death estimate was challenged at the time it was published, but subsequent data indicate that even more deaths may be attributable to medical error. Estimates of the financial impact of medical errors are no less alarming. In 2009, Donald M. Berwick, president and CEO of the Institute for Healthcare Improvement, reviewed the IOM report and noted that its impact was maximized by the inclusion of hard numbers in the number of deaths caused by medical errors. The range given (44,000–98,000 deaths each year) caught people's attention, creating interest not shown previously. He also noted that the reports have three clear messages: safety is a serious problem, the cause is not the workforce, and the problem can be fixed.[8]

The Agency for Healthcare Research and Quality (AHRQ) estimates that medical errors cost a typical large hospital about $5 million per year; all told, medical errors cost the U.S. healthcare system between $17 billion and $29 billion per year. These costs include follow-up and additional medical treatment of any adverse outcomes and any expenses related to lost income and household productivity and potential long-term or permanent disability. Virtually none of these costs can later be recouped for proactive health initiatives.[9]

Viewed in the larger context of medical errors, medication errors have become an increasing area of concern for risk management professionals. According to the IOM report, medication errors alone, either within or outside of the hospital, have been estimated to account for over seven thousand deaths a year. Moreover, a study referenced by the IOM concluded that about two out of every one hundred admissions experience a preventable adverse drug event, resulting in average excess hospital costs of $4,700 per admission or about $2.8 million in additional costs for a typical seven hundred–bed teaching hospital.[10] If these findings can be generalized, the IOM report points out, the increased hospital costs alone for preventable adverse drug events affecting inpatients are $2 billion for the nation as whole.[11]

The IOM report also enumerates and expands the categories of the types of medical errors that were reported by Leape and colleagues in 1993.[12] These categories are diagnostic, therapeutic, preventive, or related to failures of communication, equipment, or other systems. Diagnostic errors are defined as those related to error or delay in diagnosis, failure to perform indicated tests, use of outmoded tests or therapy, or failure to act on results of monitoring or testing.

Treatment-related errors are defined as those that occur in performance of an operation, procedure, or test; in administering treatment; or in the dose or method of using a drug. They may be the result of an avoidable delay in treatment or in responding to an abnormal test result or inappropriate (not indicated) care.

Preventive errors were found to include failure to provide prophylactic treatment or inadequate monitoring or follow-up of treatment.

According to AHRQ, the most common adverse events that patients experience while receiving healthcare services include medication and transfusion errors, infections, complications of surgery (including wrong-site surgery), suicide, restraint-related injuries, falls, burns, pressure ulcers, misidentification, delays, and wrong diagnosis or treatment.

Healthcare-associated infections are another important aspect of the patient safety crisis. The Centers for Disease Control and Prevention (CDC) estimate that two million patients a year are infected in U.S. hospitals, and approximately 98,000 die as a result of those infections. Based on 2002 data, healthcare-associated infections cost the U.S. healthcare system an estimated $6.7 billion annually.[13] In New York hospitals alone, for example, surgical site infections were found to be the second most common adverse event, according to the Harvard Medical Practice Study.[14] Recent studies have shown that up to 350,000 hospitalized patients acquire bloodstream infections each year at a minimum cost of about $38,703 per episode[15] and with a mean attributable mortality of 15 to 20 percent.[16]

Studies have shown that most medical errors occur in hospital intensive care units among women and children, in operating rooms, and in emergency departments. The healthcare system bears the additional costs for treatment related to medical errors. Nowhere is this more evident than in rising insurance rates and malpractice premiums. In fact, clinicians in many parts of the country have been forced to abandon their medical practices because of increasing malpractice premiums.

Finally, two of the most overlooked effects of medical errors are the unquantifiable expense of psychological damage to patients, families, and providers and the erosion of public trust in our healthcare system.

. . . .
CAUSES OF MEDICAL ERRORS

The financial and social implications of medical errors are only one aspect of the overall problem for the healthcare industry; contributing issues must be identified if they are to be adequately addressed. Closely related is the fact that risk management professionals today must have a clear understanding of the underlying causes of medical errors. According to the AHRQ, medical errors are caused by the following:[17]

- Communication problems
- Inadequate information flow
- Human-related problems
- Patient-related issues
- Organizational transfer of knowledge

- Staffing patterns and workflow
- Technical failures
- Inadequate policies and procedures

Theories of Accident Causation

Healthcare professionals are reaching out to other industries to help them understand and address the causes of medical errors. Although there may not be total agreement on how to apply non-healthcare industry strategies, everyone understands that healthcare is a complex environment in which people may suffer as a result of systems failure. Following are some of the leading theories about systems failure and how they can be applied to medical errors in a healthcare setting.

Swiss Cheese Model Two commonly used models of accident causation in the patient safety literature are found in the work of James Reason, David D. Woods, and Richard Cook. Reason's Swiss cheese model[18] makes it easy to visualize how complex systems fail due to the combination and timing of multiple small failures. Reason contends that any one failure or situation alone would be insufficient to cause an accident, but the combination and timing of small failures look much like the alignment of holes in a slice of Swiss cheese (see Figure 1.1).

A practical example of this model is an ICU nurse who floated to an oncology unit due to short staffing and administered the wrong dose of chemotherapy. In a subsequent review of the circumstances, it was learned that the ICU nurse failed to follow the standard protocol of having an experienced oncology nurse double-check the physician's order against the prepared medication before administering it to the patient. The experienced

FIGURE 1.1   Swiss Cheese Model of Accident Causation

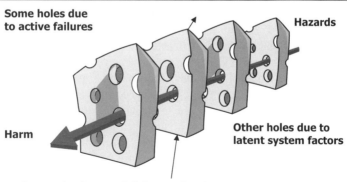

oncology nurse, who was anticipating being asked to assist with the double-check, was unexpectedly involved in a crisis and forgot to check in with the float nurse before the incident occurred. The holes in the Swiss cheese lined up, and the patient was harmed.

Active versus Latent Failures   Using the same example, the active failure was that the nurse did not comply with the medication administration policy and therefore administered the wrong dose of a chemotherapeutic agent to the patient. Other, second-layer failures, or holes in the Swiss cheese, are considered to be latent or hidden. For example, it is not immediately apparent in the circumstances of this error that the recent budget cut that led to the staffing shortage was responsible for the float situation in the first place. The inability of administrative staffing mechanisms to compensate for the budget cut is a good example of latent failure.

Blunt End/Sharp End Model   David Woods writes about a second theory of accident causation called the Blunt End/Sharp End model.[19] This model assumes that healthcare workers at the sharp end, where patient care is delivered, are affected by decisions, policies, and regulations made at the blunt end of the system. The blunt end represents, in broad terms, healthcare administration of any kind. Although this administrative end generates resources to help providers implement organizational strategy, it also generates constraints (for example, budgetary shortfalls) that further modify the environment in which the technical work takes place. Even more important, the effect of such constraints is likely to be exacerbated by the unanticipated obstacles often associated with rapidly evolving and escalating "front line" situations (see Figure 1.2). At the sharp end, providers must therefore continually adapt to complex challenges with appropriate coping mechanisms, such as letting senior management know about their perception rather than institute unsafe shortcuts, such as storing medications in their pockets as a time-saving strategy, thereby increasing the risk of medication error. Woods stresses the importance of helping providers learn and apply adaptive skills to promote safety in the health care environment.

Hindsight Bias   Richard Cook, an anesthesiologist who has extensively studied causes of, and reaction to, accidents in healthcare, notes that investigations into accidents frequently stop with identifying the human error and designating the practitioners as the "cause" of the event. Often this determination is made without any evaluation of systems or processes that might have contributed to the error. According to Cook, this limited type of investigation can lead to solutions characterized by a phenomenon he calls *hindsight bias.*[20] Such bias occurs when the investigators work backward from their knowledge of the outcome of the event. This linear analysis makes the path to failure look as though it should have been foreseeable or predictable, although this is not the case.

These theories and models raise our awareness of the complexity of the system in which patients receive care and in which providers work. They make clear that organizational leaders must become "systems thinkers" who demand in-depth analyses of safety

FIGURE 1.2   **The Sharp End/Blunt End of a Complex System**

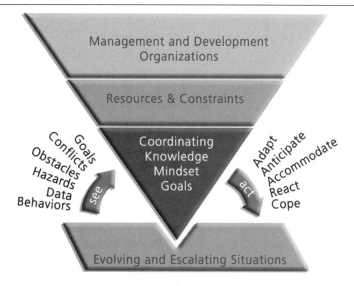

The interplay of problem demands and practitioners' expertise at the sharp end govern the expression of expertise and error. The resources available to meet problem demands are provided and constrained by the organizational context at the blunt end of the system.

Source: Woods, D.D., S.W.A. Dekker, R.I. Cook, L.L. Johannesen, and N.B. Sarter. (2010). *Behind Human Error* (2nd Edition). Ashgate, Aldershot, UK (original 1994). Reprinted with permission.

concerns. Healthcare leaders must also advocate a culture of safety that replaces punitive reactions to mistakes with an open environment that encourages staff to bring errors to light to be dissected and addressed. Only when staff members are confident that their leaders will proactively address any risks that they divulge will there be an opportunity to build safer healthcare organizations.

Creating a Just Culture of Safety

To create a culture of safety, it is important to understand the concept of *organizational culture*. Organizational culture can be described as the set of values, guiding beliefs, or ways of thinking that are shared among members of an organization. It is the feel of an organization that is quickly picked up by new members. Culture is "the way we do things around here." Culture is powerful and is likely to become particularly visible when an organization tries to implement new strategies that are not in step with the status quo. It is human nature for people to resist changing the way they do things; but it is also human nature for people to change the culture in which they live or work.

So what is the definition of a *culture of safety*? Tom Hellmich, a physician member of the Patient Safety Council at Children's Hospital and Clinics in Minneapolis, Minnesota, described it this way: "The medical culture that silently taught the ABCs as accuse, blame, and criticize is fading. Rising in its place is a safety culture emphasizing blameless reporting, successful systems, knowledge, respect, confidentiality, and trust."

In schools of medicine, nursing, and allied health, providers have traditionally been taught, through incident reporting procedures and behavior of other staff members, that when things go wrong, they should find out who did it. The focus has been on individual failures. However, in a safety culture one asks, What happened? In a safety culture, one looks at the system, the environment, the knowledge, the work flow, the tools, and the other stressors that may have affected provider behavior.

When the patient safety movement began in the United States, a nonpunitive culture was seen as a solution to medical errors. This raised concerns that people who acted recklessly would not be held accountable. Lucien Leape, the Harvard surgeon who is sometimes referred to as the father of the patient safety movement, introduced the term *just culture* and noted that having a safety culture "doesn't mean there is no role for punishment. Punishment is indicated for willful misconduct, reckless behavior, and unjustified, deliberate violation of rules . . . but not for human error."[21]

David Marx, an attorney who specializes in human resources and organizational development, also differentiates between a nonpunitive and a just response to error by describing a just culture of safety in terms of a set of beliefs and a set of duties. According to Marx, providers in a just culture must recognize that professionals make mistakes, acknowledge that even professionals will use shortcuts, and support zero tolerance for reckless behaviors. Marx adds that staff members in this culture must openly admit they have made a mistake, call out when they see risk, and participate in a learning culture in which information about mistakes and near misses is shared with others so they can prevent similar situations.[22]

Participants in a just safety culture are sensitive to risk as they try to identify where and how the next mistake might occur and then work to prevent it from happening. Staff members share information about mistakes and errors to prevent them from recurring somewhere else or to someone else, and they are constantly seeking best practices. These behaviors are characteristic of a learning organization. This type of organization also values reciprocal accountability. In other words, everyone holds everyone else accountable for patient safety. Leadership can expect staff members to call out or "stop the line" when they see risk, and the staff can expect leadership to listen and act, even if that means dealing with problem professionals who display intentionally reckless behaviors.

Patients and family members are respected partners and understand their own responsibility to keep themselves safe while in a healthcare organization. Examples of patient responsibilities may include keeping written records of medications and allergies and reminding busy healthcare workers to perform hand hygiene.

The National Patient Safety Foundation outlines several attributes of a safety culture that all healthcare organizations should strive to put into operation by implementing strong safety management systems.[23] These attributes include a culture that does the following:

- Encourages all workers (including frontline staff, physicians, and administrators) to accept responsibility for the safety of themselves, their coworkers, patients, and visitors
- Prioritizes safety above financial and operational goals
- Encourages and rewards the identification, reporting, and resolution of safety issues
- Provides for organizational learning from accidents
- Allocates appropriate resources, structure, and accountability to maintain effective safety systems
- Absolutely avoids reckless behaviors

In a just safety culture, top-down communication must be replaced by two-way communication that flows to the front line from leadership and back to leadership from those providing patient care on the front line. Similarly, silence about harmful events must be replaced with open, honest disclosure about serious patient safety events.

Communication and Teamwork

We know that the failure to communicate effectively is the root cause of many avoidable accidents. Many factors contribute to communication-related patient safety issues. The following are a few of the most important factors, accompanied by associated patient safety strategies.

Traditionally Complex Hierarchical Approach   When nurses perceive that a physician or other senior clinician is using an unsafe clinical approach, they traditionally use the chain of command to resolve the question. However, in many healthcare organizations, the chain of command is cumbersome. It may, for example, require the nurse to contact two or three people, at minimum, based on existing reporting relationships and formal interfaces between the nursing and medical staff. If patient safety is at stake, the most knowledgeable resolution must be achievable in a short time, and there is no time for the traditional chain of command. Many successful malpractice suits have involved circumstances in which a question about care or need for expert intervention was not addressed promptly.

After studying the cause of errors, the aviation industry recognized that hierarchy-associated communication failures were at the root of 70 to 80 percent of all the jet transport accidents over a twenty-year period. The industry made significant improvements in its poor safety record by using a strategy called *crew resource management (CRM) training*. One important tenet of this strategy is that every team member has a responsibility to point out a perceived risk. This places the pilot and crew on equal footing when the safety of the craft or passengers is in question.

Empirical proof of the value of such team training in healthcare has been demonstrated only in small sample studies to date, but evidence from emergency department operations and obstetric settings is proving that it reduces risk.[24] Still another strategy from outside the healthcare industry comes from manufacturing assembly lines. Some healthcare organizations have "stop the line" policies that empower everyone to respectfully call out and stop any risky process or procedure until all preventable risks are removed.[25]

Simplifying the hierarchy is a key patient safety strategy used to resolve patient safety-related communication issues. Empowering charge nurses to facilitate rapid resolution of care questions is one approach that some organizations are using.

Personal Style of Providers   Hierarchy has one additional undesirable ramification; it may legitimize intimidating behavior. One of The Joint Commission's surveyors observed that intimidation is a significant factor in wrong-site surgery. (For more information, see the discussion of the Institute of Safe Medical Practice study on intimidation discussed in Chapter 2 on medication safety.)

Solutions for addressing an intimidating personal style range from simple training to disciplinary action within the parameters of appropriate human resource protocols and medical staff bylaws. Long-term resolution often requires the strong support of senior administrative and clinical leaders. Partially in an attempt to address the issue of an intimidating personality, The Joint Commission has recently begun to require that accredited organizations formalize an approach with which to address such behaviors.[26]

At the other end of the spectrum is lack of assertiveness by frontline staff. This timidity is sometimes a response to another provider's intimidating behavior. This unassertive personal style may be equally dangerous because important issues are simply never raised. When the nurse calls a physician in the middle of the night but does not clearly explain the reason for the call, the nurse may not get the response that is needed to address the urgent clinical issue at hand.

Situational Briefing Model   One means of facilitating clear communication between providers in a crisis situation is a standardized situational briefing model. For example, the SBAR (for **s**ituation, **b**ackground, **a**ssessment, and **r**ecommendation) communication model is an approach used increasingly in healthcare settings to facilitate effective communication of issues in an impending crisis by support staff to physicians.[27]

Before using SBAR communication and calling a physician, it is important to do the following:

● Assess the patient.

● Review the chart to determine the appropriate physician to call.

● Know the admitting diagnosis.

● Read the most recent progress notes and assessments from clinicians on previous shifts.

● Have available the patient's medical record, with patient allergies, medications and IV fluids administered, and laboratory and other diagnostic test results when speaking with the physician.

The following are the essential components of SBAR communication:

1. Situation

   - State your name, position, and unit.
   - Say, "I am calling about . . ." (patient name and room number).
   - Say, "The problem I am calling about is . . ."

2. Background

   - State the admission diagnosis and date of admission.
   - State the pertinent medical history.
   - Give a brief synopsis of the treatment to date.

3. Assessment: Begin by outlining any changes from previous assessments. Include changes in the following:

   - Mental status
   - Pain
   - Respiratory rate or quality; retractions or use of accessory muscles
   - Pulse and blood pressure rate and quality; rhythm changes
   - Skin color; wound drainage
   - Neurological changes
   - Gastrointestinal, genitourinary, or bowel changes (nausea, vomiting, diarrhea, increased or decreased output)
   - Musculoskeletal weakness, joint deformity

4. Recommendation: State clearly what you think the patient needs urgently. Examples might include the following:

   - Transfer the patient to ICU or PICU.
   - Come to see the patient immediately.
   - Talk to the patient or family about the code status.
   - Ask for a consultant to see the patient now.
   - Suggest tests or laboratory studies needed (for example, chest X-ray, arterial blood gases, EKG).

If a change in treatment is ordered, the caller should ask how often vital signs should be checked and when the physician would like to be contacted again. The caller should document any changes in patient status, what intervention was completed, and whether the intervention was effective. Also documented should be any contact the caller had with the physician.

Lack of Common Language   Barriers to communication might also stem from language, ethnic, cultural, age, and gender differences. Even among providers with similar backgrounds, there might be a lack of familiarity with terminology, including jargon and abbreviations. (See the discussion of issues surrounding unclear medication orders in Chapter 2 on medication safety.) One example of a solution to standardizing communication among providers is the National Institute of Child Health and Human Development's adoption of common definitions for fetal monitor interpretation.

The Joint Commission has built into its National Patient Safety Goals several strategies to improve provider communication. These strategies include read-backs on verbal orders and critical lab values; identification of patients using two sources; site marking using the word *yes* on operative or procedure sites; checklists to verify correct patient, site, and procedure; and calling a time-out before procedures and operations begin to ensure that all healthcare team members are comfortable that safety preparations for the procedure are complete.

Other principles that can help providers avoid communication breakdowns include the following:

- The fact that one person said and understands something doesn't mean that others did.
- Communication is not accomplished unless both parties are on the same page.
- A standard structure for communication gives the right amount and type of useful information that is critical to patient safety.
- Assertiveness is necessary if a staff member has concerns about safety because patients are counting on them.
- It is necessary to ask clarifying questions if the staff member doesn't understand.
- Information about problems and mistakes must be shared appropriately to help improve systems and prevent recurrence of medical errors.

Recently, The Joint Commission took on still another important aspect of patient safety-related communication when it published standards for field review entitled "Proposed Requirements to Advance Effective Communication, Cultural Competence, and Patient-Centered Care."[28] If finalized, these standards will help address patient safety issues related to language, culture, health literacy, disease, or disability. Implementation would be expected by January 2011.

The 2010 National Patient Safety Goals can be accessed online at www.jointcommission.org. Regardless of whether healthcare organizations seek The Joint Commission accreditation, it is wise for risk management professionals to be familiar with the standards because they may arguably establish the standard of care if asserted as evidence in a malpractice case.

Human Factors and Patient Safety

Human error is reportedly responsible for most serious accidents in non-healthcare industries. For example, mistakes are responsible for 80 percent of industrial and airline accidents and 50 to 70 percent of nuclear power accidents.[29]

Human factors engineering (HFE), human factors analysis, and ergonomics are among the disciplines developed to address risk in non-healthcare industries. These fields of study have much to offer patient safety initiatives, as well.

The goal of HFE is the design of tools, machines, and systems that take into account human capabilities and limitations. To support this goal, human factors engineers research psychological, social, physical, and biological characteristics. The risk management professional and others addressing patient safety can use HFE principles to analyze the relationship between human beings and machines(equipment); it is the breakdown of that relationship that often plays a part in medical errors. Among patient safety-oriented approaches based on HFE principles are strategies that eliminate the use of dangerous shortcuts that lead to medical errors.[30] For example, staff must follow manufacturers' directions in testing defibrillators. Human factors analysis is the systematic study of the human–machine interface, with the intent of improving working conditions or operations. HFE strives to make the right thing to do the easiest thing to do. See Figure 1.3 for an illustration.

Ergonomics professionals study people at work and use those results to design tasks, jobs, information, tools, equipment, facilities, and the working environment to be safe, effective, productive, and comfortable. In healthcare, understanding how humans interface with highly complex technology and the surrounding environment is crucial to

FIGURE 1.3   Human–Machine Interface

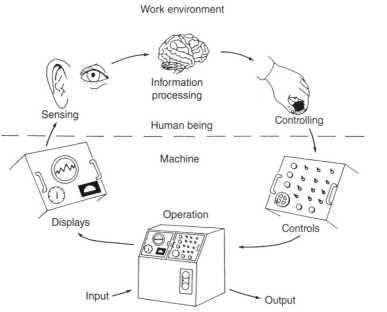

Source: McCormick, E. J., and Sanders, M. S. *Human Factors in Engineering and Design,* 15th ed. (New York: McGraw-Hill, 1982), p. 14.

preventing errors. For example, medication stations must have sufficient space around them for nurses to work without getting in each other's way at times when many nurses are preparing medications at the same time, and there must be sufficient light for nurses to see what they are doing.

To evaluate the safety of a work environment and apply human factors and ergonomics principles, the following questions should be asked:[31]

- What are the characteristics of the individual performing the work? Does the individual have the musculoskeletal, sensory, and cognitive abilities to do the required tasks? If not, can any of these gaps in ability be accommodated in the design of the task?
- What tasks are being performed, and what characteristics of those tasks might contribute to unsafe patient care? What in the nature of the tasks allows the individual to perform them safely or assume risks in the process?
- What tools and technology are being used to perform the tasks, and do they increase or decrease the likelihood of untoward events?
- Which aspects of the physical environment can be sources of error, and which promote safety? What in the environment ensures safe behavior or allows unsafe behavior to occur?

Human factors assessment should also include the following:

- Evaluating the work—what is the work-to-rest ratio?
- Evaluating the workers—what are their physical and mental capabilities?
- Evaluating the environment—are noise levels, lighting, and work flow potential barriers to successful task completion or do these factors facilitate the task? (See Figure 1.4.)

FIGURE 1.4   Components of Human Factors Assessment

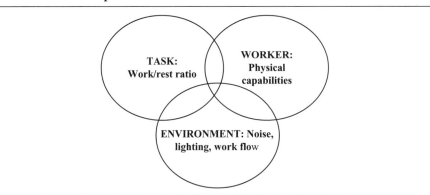

Source: Potter, P., and others. "Mapping the Nursing Process: A New Approach for Understanding the Work of Nursing." *Journal of Nursing Administration*, 2004, *34*, 101–109. Reprinted with permission.

Another illustration of the importance of evaluating the "human machine" is a recent study of the working memory of a nurse. The study found that a nurse is thinking of an average of ten things simultaneously during a work shift.[32] It is not hard to imagine errors of omission when one considers that the typical human working memory becomes taxed if asked to hold more than a seven-digit telephone number.

The mental capabilities of healthcare workers should be evaluated, as should physical characteristics such as these:

- Physical size (anthropometry)
- Endurance and fatigue (physiology)
- Force (biomechanics)
- Hand and arm coordination (kinesiology)
- Sensory characteristics (hearing, vision, touch)

Environmental issues that affect safe care delivery include the following:

- Noise, light (glare), vibration, temperature, force
- Work space or supplies layout
- Equipment–environment compatibility issues

The safety-related implications of the interface between humans and their physical environment may be illustrated, for example, by the possible desensitization of intensive care staff to the significance of one alarm in an environment in which numerous alarms sound continuously. This issue is clearly exacerbated by other employee-related safety issues such as fatigue, stress, and interruptions. Biomedical and human factors engineers should seek solutions in each individual environment.

A simpler but equally important example of the unsafe effect that comes from ignoring human factors and ergonomics principles is the poorly designed paper towel dispenser found in many hospital bathrooms. The mechanism that holds clean towels is connected to the dirty paper towel disposal unit. This design makes it easy for freshly washed hands to be contaminated by dirty towels or used tissues overflowing from the dispenser (see Figure 1.5).

Human factors and ergonomics principles can help prevent equipment-related medical errors. When used proactively, these disciplines can also mistake-proof the environment so that providers will find it hard to do the wrong thing.

Systems Thinking

Another industrial concept useful to patient safety experts is the notion of systems thinking. A system may be defined as a combination of elements organized in a structure to achieve goals and objectives. Systems may be seen as the interaction of many factors:

- Elements (personnel, equipment, procedures)
- Environment (physical, social, organizational)
- Inputs and outputs

FIGURE 1.5   Poorly Designed Paper Towel Dispenser and Disposal Unit

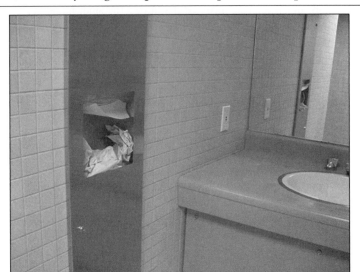

Reprinted with permission. BJC Corporate Health Services, St. Louis, MO.

● Structure

● Purpose and goals

The objectives of system evaluation must include reliability of the system and the human using it. System reliability depends on the reliability of each individual component. Components may be in series, parallel, or a combination of the two. Parallel systems are redundant and can increase reliability. Parallel redundancy is often helpful when applied to human functions because it is the human component in a system that is the least reliable.

The best way to assess the likelihood of human error is through a failure modes and effects analysis (FMEA). In FMEA, a team analyzes a process being considered in detail to determine possible system failures and then brainstorms solutions to those possible failures before the process goes into effect.

Reporting

It is impossible to reduce medical errors and adverse outcomes by focusing only on any one aspect of the healthcare system. As Dr. Richard Cook's adaptation of David Woods's blunt end/sharp end model of accident causation implies, patient safety must be analyzed from the national level, where health policy and legislation are created, down to the front line of patient care delivery.

The aviation industry illustrates the positive effect of reporting on safety. In the thirty-some years since its inception in 1976 through 2006, the Aviation Safety Reporting System

(ASRS) logged 723,427 confidential incident reports, issued over four thousand safety alert messages, and performed sixty major research studies on aviation safety. The reporting has increased 89 percent since 1988, and for calendar year 2006 the total report intake was almost 40,000 (39,964). Modeled on ASRS, the Patient Safety Reporting System was developed for the Department of Veterans Affairs (VA) as an extension of their commitment to quality and safety.[33]

The AHRQ defines *near miss* as an event or situation that did not produce patient injury, but only because of chance."[34] The effectiveness of a patient safety program can, to some degree, be measured by increased near-miss reporting because the data provide important insight into problems that need to be addressed.

The 2005 Patient Safety and Quality Improvement Act is a major step toward creation of a national voluntary system of incident reporting and medical error information. Key among the provisions of the act is the creation of patient safety organizations. These organizations are responsible for developing a network of patient safety databases that will collect and analyze voluntarily reported medical errors to identify patient safety improvement strategies. The law ensures that what is reported cannot be used against the provider in court or in disciplinary proceedings. This provision is intended to encourage providers to identify and correct medical errors. (For more information on patient safety organizations see Chapter 10 in Volume 1 of this series.)

Event Reporting Systems

In addition to providing information about individual events, event reporting systems enable the organization to prioritize resources by analyzing trends. The greatest challenge has always been the fear of punishment. This single factor is often the cause of lost valuable information that could help address system problems.

It is important for the risk management professional to be aware of common myths or unspoken rules that staff members might use to justify not reporting errors. Some examples of unspoken rules include the following:[35]

- **If I can make it right, it is not an error.** If a dose was omitted, a nurse changes the subsequently scheduled drug administration scheduled to get back on track.

- **If it's not my fault, it is not an error.** Late administration or an omission occurred when the prescribed drug was not available on the unit.

- **If another patient's needs are more urgent than accurate medication or treatment, it is not an error.** Delayed or omitted medication delivery was caused by dealing with urgent situations arising with another patient.

- **A clerical error is not a real medical error.** A nurse on a previous shift failed to document drug administration or documented in the wrong section of the record.

- **If my actions prevent something worse, it is not an error.** Nurses know that they will be busy later due to planned admissions, discharges, and so on, and administer medication early rather than risk omitting doses.

- **If everyone knows (or does it), it is not an error.** Nurses sometimes give medications early or withhold medications at night so that patients suffering from sleep deprivation can rest uninterrupted for longer periods of time.

The most common barriers to reporting include lack of knowledge about what to report or how to report, lack of trust, extra work, skepticism about the likelihood that things will change, desire to forget the event, and fear of reprisal or punishment.[36]

The most important resource to counter obstacles to reporting is a just culture of safety. If providers feel confident that their senior managers will support them, they will point out risk and report medical errors. Other strategies to facilitate reporting include the following:

- New online reporting options that include telephone hotlines or that enable staff members to input medical error data more easily and facilitate analysis

- Paper reports (if they are used) that are readily accessible by all members of the healthcare team

- Highly effective reporting programs that keep the identity of the reporter confidential

- Safety cards or other resources for patients and families to use to capture event or near-miss information

Any risk-trending analysis must assess types of errors, people, systems, and processes involved, place and time of occurrence, and risk factors identified. This information should be shared with key stakeholders and used to drive improvements that reduce risk of harm to patients (and employees).

Medical Error Reporting Requirements

After an adverse event occurs, the risk management professional and the organization's leadership must determine whether the event must be reported externally. The Centers for Medicaid and Medicare Services (CMS) has designated patient safety indicators (for example, third-degree lacerations during a vaginal birth) as incidents that must be reported by licensed organizations receiving Medicare and Medicaid funds. Furthermore, organizations that are accredited by The Joint Commission must evaluate a sentinel event and determine whether to report it; reporting these events to The Joint Commission is voluntary. The following are occurrences that are subject to review by The Joint Commission under the sentinel event policy:[37]

- The event has resulted in an unanticipated death or major permanent loss of function, not related to the natural course of the patient's illness or underlying condition or

- The event is one of the following (even if the outcome was not death or major permanent loss of function unrelated to the natural course of the patient's illness or underlying condition):

- Suicide of any patient receiving care, treatment, and services in a staffed around-the-clock care setting or within seventy-two hours of discharge

- Unanticipated death of a full-term infant
- Abduction of any patient receiving care, treatment, and services
- Discharge of an infant to the wrong family
- Rape
- Hemolytic transfusion reaction involving administration of blood or blood products having major blood group incompatibilities
- Surgery on the wrong patient or wrong body part
- Unintended retention of a foreign object in a patient after surgery or other procedure
- Severe neonatal hyperbilirubinemia (bilirubin >30 mg/dL)
- Prolonged fluoroscopy with cumulative dose greater than 1,500 rads to a single field or any delivery of radiotherapy to the wrong body region or greater than 25 percent above the planned radiotherapy dose[38]

In contrast, the following are examples of nonreviewable sentinel events under The Joint Commission's Sentinel Event Policy:

- Any near-miss event
- Full or expected return of limb or bodily function to the same level as prior to the adverse event by discharge or within two weeks of the initial loss of said function
- Any sentinel event that has not affected an individual
- Medication errors that do not result in death or major permanent loss of function
- Suicide other than in an around-the-clock care setting or following elopement from such a setting
- A death or loss of function following a discharge against medical advice (AMA)
- Unsuccessful suicide attempts
- Minor degrees of hemolysis not caused by a major blood group incompatibility and with no clinical sequelae

Most healthcare organizations have established committees that are responsible for peer review of an event that involves questionable practice or behavior of a licensed professional. These committees may consist of peers from medicine, nursing, pharmacy, or other allied health professions who review a case and determine the appropriateness of the provider's activities related to that case. The risk management professional should be formally accountable for referring an event to the organization's peer review committee as necessary.

State Requirements

There are twenty-seven adverse event reporting systems representing twenty-six states and the District of Columbia. Twenty-six of these programs are mandatory and one is voluntary. Risk management professionals must stay current with the requirements of these programs and must facilitate staff members' understanding of their implications. Similarly, risk management professionals must be aware of and facilitate federal reporting requirements such as those associated with the Safe Medical Devices Act (SMDA).

National Requirements

Despite passage of the Patient Safety and Quality Improvement Act of 2005, a national system of accountability through transparency as recommended by the IOM has not yet been created. Although twenty-six states now require public reporting of some hospital-acquired infections, the medical error reporting currently in place fails to create external pressure for change. In most cases, hospital-specific information is confidential and under-reporting of errors is not curbed by systematic validation of the reported data. Additionally, the Consumers Union notes that there has to date been no national entity empowered to coordinate and track patient safety improvements to determine if we are any better off than we were when *To Err Is Human* was published ten years ago.[39]

· · · · · · · · ·
CONCLUSION

The patient safety movement has brought numerous challenges and opportunities to risk management professionals. By collaborating with other members of an organization's management team, risk management professionals can use these new strategies to solve the ongoing challenge of medical errors.

Suggested Readings

Cook, R. *A Brief Look at the New Look in Error, Safety, and Failure of Complex Systems.* Cognitive Technologies Laboratory, University of Chicago, 1999.

Cook, R. *How Complex Systems Fail.* Revision D. Chicago: Cognitive Technologies Laboratory, University of Chicago, 2000.

Cook, R., and D. Woods. "Operating at the Sharp End: The Complexity of Human Error." In *Human Error in Medicine*, edited by Marilyn Sue Bogner. Hillsdale, N.J.: Lawrence Erlbaum Associates, 1994.

Cook, R., D. Woods, and C. Miller. *A Tale of Two Stories: Contrasting Views of Patient Safety.* Chicago: National Patient Safety Foundation, 1998.

Cook, R., M. Render, and D. Woods. "Gaps in the Continuity of Care and Progress on Patient Safety." *British Medical Journal*, 2000, 320: 791–794.

Marx, D. *Whack-a-Mole: The Price We Pay for Perfection.* Plano, TX: By Your Side Studios, 2009.

Wachter, R. M. *Understanding Patient Safety.* New York: McGraw Hill, 2008.

Woods, D., and R. Cook. "Perspectives on Human Error: Hindsight Biases and Local Rationality." In *Handbook of Applied Cognition*, edited by F. T. Durso, et al., 141–171. New York: Wiley, 1999.

Endnotes

1. Orlikoff, J., W. Fifer, and H. Greeley. *Malpractice Prevention and Loss Control for Hospitals*. Chicago: American Hospital Association, 1981.

2. *Darling v. Charleston Community Memorial Hospital*, 33 Ill.2d 326, 211 N.E.2d 253 (1965), *cert. denied*, 383 U.S. 946 (1966).

3. Joint Commission Sentinel Event Glossary of Terms, 2005, www.jointcommission.org/sentinalevents/se_glossary.htm. (Accessed November 11, 2008.)

4. Kohn, L. T., J. M. Corrigan, and M. S. Donaldson, eds. *To Err Is Human: Building a Safer Health System*. Washington, D.C.: National Academy Press, 2000.

5. P.L. 109–41 (2005)

6. Leape, L. L. and others. "The Nature of Adverse Events in Hospitalized Patients: Results of the Harvard Medical Practice Study II." *New England Journal of Medicine*, 1991, 324, 377–384.

7. Thomas, E. J., D. M. Studdert, and J. P. Newhouse. "Costs of Medical Injuries in Utah and Colorado." *Inquiry*, 1999, 36, 255–264.

8. Annual National Patient Safety Foundation Congress: Conference Proceedings, *The Journal of Patient Safety*, September 2009, 5, 131.

9. Leape, L. L. "Institute of Medicine Error Figures Are Not Exaggerated." *Journal of the American Medical Association*, 2000, 284, 95–97.

10. Bates, D. W. and others. "The Cost of Adverse Drug Events in Hospitalized Patients." *Journal of the American Medical Association*, 1997, 277, 307–311.

11. *Ibid.*

12. Leape, L. L. and others. "Preventing Medical Injury." *Quality Review Bulletin*, 1993, 19, 144–149.

13. Graves, N. "Economics and Preventing Hospital-Acquired Infection." *Emerging Infectious Diseases*, www.cdc.gov/ncidod/EID/vol10no4/02–0754.htm. (Accessed April 2004.)

14. Brennan, T. A. and others. "Harvard Medical Practice Study I." *Quality and Safety in Health Care*, 2004, 13, 151–152.

15. Stone, P. W., E. Larson, and L. N. Kawar. "A Systematic Audit of Economic Evidence Linking Nosocomial Infections and Infection Control Interventions, 1990–2000." *American Journal of Infection Control*, 2002, 30, 145–152.

16. Wenzel, R. P., and M. B. Edmond. "The Impact of Hospital-Acquired Bloodstream Infections." *Emerging Infectious Diseases*, 2001, 7, www.cdc.gov/ncidod/eid/vol7no2/wenzel.htm. (Accessed March 29, 2010.)

17. Agency for Healthcare Quality and Research. Patient Safety Initiative: Building Foundations, Reducing Risk, Chapter 2 Efforts to Reduce Medical Errors http://ahrq.hhs.gov/qual/pscongrpt/psini2.htm. (Accessed March 29, 2010.)

18. Reason, J. "Human Error: Models and Management." *British Medical Journal*, 2000, 320, 768–770.

19. D. Woods et al. *Behind Human Error*. 2nd Ed. Aldershot, UK: Ashgate, in press. Contact woods.2@osu.edu.

20. *Ibid.*

21. Leape, L. L. Presentation at Missouri Hospital Association, Patient Safety Seminar, St. Louis, Mo., 2002.

22. Marx, D. *Patient Safety and the "Just Culture": A Primer for Healthcare Executives.* Medical Event Reporting System–Transfusion Medicine (MERS-TM) New York: Columbia University, 2001, www.merstm.net/support/Marx_Primer.pdf. (Accessed March 29, 2010.)

23. National Patient Safety Foundation. *5 Attributes of a Safety Culture*, www.npsf.org/rc/mp/n-z.html. (Accessed March 29, 2010.)

24. Baker, D. P. and others. "Medical Team Training Programs in Health Care." In: *2005 Advances in Patient Safety: From Research to Implementation*, 2005, *4*, 260. Rockville, Md.: Agency for Healthcare Research and Quality, www.aptima.com/publications/2005_Baker_Gustafson_Beaubien_Salas_Barach.pdf. (Accessed March 29, 2010.)

25. *Ibid.*

26. Behaviors that Undermine a Culture of Safety: Applicable Joint Commission Standards, July 2008, www.jointcommission.org/NewsRoom/PressKits/Behaviors+that+Undermine+a+Culture+of+Safety/app_stds.htm. (Accessed December 22, 2009.)

27. Kaiser Permanente's SBAR Communication model has been adapted with permission from copyrighted material of Kaiser Foundation Health Plan, Inc., California Regions.

28. Proposed Requirements to Advance Effective Communication, Cultural Competence and Patient-Centered Care for the Hospital Accreditation Program, www.jointcommission.org/NR/rdonlyres/D44C4DE4-F5CD-4116–84AF-D5B3E8D4E94F/0/PDF1HAPProposedRequirements.pdf. (Accessed December 22, 2009.)

29. Gosbee, J. "Human Factors Engineering and Patient Safety." *Quality and Safety in Health Care*, 2002, 11, 352–354.

30. Carayon, P., C. Alvarado and A. Hundt. "Reducing Workload and Increasing Patient Safety Through Work and Workspace Design." Paper commissioned by the Institute for Medicine Commission on the Work Environment for Nurses and Patient Safety, 2003. The IOM Commission on the Work Environment for Nurses and Patient Safety commissioned nine separate working papers as background for the book *In Keeping Patients Safe: Transforming the Work Environment for Nurses*. Washington, D.C.: National Academy Press, 2004.

31. *Ibid.*

32. Wolf, L. BJC HealthCare, Patient Safety Curriculum: Human Factors Module, 2004.

33. ASRS Reporting Brief. Aviation Safety Reporting System. :http://asrs.arc.nasa.gov/overview/summary. (Accessed November 11, 2008.)

34. AHRQ PSNet Patient Safety Network Glossary, F:\AHRQ\AHRQ Patient Safety Network Glossary.htm. (Accessed November 11, 2008.)

35. Caleca, B. BJC HealthCare Patient Safety Curriculum: Importance of Reporting Module, 2004.

36. Leonard, M. Director of Patient Safety, Kaiser Permanente. Presentation. BJC HealthCare, Patient Safety Forum, St. Louis, Mo. September 2002.

37. The Joint Commission. "Sentinel Event Policy, 2007," www.jointcommission.org/NR/rdonlyres/F84F9DC6-A5DA-490F-A91F-A9FCE26347C4/0/SE_chapter_july07.pdf. (Accessed March 29, 2010.)

38. *Ibid.*

39. Jewell, K. and L. McGiffert. *To Err is Human–To Delay is Deadly*. Consumers Union's Safe Patient Project Report, May 2009. Available at: www.safepatientproject.org/safepatientproject.org/pdf/safepatientproject.org-ToDelayIsDeadly.pdf. (Accessed March 29, 2010.)

2

The Risk Management Professional and Medication Safety

Hedy Cohen
Nancy Tuohy

Before a healthcare organization's culture can truly promote safety, there must first be an unquestioning acceptance by everyone in the organization of the premise that all practitioners make errors. There must be an appreciation by the entire staff that errors are never the result of any one isolated action or deed, but rather that they result from the interaction of practitioners functioning in poorly designed systems. When an organization's leaders understand and endorse these basic principles, that organization is able to move from the pointless disciplining of individual practitioners for unintentional mistakes (a tactic that has been shown in the literature to have little effect on error reduction) to a culture of safety that is focused on identifying and addressing multifactor causes of errors. Organizations that further operationalize safety culture by using strategies such as crew resource management (CRM), thereby empowering the lowest-ranking member of a team to question more senior personnel about practice concerns, and resources such as human factors science to facilitate safer interaction between humans and machines are well on their way to becoming what is known as *high-reliability organizations.*

When it comes to medication safety, healthcare organizations have proven to be highly unreliable. In the landmark report issued by the Institute of Medicine, *To Err is Human*, it was extrapolated that more than seven thousand hospitalized patients die each year due to preventable medication errors. Although the reason for this poor safety record is multifaceted, it is historically grounded in a culture that has focused on addressing individual practitioner errors rather than the more complex and significant role of the system in which that practitioner functions. Another critical influence is the ongoing demand by consumers that organizations provide more healthcare with less money.

This chapter will delineate key issues and suggest specific strategies to enhance medication safety. To achieve success, however, healthcare organizations and their practitioners must first acknowledge and commit to addressing the many situations in which frontline practitioners work with equipment and technology that is poorly designed, ambiguous policies and procedures, and inadequate communication between management and staff. The risk management professional's role as a facilitator of senior-level commitment, as a teacher of the importance of systems—rather than individual-focused issues analysis—and as a partner to clinicians who are seeking to implement new approaches, is essential and exciting.

· · · · · · · · ·
LATENT AND ACTIVE FAILURES

The Institute for Safe Medication Practices (ISMP), a nonprofit organization dedicated to medication safety, recognizes that each unintentional medication error has its roots in multiple system failures. Although all errors are the result of active failures (which occur at the level of the frontline practitioner, with effects that are felt almost immediately), latent failures (weaknesses in the organization whose effects are usually delayed)[1] are often the most challenging causes of medical error. Active failures are sometimes characterized as *sharp-end*, and latent failures denoted as *blunt-end*. To illustrate the interaction of active and latent failures in the context of a medication error consider the following example. (The eleven active failures are underlined and the thirteen latent failures appear in *italics*.)

An infant was born to a mother with a prior history of syphilis. Despite having incomplete patient information about the mother's past treatment for syphilis and current medical status of both the mother and child, *a decision was made to treat the infant for congenital syphilis.* After consultation with infectious disease specialists and the health department, an order was written for one dose of "Benzathine Pen (penicillin) G 150,000U IM."

The physicians, nurses, and pharmacists, unfamiliar with the treatment of congenital syphilis, also had limited knowledge about this drug, which was not in their formulary. The pharmacist consulted both the infant's progress notes and *Drug Facts and Comparisons*[2] to determine the usual dose of penicillin G benzathine for an infant. However, she *misread the dose in both sources as 500,000 units/kg, a typical adult dose, instead of 50,000 units/kg.* Due to lack of a pharmacy procedure for independent double-checking, *the error was not detected.* Because a unit dose system was not used in the nursery, the pharmacy *dispensed a tenfold overdose in a plastic bag containing two full syringes of Permapen 1.2 million units/2 mL each*, with green stickers on the plungers reminding the provider to "*note dosage strength.*" A pharmacy label on the bag indicated that 2.5 mL of medication was to be administered IM, to equal a dose of 1,500,000 units.

After glancing at the medication, the infant's primary care nurse was concerned about the number of injections it would be necessary to give. (Because 0.5 mL is the maximum that providers are allowed to administer intramuscularly to an infant, a 1,500,000-unit dose would require five injections.) Anxious to prevent any unnecessary pain to the infant, the nurse involved two advanced-level colleagues, a neonatal nurse practitioner and an advanced-level nursery registered nurse (RN), who *decided to investigate the possibility of administering the medication IV instead of IM.*

NeoFax (1995 edition)[3] was consulted to determine if penicillin G benzathine could be administered IV. The *NeoFax* monograph on penicillin G did not specifically mention penicillin G benzathine: instead, it described the treatment for congenital syphilis with aqueous crystalline penicillin G, IV slow push, or penicillin G procaine IM. Nowhere in the two-page monograph was penicillin G benzathine mentioned, and no specific warnings that penicillin G procaine and penicillin G benzathine were to be given "IM only" were present.

Unfamiliar with the various forms of penicillin G, the nurse practitioner *believed that "benzathine" was a brand name for penicillin G.* This misconception was reinforced by the physician's method of writing the drug order, written *with benzathine capitalized and placed on a line above "penicillin G" rather than after it on the same line* (see Figure 2.1). It is noteworthy that many texts use ambiguous synonyms when referring to various forms of penicillin. For example, penicillin G benzathine is frequently mentioned near or directly associated with the terms "crystalline penicillin" and "aqueous suspension." *Believing that aqueous crystalline penicillin G and penicillin G benzathine were the same drug, the nurse practitioner concluded that the drug could safely be administered IV.* Although the nurse practitioner had been taught in school that only clear liquids could be injected IV, she had learned through practical experience that certain milky white substances, such as IV lipids and other lipid-based drug products, can indeed be given IV. *Therefore, she did not recognize the problem of giving penicillin G benzathine, a milky white substance, through an IV.*

Complicating matters further in this example, hospital policies and practices did not clearly define the prescriptive authority of nonphysicians. Partially as a result of this lack of clarity, the neonatal nurse practitioner assumed that she was operating under a national protocol, which allowed neonatal nurse practitioners to plan, direct, implement, and change drug therapy. Consequently, the nurse practitioner *made a decision to*

FIGURE 2.1   Chart Entry—Benzathine

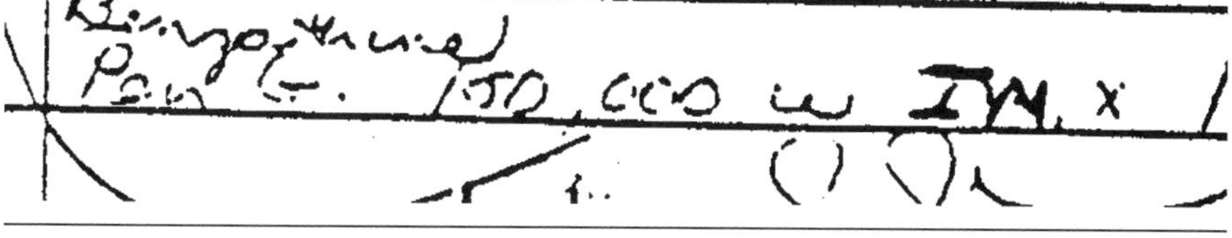

administer the drug IV. The primary care nurse, who was not certified to administer IV medication to infants, transferred care of the infant to the advanced level nursery RN and the nurse practitioner.

As they prepared for drug administration, *neither of these providers noticed the tenfold overdose or that the syringe was labeled by the manufacturer "IM use only."* The manufacturer's warning was not prominently placed. The syringe needed to be rotated 180 degrees away from the name before the warning could be seen. *The nurse began to administer the first syringe of Permapen slow IV push.* After about 1.8 mL was administered, the infant became unresponsive, and resuscitation efforts were unsuccessful.

It is important that risk management professionals focus their energies on the role of latent failures to prevent other such heartbreaking outcomes from occurring. Because the medication administration process is, in reality, a complex system, with parameters usually outside the control of the individual practitioner, most errors are rarely the fault of one individual. Thus, providing an optimal level of medication safety requires that organizations proactively recognize and correct underlying system failures before injuries to patients occur. As noted earlier, this requires a shift in focus beyond "naming, blaming, shaming, and training" of individuals.

· · · · · · · · ·
SYSTEMS THINKING

Based on the foregoing discussion, in addition to committing to a culture of patient safety and aspiring to become high-reliability operations, organizations addressing medication safety must also embrace systems thinking. This approach assesses how individual processes interrelate. Most important, it helps us understand how individual flaws in a complex system such as medication use can cause a serious error. As illustrated by Figure 2.2, we are vulnerable to system failures in our everyday life. In this example, we see how poor design may impede the process of entering a building. You want to open a door that has a pull handle. You pull the door toward you to open it, yet the door does not budge.

You pull again with no success. Then you realize that the door is to be opened by pushing, rather than pulling. Your expectation was that a door designed with a pull handle is supposed to be pulled, not pushed. This same type of misperception can occur when a nurse obtains a medication from an automated dispensing cabinet. When the medication bin is labeled with the name of a specific drug, the nurse assumes that the correct drug is in that bin. If, however, the wrong drug was inadvertently placed in the bin, an error can easily occur.

To facilitate understanding of the complex processes that interact to cause medication errors, ISMP identified ten safety-critical components of the medication-use system and categorized numerous reported errors accordingly. The following discussion of issues associated with each component provides insight into medication use-related risk. Specific risk reduction strategies are also presented.

FIGURE 2.2   Door-Pull Handle

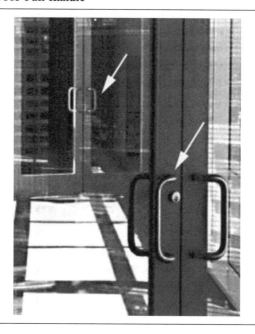

Patient Information

More than 18 percent of prescribing errors are due to inadequate patient information. Of particular concern is the lack of information about allergies and comorbidities, such as hepatic function and pregnancy status.[4] A critical related issue is that essential patient information is often unavailable to pharmacy and nursing staff prior to dispensing or administering drugs for new admissions.

Essential patient information includes the following:

- Allergies
- Diagnosis and comorbid conditions
- Renal and hepatic function
- Pregnancy and lactation status
- Age, weight (kg), height (cm)
- Full medication history (over-the-counter, herbals)
- Lab and other diagnostic results
- Clinical observations (vital signs, mentation)
- Demographics

When drugs are dispensed or administered without adequate patient information, such as lab values or key patient comorbidities, critical data that should be double-checked are omitted and risk potentially increases. For example, warfarin, an anticoagulant, is ordered on admission, but the provider ordering warfarin is unaware that the international normalized ratio (INR) is elevated. (The INR is a standardized measure of clotting time.) In another hypothetical situation, a prescriber might order a standard dosage of aminoglycide, which is contraindicated for an end-stage renal patient, because there is no available documentation of the patient's condition. Barring an emergency situation, drugs should never be dispensed unless specific clinical information has been reviewed during the ordering process. Clearly, healthcare practitioners must identify effective ways to facilitate the presence of key clinical information at this critical point in the patient's care.

A real-life example of an error due to lack of information about comorbidities involved an eighty-four-year-old woman who was transferred from a nursing home to a hospital for a coronary artery bypass graft. After surgery, her platelet count dropped by 50 percent. A hematologist was consulted, who determined that the patient was suffering from heparin-induced thrombocytopenia. Although the physician documented this diagnosis in his consultation report, it was not written elsewhere in the patient's chart, and the pharmacy was not notified. As a result, when the patient was transferred to a surgical unit two days later, nurses, unaware of the patient's comorbid diagnosis of heparin-induced thrombocytopenia, flushed her IV lines with heparin. The patient suffered a stroke six hours later and died. Although her death was probably due to the surgery, the illicit heparin administration was likely a contributing factor.

Another error that resulted from inadequate patient information occurred when a double-strength concentration of a potentially dangerous or high-alert drug was ordered for a cardiac patient in the intensive care unit (ICU). A nurse called the pharmacy and inadvertently requested that an infusion of regular insulin be prepared at twice normal strength. In carrying out this erroneous verbal order, the pharmacist failed to notice in the order entry system that diabetes mellitus was not documented as a patient diagnosis. Then, without seeing a copy of the written order, he prepared and delivered the insulin infusion. Subsequently, during ICU pharmacy rounds, he failed to obtain a copy of the physician's order or review the patient's chart to verify hyperglycemia. Without an independent double-check, the nurse administered the double-strength regular insulin infusion. As a result, the patient suffered permanent central nervous system (CNS) impairment.

Information that is of obvious and closely related importance is the patient's identity. The Joint Commission (TJC) requires that staff use two patient-specific identifiers before administering any medication. These are likely to include patient name and birth date. But accurate and complete validation of patient identification for purposes of medication administration cannot occur without comparing the patient identification to the medication administration record (MAR). Staff members should also encourage patients to state their name and show their identification bracelet before accepting any medications.

Further illustrating the importance of patient identification, medication errors also occur due to order sheets that don't have a patient's name. In one case, a potentially serious error occurred when an order for high-dose cytarabine (ara-C), a chemotherapy agent, was written on a blank order sheet that contained no identifying patient information. The order sheet was then accidentally stamped by the unit clerk with the wrong patient's name and faxed to the pharmacy. Fortunately, the patient's diagnosis of hairy cell leukemia was in the pharmacy's computer system. The error was averted when an oncology pharmacy specialist, scanning patient demographics before entering the order, realized that the high-dose cytarabine was totally inappropriate for the patient.

To enhance the collection of key patient data, all medication forms, including prescriber order forms, the MAR, and the pharmacy profile should have a designated area with pertinent prompts and sufficient space to document essential patient information. Such approaches should make it easy to capture issues such as weight fluctuation and new allergies. Healthcare organizations must educate all staff on the importance of obtaining accurate inpatient and outpatient information. Ideally, an electronic medical record (EMR) or other form of computer technology should integrate all collected data, including outpatient information.

As another safeguard, the organization should have policies and procedures in place that ensure that the pharmacist has all pertinent patient demographic and clinical information on hand prior to dispensing the medication and that the medication order received is complete with all required information, is legible, and does not pose any other concerns or questions. It is also important that high-alert medications previously not reviewed against a patient's record for allergies or other drug interactions (nonprofiled) that are available from unit stock or automated dispensing cabinets be independently double-checked before administration, except in emergency situations. An independent double-check is effective only if done in the following way: The first practitioner completes the task (calculation, pump programming, syringe verification, and so on) without sharing methods with the checking practitioner. The second checking practitioner completes the task again, without help or hints (for example, "Here's how I did this" or "This should be five units of insulin") from the first. The second practitioner then compares the results of both practitioners against the original order for accuracy before the medication is dispensed or administered.

Still other preventive strategies include keeping the pharmacy information system and computerized provider order entry (CPOE) current as drugs are added to the formulary. Additionally, all systems should contain alerts for allergies, cross-sensitivities, weight and age restrictions, and drug duplications when new medications are added to a patient's profile.

Drug Information

In recent years, there has been an explosion of new medications and innovative uses of older drugs. Keeping abreast of this constantly evolving information is a daunting, if not impossible, task. It has been noted that most medication errors occur during the prescribing and administration stages because up-to-date drug information is not available at the point of care.[5] In addition, many healthcare organizations do not have pharmacists readily available to interact, face to face, with practitioners on patient care units.[6]

Because many medication errors occur due to lack of essential drug information, ongoing staff education regarding the appropriate uses, dosages, side effects, and interactions of drugs is critical. For example, the use of the cancer chemotherapeutic agent methotrexate is well established in the oncology setting. However, providers recently began to prescribe this medication in low doses for rheumatoid arthritis, asthma, psoriasis, inflammatory bowel disease, myasthenia gravis, and inflammatory myositis. When used for these chronic diseases, such doses are administered weekly or sometimes twice a week. However, because relatively few such medications are dosed on a weekly basis, practitioners who are unfamiliar with this new clinical approach may make mistakes related to frequency of administration and to the novel dosage. In one reported case, a seventy-nine-year-old patient was to receive methotrexate for a non-cancer-related indication. The prescription was erroneously written and dispensed as methotrexate four times daily. This patient died after receiving nine doses of the medication over a seventy-two-hour period.

Prescribers, pharmacists, and nurses must never order, dispense, or administer any medication with which they are not totally familiar. Although this might be challenging for organizations that face demands for efficiency, it is essential to provide practitioners with a workload that allows adequate time to learn about their patients' medications. In yet another example of an error, a cardiac patient was admitted from the emergency department (ED) as an overflow patient to a surgical ICU unit where the staff was unfamiliar with the administration of thrombolytics. The cardiologist mistakenly ordered a loading dose of eptifibatide (used to inhibit platelet aggregation) as 180 mcg, not as 180 mcg/kg. The pharmacy was particularly busy, and the pharmacist, who was unfamiliar with eptifibatide dosing, did not read the package insert or verify the dose with the prescriber. The surgical ICU nurse, who had never administered this drug, compounded the error when she misread the prescriber's order as "180 mg." She initiated the loading dose by giving 75 mg over one hour, planning to call the pharmacy for the remainder of the dose. As the infusion was ending, another pharmacist discovered the error and the infusion was discontinued. Fortunately, the patient suffered no permanent harm.

Strategies to make drug information available at the point of care include the use of rule-based CPOE systems that provide drug information, warnings, and alerts during order input. If CPOE is not available in the organization, the use of a sound, user-friendly computerized drug information system such as Micromedex[7] or up-to-date drug information books (most recent publication and year) can provide valuable current drug information. The pharmacy computer system should also give specific warnings for those drugs that have unusual dosing schedules, such as weekly or monthly, and alerts for cumulative drug dosing. Another effective strategy is to move the pharmacist, an expert in the clinical uses of medication, from the centralized pharmacy into satellite pharmacies within patient care areas. This allows the pharmacist to establish a close working relationship with the practitioners and patients, follow the patients' clinical courses, and consult regularly with the professional staff about appropriate drug selection, dosing, and administration. It has been shown that, when the pharmacist is close to the point of care, patient outcomes are improved and errors and drug costs are significantly reduced.[8] If pharmacists are not already in place in patient care units, organizations can take a first step toward this model of care by having pharmacists make daily rounds of patient care units or enter medication orders directly at the computer terminals in patient care units. The next logical step in integrating pharmacists more closely with the care team should be to prioritize implementation of unit-based pharmacy support in key areas, such as the intensive care unit, the pediatrics or oncology units, the operating room, and the ED.

Communication of Information

Organizational barriers to communicating essential clinical patient and drug information effectively include drug information systems that do not interface with other vital patient information systems, such as the EMR and the laboratory system. Such disconnects clearly hamper the practitioner's access to information essential for safe administration, such as allergies and pertinent test results. Another closely related obstacle is the absence of computer order-entry systems. Without such systems, there is increased risk of order-related error due to illegible handwriting, missing or ambiguous information, nonconventional abbreviations, and unclear documentation of dosage.

Another barrier is a provider's flawed communication style. Of particular concern is intimidation, which contributes to about 10 percent of the serious errors that occur during administration of medication. In fact, ISMP receives many reports of lethal errors in which orders were questioned but not changed. In a survey conducted by ISMP, almost half (49 percent) of all respondents related that their past experiences with intimidation had altered the way they handle order clarification or questions about medication orders. At least once during the previous year, about 40 percent of respondents did not act on concerns about a medication order or asked another professional to talk to the pre-scriber, rather than interact with a particularly intimidating prescriber. Three-quarters (75 percent) had asked colleagues to help them interpret an order or validate its safety so that they did not have to interact with an intimidating prescriber. Also, 34 percent reported that they had found the prescriber's stellar reputation intimidating and had not questioned an order about which they had concerns. When the prescriber had been questioned about the safety of an order and refused to change it, 31 percent of respon-dents suggested that the physician administer the drug or simply allowed the physician to give the medication himself, and almost half (49 percent) felt pressured to accept the order, dispense a product, or administer a medication despite their concerns. As a result, 7 percent of respondents reported that they had been involved in a medication error during the previous year in which intimidation clearly played a role.[9,10]

To address flawed communication styles, many healthcare organizations use estab-lished protocols, consistent with human resources protocols and medical staff bylaws, to follow up with providers who are perceived to be intimidating. Additionally, TJC imple-mented new standards that require all accredited programs to address intimidation and disruptive behaviors. Furthermore, it requires organizations to include six core compe-tencies in the medical staff credentialing process, including interpersonal skills and professionalism.[11] Appropriate strategies in this regard may include the use of incident or event reports, objectively completed, to document clinically pertinent events. Of great assistance in improving communication housewide is a crew resource management approach, in which a team member with minimal stature is empowered to question team leaders. Remember that effective implementation of such strategies cannot occur without senior administrative and clinical leadership endorsement.

Another key communication issue involves verbal orders. Such orders, whether spoken in person or over the telephone, are inherently problematic because they can easily be misheard or misinterpreted. For example, there have been error reports in which verbal orders for "Celebrex 100 mg PO" were misheard to be for "Cerebyx 100 mg PO." Drug names are not the only verbal information prone to misinterpretation. Numbers are also problematic. For example, an emergency room physician verbally ordered "morphine 2 mg IV," but the nurse heard "morphine 10 mg IV," and the patient subsequently received a 10-mg infusion that caused respiratory arrest. In another situation, a physician called in an order for "15 mg of hydralazine" to be given IV every two hours. The nurse, thinking that he had said "50 mg," administered an overdose to the patient, who developed tachycardia and had a significant drop in blood pressure.

To reduce the use of verbal orders, some organizations use fax machines to communicate orders. However, fax machines are connected to telephone lines, and significant line noise can result in the loss of important information, such as portions of a drug name or even the dose. For example, the order shown in Figure 2.3 was mistaken as Flagyl 250 mg instead of Flagyl 500 mg. A related problem occurs when prescribers write on the very edge of the order form, making it impossible for some fax machines and scanners to read the entire order. Thus an order for "Lomotil QID PRN" may appear as Lomotil QID, as if the *PRN* were never written.

Verbal orders must be eliminated, except in emergency and sterile situations. Such orders are especially inappropriate when potentially lethal drugs, such as chemotherapy agents, are prescribed. To further decrease the risk of verbal order-related errors, healthcare organizations should adopt yet another crew resource management principle. This particular strategy concerns the standardization of communication. Here are approaches that might help achieve standardization of verbal orders.

- Verbal orders should only be accepted for emergency treatment. When the prescriber is present, a verbal order should never be accepted.

FIGURE 2.3 Faxes Aren't the Problem

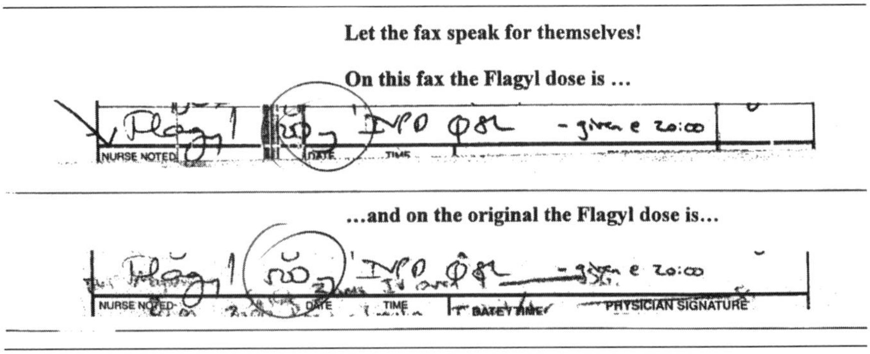
Let the fax speak for themselves!
On this fax the Flagyl dose is ...
NURSE NOTED
DATE
TIME
...and on the original the Flagyl dose is...
NURSE NOTED
DATE
TIME
PHYSICIAN SIGNATURE

- When accepting a verbal order, a staff member should write down on the patient's chart or an order form with the appropriate identifying information the order as it is being given.

- When verbal orders are allowed, prescribers must enunciate the order clearly, and the receiver should always repeat the order to the prescriber to avoid misinterpretation.

- The person receiving the order should read back the entire order to the prescriber, including the patient's name and second identifier.

- As an extra check, either the prescriber or receiver should spell unfamiliar drug names, saying "T as Tom," "C as Charley," and so forth. Pronounce each numerical digit separately, saying for example, "one six" instead of "sixteen" to avoid confusion with *sixty*.

- The receiver must ensure that the verbal order makes sense when considered in conjunction with the patient's diagnosis and should ask the prescriber for the drug indication when necessary. The order should also be documented in the patient's medical record as soon as possible.

- For telephone orders, the recipient must obtain a telephone number for the prescriber in case it is necessary to call back with follow-up questions.

- Limit verbal orders to formulary drugs, because staff members are more likely to misunderstand drug names and dosages with which they are unfamiliar.

- Limit the number of personnel who routinely receive telephone orders to reduce the potential for unauthorized orders.

Still another issue is poor communication of medical information at care transition points. According to the Institute for Healthcare Improvement (IHI), miscommunication when the patient moves from one care environment to another is responsible for about 50 percent of all medication errors and up to 20 percent of adverse drug events in numerous healthcare organizations across the country.[12] One illustration of this type of error is a patient who was transferred from one hospital to another and received a duplicate dose of insulin because the receiving nurse did not know that the medication had been given before transfer. In another case, enalapril 2.5 mg IV was administered to a patient after transfer from a critical care unit to a medical unit. The drug had been discontinued upon transfer, but the orders had not yet been transcribed. Yet another error occurred when, before discharge, the patient's Lexapro was increased to 10 mg daily, but the discharge instructions erroneously called for 5 mg daily. When the error was noticed, a pharmacist called the patient and learned that she had been cutting her newly prescribed 10-mg tablets in half.

TJC standards now require that healthcare organizations address medication reconciliation. Particularly helpful is documentation of this process that assesses and addresses medication duplications and incompatibilities at vulnerable points of transition, such as admission, transfers between care settings, and at discharge.

Finally, to facilitate communication about medication orders, it is important that written and computerized medication orders include the generic and brand names of the medication, without abbreviations. There are literally thousands of drug pair names that sound and look similar, so detailed information helps prevent these medications from being mistaken for one another. In addition, medication should never be prescribed by volume, number of vials, or ampules. When such orders are received, the staff should seek clarification immediately.

Labeling, Packaging, and Drug Nomenclature

Improper hospital drug labeling and failing to keep drugs in packaging until administering them contribute to medication errors. Additionally, the pharmaceutical industry has sometimes unwittingly undermined the safe use of medication by marketing drug names that look alike and sound alike, using confusing labeling, or providing drugs to healthcare organizations in nondistinct or ambiguously marked packages. In reports submitted to MedMarx® (a subscription-based reporting program sponsored by Quantros), nearly thirty-two thousand medication errors over a thirty-nine-month period occurred among look-alike or sound-alike drugs due to packaging or labeling. Approximately 2.6 percent of these errors were classified as harmful.[13]

Labeling   Confusing labeling, sometimes associated with manufacturer's use of similar colors, font sizes, and layout to achieve a product image, can also result in errors. For example, the drug Temodar (temozolomide) has reportedly been the subject of numerous dispensing and administration errors because labeling leads staff members to misinterpret capsule strength. This alkylating agent is available in 5-, 20-, 100-, and 250-mg capsules. The strength is stated directly beside the quantity of capsules (Figure 2.4). One who reads the number of capsules right next to the strength might reasonably conclude that the total number of capsules in the bottle is equal to the strength, for example, 20 capsules equals 100 mg, rather than 20 capsules, each containing 100 mg. Adding to the confusion is similarity between the strength of the dosage and the number of capsules

FIGURE 2.4   Capsule Quantity Is Often Confused with Product Strength

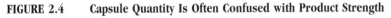

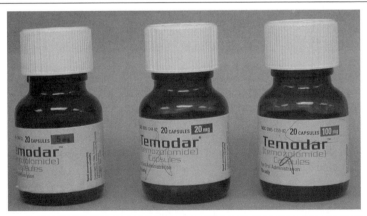

in the bottle. Capsules in strengths of 5 mg and 20 mg are often dispensed in packages that contain either five or twenty capsules. The FDA pointed out that this confusing packaging and labeling can lead to serious, even fatal, errors.[14]

One potentially serious error was reported in which a prescription for oral Temodar 60 mg daily was written for a patient with a brain tumor. The pharmacist dispensed the dosage from a 100-mg bottle containing twenty capsules, and simply misread the label. The pharmacist was under the impression that twenty capsules were equal to 100 mg, so he concluded that each capsule contained 5 mg and dispensed twelve capsules to make up a 60-mg dose. Fortunately, the patient's mother caught the error when she was filling the patient's pillbox before any of the medication was given.

To address these issues, the manufacturer submitted a redesigned label to the FDA for approval.

To proactively address label confusion such as this, organizations may affix name and strength alert stickers on products that have potentially confusing labels and highlight the differences with a pen or highlighter. The staff should also employ at least two independent checks in the dispensing and administration processes for these medications. Organizations also might consider implementation of point-of-care bar coding technology, which, for example, requires the provider to scan the patient's name band along with the drug package before administering the drug. Other invaluable devices are smart infusion pumps that contain drug libraries to further enhance safe administration of such drugs.

Packaging   Like confusing dose information, look-alike packaging is of great concern. Related errors generally involve assumptions by staff members that a medication that sounds similar to the one they are ordered to give is appropriate, or they pick up a wrong vial or other dispensing device because it looks like the medication they are ordered to give. In one example, a woman who was thirty-one weeks pregnant received Methergine (methylergonovine) instead of terbutaline (Brethine), which resulted in the emergency premature cesarean-section delivery of her baby. Similar sounding names and similar-looking packaging contributed to the error (Figure 2.5). Fortunately, mother and child were unharmed.

Another look-alike medication issue involves respiratory therapy inhalation drugs, such as ipratropium (Atrovent) and levalbuterol (Xopenex), which are packaged in disposable, clear plastic containers with raised, embossed labels that are difficult to read. Compounding the risk, respiratory therapists often pocket several of each of these medications, to be more efficient. Of additional concern, other products, such as ophthalmic solutions and preservative-free medications such as Xylocaine, are also illegibly packaged in small plastic vials. See Figure 2.6.

To minimize confusion associated with look-alike packaging, healthcare organizations should, whenever possible, consider using equivalent products from different manufacturers. Organizations should also avoid storing look-alike products near one another in unit stock and automated dispensing cabinets.

Applying auxiliary labels might help distinguish similar-looking packages. Additionally, the use of *tall man* lettering might help to visually differentiate drug names on

FIGURE 2.5   Merthergine versus Brethine

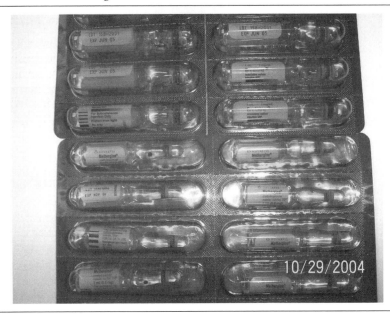

FIGURE 2.6   Mix of Ophthalmic and Respiratory Solutions

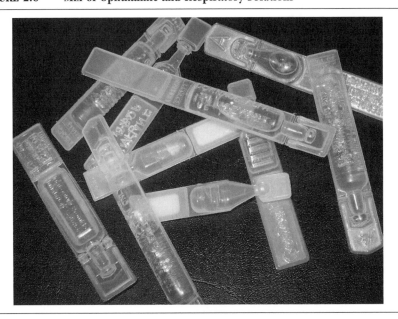

similar-looking packages. Tall man lettering uses capital letters within a drug name to highlight the letters of a name that differentiate two similar names. For instance, hydrALA-ZINE and hydrOXYzine. In 2001, the U.S. Food and Drug Administration's (FDA's) Office of Generic Drugs requested manufacturers of sixteen look-alike name pairs to voluntarily reformat the appearance of these drug names on their packaging, and tall man lettering was used extensively in this effort. This was a voluntary program, thus not all manufacturers complied. Facilities, however, may choose to employ tall man lettering on auxiliary labels, shelf and bin labels, or medication administration records.

Yet another packaging-related issue that contributes to errors involves the removal or discarding of packaging before the drug is administered. Although most drugs are packaged as unit doses, this does not ensure that medications will remain labeled until they reach the patient's bedside. Often, nurses prepare drugs at a central location, removing pharmacy or manufacturer drug packaging and labeling and placing the open medication in cups for administration. Thus, the chance for errors, especially administering a medication to the wrong patient, is greatly increased. Institutions should require that the drug remain labeled throughout the drug use process, up to the point of administration. Using barcode technology might make this easier. Until this technology is instituted nationwide, however, it might be valuable to convene staff focus groups to identify and address the reasons that providers remove drug packaging and labels before administering drugs.

Nomenclature   Errors in identifying medication sometimes occur when providers refer to medication by a shorter name. Other reasons for misidentification include confusion due to the indiscriminate use of brand and generic names, in combination and separately, in written and computerized orders. Sometimes confusion results from a *line extension,* when the manufacturer substantively changes the drug, but changes only the suffix of the name, to better market the progeny of a successful pharmaceutical. To address such confusion, ISMP recommends that both brand and generic names be documented in ordering and transcribing and that the indication for the medication be included.

One example of potential omission related to nomenclature was generated by a mix-up between the sound-alike medications, Cerebyx and Celebrex. In this case, Cerebyx (fosphenytoin) 100 mg IV TID, an anticonvulsant, was listed on a patient's MAR from a transferring hospital. The admitting cardiologist at the receiving hospital was unfamiliar with Cerebyx and misread the drug as Celebrex (celecoxib), a pain medication, even though he knew it was not available in a parenteral form. He did not order the drug because the patient was not having pain. When a pharmacist reviewed the orders along with the old MAR and investigated, he was able to correct the order, thus preventing an omission error. Although often not considered as serious a potential threat to patient safety, patients can be harmed as much by the omission of a drug as from an erroneous dose.

In another issue related to nomenclature, Pamelor (nortriptyline), an antidepressant, was misheard as Tambocor (flecainide), an antiarrhythmic, and the prescription was dispensed as such. Although the patient took this erroneous medication for one month and experienced fatigue, he fortunately suffered no cardiovascular symptoms.

In yet another example, a pharmacist received an order for Gabitril (tiagabine), which is used for seizure disorders. He entered the order correctly, but the patient still received the wrong drug because the pharmacy mistakenly dispensed Zanaflex (tizanidine), a drug used for muscle spasticity. Tiagabine and tizanidine were stored alphabetically by generic name in the pharmacy, separated by only one space on the shelves. Both drugs are also available in 2-mg and 4-mg strengths. The error occurred despite a bright-orange warning sticker stating "Name Alert" on the tizanidine supply. The potential for error was increased because the hospital had repackaged the drugs in unit doses using only the generic names. Fortunately, in this case a nurse detected the difference before administering the drug.

Nomenclature-related safety issues have resulted in the United States Pharmacopeia's (USP) adoption of a resolution to encourage the use of generic names alone for new single-active ingredient products marketed after January 1, 2006. However, a single drug name—generic or brand—would not prevent all such mix-ups. Examination of the drug pairs delineated in TJC's National Patient Safety Goal, requiring accredited entities to annually review a list of pertinent look- and sound-alike drugs, reveals that nine of ten problem pairs involve similar generic names.[15]

Trademark extensions are another risk issue. There are no standard meanings for various suffixes such as XL, ER, and SR that follow drug names. The line of Wellbutrin (bupropion) products has been of particular concern in this regard. Twice in one week, a hospital psychiatrist ordered Wellbutrin XL 300 mg, but two tablets of Wellbutrin SR 150 mg were dispensed. The pharmacists filling the orders were unaware of the new XL formulation, and poor physician handwriting made it difficult to discern the XL portion of the drug name. In another reported case, a prescriber wrote Wellbutrin XR (instead of either XL or SR) 150 mg daily. The pharmacist could have looked at the once-daily frequency and concluded that it must be the XL product. However, he reviewed the profile and found that the patient had, in fact, been taking Wellbutrin SR daily, so that is what he dispensed. Unfortunately, the physician actually meant to prescribe the XL formulation.

Different forms of a drug can also be confused. For example, significant harm may occur when liposomal and conventional products are mixed up. In one case, liposomal doxorubicin (Doxil) and conventional doxorubicin (brand names include Adriamycin and Rubex), both packaged in 20-mg vials, were stored together in the same drawer in a pharmacy refrigerator. Although both drugs are chemotherapeutic agents, their actions are very different. The patient involved received an IV push injection of 75 mg of Doxil, rather than the conventional doxorubicin that was intended. The patient's reaction was not serious, but other reports indicate that similar incidents have resulted in severe side effects and even death.

To reduce drug mix-ups related to nomenclature, it is important that providers seek clarification if the drug being ordered does not seem to match the patient's condition. Additionally, institutions should require both the brand and generic names in all documentation, including orders, and on pharmacy labels.

Drug Storage, Stocking, and Standardization

The traditional floor stock model of medication storage and stocking has been phased out in most U.S. hospitals. Formerly, a nearly complete pharmacy was maintained on every unit in a hospital or nursing home, which increased the probability of errors. Acting alone, the nurse typically interpreted and transcribed a physician's order, chose the proper container from hundreds available on the shelves, prepared the correct amount, placed the dose in a syringe or cup, labeled it, took it to the patient, administered it, and verified that the dose had been administered. The obvious lack of check systems has led to the elimination of this medication administration model in most organizations.

Errors are still likely to occur, however, in organizations that employ a modified floor stock model on nursing units, even if there are just a few stock bottles for nurses to manage. The chance of error under these circumstances increases if drugs are stored on units (or in the pharmacy) by alphabetical name or if the unit fails to sequester high-alert drugs (such as neuromuscular blockers).

Technological solutions are helpful only to a point. For example, even when unit stock is placed in automated dispensing cabinets, problems still might occur if there are not enough cabinets or if poor workspace planning results in nurses crowding the cabinets at times when many patients require medications simultaneously. Under such circumstances, staff members often try to circumvent an inefficient work environment by storing medications in their pockets. Also of concern is the partial implementation of technological solutions—for example, if the pertinent technology does not integrate with other documentation systems in-house or fails to encompass safety features such as patient profiling and on-screen alerts.

Indeed, if automated dispensing cabinets (ADCs) store a wide assortment of medications or excessive quantities of a single medication, yet do not interface with the pharmacy's computer-based profiling system, the risk of error actually increases. Pharmacy profiling allows a pharmacist to review each medication order and screen it for safety before the drug can be removed from the cabinet. Without this safeguard, nurses might not be alerted to unsafe doses, potential allergic reactions, duplicate therapy, contraindications, drug interactions, or other important information that could make the drug, dose, or route of administration unsafe. Additionally, medications in ADCs are not always limited to the dosage that is necessary for a patient. Also, manufacturer-generated unit dose medication is not often labeled with the individual patient's dose. These issues resulted in the death of a patient who received 10 mg of colchicine IV (before this preparation was removed from the market in 2008). The physician had prescribed "colchicine 1.0 mg IV now," but the decimal point was hidden on the line of the order form and the use of an unnecessary trailing zero led to misinterpretation. However, the error reached the patient primarily because there was an excessive quantity of colchicine in the ADC. Ten ampules of colchicine (1 mg each) were available in the ADC; thus the nurse had enough ampules to prepare the overdose.

Safety procedures for automated dispensing cabinets are essential error prevention tools. For example, without a protocol that addresses proper storage, drugs may be placed erroneously in compartments of a cabinet that has been labeled for other medications. Procedures should also require that no medication be routinely available to administer to patients without appropriate order screening by the pharmacist. This includes initial doses of medication. Particularly dangerous drugs should be dispensed directly from the pharmacy.

Device Acquisition, Use, and Monitoring

Practitioners involved in the medication-use process often employ one or more drug-administration devices to administer a specific drug. Historically, many devices, such as infusion pumps, were designed without the benefit of human factors engineering. Human factors engineering and human factors ergonomics are the "scientific disciplines concerned with the understanding of interactions among humans and other elements of a system, and the profession that applies theory, principles, data, and other methods to design in order to optimize human well-being and overall system performance."[16] This definition was adopted by the International Ergonomics Association in August 2000. Failure to take human factors principles into consideration when designing medication delivery devices can contribute to patient harm.

For example, the misuse of infusion pumps and other parenteral device systems is the second-leading cause of serious errors during drug administration.[17] A classic human factors–related problem that involves infusion pumps is the free flow of medication into a patient due to the lack of free-flow protection on intravenous (IV) pumps. Before TJC implemented a standard that required free-flow protection on pumps, such errors occurred when practitioners forgot to slide the clamping mechanism closed when they removed the infusion tubing sets from the pump. As the issues associated with infusion pumps illustrate, reliance on human vigilance in the operation of a device is inherently prone to error. All devices should be designed to compensate for normal error-causing human behavior, such as momentary lapses in attention and fatigue.

Even with the presence of more recent equipment in the clinical setting, errors may still occur. For example, the design of infusion pump keypads makes it easy for tenfold dosing errors to occur. Specifically, the close proximity of the zero and decimal point keys on some IV pumps, and multiple-function keys, such as an up arrow that also serves as an enter key, has led nurses to misprogram pumps with rates that can cause overdose. The newest pumps, called *smart pumps*, may include a computerized drug library of preset dose limits that alert nurses to programming errors, but many older pumps without such features remain in use.

Other problems involving IV infusion pumps include the following:

- Infusion pumps being turned off accidentally by users or when physically bumped against other objects
- Lack of visible or audible warning alarms when the syringe or cassette is not properly loaded, resulting in overdosing or underdosing of medication
- Confusing tubing on pumps when multiple lines are used

- The inadvertent setting of a drug or solution at the primary IV rate instead of at the intended secondary rate
- Decimal point errors, such as keying in the infusion rate at ten times the intended rate (for example, 44.5 mL/h instead of 4.5 mL/h and 88 mL/h instead of 8 mL/h)
- Dosage calculation errors
- Keying in the volume of the drug to be infused as the infusion rate (for example, a volume of 500 mL heparin mistakenly entered as a rate of 500 mL/h)
- Selecting the wrong drug, strength, and/or concentration from the smart pump library

It is particularly essential from a safety perspective that special precautions be taken with patient-controlled analgesia (PCA) pumps. When used as intended, PCA reduces the risk of oversedation by allowing patients to self-administer more frequent but with smaller doses of analgesia through an infusion pump. However, because this therapeutic intervention combines inherently error-prone devices and narcotics, serious, unintended outcomes have frequently occurred.

Fortunately, by identifying specific issues, risks associated with this technology can be reduced. Table 2.1 summarizes some of the issues surrounding the use of PCA pumps and appropriate solutions.

TABLE 2.1   PCA Problems and Safety Recommendations

Problem	*Description*	*Safety Recommendation*
PCA by proxy	When another person (health professional, family member) administers a dose of medication instead of the patient's dosing himself or herself. It can lead to oversedation, respiratory depression, and death. Patients are to control the PCA so that a sedated patient cannot press the button, thereby overdosing.	Warn patients, family members, and visitors about the dangers of PCA by proxy. Place warning labels on activation buttons that state "FOR PATIENT USE ONLY." Keep PCA flow sheets at the bedside to document PCA doses and patient monitoring.
Improper patient selection and education	Only patients who have the mental alertness and sufficient cognitive, physical, and psychological ability should use a PCA. It can lead to inadequate pain control or oversedation. Teaching patients during the immediate postoperative period is ineffective if the patient is too groggy to understand. This has often led to poor pain control in the first 12 hours following surgery.	Check patient allergies, which should be visible on the MAR, before initiating PCA. Educate patients preoperatively about PCAs. Establish patient selection criteria. In general, infants, young children, and confused patients are not suitable candidates for using a PCA pump.

(Continued)

TABLE 2.1   PCA Problems and Safety Recommendations (*Continued*)

Problem	Description	Safety Recommendation
Inadequate patient monitoring	Patients using a PCA pump must be frequently and appropriately monitored. The level of consciousness achieved from physical stimulus is only a temporary way to monitor for toxicity. When the physical stimulus is removed, patients can quickly fall back into an oversedated state. Pulse oximetery alone can give a false sense of security because oxygen saturation is usually maintained even at low respiratory rates.	Ensure that nurses recognize the signs and symptoms of opiate toxicity. Have oxygen and naloxone readily available. Teach the need to assess using minimal verbal or tactile stimulation. Establish a standard pain assessment scale. At minimum, evaluate pain, alertness, and vital signs, including rate and quality of respirations, every 4 hours. More frequent monitoring should be done in the first 24 hours and at night, when hypoventilation and nocturnal hypoxia may occur. Keep PCA flow sheets at the bedside to document PCA doses and patient monitoring. Monitor the use of naloxone to identify adverse events related to PCA.
Drug product mix-ups	Many opiates used for PCA have similar names and packaging leading to selection errors. Morphine and meperidine have been packaged in similar boxes. Use of floor stock of opiates in PCAs has led to significant overdoses.	Require independent double-checks for patient identification, drug and concentration, pump settings, and the line attachment. Establish one concentration for each opiate used for PCA. Separate the storage of hydromorphone from morphine. Affix prominent warning labels on nonstandard concentrations. Use commercially prefilled syringes/bags/cassettes. Require the pharmacy to review all PCA orders before initiation. Alert all clinicians to drug shortages and provide clear alternate dosing instructions.
Practice-related problems	Misprogramming the PCA is the most frequently reported practice-related issue. Other problems include incorrect transcription of orders, miscalculation of dose or rate of infusion, and IV admixture errors.	Require independent double-checks for patient identification, drug and concentration, pump settings, and the line attachment. Limit PCA pumps to a single model to promote proficiency. Provide laminated instructions attached to each pump. Program pumps to require a review of settings before infusing.

(*Continued*)

TABLE 2.1   PCA Problems and Safety Recommendations (*Continued*)

Problem	*Description*	*Safety Recommendation*
Device design flaws	Many PCAs are not intuitive in their design, making programming problematic. Many PCAs have default programming for medication concentrations such as 0.1 mg/mL or 1 mg/mL, but a higher concentration may be used in the device, leading to overdoses and deaths. Other drug delivery problems include lack of requiring review of programming before starting the infusion and free flow of medication as a result of syringe or cassette breakage. Patients may also confuse the PCA button with the nurse call button, resulting in overdosing and frustration.	Establish default settings of zero for all opiates. Connect PCA to a port close to the patient (to avoid dead space) and prominently label the infusion line to avoid mix-ups. Require pumps to be programmed in milligrams per milliliter and micrograms per milliliter (mg/mL and mcg/mL), not just milliliters. Program pumps to alert users and stop PCA if a syringe or bag is empty or damaged. Limit PCA pumps to a single model to promote proficiency. Provide visual and auditory feedback to patients when the button is pressed.
Inadequate staff training	Nurses may not receive effective training or may not retain proficiency when PCA pumps are used infrequently or if multiple types of PCAs are used. Prescribers may not undergo verification of proficiency with this form of pain management, resulting in improper medications and dosing.	Ensure training is timely and comprehensive and that annual competency testing is required. Require independent double-checks for patient identification, drug and concentration, pump settings, and the line attachment. Limit PCA pumps to a single model to promote proficiency. Provide laminated instructions attached to each pump.
Order communication errors	Mistakes are made in converting an oral opiate dose to the IV route. Most problematic is hydromorphone. Concurrent orders for other opiates while a PCA is in use have resulted in opiate toxicity.	Design standard order sets to guide drug selection, doses, and lockout periods; patient monitoring; and precautions such as avoiding concomitant analgesics. Limit verbal orders to dose changes only. Require independent double-checks for patient identification, drug and concentration, pump settings, and the line attachment. Use morphine as opiate of choice, use hydromorphone for patients needing very high doses, reserve meperidine for patients allergic to morphine and hydromorphone.

PCA, patient-controlled analgesia.

PCA Problems and Safety Recommendations

Nurses, biomedical engineers, and others should plan and monitor the effectiveness of infusion pump deployment. A first step is to provide nurses and other users with input into selection of all new pumps. All IV pumps should be tested for free-flow protection, and any that fail (medication flows freely from the tubing as the set is removed) should be removed from service. By limiting standard hospital IV pumps to a single model and specialty pumps, such as syringe and PCA pumps, to clinical areas in which the staff is fully competent in their use, the proficiency of all nurses using these devices can be maximized. Attaching laminated instructions and safety checklists to each pump raises awareness and reinforces key safety measures. Each provider who uses a pump should also be required to label all tubing and have a partner assist with independent double-checks for patient identification, drug and drug concentration, pump settings, and line attachment.

Above all, an independent double-check that verifies dose and rate settings is critical. This is because the settings on PCA pumps often default to a standard concentration, which requires the operator to change the settings if a nonstandard concentration is used. Even when the staff has expertise in the proper use of these drug delivery devices, serious dosing errors have been associated with improper flow rate settings. Thus, PCA pump settings should be programmed by one individual and checked independently by another before administering medication. Settings at the time of administration should be documented based on this independent check.

Other medication administration devices can also cause errors in a healthcare setting. For example, the wrong reservoir in implantable medication delivery devices has reportedly been filled with medication, causing patient death. Also, patients are often admitted to the hospital with implantable devices, such as insulin pumps, yet no instructions are available to assist nurses with the use of these devices.

Additional misuses of medication-related devices, often with serious outcomes, include the inadvertent connection of intravenous tubing to devices not intended for medication delivery. In one case, a nurse accidentally connected the blood pressure (BP) monitor tubing to a needleless IV port. Propofol, which is white and opaque, had been infusing through the patient's IV line. Thus, the IV tubing and its port looked very similar to the white length of tubing and connector on the BP cuff (Figure 2.7). In another, similar case, an agitated patient died when he removed the tubing from his BP cuff and attached it to his IV line.

In another tubing-related event, a young child died when her oxygen tubing was mistakenly connected to her IV line. The child had been receiving medication via a nebulizer to treat asthma. While still attached to a wall outlet, the oxygen tubing became disconnected from the nebulizer fluid chamber (Figure 2.8).

The situation worsened when the staff member who discovered the disconnected oxygen tubing accidentally reconnected it to the injection port on a Baxter Clearlink Needleless Access System IV tubing Y-site. Although oxygen tubing does not have a Luer connector, the staff member managed to make the connection with the Baxter Clearlink valve work by applying considerable force (Figure 2.9). The oxygen tubing disconnected

FIGURE 2.7   Tubing Lines

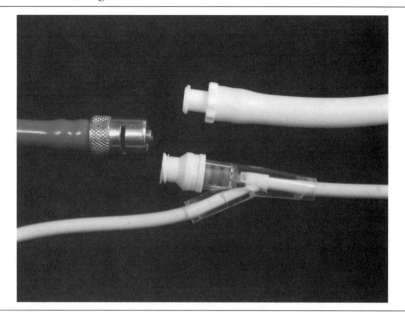

from the IV tubing in seconds, but not before the pressure of the compressed oxygen supply forced the needleless valve open and allowed air into the tubing. The child died instantly.

Other, similar issues have occurred when medications have inadvertently been delivered into the balloon inflation ports of endotracheal tubes, gastrostomy tubes, and Foley catheters instead of into the intended intravenous catheter. In each case, the balloon expanded when the medication was injected, causing harm to the patients.[18]

A more recent issue underscores the importance of vigilance in the use of color-coded tubing and devices. Oral Keppra (levetiracetam) liquid was inadvertently administered intravenously into a Bard PowerPICC (peripherally inserted central catheter) line instead of through a percutaneous endoscopic gastronomy (PEG) tube, as was clinically indicated. Even though the medication was dispensed in an oral syringe that did not easily connect to the hub of the intravenous line, the provider held the syringe against the opening for injection. The experienced nurse probably became confused by the purple color-coding system used by the enteral feeding tube manufacturer, Covidien, because the purple color is identical to the color used for the Bard PowerPICC. Although purple is not the official color for enteral feeding devices or PICC lines in the United States, it is considered the official color for such devices in the United Kingdom.[19]

As these examples illustrate, it is essential that healthcare organizations review existing medical equipment used in their facilities for potential misconnections. Each practitioner who connects or reconnects tubing should be required by policy to

FIGURE 2.8   IV Tubing to Oxygen

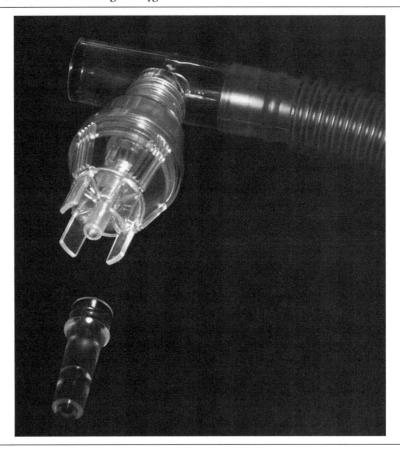

FIGURE 2.9   IV Misconnect

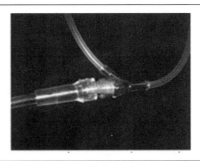

completely trace the tube from the patient to the point of origin before connecting the tubing. Appropriately labeled IV lines help alert the staff that they may be about to access the incorrect line accidentally. Additionally, before introducing new tubes, catheters, and connectors, an interdisciplinary team should use failure mode and effect analysis (FMEA) to identify potential issues related to connectivity with other medical equipment.

As previously noted, medication safety is enhanced when healthcare organizations involve end users in the product selection process. Building on this principle by using a standardized evaluation process for devices and looking for areas of potential failure before the device is acquired might help the organization avoid future errors. A suggested approach for evaluating infusion pumps is presented in Box 2.1. The same process can be adapted for use for any new medical device.

Patient Monitoring

Connected to each medical device or piece of equipment is a patient. For therapeutic interventions to succeed, practitioners must continually assess their effectiveness by monitoring the patient based on predetermined parameters such as vital signs and including such criteria as for neurological assessment, quality of respirations, and lab results. In addition to proactively defining key parameters as part of established protocols, order sets, and flow sheets, healthcare providers also might need to incorporate these parameters in computerized monitoring systems.

Documentation of monitoring is critical, and all associated forms (for example, diabetic flow sheets, PCA flow sheets, and sedation flow sheets) should be used at the bedside, with the information remaining there for quick reference, whether documentation is entered on a paper graphic or into a computerized record. Appropriate antidotes and resuscitation equipment should also be readily available at the bedside, and their presence should be noted in the record. Subsequent chart audits should contrast documentation of patient monitoring with outcomes to identify patterns in untoward care results and identify opportunities for improvement.

Environmental Stressors

In an ideal healthcare setting, medications would be prescribed, transcribed, prepared, and administered in an environment free of distractions, with comfortable surroundings, adequate physical space, and good lighting. Practitioners would come to work rested and could take rest and meal breaks to maintain focus and attention. In reality, hospital workers are constantly exposed to noise, interruptions, and nonstop activity. The process of order transcription is particularly vulnerable to distraction, because it usually occurs in an environment in which unit secretaries, nurses, and pharmacy personnel are answering telephones and talking with other providers and patients. A study confirms that simple slips due to distractions are responsible for almost three-quarters of all transcription errors.[20] Some strategies that might minimize such distractions include overlapping of staffing coverage during peak activity times and encouraging fax or e-mail communications to the nursing station instead of making telephone calls.

BOX 2.1   Using FMEA to Predict Failures with Infusion Pumps

BASIC FUNCTIONALITY—HOW WELL DOES THE PUMP PERFORM THE REQUIRED TASK?

- Is this the correct pump to use to perform the desired task(s)?
- Can the pump deliver the volume/increments needed under the correct pressure?
- Are any features incompatible with the environment in which it will be used (size, weight, number of channels)?
- Will the pump deliver medications in the concentrations most typically used?
- What tubing and other supplies are required for the pump to perform effectively and safely? Are they interchangeable with other pumps? Could interchangeable tubing be used for this pump, rendering it unsafe?
- Are users alerted to pump-setting errors? Wrong patient errors? Wrong channel errors? Wrong medication/solution errors? Mechanical failure?
- Does the pump have memory functions for settings and alarms with an easily retrievable log? If the pump is turned off, does it retain settings for a period of time?

USER-MACHINE INTERFACE—HOW EASY AND INTUITIVE IS IT FOR PEOPLE TO USE THE PUMP?

- What functions do users expect the pump to have?
- Are the programming steps minimal?
- Are the touch buttons used for programming clearly labeled, logically positioned, and the proper size?
- Are the screens readable, with proper font size, lighting, contrast, and other cues to enhance performance?
- Do the units of medication delivery (e.g., mcg/kg, mcg/kg/min) match current practices?
- Do the medications, units of delivery, and strengths appear in a logical sequence for selection?
- Is there any information that defaults to a predetermined value? If yes, is it safe?
- Is it easy to install and prime administration sets and to remove air in the line?
- Are the special features, such as drug/dose calculations and dose alerts, helpful and easy to use?
- Are the screens free of abbreviations, trailing zeros (e.g., 1.0 mg), and naked decimal points (e.g., .1 mg)?
- Do the alarms clearly guide staff to the problems? Is it possible to permanently disable audible alarms or set them too low to be heard?
- If the infusion rate is changed, but not confirmed, does the device continuously alert the user that the solution is infusing at the old rate?
- Could the administration settings be mispositioned during installation or accidentally dislodged, separated, or removed by patients?
- Does the administration setting prevent gravity free-flow of the solution when it is removed from the pump?
- Is the device tamper resistant?
- Does the pump fit into the typical work flow?
- How does the pump compare to the pumps now in use?

Interruptions during any step in the medication-use process can have devastating consequences. In one example, an ED patient died after receiving a 10-mg dose of hydromorphone when morphine 10 mg was ordered. As the ED nurse was selecting the drug, she was temporarily distracted by another of her patients who was attempting to climb off the end of the stretcher. She quickly placed a vial of hydromorphone in her pocket while she attended to the second patient, interrupting her normal routine of checking the medication and documenting the sign-out on the narcotic record. After settling the agitated patient, she resumed medication administration to the first patient, inadvertently omitting the step of signing out the narcotic. After receiving 10 mg of hydromorphone, when 2 mg is the usual intramuscular dose, the patient was discharged. He subsequently suffered a respiratory arrest in the family car and could not be resuscitated.

Fatigue can also contribute to medication errors. Research conducted by the Anesthesia Patient Safety Foundation documented anesthesiologists' performance failures when fatigued.[21] One group of researchers observed the incidence of a phenomenon called micro-sleeps in a study of anesthesiologists who were in a sleep-deprived condition. In videotapes of simulated surgical procedures, the researchers identified behaviors indicative of micro-sleeps during 30 percent of the four-hour cases.[22] Micro-sleeps are intermittent lapses in consciousness, lasting seconds to minutes. The person's eyes are open, yet the person is not cognizant of surroundings, cannot process information, and, once fully conscious again, is unaware that the lapse has even occurred![23]

Research has also shown that the risk of nurses making medication-related errors is increased significantly when they work longer than twelve hours in a shift, when working overtime, or when working more than forty hours in one week.[24] Performance of a fatigued healthcare worker has been shown to equal that of a person with a blood alcohol level of 0.1 percent, which is over the legal limit for driving in many states.[25] See Box 2.2 for a list of the effects of fatigue.

Addressing safety issues associated with fatigue requires that the institution support a culture in which admission of fatigue is accepted and rewarded. To achieve this environment, the management and the staff must be educated about the risks associated with fatigue and the research-based approaches to optimize performance in the face of fatigue, especially with regard to night shift workers. Based on organizational commitment to address this important problem, healthcare organizations should examine staffing patterns to ensure adequate rest and recovery opportunities for their employees. Contingency plans should be developed to manage staffing needs if personnel appear to be or consider themselves too fatigued to work safely. It is important to ensure that staff members can take fifteen- to thirty-minute rest breaks away from the work area and a meal break during each shift. Other interventions to consider are providing for short planned naps in the workplace and offering light therapy to reduce the effects of fatiguing schedules and disrupted circadian rhythms.[26]

To address all of these environmental impediments to medication safety, organizational leaders should aim to foster a "sterile cockpit" similar to that used by the airline industry to promote safety. In a sterile cockpit environment, pilots and flight crew are

BOX 2.2   Effects of Fatigue

- Slowed reaction time
- Reduced accuracy
- Diminished ability to recognize significant but subtle changes in a patient's health
- Inability to deal with the unexpected
- Lapses of attention and inability to stay focused
- Omissions and neglect of nonessential activities
- Compromised problem-solving and decision-making abilities
- Impaired communication skills
- Inability to recall
- Short-term memory lapses
- Reduced motivation
- Irritability or hostility
- Indifference and loss of empathy
- Intrusion of sleep into wakefulness
- Decreased energy for successful completion of required tasks
- Decreased learning of new activities
- Reduced hand-eye coordination

Source: From L. M. Linde and M. Bergstrom, "The Effect of One Night without Sleep on Problem-Solving and Immediate Recall," *Psychological Research.* 1992, 54(2):127–36; S. Howard, "Fatigue and the Practice of Medicine," *Anesthesia Patient Safety Foundation Newsletter.* Spring 2005; 20(1): 1–4.

specifically prohibited from participating in distracting activities while performing critical duties. The Federal Aviation Administration written policies (Sec. 121.542) state:

(a) No certificate holder shall require, nor may any flight crewmember perform, any duties during a critical phase of flight except those duties required for the safe operation of the aircraft. Duties such as company required calls made for such nonsafety related purposes as ordering galley supplies and confirming passenger connections, announcements made to passengers promoting the air carrier or pointing out sights of interest, and filling out company payroll and related records are not required for the safe operation of the aircraft.

(b) No flight crewmember may engage in, nor may any pilot in command permit, any activity during a critical phase of flight which could distract any flight crewmember from the performance of his or her duties or which could interfere in any way with the proper conduct of those duties. Activities such as eating meals, engaging in nonessential conversations within the cockpit and nonessential communications between the cabin and cockpit crews, and reading publications not related to the proper conduct of the flight are not required for the safe operation of the aircraft.

(c) For the purposes of this section, critical phases of flight includes all ground operations involving taxi, takeoff and landing, and all other flight operations conducted below 10,000 feet, except cruise flight.[27]

Because a failure in any step of the complex medication use process could lead to a medication error and patient harm, every step equates to an aircraft's critical phase of flight. Distractions, interruptions, and competing activities should be eliminated or minimized. Managers and staff members should focus on creating and supporting an environment that allows concentration on the critical task at hand.

Competency and Staff Education

Many practitioners have limited awareness of error-prone situations, even those that are well-documented in their own organization or published in professional literature. Without this information, these staff members are likely to make similar errors. With the information, staff members can help the organization identify ways to prevent such errors from occurring. Upon joining the medical staff, and regularly thereafter, staff members should be provided with current information about errors that have occurred within the organization as well as those that occur elsewhere. Healthcare organizations should also develop a medication safety test for providers who will administer medications. Included should be questions that address problem-prone areas such as morphine and insulin dosing and the use of cross-allergenic medications such as Toradol and aspirin.

Medication Competency Tests

Anecdotal evidence from ISMP shows that many medication competency tests currently used are outdated. For example, the questions on such tests often contain, and thus legitimize, dangerous abbreviations and dose designations. They also test obsolete approaches, such as conversion from apothecary units (formally eliminated in 2001 by the American Society of Health-System Pharmacists) to metric units.[28]

In addition to updating the content, it is essential that such tests go beyond mere calculation and memorization of drugs and doses to critical thinking. Medication competency tests should incorporate questions about safety issues such as lab values associated with drug use, appropriate monitoring of patients, and correct patient identification procedures. They should address such issues as identifying high-alert medications and the special precautions that are essential to use with these drugs. It is, of course, important to have staff members explain the correct procedure for an independent double-check, and they should also be able to describe appropriate and inappropriate therapy for patients, based on medical history.

When administering a medication competency test, allow the practitioner who is unsure of an answer to use medication resources (books, Internet or intranet, other practitioners). With this approach, all questions should be answered correctly and any wrong response should be thoroughly discussed with the test taker.

Although staff education is vitally important, it cannot be successful as the single safety strategy; it must be provided in conjunction with other approaches. One case that illustrates the importance of this principle involved a nurse who successfully completed her medication competency test but later administered a dose of pronestyl after checking the pronestyl level but not the NAPA level. (NAPA is a metabolite of pronestyl that has the same pharmaceutical effect as pronestyl.) The NAPA level was elevated; therefore, the medication should have been held and the prescriber contacted. The nurse was unaware of the need to check the NAPA level before administrating this drug.

Simply drafting a policy or including a question on a competency exam about NAPA levels and pronestyl administration is likely to be ineffective in addressing this situation without the accompanying use of such resources as auxiliary warnings printed on MARs to check NAPA levels and hard stops. A hard stop prevents the practitioner from proceeding with an order unless a current lab value or other patient data (weight, allergy status, and so on) is entered. In this case, a hard stop would probably take the form of a note that appears on the provider order entry screen, requiring the user to check (or enter) the NAPA lab result before administration of the drug. A hard stop requiring lab value entry could also be implemented in bedside barcode drug administration software. Tools such as these compensate for natural lapses in human concentration and memory in ways that education alone cannot.

Patient Education

An alert and knowledgeable patient can serve as the last line of defense in preventing medication errors. For example, patients who have been educated about the need for proper identification prior to procedures or medication can alert staff members when their armband has not been checked. Also, when patients are aware of the usual times for drug administration, they can remind staff members that their medication is due to help prevent drug omission errors. To fulfill this role in preventing errors, patients must receive ongoing education by physicians, pharmacists, and nurses about drug brand and generic names, indications, usual and actual doses, expected and possible adverse effects, drug or food interactions, and how to protect themselves from errors. Although this education takes additional staff time, it can pay significant dividends in patient safety.

Even patients who have merely been encouraged to ask questions and seek satisfactory answers can play a vital role in preventing medication errors. A tragic example of a case in which a staff member did not heed the patient's questions involved an informed patient at the Dana Farber Cancer Institute who told her healthcare practitioners that she felt that something was wrong after two days of cancer chemotherapy. Numerous times both the patient and her husband requested that the staff check her chemotherapy orders for accuracy because she was experiencing different side effects from her previous courses of therapy. Without a thorough investigation of their concerns, the patient's practitioners reassured the patient and her husband that the medication she was receiving was correct. Unfortunately, she received an entire course of chemotherapy every day for four days. It is impossible to say whether the patient would have survived if the error had been detected earlier, but there is no doubt that those four days of chemotherapy were the direct cause of her death.

The way in which patients are educated about their medication is also critical. Simply handing a drug information sheet to a patient is often not sufficient, as patients might misunderstand or be frightened by the information concerning the risk of taking the medication. Also, one study claims that nearly 50 percent of the population has either low or limited literary skills. This figure represents approximately 90 million adults.[29] Thus, practitioners need to assess whether patients fully understand their medications by asking what they are taking and verifying that patients understand why these medications are being given. For patients receiving multiple drugs and those who are receiving medications with a narrow therapeutic index, the healthcare organization should consider involving a pharmacist in patient education during the admission process, during treatment, and at discharge.

. . . .

A PRIORITIZING APPROACH

To help the organization address risk and improve safety of medication use, it is critical that the risk management professional be aware of strategies for prioritizing issues and interventions.

Some medication safety strategies are more effective, or have more leverage, than others. Leverage involves the relationship between input and output. Where the amount of force (input) necessary to make a significant change (output) is small, the action is one of high leverage and is considered more favorable and effective in producing change. Leverage is considered to be highest when it meets ISMP's first principle of error reduction: reducing or eliminating the possibility of errors. The second principle of error reduction, possessing moderate leverage, is to make errors visible. The third is to minimize the consequences of errors after their occurrence. These principles provide a framework for developing error reduction strategies. The error reduction strategies in Figure 2.10 are presented in rank order of leverage, highest to lowest.

FIGURE 2.10   Rank Order of Error Reduction Strategies

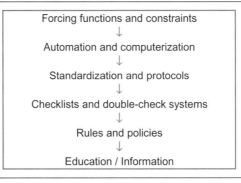

Forcing functions and constraints
↓
Automation and computerization
↓
Standardization and protocols
↓
Checklists and double-check systems
↓
Rules and policies
↓
Education / Information

An example of a constraint is supplying epidural tubing without any ports that might allow accidental injection of intravenous drugs. Forcing functions are strategies that do not allow an action to occur unless certain conditions are met, potentially preventing an error. (The terms *forcing function* and *hard stop* are often used interchangeably.) Computerized or automated devices can act as forcing functions; for example, the provider might be prevented from entering a drug order unless patient weight is entered or might be unable to access an automated dispensing drawer unless the drug in that drawer is in the patient's pharmacy profile.

Automated devices may also alert the user in the event of a negative outcome, thereby making an error visible (for example, alarms on infusion pumps, patient monitors). Although the result might be after the fact and therefore is lower in leverage, automated alerts can also prompt drug orders for antidotes and reversal agents, thereby minimizing the consequences of an error. Rules, policies, and education are important components of error reduction strategies, but they have very limited leverage in creating real change.

Another important prioritizing strategy is to categorize certain medications and patient populations as *high alert* or *high risk*. High-alert medications are those that pose the greatest risk of causing significant harm when misused. Classes and categories of medications considered to be high alert are as follows:

- Adrenergic agonists, IV
- Adrenergic antagonists, IV
- Anesthetic agents, general, inhaled, and IV
- Antiarrhythmics, IV
- Antithrombotic agents
- Cardioplegic solutions
- Chemotherapeutic agents, parenteral and oral
- Dextrose, hypertonic, 20% or greater
- Dialysis solution, peritoneal and hemodialysis
- Epidural and intrathecal medications
- Hypoglycemics, oral
- Intropic medications, IV
- Liposomal forms of drugs
- Moderate sedation agents, IV
- Moderate sedation agents, oral, for children
- Narcotics/opiates, IV, transdermal, and oral
- Neuromuscular blocking agents
- Radiocontrast agents, IV
- Total parenteral nutrition solutions

Specific high-alert medications include the following:

- Colchicine injection
- Epoprostenol (Flolan), IV
- Insulin, subcutaneous and IV
- Magnesium sulfate injection
- Methotrexate, oral, nononcologic use
- Opium tincture
- Oxytocin, IV
- Nitroprusside sodium for injection
- Potassium chloride for injection concentrate
- Potassium phosphates injection
- Promethazine, IV
- Sodium chloride for injection, hypertonic (greater than 0.9% concentration)
- Sterile water for injection, inhalation, and irrigation (excluding pour bottles) in containers of 100 mL or more

High-risk patients are those at risk of suffering significant harm if they experience a medication error, such as the following:

- Patients with renal/liver impairment
- Pregnant/breast-feeding patients
- Neonates
- Elderly/chronically ill patients
- Patients on multiple medications
- Oncology patients

The terms *high alert* and *high risk* do not mean that errors occur more frequently with these medications or to these patients; it simply means that the resulting harm is more difficult to ameliorate. Such categories help the healthcare organization properly prioritize error reduction efforts.

Because risk reduction efforts must begin at the highest leverage point, where the most effectiveness can be gained from minimal actions, prioritization is critical to maximizing the organization's resources, including staff time.

Additionally, certain subprocesses within the medication use process may be considered more error-prone than others, such as the following:

- Patient-controlled analgesia, epidural analgesia
- Use of automated dispensing equipment
- Preparation of complex products in the pharmacy with automated compounders
- Administration of enteral feedings in patients with IV catheters in place
- Obtaining accurate allergy information

These processes should be examined in detail, with attention to various ways that things could go wrong at each step and the potential for patient harm that might result from a failure at each process step. A more formalized examination entails a failure mode and effects analysis (FMEA). ISMP offers a sample FMEA on the error-prone process of patient-controlled analgesia on its Web site at www.ismp.org/Tools/FMEAofPCA.pdf.

Yet another high-priority activity that should involve the risk management professional is performing due diligence regarding a new clinical activity. In some settings, competition with other organizations results in rapidly expanding services. Neonatal intensive care, organ transplants, open-heart surgery, home care infusion, and oncology units are but a few examples of the areas currently experiencing growth. Often, in such situations, there has been little time to properly prepare for the new activity by reorganizing workflow and providing staff education.

It is critical that appropriate planning take place and that medication use issues receive a high priority. In one unfortunate situation, soon after a hospital established a new pediatric emergency service, a pharmacist was called to supply the unit with ketamine injections to sedate children during procedures in the ED. Ketamine is available in vials with concentrations of 10 mg/mL, 50 mg/mL, and 100 mg/mL. The pharmacy sent five 100 mg/mL vials to the unit. Before long, a four-year-old patient came to the ED for suturing of a wound. A physician who was accustomed to using vials of ketamine that were 10 mg/mL did not notice the 100 mg/mL concentration and inadvertently administered the total contents of the 500 mg vial instead of the 50 mg pediatric dose. The child suffered a respiratory arrest but was successfully resuscitated. During the review of the error, the pharmacy staff readily admitted that they were not well informed about the use of ketamine for ambulatory sedation in pediatric patients and therefore were unsure about which concentration to supply. It was also determined that no one in the pharmacy department had prior pediatric care experience.

When a new service or expansion of an existing department is contemplated, senior management must ensure that all staff members are provided with timely communication. A FMEA should take place to discover potential areas of weakness and explore steps that are needed to promote safety. Staff orientation and proper education for new services must be planned as early as possible, but close enough to the start of the new service to maintain an appropriate skill level. In addition, consideration must be given to staffing levels, which might need to be increased (even if temporarily) in proportion to the new workload. The risk management professional can play an invaluable role in facilitating senior administrative support of necessary planning.

Error Reporting and Follow-Up

Each practitioner must firmly believe that errors may be reported without disciplinary action and that the organization will use the incident report to evaluate the medication delivery system. In one case, a nurse was afraid to report a serious medication error to her manager because of her concern that this would blemish her record. She feared that the next time she committed an error she might be suspended or even fired. The nurse contacted ISMP because she was afraid to ask anyone at work if her patient, who was scheduled for an invasive procedure later that day, could be adversely affected from an inadvertent overdose of heparin. Although it seemed unlikely that the increased amount of heparin would have an effect several hours later, ISMP encouraged her to report the error because the physician might choose to postpone the procedure as a precaution. It was later learned that, because of her fears, she did not inform anyone of the incident. Therefore, any opportunity for preventing patient harm or addressing the system issues that caused this error was lost.

Although no one would condone this nurse's decision, it is easy to understand the mind-set behind it. If practitioners do not see any benefit associated with reporting, there is no incentive to report. Moreover, if they perceive a danger to themselves, they will be discouraged—and may discourage others—from reporting.

Patient safety cannot be promoted in any organization without open communication about errors. Risk management professionals have the opportunity to encourage such openness and maximize the value of reporting. Practitioners can be motivated to report if they are clear that the purpose of reporting is proactively aimed at protecting their patients from future harm.

· · · · · · · ·

CONCLUSION

It is fundamental that risk management professionals and the multidisciplinary team they are part of accept ownership of the medication-use process and enthusiastically embrace the opportunity to improve patient safety. Although they may celebrate a safety week or safety month, organizational leaders must also demonstrate around-the-clock commitment to medication safety. Risk management professionals can facilitate senior management support of the financial commitment and time required to train staff members in communication skills and implement a physical environment that promotes safe and effective medication use processes. Critical to achievement of this goal is a thorough understanding of exactly how the components of these processes interact, taking into account the varied perspectives of practitioners and the complexity of their patients.

Endnotes

1. Reason, J. *Managing the Risks of Organization Accidents*. Aldershot, U.K.: Ashgate, 1990; 1–19.

2. *Drug Facts and Comparisons*. St. Louis, Mo.: Wolters Kluwer Health. For ordering information visit: www.factsandcomparisons.com/index.aspx. (Accessed April 9, 2010.)

3. NeoFax. Raleigh, N.C.: A Thomson Reuters Product, Acorn Publishing, 1995. For online ordering information visit: www.micromedex.com/products/neofax/. (Accessed April 9, 2010.) NeoFax is a neonatal drug information resource available electronically and in print.

4. Leape, L. L., D. W. Bates, D. J. Cullen et al. "Systems analysis of adverse drug events." *JAMA* 1995; 274:35–43.

5. *Ibid.*

6. Institute for Safe Medication Practices. *2004 ISMP Medication Safety Self Assessment for Hospitals*. Huntington Valley, Penn: Institute for Safe Medication Practices, 2004.

7. Thompson Reuters MicroMedex [database online]. Available at: www.micromedex. com/. (Accessed November 14, 2009.)

8. Leape, L. L., D. J. Cullen, M. Clapp et al. "Pharmacist participation on physician rounds and adverse drug events in the intensive care unit." *JAMA* 1999; 282:267–270.

9. Institute for Safe Medication Practices. "Intimidation: Practitioners speak up about this unresolved problem (Part I)." *ISMP Medication Safety Alert!* 2004; 9(5). Available at: www.ismp.org/Newsletters/acutecare/articles/20040311_2.asp. (Accessed November 14, 2009.)

10. Institute for Safe Medication Practices. "Intimidation: Mapping a plan for cultural change in healthcare (Part II)." *ISMP Medication Safety Alert!* 2004; 9(6).

11. More information on TJC credentialing requirements is available at: www. jointcommission.org/SentinelEvents/SentinelEventAlert/sea_40.htm. (Accessed November 10, 2009.)

12. "Reconcile Medications at All Transition Points." Institute for Healthcare Improvement. Available at: www.ihi.org/IHI/Topics/PatientSafety/MedicationSystems/Changes/Reconcil e+Medications+at+All+Transition+Points.htm. (Accessed November 14, 2009.)

13. "Look-alike/sound-alike drug products affect cognition." USP CAPSLink [serial online]. May 2004; 1–5. Available at: www.usp.org/pdf/EN/patientSafety/capsLink2004–05–01. pdf. (Accessed November 14, 2009.)

14. Holquist C., and J. Phillips. "FDA Safety Page: Fatal medication errors associated with Temodar." *Drug Topics* 2003; 7:42.

15. Joint Commission on Accreditation of Healthcare Organizations. "Most problematic look-alike and sound-alike drug names for specific health care settings." Available at: www.jointcommission.org/NR/rdonlyres/C92AAB3F-A9BD-431C-8628– 11DD2D1D53CC/0/LASA.pdf. (Accessed November 14, 2009.)

16. International Ergonomics Association. "The discipline of ergonomics." Available at: www.iea.cc/browse.php?contID=what_is_ergonomics. (Accessed November 14, 2009.)

17. Cohen, M.R. and J.L. Smetze. "One Organization's Advocacy Effort for Error Prevention: The Institute for Safe Medication Practices." Chapter 42 in *The Patient Safety Handbook*, eds. B. Youngberg and M. Hatlie. Sudbury, Mass: Jones & Bartlett, 2004, p. 653.

18. Institute for Safe Medication Practices Canada. "Devices with inflation ports–Risk for medication error-induced injuries." *ISMP Canada Safety Bulletin*. May 2004; 4(5).

19. "Purple is not an official standard for either enteral feeding equipment or PICC Lines" *ISMP Medication Safety Alert!* 2009; 14(11).

20. Cohen and Smetzer, *op. cit.*

21. Anesthesia Patient Safety Foundation Newsletter. Spring 2005; 20(1):1–24.

22. Howard, S. K., D. M. Gaba, B. E. Smith et al. "Simulation study of rested versus sleep-deprived anesthesiologists." *Anesthesiology* 2003; 98:1345–1355; discussion A.

23. Rosekind, M. R., P. H. Gander, L. J. Connell et al. *Crew Factors in Flight Operations X: Alertness Management in Flight Operations*. NASA Technical Memorandum no. 1999–208780. Moffett Field, Calif.: NASA 1999.

24. Rogers, A. E., W. T. Hwang, L. D. Scott et al. "Hospital staff nurse work and patient safety." *Health Affairs* 2004; 23:1–11.

25. Dawson, D., and K. Reid. "Fatigue, alcohol and performance impairment." *Nature* 1997; 388:235.

26. Gillberg, M., G. Kecklund, and T. Akerstedt. "Relations between performance and subjective ratings of sleepiness during a night awake." *Sleep* 1994; 17(3): 236–241.

27. Code of Federal Regulations. 14CFR121.542. Title 14: Aeronautics and Space, Chapter I: Federal Aviation Administration, Department of Transportation, Part 121: Operating requirements: Domestic, flag, and supplemental operations, Subpart T: Flight Operations, Section 121.542: Flight crewmember duties. Doc. No. 20661, 46 FR 5502, Jan. 19, 1981. Revised as of January 1, 2003

28. American Society of Health-System Pharmacists. AHSP Position number 8613. Policy Positions, Statements and Guidelines. Available at: www.ashp.org/Import/ PRACTICEANDPOLICY/PolicyPositionsGuidelinesBestPractices/BrowsebyTopic/ PharmaceuticalIndustry/PolicyPositions.aspx#8613. (Accessed November 14, 2009.)

29. Kirsch, I. S., A. Jungeblut, L. Jenkins et al. Executive summary of adult literacy in America: A first look at the results of the national adult literacy survey. Executive summary. National Center for Education Statistics, U.S. Department of Education. Available from: http://nces.ed.gov/pubs93/93275.pdf. (Accessed April 9, 2010.)

3

The Risk Management Professional and Biomedical Technology

Sally T. Trombly

Biomedical technology should be part of an enterprise risk management (ERM) program in every healthcare organization, and the risk management professional should play an active role. Key biomedical technology-related issues for which the risk management professional can provide expertise include patient safety, staff education requirements, and resource implications. Equally important is the risk management professional's input on the potential effects of decisions on biomedical technology in relation to existing patient care needs, new services planned or desired, and the effect of each of these on the system or facility's overall strategic plan, financial resources, and its workforce.

STRATEGIC CONSIDERATIONS

The risk management professional can help an individual facility or healthcare system make correct decisions about the acquisition and use of biomedical technology.

Simply because a piece of medical equipment or new type of biomedical technology carries risk is no reason to forego purchase; likewise, just because something is new is no reason to obtain it. An apparent increase in resource use (such as training time or changes in allocation of staffing) can ultimately result in increased overall efficiency, benefits to patient care outcomes, and increased satisfaction for both staff and patients.

To effectively contribute risk benefit analyses regarding purchase of biomedical technology, the risk management professional must participate in the strategic planning and evaluation process from the onset, not just after decisions have been made, equipment has been acquired, or problems have occurred.

· · · · · · · · ·
RISK MANAGEMENT INPUT

When pursuing new ventures that involve biomedical technology, the choice of equipment is likely to be senior management and governing body decisions. Risk management input at the beginning of the process can contribute to more effective decision making. It also gives the risk management professional early notice of areas that might require additional risk management attention if the potential venture becomes a reality. For biomedical technology–related needs of existing services, the risk management professional can offer useful insights from past patient care situations and previous experiences with vendors. The risk management professional also might have current information on devices with enhancements that facilitate patient safety, for example, smart pumps (intravenous pumps that help prevent medication dosage and rate errors). Progressive institutions are beginning to recognize the value that risk management can bring to strategic planning and decision-making processes. As this trend grows, the ability of the risk management professional to effectively operationalize the institution's biomedical technology decisions and reduce the potential for risk exposure related to biomedical technology should become more widely recognized.

· · · · · · · · ·
FINANCIAL CONSIDERATIONS

As part of the biomedical technology due diligence process, the risk management professional should be involved in assessing the available options and fiscal effect of decisions concerning whether to buy, lease, or enter into a consignment arrangement for medical devices. Each of these options for obtaining such devices has ramifications for subsequent operations. These ramifications extend far beyond the fiscal concerns of capital costs, the budgeting process, and ongoing funding and allocation of biomedical technology costs. For example, there might be varying regulatory mandates, depending on which party actually owns the piece of biomedical technology at a specific time. Adverse events and equipment recalls made by the manufacturer or the federal government trigger reporting requirements by specific areas. Without risk management coordination, there might be unnecessary confusion within the institution over the division of mandated responsibilities. Considering these factors during the decision-making process can help identify the potential effects of short- or long-term fiscal options. This information can also provide useful background information for those involved in the subsequent contract negotiations relating to biomedical technology equipment.

·········
CONTRACTS WITH VENDORS

In addition to the traditional elements of healthcare contracts (see Chapter 17, A Contract Review Primer, in Volume 1), contracts concerning biotechnology-related equipment should also clearly delineate the following:

- Responsibilities of each party regarding preventive and ongoing maintenance of the particular type of biomedical technology or medical equipment.

- Guarantee of equipment uptime or prompt provision of a substitute acceptable to the healthcare organization (and identification of any associated costs) for biomedical equipment critical to patient care.

- Circumstances under which a piece of biomedical equipment may be deemed to be unsatisfactory by the institution and remedies available, such as a full or partial replacement by the vendor or return for credit, and identification of the associated responsibilities of each party in this situation (comparable to a lemon law process for automobiles).

- Conditions under which credits toward future updates or trade-in are available.

- Provisions for an annual assessment of the vendor's service and support by the institution, with the ability to make recommendations for vendor improvements as necessary.

- Procedures for the vendor to notify the institution regarding product hazards identified or recalls instituted and the follow-up responsibilities assigned to each party.

- Allocation of mandated reporting responsibilities for biotechnology used on a consignment basis.

- Institutional requirements or restrictions on representatives of the vendors who visit staff or departments in facilities (such as sign-in processes, identification badges, limitations on access to certain areas, and so on). When a vendor representative is present in the operating room or special procedure area, additional requirements apply, including the need for the operative consent process and form to reflect patient awareness of the vendor's presence.

- Responsibilities of each party under the federal privacy and security regulations under HIPAA and/or Health Information Technology for Economic and Clinical Health Act (HITECH) (see Chapter 16, Volume 3, on HIPAA). These may arise in several areas. First, if the biotechnology equipment (or its associated software) uses individually identifiable health information, a written business associate agreement (as defined by the HIPAA regulations and meeting the requirements of 45 C.F.R. 164.504 (e) (1)) must be incorporated into the contract or executed as a separate agreement or addendum between the parties. Second, the Food and Drug Administration's (FDA) regulations involving reporting, tracking, and recall policies for biomedical technology may require disclosure of individually identifiable health information subject to the disclosure requirements of HIPAA (see 45 C.F.R. 164.512(b) (1) (iii)). Finally, safeguarding the security of individually identifiable health information collected by a biomedical device's software and system components from reasonably anticipated threats or vulnerabilities is required under the security portion of the HIPAA regulations (see 45 C.F.R. 164.306). This presents challenges for a variety of healthcare devices, such as imaging systems that obtain, archive, and communicate across an institutional network; various types of patient monitoring systems; and laboratory information systems connected to clinical laboratory analyzers. Although manufacturers have significant responsibilities in this area, healthcare organizations need to be knowledgeable partners to make the process successful and help avoid problems.

BULK PURCHASING ARRANGEMENTS

Purchasing arrangements among healthcare organizations have become much more common in recent years. The ability to aggregate several smaller requests into larger volume purchases can offer significant benefits in terms of efficiency and potential cost savings due to greater bargaining power among the participants in these programs. When applied to biomedical technology-related equipment purchases, such arrangements can also enhance safety by promoting organizational efforts toward equipment standardization where applicable, much as healthcare entities have done with implementation of drug formularies. From a risk management perspective, the key considerations in purchasing arrangements are the selection of biomedical technology items suited to the medical care needs of patients and the safe and efficient use of such items by clinicians and staff. The healthcare organization can enjoy significant benefit when these objectives are achieved, combined with the cost savings realized through group purchasing organizations.

STAFF TRAINING

Staff training is crucial to the successful management of risk exposures that result from the interaction of humans and biomedical technology. The need for staff training in general and cross-training to meet particular needs is not limited to permanent personnel of the facility. The increased use of clinical staff from per diem pools and commercial companies that provide individuals for short- or long-term assignments raises significant orientation and training challenges for healthcare facilities. However, the public expects that all staff authorized by a healthcare facility to use a piece of biomedical technology will be competent to do so, regardless of the individual's employment status.

The institution must be prepared to meet the full spectrum of biomedical technology training needs, from initial training in the use and support of a new piece of equipment, to ongoing in-service training, to individualized remedial training when indicated. Depending on the complexity of the biomedical technology in use at a particular site, staff and the facility's clinical providers may require education about the equipment.

Appropriate training of frontline staff nurses and other clinical staff with direct patient care responsibilities, such as respiratory therapists, is a critical factor in successful use of the complex biomedical equipment necessary for today's patient care needs. Institutions should have basic competency requirements that must be met before certain types of equipment can be used in a particular clinical setting. These skills should be part of orientation for new frontline clinical staff as well as more experienced professionals joining the organization. Expertise in the use of one particular manufacturer's medical device model may not necessarily transfer to another apparently comparable device.

At the other end of the spectrum of biomedical training needs, all staff who interface with patient care equipment must be clear on their responsibilities, however simple. For example, inadvertent unplugging of an intravenous pump by untrained staff can result in shut-off due to battery depletion, which sometimes goes unrecognized, with potentially serious patient care ramifications. It is also important for those whose job duties relate to maintenance or calibration, such as biomedical engineering personnel and those responsible for routine cleaning, disinfecting, or sterilization of certain medical devices to have appropriate ongoing training and education.

· · · · · · · · ·
TRAINING NONMEDICAL USERS

Consider the need for awareness training regarding biomedical technology for users such as patients, families, and nonmedical personnel. This need is not limited to hospital-based sites. It also applies to leased settings in which healthcare organization employees provide ambulatory healthcare services but the building owner furnishes the janitorial staff. The public is increasingly aware of biomedical devices such as automatic external defibrillators (AED) in airports and businesses, and television series that feature scenarios using such biomedical technology have become popular. This familiarity can encourage a cavalier attitude among laypeople about the significant realities involved in biomedical technology. For example, in at least one reported case, a death occurred when a worker in a janitorial service "playing with a defibrillator" placed the paddles on a coworker's chest.[1] Similarly, harm to workers may occur if housekeeping staff are not trained in MRI precautions. (Please see Chapter 11 on patient safety in radiology in this volume.)

Situations that involve unauthorized access to, or handling of, biomedical devices by noninstitutional personnel are not new. When protective containers for used needles and other sharps came into widespread use, there were instances of children trying to access containers that were within reach. The red plastic brick-shaped sharps containers resembled a popular building block for children. Children have also been involved in potentially serious incidents with electric beds during upward or downward movement of the bed. Recommendations made by ECRI Institute, a health services research organization dedicated to safe and effective patient and resident care, in their "Playing with Medical Devices Can Be a Deadly Game"[2] include

- educating the facility's nonmedical personnel and the clinical staff about the dangers of misusing medical devices and the range of problems that could arise from improper use by any person;

- reminding the staff to remain alert for any evidence of tampering when setting up a medical device;
- reviewing the location of medical devices in the facility and, to the extent possible, storing them in an area accessible only to appropriate medical personnel;
- considering the availability of safeguards against tampering when selecting new medical devices.

. . . .

OPERATIONAL FACTORS

A systematic biomedical technology management process helps ensure that an institution uses its resources to benefit its patient base, meets applicable regulatory edicts, and reduces the likelihood of adverse outcomes and potential liability exposure. Management processes may vary with the type and complexity of both the biomedical technology and the care setting, but should include adequate risk management systems and structures to identify and resolve actual or potential problems generated by the biomedical technology in use. The core business practices that relate to biomedical technology must address applicable federal and state mandates or reporting requirements imposed by these governmental entities or relevant accrediting bodies. The risk management processes and supporting materials also need to recognize and respond to the realities of implementation, such as the following:

- Reporting of adverse events or near-misses
- Follow-up on reports of problems or concerns raised by the staff
- Preventive maintenance or repair of biomedical equipment
- Recalls instituted by a manufacturer or the FDA
- Inventory control and tracking of biomedical-related equipment
- Institutional decisions regarding reuse or reprocessing
- Disposal of biomedical equipment that is no longer needed by the facility

. . . .

REALITIES OF IMPLEMENTATION

As discussed in Chapter 6, Volume 1, on early warning systems for the identification of organizational risk, the timely identification and analysis of potential risk exposures is a key component in a risk management program, no matter where the care is being rendered. Although the mandatory reporting requirements of the Safe Medical Device Act (SMDA) (refer to Chapter 1, Volume 3, on statutes, standards, and regulations) might not apply in certain types of healthcare settings, the risk management professional still needs to be aware of issues and concerns about biomedical technology. Even if these issues might not need the same type of formal review and reporting as those in an SMDA-mandated setting, the requirements provide guidance in setting up appropriate internal review systems. Patient care is increasingly moving to non-hospital-based settings, and the scope of services in physicians' offices and the few other locations in which SMDA compliance is not mandatory is continually expanding. Inconsistencies in practice and processes across multiple affiliated locations that are promoted to the public as a coordinated delivery system for healthcare create potential risk exposures. Reducing variation among such locations presents an ongoing challenge for the risk management professional.

· · · · · · · · ·
REPORTING AND FOLLOW-UP OF ADVERSE EVENTS AND NEAR MISSES

The advent of the SMDA, effective in 1991, and its refinements in 1997 and 2000, placed new emphasis on the responsibility of healthcare facilities to report medical device–related incidents to the device manufacturer and to the FDA and to track various types of biomedical technology, particularly certain devices implanted in patients. Although much of the SMDA's focus is on mandatory requirements, voluntary reporting of concerns and near misses plays an important role in timely identification of product design concerns that could lead to user errors and potential patient care problems. Additional information is available at www.fda.gov/MedicalDevices/DeviceRegulationandGuidance/PostMarketRequirements/HumanFactors/ucm124851.

Healthcare facilities need a systematic internal process to document, analyze, and follow up on incidents that may be related to biomedical technology. This is critical to achieving basic goals of the risk management program, such as promoting safe patient care, avoiding injury to the staff using biomedical technology, and reducing the likelihood of potential liability exposure from an adverse event that involves the biomedical technology. Developing a flowchart specific to the institutional structure can help clarify the process and serve as a training tool for the staff. For example, Exhibit 3.1 in this chapter provides a road map for the risk management professional to use to document the review and decision process required to determine whether external reporting is indicated. Additional resources and information about the medical device reporting requirements are available online from the FDA www.fda/gov/MedicalDevices/Safety/ReportaProblem/default.htm.

When a medical device is potentially involved in an unanticipated outcome for a patient, it adds a new dimension to the risk management follow-up. It is important to have institutional processes in place so that, no matter what the day or time, identification and preservation of what may be potential evidence can take place. A healthcare facility might not always have available on-site or on-call risk management and biomedical or clinical engineering staff, so there should be a plan in place to handle these circumstances. Areas that the institution's processes should address include the following:

- Identification of institutional personnel to contact and information on how to reach them (or a designated alternate) during off-shift hours and on regular workdays.

- Protocols to identify, preserve, and impound the medical device, associated components and packaging. The medical device itself must be clearly labeled or tagged as out of service and not to be used, and it should placed in a secured area. The protocols should also include directives not to change any existing control settings, turn off or unplug the device, remove a battery, or otherwise do anything that might hinder retrieval by biomedical or clinical engineering of error codes that might be stored in the device's memory. Clearly identify when cleaning or processing the medical device should be delayed because it might have an adverse effect on subsequent investigation.

EXHIBIT 3.1   ECRI Institute's Medical Device Reporting Decision Pathway

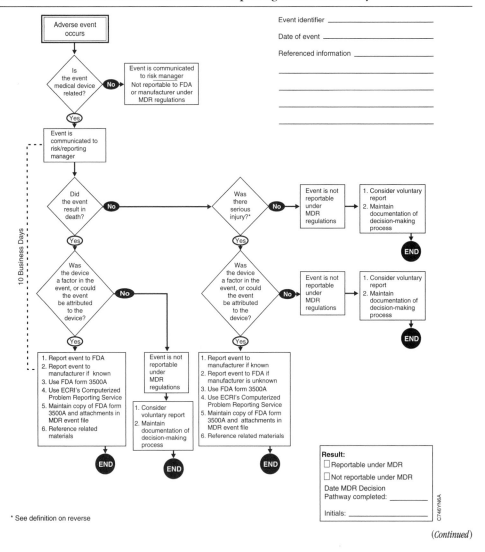

* See definition on reverse

(Continued)

EXHIBIT 3.1   ECRI Institute's Medical Device Reporting Decision Pathway (*Continued*)

Instructions for Using ECRI's MDR Decision Pathway

The ECRI MDR Decision Pathway should be used to document your deliberations when deciding whether an adverse event is reportable under the MDR regulations. The pathway may be duplicated as often as you wish. Maintain MDR Decision Pathways for a minimum of two years from the date of the event. You may also wish to include a copy of the pathway and these instructions in your MDR policies and procedures.

Complete the pathway as follows:

1. Fill in the event identifier as prescribed by policies and procedures. **Do not** use the patient's name, clinician's name, or any social security number as an identifier.

2. Fill in the date of the event.

3. List other referenced materials related to the adverse event (e.g., engineering reports, medical records, incident reports, patient files).

4. Highlight the path followed to reach your conclusion of whether or not the event is reportable under the MDR regulations.

5. Check off the appropriate box indicating whether or not the event is reportable under MDR regulations.

6. Submit voluntary reports as desired to ECRI's Problem Reporting Program, 5200 Butler Pike, Plymouth Meeting, PA 19462-1298, phone: (610) 825-6000, fax: (610) 834-1275; the manufacturer; and/or to FDA on MedWatch Form 3500 (the voluntary reporting form).

7. Fill in the date the MDR Decision Pathway was completed.

8. Fill in the initials of the person completing the pathway.

Serious Injury Considerations for MDR Deliberations

1. Was the injury or illness life-threatening?   ❑ yes ❑ no

2. Did the injury or illness result in permanent* impairment of a body function or permanent damage to a body structure?   ❑ yes ❑ no

3. Did the injury or illness necessitate medical or surgical intervention to preclude permanent* impairment of a body function or permanent damage to a body structure?   ❑ yes ❑ no

Permanent means irreversible impairment or damage, excluding trivial impairment or damage.

Source: ECRI Institute, "Decision Tree for Evaluating Single-Use Devices for Reuse," from pages 44–45 of ECRI Institute's special report, *Reuse of Single-Use Medical Devices: Making Informed Decisions.* Copyright ECRI Institute, 1997. www.ecri.org.

- Maintenance and documentation of a complete chain of custody for the medical device and any associated components or packaging. A paper trail should track the who, what, and where of the items originally impounded and the subsequent transfer(s) of control and custody of any or all of these items (whether internal or external) that might occur. The degree of thoroughness in handling and documenting these steps can be a significant factor if litigation ensues.

- Interactions with the manufacturer of the medical device. In most situations, the healthcare facility is the owner of the medical device involved, and it has a duty to protect its own interests. When a potentially significant problem or adverse patient care outcome is reported to a manufacturer, the company's first response is likely to be an attempt to regain possession of the medical device, ostensibly for testing purposes. A healthcare facility may be offered a refund, exchange, or comparable new product in return. However, because the healthcare facility and the manufacturer might ultimately become defendants with differing interests if litigation results, the decision to send the manufacturer the medical device involved should not be made lightly. This is particularly true where death or serious injury resulted and the health-care facility might ultimately need to have an outside evaluation of that medical device for potential liability purposes. When injury is minimal and litigation seems less likely, completion and documentation of the facility's own investigation and testing and any independent evaluation of the medical device should be completed before deciding whether to send the medical device to the manufacturer for its own testing. Expectations for return of the device should be explicitly documented in correspondence with the manufacturer. Complete documentation of all aspects of the process and transfer must be maintained, including chain of custody tracking.

· · · · · · · · ·

TRACKING BIOMEDICAL DEVICES

The FDA has authority to require manufacturers to track certain classes of medical devices from manufacture down to the level of specific patients who use them. The FDA's goal with this requirement is to ensure that manufacturers remove potentially dangerous or defective medical devices from the market or notify individual patients of significant medical device problems in a timely manner. This authority is in addition to the FDA's authority to order mandatory recalls and require manufacturers to notify healthcare professionals and patients regarding situations in which the FDA determines that there is an unreasonable risk of substantial harm associated with a particular medical device.

The FDA also has the authority to change the list of devices that it requires manufacturers to track, and it has done so periodically. The current list and other information related to tracking is available at http://www.fda.gov/MedicalDevices/DeviceRegulationandGuidance/GuidanceDocuments/ucm149673.

Items tracked include several medical devices that are implanted in patients and another category of biomedical technology equipment that is tracked when used outside a healthcare facility. The responsibility for developing a written standard operating procedure to track a device rests with the manufacturer, but the healthcare facility and individual practitioners are involved in implementing the process, complying with documentation requirements, and maintaining the appropriate records. Healthcare facilities need to be aware that, for implants on the FDA's list, the manufacturer is responsible for tracking the device implanted in the patient and updating the patient's address as necessary. Because the manufacturer should specify in its operating procedure how that updating is to occur, healthcare facilities should make sure they know about (and agree with) any responsibilities the manufacturer may place on them to furnish information in the future.

· · · · · · · · ·

RECALLS OF BIOMEDICAL DEVICES

Healthcare facilities need effective policies and procedures for handling reports of hazardous conditions or recalls that involve biomedical technology–related devices. For hospitals accredited by The Joint Commission (TJC), this requirement is specified in the commission's standards. Recalls may be instituted by the manufacturer (voluntary recall) or by the FDA (mandatory recall) under authority granted to the agency by the SMDA.

Manufacturers initiate most of the recalls involving medical devices, but the FDA plays an active role in the process. By law, the manufacturer must notify the FDA that it is recalling a medical device and submit progress reports to the agency. The initial report must be made to the FDA within ten working days for recalls that involve defective products that could cause serious health problems (for example, a defective artificial heart valve). The FDA reviews the manufacturer's proposed recall plan to determine whether it is adequate and may recommend changes. If the FDA recommends modifications to the recall plan and the manufacturer declines the advice, the FDA can issue its own recall order.

Ordering a recall is only the first step in what can be a tedious and perhaps complicated process in healthcare institutions. Recall notices from a manufacturer can go unnoticed if they are sent to an incorrect address or labeled with the wrong department name. Thus hospitals that frequently use various addresses for different areas on the facility's campus should develop a reliable internal notification system. Beyond issuing recall notices to facilities using the device, manufacturers are not required to publicize that they are recalling a medical device and may choose not to do so.

It is easy to see why medical device recall notices can fail to reach the individuals who need to know about them. Risk management professionals should take steps that improve the odds that the information will get to the right place in a timely manner. Those actions include the following:

- Designate a central collection point for recall notifications and instruct staff about their responsibility to immediately forward information that might come to them to that collection point.

- Require faxing of all recall notifications to that central collection point as part of vendor contracts and purchase orders.

- Determine available options for tracking the type and location of medical devices in the institution and for maintaining an accurate inventory of medical and surgical supplies. In some institutions, purchasing may have designated buyers for certain areas (such as the operating room), and these individuals can play a key role in the recall process.

- Designate an ad hoc group that includes clinical, biomedical, risk management, patient safety, purchasing, and other administrative representatives who can be quickly convened to consider options, alternatives, and ramifications for patient care and recommend a course of action when removal of a medical device from service is necessary.

- Identify an individual or group to coordinate the recall process and related activities, such as ongoing monitoring of FDA and industry information and selected Web sites related to biomedical technology.

··········

REPROCESSING OF SINGLE-USE MEDICAL DEVICES

Whether to reprocess medical devices labeled as single-use by the manufacturer has been an ongoing issue in the healthcare environment. These medical devices can be very expensive to purchase. In some cases, the packaging on the device might have been opened during a procedure without the device itself having been used on a patient. Many healthcare institutions have stopped doing their own reprocessing altogether in light of the many requirements now placed on this practice by the FDA; however, the debate surrounding "open but unused" single-use devices continues. Current information and guidance is available at www.fda.gov/MedicalDevices/DeviceRegulatonandGuidance/ReprocessingofSingle-UseDevices/default.htm.

··········

DISPOSAL OF BIOMEDICAL TECHNOLOGY–RELATED DEVICES

What factors help determine that a piece of biomedical technology is becoming obsolete and replacement, retirement, or disposal should be considered? Guidelines from the American Society of Anesthesiologists[3] regarding anesthesia machines offer some broad categories that an institution can use as a starting point. These include

- lack of essential safety features;
- presence of unacceptable features, such as multiple controls for the same function;
- maintenance problems that potentially affect patient safety, such as a lack of available replacement parts;
- increased potential for human error when compared with newer technology with more safety features.

When healthcare institutions upgrade or otherwise replace items of biomedical technology, they may be faced with a decision about what to do with the piece of equipment currently in use. In some cases, eventual disposal might have been addressed as an aspect of the purchase arrangement. In other situations, trade-in options might be associated with the contract for the new device being purchased.

Disposal concerns, in general, fall into two categories: (1) divestiture, including the sale or donation of a healthcare facility's equipment to another entity, group, or individual, or abandonment or destruction of the equipment, and (2) an acquisition of a piece of biomedical equipment that is being disposed of by another facility. It might seem altruistic to recycle and pass on unneeded or outmoded equipment to others or to preserve institutional resources by acquiring a used piece of biotechnology. However, the potential for allegations that an adverse outcome is linked to the newly divested or acquired piece of equipment makes it essential that the healthcare organization evaluate related risk as part of the decision-making process. There are many potential exposures, including the following:

- The selling or donating entity could find itself being considered part of the distribution chain, with a potential for product liability exposure.

- Compliance with FDA-mandated medical device tracking and documentation requirements may be associated with the disposal.

- Issues involving the existing condition of the biomedical equipment, its remaining useful life, and warranty concerns may arise for parties on both sides of the transaction.

- Whether the pertinent device was donated or sold could become a factor in how the biomedical equipment recycling or transfer to another entity is viewed if something adverse subsequently occurs.

- If biomedical equipment is to be scrapped, it should be rendered unusable, and computer-related or potentially hazardous components and materials should be removed and disposed of properly.

There are national and international organizations that are willing to facilitate the recycling, donation, and independent transfer of medical equipment. Recycling and appropriate sharing of biomedical equipment technology and resources should not be prohibited; however, consideration of the pros and cons in the particular situation should address risk management issues.

· · · · · · · · ·
THE FUTURE OF PATIENT SAFETY AND BIOMEDICAL TECHNOLOGY

Patient safety will continue to affect biomedical technology and vice versa. The movement of biomedical technology from the hospital setting, to the ambulatory setting, to the community at large will change the way the public views the risks and benefits of medical equipment and biomedical technology as a whole. This change is already being seen in the widespread movement of defibrillators from hospitals to ambulances, to businesses and organizations, and even to individuals as defibrillation becomes increasingly automated.

Risk management professionals have many issues to consider as the role of biomedical technology within the community continues to expand.

- Does your institution provide preventive maintenance services (either at no cost or for a fee) to community services, such as local fire department or community ambulance services, that have the regular type of cardiac defibrillators or to businesses and nonprofit agencies that have the automatic ones (AEDs) on-site?

- If so, what formal agreements do you have with the participants, and does your professional liability insurance carrier need to be aware of this activity?

- Do you have physicians or other healthcare providers who provide medical oversight to such programs?

- If so, are they covered under the present institutional or their own individual professional liability insurance programs? Are there state statutes regarding such activities (and do they provide any immunity from litigation or damages for these activities)?

Risk management professionals will continue to need ways to keep abreast of new developments in the biomedical technology arena. One way to address this task is to sign up for selective e-mail notifications from the FDA (www.fda.gov/AboutFDA/ContactFDA/StayInformed/GetEmailUpdates/default.htm) about particular areas of interest or relevance to the facility. Information available through this site includes materials useful to the medical device industry, healthcare providers, and consumers.

Suggested Readings

Feigel, D., S. Gardner, and M. McClellan. "Ensuring Safe and Effective Medical Devices." *New England Journal of Medicine*, 2003, 348(3): 191–192.

Healthcare Information and Management Systems Society (HIMSS), "Medical Device Security." www.himss.org. (Accessed July 2009.)

Porto, G., "Safety by Design: Ten Lessons from Human Factors Research." *Journal of Healthcare Risk Management*, 2001, 21(3): 43–50.

U.S. Food and Drug Administration. "Device Advice (Self-service site for medical device information)." www.fda.gov/MedicalDevices/DeviceRegulationandGuidance/default.htm. (Accessed July 2009.)

U.S. Food and Drug Administration. "Incorporating Human Factors Engineering into Risk Management," July 2000. www.fda.gov/MedicalDevices/DeviceRegulationand Guidance/GuidanceDocuments/ucm094460.htm. (Accessed July 2009.)

U.S. Food and Drug Administration. "Information for Healthcare Organizations about FDA'S 'Guidance for Industry: Cybersecurity for Networked Medical Devices Containing Off-The-Shelf (OTS) Software.'" www.fda.gov/MedicalDevices/DeviceRegulationandGuidance/GuidanceDocuments/ucm077812.htm (Accessed July 2009.)

Endnotes

1. "Playing with Medical Devices Can Be a Deadly Game." *Health Devices* 2002; 31(7) 2002:269–270.

2. *Ibid.*

3. "Guidelines for Determining Anesthesia Machine Obsolescence." *American Society of Anesthesiologists* , June 2004. Available at: www.ASAhq.org. (Accessed July 2009).

4

Informed Consent as a Loss Control Process

Fay A. Rozovsky

Securing the informed consent of a patient marks the culmination of an important step in the care provider–patient relationship. *Consent*, the act of agreeing to a specific diagnostic test or treatment, is not merely the completion of a form but is rather a communication process[1] based on an effective discussion. The communication usually occurs between a care provider and a patient, but sometimes a surrogate is responsible for making such decisions on behalf of the patient. Consent to treatment is like a contract for agreed-upon services by the care provider in exchange for valuable consideration (payment) by the patient or payer.[2]

In other ways, however, consent to treatment is different from other contracts. It is the bond that holds together the ongoing healthcare provider–patient relationship. It is the platform for communication between patient and care provider that starts at the outset of the care-giving relationship and ends with the completion of treatment. It is also the backdrop for disclosure of both anticipated and unanticipated outcomes of tests or treatments.[3] Consent to treatment is marked by extensive case law and is guided by federal and state statutes and regulations that set forth not only the broad parameters for a valid treatment authorization[4] but also requirements for specific diagnostic interventions and surgery. Consent to treatment is also the subject of the *Interpretive Guidelines*[5] published by the Centers for Medicare & Medicaid Services (CMS) used to guide state surveyors in conducting validation and compliant-based surveys of hospitals and other types of healthcare facilities. At the state level, a host of laws set forth specific consent requirements for a myriad of healthcare needs, including genetic testing, HIV testing, breast cancer surgery, abortion, and end-of-life choice making.

Despite all the judicial interpretations, statutes, and regulations, consent (or the lack of it) remains a persistent basis for claim in health professional liability lawsuits. This is true whether the consent claim is ancillary to other tort allegations or is a stand-alone basis for action. Additionally, attempts continue to be made through litigation to impose a consent responsibility on healthcare organizations.

Consent litigation has moved beyond negligence claims and intentional torts, such as battery, to new levels of legal argument. These include breach of contract in situations in which patients argue that the caregiver guaranteed a specific outcome and claims based on misrepresentation, deceit, or fraud. Due to state-based legislation governing unfair and deceptive trade practices, caregivers can find themselves on the receiving end of litigation that relies on such laws in lawsuits involving misrepresentation. Unlike traditional negligence litigation, consent claims based on misrepresentation may involve punitive damages.

Some state legislation ties consent litigation to laws that govern unprofessional conduct. This is an interesting risk management issue. Not only would a caregiver be exposed to either a traditional negligent consent claim or a consent allegation involving an intentional tort, but the state professional licensing body might also pursue an investigation or hearing for unprofessional conduct based on the same set of facts and circumstances. Defending on more than one front means that the caregiver has more risk exposure than was present in years past.

From a risk management perspective, it is disturbing that consent litigation persists. As a communication process and an integral part of the care provider–patient relationship, a successful consent process can be used to pinpoint and address at-risk situations. To appreciate management of the consent process as a loss control or risk management technique requires an understanding of the elements of a valid treatment authorization, of the right to make an informed refusal-of-care decision, and of common problem areas that involve minors or patients whose capacity to make treatment choices is in doubt. At the same time, the risk management professional should be familiar with recurrent problems such as those emanating from compulsory treatment situations, behavioral health settings, ambulatory care, and the absence of appropriate documentation of the consent process.

Consent-to-treatment responsibilities belong to the care provider who is to conduct the proposed test or treatment. This responsibility is as true for physicians performing office-based surgical procedures as it is for surgeons performing operations in a hospital or ambulatory surgery center. Similarly, it is a responsibility that is as applicable to clinical psychologists in the outpatient setting as it is for dentists or ophthalmologists in the office setting. In other words, consent to treatment is part of the core responsibilities of a broad range of care providers.

That consent is the responsibility of the care provider who is to perform the test or procedure does not diminish the important role that other healthcare professionals may play in the communication process. Thus a nurse may ask a series of key questions designed to elicit risk factors and then share any issues identified with a physician. Such information, gleaned from the history-taking component of the consent process, may alter what might have been the plan of care for the patient. However, the ultimate responsibility for the consent process rests with the physician, dentist, or other individual who will provide the treatment.

Educating providers about their respective roles and responsibilities is a function that is well suited to risk management professionals. Treating consent as a tool to avoid liability exposure, the risk management professional can also use it as a means of facilitating greater trust among patients and care providers in healthcare systems that undergo dynamic change.

This chapter identifies the contemporary legal sources of influence for the consent process. It describes the basic elements of the consent-to-treatment process from both a clinical and enterprise risk management perspective. It also discusses the principal exceptions to the consent process and suggests measures that can be taken to avoid liability exposure with regard to consent to treatment. This chapter also describes the expanding nature of the consent process as a pivotal tool in the financial and regulatory aspects of healthcare delivery. Finally, the chapter discusses the use of the consent process as a patient safety tool for both avoiding liability exposure related to basic principles of informed consent, and following tests or treatment, a framework for disclosing the outcomes of care.

· · · · · · · · ·
INFLUENCE OF LEGAL DECISIONS ON THE CONSENT PROCESS

Case law has long been an impetus for consent to treatment in the United States. Although many judicial opinions have been credited with helping to create the framework for consent law, perhaps the most famous is a New York decision by a judge destined to be a distinguished member of the United States Supreme Court, Mr. Justice Benjamin Cardozo. In affirming a judgment for a hospital, Justice Cardozo wrote: "Every human being of adult years and sound mind has a right to determine what shall be done with his own body."[6]

Cardozo, an eloquent jurist, was not the only judge to write opinions on the subject of informed consent. Indeed, some decisions on this subject predated the above-quoted Scholendorff case,[7] and other landmark cases continued to emerge from the late 1950s through the early part of the 1970s.[8]

Along with case law, state legislatures have enacted statutes that address consent to treatment. This mosaic of state legislation is fascinating to review and is definitely an important influence in shaping contemporary consent law. For example, some states have enacted laws delineating broad requirements for consent to treatment whereas others have turned these components into elements of a negligent consent claim under statutory law. Some jurisdictions have enacted age-specific consent laws. Thus a minor may be deemed capable of giving consent to donate blood at age seventeen in one state and in another jurisdiction, legislation may set a different age threshold for a young person to give such consent. For risk management professionals the key is to become familiar with consent law in their respective jurisdictions.

Another influence can be found in federal legislation and regulations. Examples include federal requirements on informed consent that date back to the 1970s in the area of human research[9] and more contemporary legislation and regulations that address "patient dumping" under the Emergency Treatment and Labor Act (EMTALA) and its accompanying rules.[10]

Other federal sources of influence that promote consent as a process include provisions that are not part of laws or regulations directly related to patient care. Instead, these regulations are designed to protect and promote civil rights. For example, the regulations under the 1964 Civil Rights Act that bar discrimination on the basis of race, color, or national origin also affect consent practices. Hospitals and other healthcare organizations that provide services to recipients of federally assisted programs must take reasonable steps to provide information in appropriate languages to such persons.[11] This means that non-English-speaking patients enrolled in federally assisted programs enjoy some language service–related protection. Failure to meet such requirements could subject a healthcare organization to enforcement activities under the auspices of the U.S. Department of Justice, Office of Civil Rights (OCR). The guidance document that supports the Civil Rights Act addresses the needs of those with limited English proficiency (LEP) and the cultural needs of those seeking treatment more specifically.[12]

The Civil Rights Act is part of a body of legislation and regulations that address compliance with standards set by the federal government. Some of these standards involve clinical care and consent to treatment. The Patient Self-Determination Act, which deals with advance directives, offers yet another illustration of federal requirements linked to delivery of clinical care.[13] Another example includes the Conditions of Participation (CoPs) for healthcare facilities receiving Medicare and or Medicaid dollars. The provisions for hospitals state in part that

> [p]atients or their representatives (as allowed under state law) have the right to make informed decisions regarding their care. Patients' rights include being informed of their health status, being involved in care planning and treatment, and being able to request or refuse treatment.[14]

Healthcare organizations involved in corporate compliance activities purport to adhere to such requirements. Evidence of nonconformity with the CoPs, EMTALA, or the Civil Rights Act of 1964 might constitute noncompliance under the entity's corporate standards of conduct. The subsequent failure to take corrective action for nonconforming consent practices may cast doubt on the effectiveness of the corporate compliance plan. In some instances involving billing or coding issues or patient complaints, it might trigger a regulatory investigation. Hence, corporate compliance, a voluntary program for healthcare organizations, might actually be a "federal driver" in the area of informed consent. Refer to Chapter 4 in Volume 3 for further information on corporate compliance.

As noted elsewhere in this book, there are very specific federal requirements governing consent to participate in human subject research trials.[15] Consent requirements have been set for organ procurement and transplantation[16] and for long-term care facilities.[17] These are important requirements that are quite specific in their application. Additionally, the HIPAA Privacy Standards provide direction for securing not a consent but rather an acknowledgement of a privacy notice with respect to certain uses of protected health information (PHI).[18]

Some federal agencies or departments have developed informational tools that can be used to facilitate the consent process. For example, the Centers for Disease Control and Prevention (CDC) have developed a series of informational tools to explain the benefits and possible side effects of childhood immunization.[19]

Beyond legislation and regulations, guidance documents have also been issued by the Office of Civil Rights of the Department of Health and Human Services. Such guidance does not have the full weight or authority of legislation or regulations. Nevertheless, it provides important insight into the regulatory mindset regarding two important factors that are integral to an effective consent: linguistic capability and culture.

The Office of Civil Rights of HHS characterizes the linguistic issue in terms of LEP.[20] With respect to cultural issues, the government has coined the term *CLAS*, an acronym that stands for culturally and linguistically appropriate services.[21] Whereas the LEP documentation is in the form of policy guidance, the CLAS information reflects actual standards. The point is that the government has determined that deficiencies in language accommodation and cultural sensitivity have a direct influence on the quality of communication. In the healthcare area, this includes the consent process.

In April, 2007, CMS revised the *State Operations Manual* (*Interpretive Guidelines*) used by state surveyors to assess compliance with the Conditions of Participation in Medicare and Medicaid. These revisions offer regulatory insights into what CMS described as a "well-designed informed consent process" and a "well-designed informed consent form." (See Exhibit 4.1.)

Like other guidance described earlier, the Interpretive Guidelines do not have the effect of law. Still, from a risk management and consent perspective, the content is important for two reasons. First, the content might influence court decisions, especially in those situations in which a judge is discussing regulatory intent. Second, the Interpretive Guidelines offer a window on regulatory compliance. The guidelines are the equivalent of a road map that tells a hospital what to anticipate in terms of a validation or complaint survey. From another perspective, the Interpretive Guidelines serve as a blueprint for hospital operations. The same holds true in the consent arena. Designing consent policies and procedures to meet such guidance helps avoid regulatory risk exposure.

The cadre of federal legislation, rules, and regulations that shape patients' rights and responsibilities create legal concerns and risk exposures. The sanctions can be quite serious, including decertification from federal funding programs, civil monetary penalties, and in the case of corporate compliance, imposition of a corporate integrity program. As suggested later in this chapter, the evolving link between financial reimbursement and so-called never events may also turn on the effective use of the consent process.

Another consideration is that any reimbursement from insurance coverages for defense costs associated with a regulatory proceeding may be limited, and insurers will not reimburse healthcare organizations for criminal fines at all. Hence, there is a substantial financial loss exposure that stems from the federal drivers of consent. Coupled with potential fallout from adverse media coverage, such loss of reputation and money merits innovation in using the consent process as a loss control tool. Getting to this point

EXHIBIT 4.1   Informed Consent Forms

A properly executed informed consent form should reflect the patient consent process. Except as specified for emergency situations in the hospital's informed consent policies, all inpatient and outpatient medical records must contain a properly executed informed consent form prior to conducting any procedure or other type of treatment that requires informed consent. An informed consent form, in order to be properly executed, must be consistent with hospital policies as well as applicable state and federal law or regulation. A properly executed informed consent form contains the following minimum elements:

- Name of the hospital where the procedure or other type of medical treatment is to take place

- Name of the specific procedure, or other type of medical treatment for which consent is being given

- Name of the responsible practitioner who is performing the procedure or administering the medical treatment

- Statement that the procedure or treatment, including the anticipated benefits, material risks, and alternative thera-
pies, was explained to the patient or the patient's legal representative (Material risks could include risks with a high degree of likelihood but a low degree of severity, as well as those with a very low degree of likelihood but high degree of severity. Hospitals are free to delegate to the responsible practitioner who uses the available clinical evidence as informed by the practitioner's professional judgment the determination of which material risks, benefits and alternatives will be discussed with the patient.)

- Signature of the patient or the patient's legal representative

- Date and time the informed consent form is signed by the patient or the patient's legal representative

    If there is applicable state law governing the content of the informed consent form, then the hospital's form must comply with those requirements.
    A well-designed informed consent form might also include the following additional information:

- Name of the practitioner who conducted the informed consent discussion with the patient or the patient's representative

- Date, time, and signature of the person witnessing the patient or the patient's legal representative signing the consent form

- Indication or listing of the material risks of the procedure or treatment that were discussed with the patient or the patient's representative

- Statement, if applicable, that physicians other than the operating practitioner, including but not limited to residents, will be performing important tasks related to the surgery, in accordance with the hospital's policies and, in the case of residents, based on their skill set and under the supervision of the responsible practitioner

- Statement, if applicable, that qualified medical practitioners who are not physicians who will perform important parts of the surgery or administration of anesthesia will be performing only tasks that are within their scope of practice, as determined under state law and regulation, and for which they have been granted privileges by the hospital

Source: Interpretive Guidelines §482.24(c)(2)(v), *State Operations Manual,* Appendix A, Survey Process for Hospitals, (Rev. 47, 06–05–09).

requires the risk management professional to have a firm knowledge of the basic elements of the consent process.

· · · · · · · · ·

ELEMENTS OF CONSENT TO TREATMENT

Although laws vary from jurisdiction to jurisdiction, several elements generally are recognized as integral to the consent process. These elements involve not only what information should be disclosed to the patient or surrogate decision maker but also the qualifications for who may authorize or decline treatment. These factors apply to so-called elective care situations in which there is sufficient time to obtain relevant history and to exchange pertinent information.

The law presumes that an adult is capable of making a treatment choice. Sometimes this ability to consent is extended to minors, including minors who are emancipated, living independently from their parents or guardians. In other cases, the law has carved out certain treatment-specific exceptions that enable even unemancipated minors to authorize treatment. For example, minors who seek treatment for substance abuse, sexually transmitted diseases, and other sensitive issues may be authorized to obtain care without consent of a guardian or parent. In other situations, these procedure-specific laws enable minors to donate blood. These laws depend on the criteria found in a specific state. Some set age thresholds for when a minor is legally capable of making such decisions. In others, although there is no requirement to obtain consent from a guardian or parent, leeway is given to the caregiver to notify parents in some instances.

Sometimes the law removes the right of an individual to give or decline consent to treatment. For example, a court determination may be made for a specific situation, such as court-ordered treatment for a highly communicable and deleterious disease such as tuberculosis, on a temporary or permanent basis, where a finding is made that the individual can no longer make treatment choices. When a court appoints a guardian to make healthcare decisions on behalf of the patient, it signifies a judicial determination that the person is legally incapable of making treatment choices. From a practical standpoint, however, many caregivers still involve the patient in the dialogue to the extent that is practical. The rationale is that the patient might have important information about prior treatments, allergies, and so on that could influence the care plan recommended for the individual.

The law also assumes that every individual has the requisite mental capability to make a treatment decision. In essence, it is a belief that the person can weigh the pros and cons of recommended and alternate care to make a treatment choice. The law recognizes, however, that patients may lack such ability due to injury, egregious pain, the influence of medication, illegal drugs, or alcohol abuse. The law will not tell a caregiver who is and who is not mentally capable of making a treatment choice. This necessitates a case-by-case determination by the caregiver. Sometimes the results can be surprising. For example, a person may have a blood alcohol level that is over the legal limit for driving under the influence, yet the individual has the ability to make cogent treatment choices. From a risk management standpoint, it is important to work with caregivers to develop practical criteria for making such a determination and designing a framework for documenting such an assessment. This is especially important in cases fraught with ethical implications. Care providers might be very much opposed to a patient's decision, yet they are legally and morally obliged to respect it. A clinical impression of mental incapacity may serve as a pretext to overruling the patient's choice. Such a paternalistic approach must be avoided. Risk management professionals engaged in consent education programs often appropriately reinforce the point that care providers must not insert their values in place of those of their patients. Also reinforced in these programs is the need to respect patients' rights and to consult ethics committees in difficult cases.

Aside from a person's legal capability and mental capacity, many jurisdictions have delineated the fundamental elements of what should be disclosed to the person making a treatment choice. These elements include the following:

- A disclosure of the nature and purpose of the proposed test or treatment
- A description of the probable risks and benefits of the test or treatment
- An explanation of alternate tests or treatment and the probable risks and benefits associated with these options
- An explanation of the probable risks and benefits of forgoing proposed or alternate tests or treatment
- An opportunity to ask questions and receive understandable answers
- An opportunity to make a decision free of coercion and undue influence

As a practical starting point, the consent conversation must be geared to the comprehension level of the patient. Medical jargon is unacceptable for most patients. However, talking down to a patient to the point that the patient is insulted or turned off is equally unacceptable.

The degree or extent of disclosure is a matter of sharp legal differences of opinion. The majority position, the patient need standard, requires disclosure of material or significant information that a reasonable person, in the same or a similar position as the patient, would want to know so as to make a treatment choice. The minority perspective is based on what the medical community believes the patient should know.

Whether the risk management professional works in a jurisdiction that follows the patient need or the medical community standard, the risk management stand is to furnish relevant, understandable information that will prevent or eliminate any misinformation or misunderstanding. In practical terms, this means conveying to patients information regarding the following:

- The risk of death, disability, disfigurement, or major change in lifestyle
- The degree of pain, dysfunction, or discomfort associated with the test or treatment
- The time commitment associated with proposed and alternate treatments, including rehabilitation, physical therapy, or long-term medication management
- The urgency to undergo the test or treatment
- The consequences of deferring the test or treatment

Many care providers find it difficult to discuss certain types of risk information with patients.[22] Known risks should be discussed with the patient. Generally speaking, remote risks need not be disclosed, except in a few well-defined situations. If there is a risk of death, albeit remote, associated with a contemplated procedure, such risk should be discussed. The risk of death from general anesthesia is a frequently cited example. The anesthesiologist or nurse anesthetist is obliged to disclose to the patient that death is a possibility, albeit a remote one. In this instance, the risk management point to convey to care providers who are uneasy about such discussions is that their effectiveness rests on two important elements: what is said to the patient and how the message is delivered.

Remote risks can be put in an appropriate context to enable patients to make informed choices. From a risk management standpoint, the use of statistics should be discouraged in this regard because many patients do not have a framework for understanding what a 15 percent risk of death from anesthesia or surgery really means.

Another area of friction in consent involves the concept of *common knowledge*. In essence, care providers may believe it acceptable to assume that most patients understand certain risks as being part and parcel of a recommended test, procedure, or medication management regimen. Assuming too much in terms of common knowledge may lead to untoward risk, especially when the consent process involves patients who do not share the same cultural grounding as the care providers. Add to the situation linguistic barriers, or in the case of written information, deficiencies in health literacy, and the prospect of a dysfunctional consent process increases.

· · · · · · · · ·
EXCEPTIONS TO THE GENERAL RULES OF CONSENT

The requirements for a valid consent to treatment are not absolute. Indeed, the law recognizes several exceptions to the rule, including exceptions for emergency treatment, impracticality of consent, therapeutic privilege, compulsory treatment situations, and the recently recognized psychiatric or mental health advance directive.[23]

Emergency Treatment Exception

The emergency treatment exception is well recognized in case law and in legislation.[24,25] Although the specifics vary from jurisdiction to jurisdiction, the basic criteria are the same:

- The patient presents with a life-threatening illness or injury that requires immediate attention.

- The patient is unable to either communicate or take part in a communication process.

- There is no time to secure a treatment authorization from someone else who might be empowered by law to act on the patient's behalf.

When these criteria are met, the law implies a treatment authorization on behalf of the patient for such diagnostic tests or treatments as are medically necessary to alleviate a life-threatening event. In doing so, the law assumes that if patients were capable of participating in the consent process, they would readily agree to the course of treatment provided.

The emergency treatment exception authorizes only care that is medically necessary to rectify the urgent situation. Medically necessary care can be quite expansive, including removal of organs, amputation of limbs, and the causing of a miscarriage. However, it does not authorize a care provider to perform tests or treatments that are not immediately required. Thus, a surgeon might be within the scope of the emergency exception in removing a patient's ruptured spleen, but not in removing a pigmented nevus on that patient's abdomen.

From a risk management perspective, it is important to understand that the law will not sanction the application of the emergency exception when a patient is temporarily incapacitated by a preoperative medication and there is neither a life- nor health-threatening event that requires urgent surgical intervention. A competent patient in the midst of a health-threatening event still enjoys the right to refuse treatment. The emergency exception does not preempt the competent patient's right to refuse treatment.

Caregivers often have difficulty accepting the fact that a competent person may decline life-saving care when confronted with the potential of death or serious harm from a heart attack, stroke, allergic reaction, or asthmatic attack. As health professionals trained to save life, they feel that the better approach is to intervene to provide treatment. In doing so, they minimize the power of the law and the significance of the principle of individual choice making. Judges and juries alike are apt to react quite negatively in cases in which the patient had made clear a choice not to undergo treatment when confronted with a life- or health-threatening event. In such instances, the risk is one of a battery claim in which there need not be proof of actual harm to the individual.

Today, the right to refuse life-saving care is closely connected with end-of-life decision making. Although there is a substantial amount of overlap between the two topics, it should be understood that the competent patient can decline treatment designed to save life or health without any requirement that the situation involve a terminal illness. This is particularly important in EMTALA-style cases and emergency department treatment decisions.

Risk management professionals know that most emergency cases are not black-and-white episodes. Indeed, many cases are filled with shades of gray that necessitate uncovering factual information to verify that a true emergency does exist. To this end, several steps can be taken to minimize inappropriate use of the exception, including the following:

- Clinical pathways for declaring an emergency
- Decision trees for declaring an emergency
- Education on the emergency treatment exception for new hires and in-service for regular staff
- Mandatory training and in-service for contracted employees of the emergency and urgent care departments
- Documentation to substantiate the declaration of an emergency
- Documentation to substantiate compliance with a patient directive declining treatment in an emergency

IMPRACTICALITY OF CONSENT

A variation on the emergency exception is impracticality of consent.[26] Although it is not well-defined in law, it reflects many of the treatment situations found in emergency departments and urgent care centers. Like the true emergency situation, the patient presents with a life-threatening or health-threatening event that requires immediate treatment. However, unlike the true emergency situation, the patient is able to communicate with the treatment team. The urgency of the situation, however, precludes the opportunity for a full discussion of the indications for treatment, an explanation of care, probable benefits, probable risks, and treatment alternatives.

From a risk management perspective, consent policies and procedures should include a framework for managing impracticality of consent. Care providers should be oriented to managing impracticality of consent situations, including the following:

- Situations in which the exception is applicable, for example, patients who present in shock due to a bee sting, gunshot wound, allergic reaction, and who are capable of communication

- What questions to ask of such cognitive and communicative patients, for example, details of current medications, allergy or drug sensitivity history, and so on

- What information to share with the patient, for example, what the team will be doing to address the life-threatening or health-threatening event

- Answering patient questions as the situation permits, noting that after the immediate event is over, a more detailed discussion will take place with the individual

- Documentation of the reason(s) for using the impracticality of consent exception

Therapeutic Privilege Exception

In comparison to the emergency treatment provision, the therapeutic privilege exception is a far more nebulous concept. This exception usually applies in narrowly drawn circumstances in which the disclosure of certain information is believed to cause the patient a risk of significant harm (likely to be psychogenic or psychobiological in nature).

To invoke the therapeutic privilege exception, certain criteria must be met. These include a full assessment of the facts and circumstances of the patient's case and condition and a medical opinion that a full disclosure of information will have a significant or seriously adverse effect on the patient.[27] Typically, this is done in accordance with well-delineated policy and procedure in the healthcare organization. Many healthcare entities require that the assessment be performed by a person expert in psychiatry. To be certain that the evaluation is objective, the person making the assessment is one who is not otherwise involved in the care and treatment of the patient. If the second opinion confirms the need for therapeutic privilege, this assessment is documented in the medical record along with the rationale for it.

From a risk management standpoint, caregivers are often encouraged to document what they did disclose to the patient in the therapeutic privilege context in addition to what was not revealed in the discussion. This may be done as a concurrent note in the medical record. If it is determined after the test or treatment that the patient's status is such that untoward harm is not likely to occur as a result of the disclosure, the caregiver may explain to the patient why information was withheld and the nature of the details that had not been imparted earlier. The fact that such a discussion took place should also be documented in the medical record.

The therapeutic privilege exception does not negate the obligation to inform the patient. Rather, it grants the care provider leeway in the degree of disclosure surrounding those details that are apt to cause harm to the patient. From a risk management perspective, the exception requires careful application and detailed documentation to verify that it was used appropriately.

Compulsory Treatment Exception

The compulsory treatment situation is another type of exception from the general rules of consent. In essence, the law makes a value judgment that the rights and liberties of the individual must give way to the greater good and health of the community. As such, the compulsory treatment exception is largely rooted in public health legislation, empowering officials to quarantine, test, or treat individuals with infectious illnesses.[28] Concerns about H1N1 A influenza, severe acute respiratory syndrome (SARS), and other pandemic occurrences offer illustrations of situations in which state public health officials may exercise authority under legislation for compulsory treatment decision making.

Even in the context of this exception, however, there are safeguards to obviate inappropriate use of public health legislation as a mechanism for circumventing the law of consent to treatment. As described earlier, even if a person comes within the category of compulsory treatment, patient safety and good clinical judgment play an important role in treatment. Thus, a prudent care provider would ask questions to determine if the patient is taking medication that renders the public health treatment ill advised or if the patient has an underlying allergy that points toward an alternative form of care. The key point is that even in the exercise of this exception, effective communication is important.

· · · · · · · · ·
EFFECTIVE COMMUNICATION IN THE CONSENT PROCESS

Communicating in practical terms that the patient can understand may involve using several communication channels. In addition to face-to-face verbal explanations, media may include video displays, interactive computer programs, and printed items such as brochures, pamphlets, or information sheets. From a risk management perspective, the key point is that the message conveyed in all the media must be consistent because discrepancies create an opportunity for a plaintiff to challenge the integrity of the consent process. It also is important to remember that multimedia resources, though useful tools, are ancillary to the care provider–patient communication that underpins the consent process.

In today's Internet society, communication is a serious issue in terms of informed consent. Patients access the Web and may find a host of sites that offer information pertinent to their healthcare needs. Some of the Web sites are legitimate locations that contain valid information. Other sites, such as blogs or video material posted on YouTube, however well-crafted by well-intentioned individuals, contain personal observations or life experiences that cannot be validated or replicated for others. This is also true of medical blogs and consumer mailing lists dedicated to specific illnesses. Reliance on such information could lead to imprudent health choices by patients.

Why do patients surf the Web if their caregivers are furnishing them with salient information? The answer is that there is a level of distrust among today's healthcare consumers and a concern that they are not getting the full story. They may believe that they should do their own independent research lest they rely on inadequate information in making treatment decisions. Marketing by self-help and health information Web sites promotes such activity.

Confronted with a multitude of pamphlets, brochures, booklets, information sheets, and video material, there is a danger that patients may be confused rather than informed in making choices. Add to this abundant Internet material that contradicts or casts doubt on details provided by caregivers, and the patient shifts from confused to doubtful or uncertain. Patients are primed to confront caregivers with challenges demanding to know why they were not told about risks or treatment alternatives they found on the Internet. Indeed, enterprising plaintiffs' counsel will use such information to raise questions about the completeness of the informed consent process.

The role of the risk management professional is to restore order to consent as a communications process. This may involve preemptive practice assessments including the following:

- Inventory of media used for conveying information to patients
- Consistency of information disseminated to patients, including information sheets, brochures, and pamphlets
- Reviewing content of patient information Web sites sponsored by the healthcare entity
- Providing sanctioned Web addresses to patients
- Warnings that some Web addresses, blogs, and mailing lists may contain information that is not scientifically proven or valid and to exercise caution in relying on treatment details at these sites

Patients today are also hearing more and more about complementary and alternative medicine (CAM). Some people use herbal supplements or remedies to treat mood swings, joint pain, and the symptoms of menopause. The failure to acknowledge this practice may lead to misdiagnosis or treatments with severe adverse results. The contemporary risk management consent toolkit contains salient questions to ask during the communication process to elicit information regarding such treatment practices. Once the information is in hand, appropriate treatment plans can be recommended to the patient. For more information on CAM, refer to Appendix 15.1 in this volume.

Another communication-related consideration is the choice of messenger. Ideally, the person who is to perform the test or treatment should secure the patient's authorization. This step does not involve the administrative or clerical act of securing the patient's signature on a treatment authorization. Rather, the focal point of the consent process is on the communication exchange, the solicitation of critical information from the patient, and the dissemination of relevant details in return. Another care provider is less likely to complete a successful consent process due to being less familiar with the patient's history, needs, and desires. Thus, relying on another to fulfill this task might create information gaps that culminate in consent claims.

The growth in computer-based communication has been seen by some as an opportunity to enhance the consent process. Interactive computer software can help the technically savvy patient delve deeply into factors important to him or to her regarding a range of treatment options. Such asynchronous learning may lead the patient to ask a series of follow-up questions that should be addressed by a care provider in an office or clinic visit.

Still others have developed Web-based programming that presents patients with information to help him or her make treatment choices. Often accompanied by colorful graphics, the Web site reduces to as common a level as possible significant information that a person would want to know in order to make a treatment choice.

Computer-generated tools and Internet-based technologies, like handwritten or hard copy illustrations are assistive in nature. The information is *not* a substitute for two-way communication between a care provider and patient. That such tools might be used in this way, as a consent expedient, can create a serious risk exposure in terms of the completeness of the consent process.

Sometimes missing in the communication aspect of informed consent is confirmation of the successful exchange of information. A consent form is evidence of the process; however, it typically provides little to substantiate that decisions were made with an understanding of benefits, risk, alternatives, opting for alternative and complementary therapy, and the consequences of declining all care.

The confirmation aspect of communication can occur in several ways. Establishing a consistent protocol of questions that substantiates a confirmation of communication is one method. Making it a usual and customary practice might suffice in some states. However, a better approach is to use a checklist or some other form of documentation. Posing confirmatory questions is a useful risk management tool. Rather than asking patients, Do you understand what I have been saying?, a preferable approach is to use open-ended statements such as, Tell me in your own words what you understand to be involved in the operation. A patient's response with appropriate answers is a confirmation of the communication process. From a risk management standpoint, the use of a confirmatory dialogue is important in especially risk-prone situations, including those in which the patient has communication challenges that must be accommodated by use of devices (language boards, TTY, teletype) or interpreters. Documenting that the patient gave knowledgeable responses to such questions affirms that the communication was effective. A similar process may be used with surrogate decision makers.

Informed Refusal of Care

Although most healthcare professionals recognize the importance of informed choice in leading to a patient's agreement to some type of diagnostic test or treatment, the same level of recognition is not always present in regard to informed refusals of care. Because the law has given particular recognition to the need for patients to decline tests or treatment on the basis of informed choice making,[29] informed refusal is an important concept.

The leading case on this topic involved a patient in California who repeatedly declined recommendations from her primary care physician to undergo a pap smear.[30] Ultimately, she died of cervical cancer, leaving two minor children as survivors. The children sued the primary care physician for lack of informed refusal of care, successfully persuading the court that it was not sufficient for a care provider simply to recommend a diagnostic test. Instead, they argued, the duty to inform goes further, requiring the care provider to ensure that a patient's decision to refuse or decline tests or treatment is an informed decision.[31]

This California case has become a legal benchmark. To the extent that it is practical to do so, care providers need to discuss with their patients the consequences of declining tests or treatment and to document this phase of the consent process. Use of this approach makes patients hard-pressed to claim later that a decision to forgo tests or treatment was based on inadequate disclosure of information. It is also important to note that informed refusal of care has applications beyond routine care in the physician's office. It is equally applicable in emergency department (ED) settings in which decisions to forgo transfer to another facility or to decline admission for care have profound legal implications under EMTALA provisions of applicable federal and state law.

For an informed refusal of care to be valid, the patient must be legally and mentally capable of making a choice. When the patient does not meet these criteria, a duly authorized surrogate decision maker may make the determination. Like the patient, the surrogate decision maker must be properly informed about the consequences of a refusal of care.

Once the patient (or surrogate decision maker) has made an informed choice to refuse care, it is incumbent upon care providers to respect that determination.[32] Care providers sometimes find this concept difficult to apply. Nevertheless, the law does not permit them—however well-intentioned they may be—to substitute their values and beliefs regarding what is best for those of their patients. Furthermore, the law expects that in providing patients with the requisite degree of information needed to make a treatment choice, care providers will deliver the details about the pros and cons of treatment evenhandedly. Failure to do so creates a needless risk of exposure for lawsuits based on lack of informed refusal of care.

RIGHT TO WITHDRAW CONSENT

Patients have the right to withdraw a treatment authorization. From a risk management standpoint, it is important to ask when a patient can make such a decision. A Wisconsin ruling offers an answer on the issue of a change of mind in the informed consent process.[33]

A patient, pregnant for the third time, was informed by her doctor that although she had previously undergone caesarean deliveries, she should have a vaginal delivery this time. The doctor suggested that, if medically necessary, a caesarean section would be performed. During admission, the patient signed both a consent form for a vaginal delivery and another regarding a caesarean section. Several hours later, when the doctor came in to see the patient, she told him she wanted to have a caesarean section. The doctor responded by encouraging her to stick to the original delivery plan. When the patient's labor was not proceeding as had been anticipated, the doctor broke the amniotic sac to accelerate the process. The patient suffered such severe abdominal pain that the medication did not work. Once again, the patient informed the doctor that she had changed her mind and that she wanted a caesarean section. The doctor indicated that if he acceded to all such requests, all deliveries would be accomplished by caesarean section.

When the baby's heart rate dropped, an emergency caesarean section was performed. The outcome was poor. The mother's uterus had ruptured and the lack of oxygen left the child with spastic quadriplegia, unable to speak and unable to move below her neck.

In remanding the case for a determination of damages, the Supreme Court of Wisconsin reasoned that once a medical procedure has commenced, the patient does not relinquish the right to withdraw consent to treatment. Much depends on the circumstances of each case and the specific treatment alternatives in deciding at which point there is no turning back. In this case, caesarean section was an alternative form of delivery; therefore, the patient was able to withdraw her consent to vaginal childbirth. By changing her mind, the patient set in motion a responsibility to complete a new informed consent discussion.

This change of mind case points out a critical component of risk management training on informed consent. It is imperative to sensitize caregivers to recognize consent speed bumps put in place by patients or substitute decision makers. As long as the point of no return has not been reached and there are treatment options, the patient has the right to opt out of an agreed-upon course of care.

· · · · · · · · ·
SPECIAL NEEDS PATIENTS AND THE CONSENT PROCESS

Many states have singled out specific categories of patients for special consideration under the law of consent to treatment. These categories include minors, elderly patients, mentally disabled or challenged persons, and those undergoing tests or treatment for certain diseases, such as breast cancer or blood transfusion therapy.

Care should be exercised in generalizing about the requirements for consent with regard to specific patient groups or types of tests or treatment. Much of the law is quite state-specific, necessitating specific legal advice and policies and procedures to address these matters.

Although state law is quite specific in this area, it is important to keep in mind the basic requirements for a valid consent process. The law presumes that a patient possesses both legal competency and mental capability to make a treatment choice. Only in certain specific situations does the law require a different approach to the consent process. Such requirements typically go into effect when

- legislation varies the general rules of consent;
- court orders require specific treatment or bar certain care; and

- the facts of a given consent trigger the need to determine legal competency or mental capacity to make a treatment choice.

Aside from the law, there are very practical reasons for managing the consent process differently with certain categories of patients. These reasons include

- auditory, speech, or visually impaired patients;
- culturally sensitive consent situations; and
- linguistic barriers between patients and care providers.

Yet another cohort of patients who may need special consideration may not be found in statutes or regulations. They may not have physical or intellectual challenges that impede decision making. Instead, this is a group of patients who have such complex medical needs and who face a wide range of options that they need a consent process managed over a series of meetings.

Preliminary screening of patients can eliminate the risk that the process will unravel due to the patient's inability to hear, speak, or see sufficiently to engage in a valid consent process. Indeed, this risk can be obviated by telling patients at the outset that the care provider or facility is sensitive to such needs and encourages patients to disclose them. By the same token, care providers should be trained in methods that help detect those patients who need assistive devices, such as TDD (telephone devices for the deaf) or TTY (teletype). From a patient safety perspective, an effective consent process may benefit from use of a consent time-out. (See Exhibit 4.2.) This approach contemplates the use of a consent time-out checklist to document the resolution of identified patient or surrogate-specific needs regarding consent. The checklist should be signed, timed, and dated by the care provider and then made a part of the consent documentation process. From a risk management perspective, the tool can help avoid flawed consent processes. It can also be used as evidence of a valid consent to treatment.

Most healthcare entities are required by the American With Disabilities Act to make reasonable accommodation to meet the needs of patients with a disability that could impair the consent process.[34] Some states have gone further, requiring the use of interpreters for those who confront a linguistic barrier to an effective consent process.[35] These laws have heightened awareness about informed consent–related regulatory compliance. This increased emphasis on compliance is also reflected in the federal initiatives dealing with LEPs, discussed earlier.

Cultural sensitivity is also an important consideration.[36] Although sometimes difficult to embrace in policy and procedure, cultural sensitivity reflects an awareness of what is disclosed to a patient and by whom. For example, discussion of urogenital anomalies or surgery by a male clinician with a female patient can be culturally charged and can cause the consent process to become derailed. In other situations, the cultural and language-based context of patients from other countries may make it difficult for them to understand such things as the meaning of over-the-counter medications, home remedies, and so on. Good risk management in this regard demands identification of the cultural needs in the catchment area served by the healthcare organization. In addition, the consent policy and procedure should be flexible enough to accommodate the needs of

EXHIBIT 4.2   Sample Consent Time-Out Tool

This tool is designed to help care providers evaluate communication needs and capabilities of patients and surrogate decision makers prior to embarking on a consent process. The term *surrogate* may be substituted in the tool where the words *patient* or *patient's* are found in the text. The tool prompts care providers to ask questions in a manner that is respectful of the dignity of the patient. For example, instead of asking, "Are you hard of hearing?", the tool rephrases the inquiry as, "Do you have problems hearing me? Would it help if I spoke in a lower tone of voice or a higher tone for you?" This time-out tool also contemplates participation of others in the consent process, including interpreters, family members, and cultural brokers.

Introduction: **Do not** assume it is correct to shake hands with the patient. A handshake may not be permissible in the patient's culture. However, it is appropriate for the caregiver to introduce himself or herself. A caregiver may ask if it is acceptable to shake hands if he or she is unfamiliar with the patient's cultural background.

AUDITORY NEEDS

Evaluate the patient's ability to hear by asking questions that require more than a "yes" or "no" answer. **Do not** *rely on the person shaking his or her head up and down or to the side to serve as a substitute for an answer.*

Ask relevant questions. Consider the following:

- "I want to be certain that you can understand what I am saying."
- "Can you hear me?"
- "Would it help if I raised my tone of voice or if I lowered it? Are you accustomed to using TTY or other devices to help you in communication? Do you use American Sign Language?"

VISUAL NEEDS

Evaluate the patient's ability to visualize material used in the communication process.

Ask relevant questions. Consider the following:

- "Can you see the information on the chart?"
- "Would it help if there was better lighting?"
- "Would it help if the information was enlarged for you?"
- "Are you accustomed to using a reading machine to help you see?"
- "Are you comfortable having someone read aloud printed information?"

SPEECH NEEDS

Determine what is the most practical and effective means for communicating with a speech-impaired patient or surrogate.

Ask relevant questions. Consider the following:

- "I know that you have difficulties speaking. Would it be helpful for you to use an assistive device? By nodding (or eye blinking) please indicate if you would prefer:"
- A message board?
- Typing on a keyboard?
- Using eye-blinking code?
- A voice simulator?

PHYSICAL NEEDS

Evaluate the patient's comfort. If a disabled person is more comfortable sitting in a customized wheelchair, think about letting him or her remain seated in this way instead of transferring the individual to an examining table or a seat that provides little support. Physical discomfort can impede the ability of the person to communicate effectively. Also consider the person's ability to sign documents.

(*Continued*)

EXHIBIT 4.2   Sample Consent Time-Out Tool (*Continued*)

Ask relevant questions. Consider the following:

- "We have a number of things to discuss. Where are you most comfortable?"

- "Would you prefer to remain seated in your wheelchair?"

- "I note from your history that you have difficulty signing documents. Have you been given an adaptive device to assist you? Has another arrangement been made for obtaining your signature or a surrogate's signature?"

COGNITIVE NEEDS

Some patients process information at a much slower pace than others. Injury, stroke, or the impact of medication may slow cognition. The fact that the person is slow to absorb information or to respond does not mean that he or she is incapable of communicating. Instead, it means that the pace of the communication must be adapted to the patient's requirements.

Ask questions to help evaluate cognitive ability. If it is determined that a slower pace is in order, consider a few shorter communication sessions that build one upon the other. For example:

- "How are you doing today?"

- "I think it would be helpful to pick up where we left off the other day. First, tell me what you remember of our conversation?" (If it is spotty or inaccurate, gently provide reminders and verify through additional questions that the person understands the information.)

- "That is a great summary of what we discussed. Now let me provide some additional information." At the end of the session say, "Before you leave I have a question for you. Can you tell me what you understand from what we discussed today?" (If it is spotty or inaccurate, gently provide reminders and verify through additional questions that the person understands the information.)

LANGUAGE NEEDS

Evaluate the patient's linguistic ability by asking questions that require more than a "yes" or "no" answer. **Do not** *rely on the person shaking his or her head up and down or to the side to serve as a substitute for an answer:*

Ask relevant questions. Consider the following:

- "Tell me, what brings you to the clinic today?" If the person does not understand or [he or] she has trouble responding clearly, continue with follow-up questions.

- "Would you be more comfortable speaking in a different language? Please let me know. I want you to be comfortable."

- "Will you permit me to use a translator?" In lieu of a question, consider a statement: "I have to tell you that I would be more comfortable if I had an interpreter to help me."

- Ask relevant questions through the interpreter to be certain that the patient understands.

CULTURAL REQUIREMENTS

Refer to the Cultural Advance Directive or ask relevant questions to determine if it would be helpful to have a cultural broker or representative participate in the consent communication.

HEALTH LITERACY NEEDS

Evaluate whether the patient or surrogate has literacy challenges.

Ask relevant questions:

- "I understand that English is not your preferred language for verbal communication and that you want to speak in (*name of language and dialect*). Do you have similar needs when it comes to reading health information?"

- "Do you prefer to have someone read health information to you in (*name of language and dialect*)?"

(*Continued*)

EXHIBIT 4.2   Sample Consent Time-Out Tool (*Continued*)

FAMILY PARTICIPATION NEEDS

Sometimes patients are anxious or afraid. Sometimes family members also may help facilitate the discussion or shed light on symptoms or care plan compliance. With permission, family members should be encouraged to participate in the discussion.

Ask the right questions. Consider the following approach:

- "Would you be more comfortable if your spouse sat in for our conversation?"

- "In my practice, I welcome the opportunity for a patient's loved one to sit in for the conversation. Would you like to have your adult daughter be with us today?"

- "Is it acceptable to you if your daughter takes an active role in the discussion?"

FUNCTIONAL LEARNING NEEDS

To facilitate an effective consent process, it is useful to identify the ways in which the patient or surrogate absorb information. Some are more visual; others prefer more auditory input.

Ask the right questions. Consider the following approach:

- I want to make certain that you have the opportunity to learn about the proposed (test or treatment). We shall discuss the recommendations. Tell me, would you prefer information provided in

- interactive computer programs?

- video media such as a DVD or VHS tape?

- online programming over the Internet?

- recorded speech

- reading information in a book or brochure

RECOMMENDED ACCOMMODATIONS:

_____

| Caregiver Signature | Time | Date |

Source: F. A. Rozovsky, "Consent Time Out," *Dialogues in Healthcare: Strategies for Effective Communication.* July 2008, 2(7). Reprinted with permission. All rights reserved.

patients who object to such discussions. The content for such a policy and procedure may be influenced to some extent by the CLAS standards described earlier.

Another important class of patients has been singled out for special consideration in obtaining informed consent. A number of states have enacted laws that empower patients to execute an advance directive for mental health services. Like the advance directives that take effect when a patient is incapacitated due to the effects of injury, coma, anesthesia, or terminal illness, the psychiatric advance directive comes into effect when a mental health patient is unable to participate in treatment decision making. The statutes vary from state to state, but the goal is the same: afford mental health patients the opportunity to delineate treatment choices or preferences while they are capable of making such decisions. The statutes typically include some limitations on what a person may or may not request. Nevertheless, the exception is an important one from a risk management standpoint.

Having such tools in place can avoid a lot of confusion, misunderstanding, and delays in care in the middle of a psychiatric event. The use of a psychiatric advance directive may also obviate the need for going to court and seeking a court order or the appointment of a person to act on behalf of the patient. As such, it is a tool that should be considered in consent policy and procedure development. The use of the psychiatric advance directive requires orientation and in-service training for those likely to encounter patients with such documents, including personnel in the emergency department, urgent care, and behavioral services. Because the psychiatric advance directive was singled out for discussion in the preamble discussion to the Patient's Rights Standards under the Conditions of Participation for Hospitals in Medicare and Medicaid,[37] it is a topic that also merits review from a regulatory compliance perspective.

Although the law views consent as a process between patient and care provider, it is not uncommon for family members to be involved in the discussion. Family involvement is not necessarily a sign that the patient distrusts the care provider. Indeed, family members may facilitate the process by furnishing additional details that the patient is unable to recall. Furthermore, from a loss control perspective, family involvement affords an opportunity to set expectations and establish a strong relationship. This rapport may be beneficial in short-circuiting potential litigation if untoward consequences result from tests or treatments.

The benefit of family involvement is reflected in the ASHRM white paper, "Perspective on Disclosure of Unanticipated Outcomes of Care."[38] Consistent with The Joint Commission's (TJC's) Patient Safety Standard on disclosure of treatment outcomes, the disclosure should be directed to the patient, and when practical, the family.[39] As discussed in the ASHRM white paper, having a rapport with the patient and patient's family is important. The communication component of the consent process helps set the context for discussing adverse and unanticipated outcomes of care.[40] (For further discussion on this topic, see the ASHRM Disclosure Monograph Series available at www.ashrm.org)

From a risk management standpoint, it is critical that consent policy and procedure recognize state-specific exceptions and delineate an appropriate, practical process for securing a treatment decision in these matters. The same holds true for involving the family in the consent process, taking into account patient confidentiality and HIPAA Privacy Standards requirements (please see Chapter 16 on HIPAA in Volume 3 of this series). This approach can avert needless risk exposure and potential litigation.

For patients with complex needs, another risk management consideration is documenting various exchanges with care providers. For example, consider the needs of a 37-year-old single parent who was just diagnosed with stage III prostate cancer. Can he really "hear" the care provider after receiving such an ominous diagnosis? Would it not be better to discuss treatment options over a series of brief meetings either in person or by telephone? At the outset of each session, the care provider can complete a "systems check," validating what the patient remembers of the previous discussion, setting an agenda for the current discussion, and then completing the conversation with a recap. This consent ladder approach would include documentation following each encounter and can help to solidify patient understanding. From a risk management standpoint, this approach also diminishes the risk of litigation based on a lack of understanding.

CONSENT REQUIREMENTS ALONG THE CONTINUUM OF CARE

Consent to treatment has long been associated with hospitals. For many years, *consent* has been viewed as a forms-driven necessity to prove in writing that the patient agreed to a specific treatment. In reality, consent as a process should take place in physicians' offices, clinics, ambulatory care and day surgery centers, and behavioral health units. Consent as a process is very much a part of long-term care, end-stage renal dialysis, and hospice care.

The essential elements for consent to treatment remain the same along the continuum of care. However, some differences merit recognition from a risk management perspective. For example, in the end-stage renal dialysis setting in which patients may present for repetitive care three times a week, there need be only one consent process. This process is completed at the outset of care. During each repeat visit, screening questions are posed to rule out treatment and rule in the need for an assessment of the patient. Questions posed may include the following:

- Did you follow your renal diet?

- Did you take your medications? Have you added any over-the-counter medicines, herbs, vitamins, or supplements since your last visit?

- Have you seen any other care providers, including dentists, who added new medications to your treatment regimen? If so, what medications were added?

- Have you had any complications, such as fever, chills, nausea?

- Have you experienced any problems with the cannula site, such as redness, soreness, or swelling? (The care provider doing the screening will also examine the cannula site.)

If there have been changes that shift the risk-benefit analysis on which the initial consent was based, the situation calls for a new consent process. This risk management approach to consent can avoid untoward consequences in repetitive treatment settings while obviating the need for a new consent process each time the patient presents for care.

Other settings of care might warrant very specific consent procedures. For example, some states require a specific consent for patients involved in telemedicine treatment.[41] In this type of treatment setting, the patient is in one location while the care provider interpreting an X-ray, CT scan, or MRI is located in another state or country. Because the doctor is not on location and the information is being transmitted electronically, it necessitates a different type of consent process.

Friction may occur between physicians and healthcare facilities regarding the proper location of the consent process. Surgeons may spend considerable amounts of time discussing surgical procedures. This discussion typically takes place in the surgeon's office or clinic. The patient may execute a consent document in the office or clinic. At the day surgery center or the acute care facility, the patient is asked to sign an additional consent for the procedure. Not only is this confusing for the patient, it presents a risk management concern. Many times the content of the facility-based consent document is inconsistent with what the patient signed in the care provider's office or clinic. Rather than cementing the treatment authorization process, this duality of consents serves as the basis for confusion. In some situations, when there is marked variation in the content of the two consent forms, the integrity of the consent to treatment may be eviscerated.

In the current version of the well designed consent process found in the State Operations Manual, CMS has anticipated this issue. It recognizes the value of the medical staff approving a well-crafted consent process that is completed in the medical office and then confirmed at the hospital.[42] If the patient's understanding of the procedure varies from the information completed at the medical practice, or if the patient's condition has changed, this serves as a red flag to warn that the process is incomplete. Since the history and physical (H&P) process completed at intake is done as a consequence of other federal regulations,[43] it serves as a type of consent speed bump that helps determine whether or not the patient's health status has changed so significantly or materially that the office-based consent is now in doubt.

· · · · · · · · ·
BREAKDOWN IN THE CONSENT PROCESS

Traditionally, consent litigation was premised on battery, an intentional tort that did not require proof of actual harm. However, in most states, patients can now sue on several different legal theories for ineffective informed consent. These include the following:

- Negligent consent: An unintentional tort that requires actual injury emanating from failure to follow appropriate standards for completing the consent process, resulting in causally linked and reasonably foreseeable harm

- Misrepresentation or deceit: The failure to honestly disclose important information or the act of presenting details in a way that misstates such details, resulting in an authorization that otherwise would have been withheld by the patient. In many jurisdictions, this type of claim carries with it the prospect of punitive damages

- Breach of contract: A claim premised on traditional notions of contract law in which the patient asserts that the care provider guaranteed or promised a certain result that was not achieved. This is most likely to happen in elective procedures involving plastic surgery, orthodontics, or other restorative fields of medical or dental care

- Battery: The traditional basis for claims involving an unauthorized test or treatment. Battery also can be asserted in cases in which a patient has withdrawn consent and the care provider nonetheless proceeds with the test or treatment

- Corporate liability: Perhaps the least likely basis for a consent claim, but nevertheless a source of consternation for healthcare risk management professionals. Traditionally, consent responsibilities have been reviewed as a duty of care of the attending care provider. However, to the extent that healthcare facilities intrude into and impose conditions and requirements upon the consent process, the risk of corporate liability for defective consents has increased. Corporate liability may also follow from constructive notice of a flawed consent process that was known to an allied health professional who did not follow healthcare facility policy and procedure and inform a supervisor of the problem. Coupled with a healthcare facility's mission statement, bylaws, and policies and procedures that speak to the institution's responsibility to safeguard patient care and well-being, the groundwork may be in place for such a claim to be made.

- Licensure action: The failure to follow applicable laws and regulations in the consent process may form the basis for a complaint based on unprofessional conduct under state licensing laws. This may occur as an administrative proceeding stemming from the same set of facts that forms the basis for civil litigation.

- Compliance action: The Conditions of Participation for Hospitals in Medicare and Medicaid include patients' rights standards (COPs).[44] It is possible that a serious breach of the compliance standards relative to the patient's role in care planning and treatment decision making may trigger regulatory scrutiny. In some instances this might involve allegations of regulatory noncompliance or a breach of the Conditions of Participation. Because this may affect Medicare and Medicaid certification, it is a matter that should be taken seriously.

The issue of "never events" and consent to treatment presents yet another type of fallout from failed consent processes. Consent forms have been seen by patient safety advocates as a key tool to include in the surgical time-out process. The World Health Organization (WHO) Surgical Safety Checklist is a good illustration.[45]

In August 2007, in the Preamble to the Inpatient Prospective Payment System (IPPS) Rule for Hospitals, CMS made it very clear that there would not be any reimbursement for what it termed, "wrong surgery."[46] CMS reinforced this point in 2009 when it issued a three-pronged National Coverage Determination (NCD):

Effective January 15, 2009, CMS will not cover a particular surgical or other invasive procedure to treat a particular medical condition when the practitioner erroneously performs: (1) a different procedure altogether; (2) the correct procedure but on the wrong body part; or (3) the correct procedure but on the wrong patient. Medicare will also not cover hospitalizations and other services related to these noncovered procedures as defined in the Medicare Benefit Policy Manual (BPM), chapter 1, sections 10 and 120 and chapter 16, section 180."[47]

CMS recognized the National Quality Forum on this issue, stating that:

In 2002, the National Quality Forum (NQF) published "Serious Reportable Events in Healthcare: A Consensus Report," which listed 27 adverse events that were "serious, largely preventable and of concern to both the public and healthcare providers." These events and subsequent revisions to the list became known as "never events." This concept and the need for the proposed reporting led to NQF's "Consensus Standards Maintenance Committee on Serious Reportable Events," which maintains and updates the list which currently contains 28 items. Among surgical events on the list is "Wrong surgical procedure performed on a patient." Similar to any other patient population, Medicare beneficiaries experience serious injury and/or death if wrong surgeries are performed and may require additional healthcare in order to correct adverse outcomes resulting from such errors.[48]

The expanse of the NCD is made clear by the definition provided for *related services*. As stated in the NCD,

- related services do not include performance of the correct procedure;
- all services provided in the operating room when an error occurs are considered related and therefore not covered;
- all providers in the operating room when the error occurs, who could bill individually for their services, are not eligible for payment;
- all related services provided during the same hospitalization in which the error occurred are not covered; and
- following hospital discharge, any reasonable and necessary services are covered regardless of whether or not they are related to the surgical error.[49]

A central focus of the CMS National Coverage Determination is the consent for surgical and other invasive procedures:

> A surgical or other invasive procedure is considered to be the wrong procedure if it is not consistent with the correctly **documented informed consent** for that patient. …
>
> A surgical or other invasive procedure is considered to have been performed on the wrong body part if it is not consistent with the **correctly documented informed consent** for that patient including surgery on the right body part, but on the wrong location on the body; for example, left versus right (appendages and/or organs), or at the wrong level (spine).[50]

CMS noted in the same document that it is unlikely that a facility or care provider will be able to shift the financial burden to the Medicare beneficiary for the erroneous surgery or invasive procedure.[51] Given the trend among many private payers on the issue of never events, it is quite possible that they too would deny any Medigap coverage for wrong surgical or invasive procedures.

The NCD policy ties the consent process to financial reimbursement in a way that goes far beyond the hospital. It applies to care providers involved in surgical or invasive procedures involving wrong patient, body part, or procedures. The NCD uses any deviation from the requirement that consent of the patient be correctly documented as a major component of its framework for coverage determination.

From a risk management perspective, the NCD may also facilitate litigation based on professional liability. If the reason for denial of coverage is a departure from a correctly documented informed consent resulting in a wrong surgery or wrong invasive procedure, the stage may be set for a claim against a care provider. Furthermore, if a hospital knew or ought to have known through its agents and employees that there was such a deviation, the foundation may be in place for a liability claim against the hospital. The likelihood of such a claim is apt to increase as hospitals use the WHO Surgical Checklist, or a version of it, as a mechanism to prevent wrong surgery or wrong invasive procedures. Since the preoperative time-out measures encompass a verification of consent, one can see how a plaintiff's attorney could assert that a failure to follow established policy or protocol resulted in foreseeable harm.

Should there be a concern about a facility having a number of these wrong procedures, it is quite possible that it would trigger regulatory scrutiny by a state agency on behalf of CMS. The same may be true of accrediting bodies. The point is that a Medicare consent failure involving a wrong procedure, wrong body part or wrong patient may culminate in a series of risk management concerns. It is not simply a matter of negligent consent. Rather, it underscores the importance of an enterprise risk management approach to consent to treatment.[52]

Notwithstanding these developments regarding the National Coverage Determination and consent, the most likely basis for a claim is negligent consent. It may be asserted as an ancillary claim in a professional liability lawsuit or may proceed as a separate basis for claim. The point to remember is that consent is a viable basis for litigation. With the prospect of punitive damages for battery or misrepresentation,[53] consent is an issue ripe for effective risk management treatment.

· · · · · · · · ·
RISK MANAGEMENT AND CONSENT TO TREATMENT

From a risk management perspective, several measures can be taken to avoid liability exposure involving consent to treatment. Many of these measures go to the core of patient safety initiatives. Such measures involve the following:

- Consent policies and procedures
- Consent clinical algorithms or pathways
- Consent risk identifiers
- Education
- Documentation

Each of these measures is discussed in the following sections as a component of a comprehensive approach to consent as a loss control mechanism. Taken together, these measures represent a practical, hands-on approach to lessening the risk of consent-related litigation.

Consent Policies and Procedures

Consent policies and procedures are central to a loss prevention program; they should be comprehensive, yet practical. The content should address frequently encountered problems, providing healthcare professionals and management with reasoned, legally appropriate responses. Consent policies and procedures should address all aspects of healthcare delivery reflected in healthcare organizations. Thus, a hospital network that merges with a group of nursing homes or that purchases a home infusion company needs to expand its consent policies and procedures to address the additional informed consent requirements of the new additions.

Certain basic components should be reflected in the consent policies and procedures. Some issues to address include the following:

- Definitions
- Requirements for a valid consent to treatment
- Recognized exceptions to the requirements for consent to treatment
- Assessment for legal and mental capacity to give consent
- Admission requirements
- Patient self-determination requirements
- Surrogate decision makers
- Requirements for a valid consent to participate in human experimentation
- EMTALA consent requirements
- Managed care consent requirements, for example, assuring that a patient receives information on all treatment options, regardless of whether reimbursement is available from the managed care organization (MCO)
- Documentation requirements
- Handling specific situations
- Anesthesia consents
- Advance directives
- Do-not-resuscitate orders
- Organ procurement
- Authorizations for autopsies
- Handling refusals of care
- HIV testing
- Requests not to use certain types of care, such as blood transfusion therapy

As with other policies and procedures, the content should be field-tested to ensure that it is practical and understandable to end users. Furthermore, it should be reviewed and updated periodically to ensure that any changes in federal or state law and regulations, including judicial decisions, are reflected in the policies and procedures.

Consent Algorithms

Based on a clearly written policy and procedure, clinical pathways or algorithms can help achieve compliance with consent requirements. For example, in the emergency department such an approach might be as illustrated in Figure 4.1.

The pathway must permit individual variations. Such variations should be documented to explain why the process was not followed. Follow-up action should also be

FIGURE 4.1   Patient Presents

Unconscious	Conscious
Life or health-threatening event	Life or health-threatening event
YES↓	YES↓
Criteria met for emergency exception	Follow impracticality pathway
YES↓	↓
Scope of emergency intervention defined	No time to secure consent from legal surrogate. Follow nonemergency care consent pathway.
YES↓	↓
Emergency exception documented	Impracticality exception documented

taken to address noncompliance with the pathway to reduce potential liability risk and patient safety concerns.

Consent Risk Identifiers

A comprehensive loss program should include monitoring for consent risk exposures. A broad approach to such monitoring includes using quality outcome data, patient satisfaction information, and the results gleaned from incident reports, loss runs, and litigation files. In addition, personnel should be encouraged to report consent risk situations, including disputes among family members regarding appropriate treatment for an incompetent relative, managed care–linked EMTALA problems in the ED, and refusals of care from questionably capable individuals. Effective patient history screening is a potent tool in identifying potential consent problems. For example, a patient or family member who presents with conflicting history information might be withholding important data that could affect the risk-benefit analysis of one form of care over another. This can happen with placement of an elderly person in an institutional care setting, when the relative selectively discloses information in the hope that the elderly patient will be situated in an assisted-living environment rather than a nursing facility or skilled nursing facility.

In other situations, the information disclosed by the patient or relative might reveal unrealistic expectations of care or treatment outcome. This, too, is a risk-prone situation that should be addressed appropriately.

In some instances, potential pitfalls may be found in the way the sequence of consent processes is designed to work. For example, consent documentation for surgery might include a provision for patients to be informed of the option to participate in autologous blood donation and storage programs. If the notification is dated the same day or the day before an elective surgical procedure, the result is that the patient was not notified or informed of the autologous blood program until it was too late to participate in this transfusion plan, providing glaring evidence of an inadequate consent process.

Traditionally, incomplete consent documentation has been viewed as a sentinel indicator of risk. Although such incomplete documentation is certainly a valid consent risk identifier, it does not relieve a healthcare entity of the need to ferret out other, perhaps less obvious risk exposures in the processes.

Education

Risk management professionals should never assume that healthcare professionals know how to properly secure a valid consent to treatment. Healthcare professionals can learn a great deal through clinical mentoring, including a discussion of inappropriate methods for communicating information to patients and recording a treatment authorization. To lessen the likelihood of liability exposure, it is prudent to address the proper way to secure a valid consent to treatment in orientation and regular in-service education.

Education efforts regarding informed consent have become far more expansive in recent years. With hospitals and other healthcare entities taking on increased roles in home healthcare, hospice, long-term care, subacute care, and ambulatory care, the horizon has broadened with respect to who must and actually does obtain consent to treatment; therefore, it is important for the risk management professional to think broadly about who needs education on consent to treatment processes and practices.

Documentation

Consent documentation is important as a mechanism to record in writing the scope of a treatment authorization. It is not a replacement for the consent process. Consent documentation should incorporate language and terms that are consistent with recognized standards for health literacy. Selecting the best method or methods for documenting consent is a collaborative activity involving care providers, legal counsel, and the risk management professional.

Some healthcare entities prefer the long-form consent, which delineates risks, benefits, alternatives, and additional information. Others prefer the short-form consent, which indicates only that a valid consent transaction occurred. A third approach calls for a detailed note in the patient record, with or without execution of a specific consent form. The note should record the time and date of the transaction and should be signed by the provider who informed the individual and secured the authorization. This customized approach is considered to be more credible and genuine than a standard boilerplate consent form. A fourth method is the checklist consent form, which has categories that are checked off by the care provider who secures the patient's consent. Once the consent process is completed, the form is signed by the provider and, in some locations, the patient. The form, designed to meet state law requirements, provides ample room for the care provider to detail the probable risks, probable benefits, and treatment alternatives for the patient, along with the risks of forgoing care. This approach is seen as a compromise between the traditional long-form consent and the detailed note in the record. Because it is streamlined and allows the document to be customized to a specific patient, the checklist consent form may be seen as a reasonable approach to record the consent process. Regardless of the method chosen, it is important that the process is consistent with applicable federal and state laws governing documentation.

The importance of the format of a consent form has been the subject of significant debate. Consent documentation that uses a small font might be setting the stage for risk exposure if the print is so small that it cannot be read easily by the patient or surrogate decision maker. Indeed, provision has been made in the *Medicare Carrier Manual* for suggesting that the Advance Beneficiary Notice (ABN) be printed in 12-point type.[54] Taking the lead from Medicare, it is important to develop a format that is easily read by the intended recipient. This might mean field-testing different document styles and fonts to find the one that is best for the service population. Although the form does not replace the consent communication process, if the supporting documentation is unreadable, it does little to substantiate that an effective consent process did, in fact, occur.

Another issue that often comes up with consent documentation is the matter of signatures on traditional consent forms. There are different signatures for different purposes. The physician usually signs traditional documents to verify completion of the consent process. If evidence disputes that the process was completed properly, the signature could be used against the practitioner. On the other hand, a signature by a nurse who witnesses the consent process does not attest to the content of the consent process, but rather only provides evidence that the consent process actually took place.

Consent forms, whether the documents are traditional in format or more innovative, do not replace the basic informed consent discussion requirements described in this chapter. Consent is a communication process, not a form. Written evidence that supports a successful consent process is important for purposes of billing, continuity of care, and legal defense to a consent claim. Whatever method of consent documentation is selected, the key is to use it consistently. Failure to do so might signal potential risk concerns, bringing into question why consent was not documented in a specific manner in a given case. It is important to engage healthcare professionals in the design and development of the documentation system to ensure that they will cooperate and use the documentation format effectively.

The Consent Patient Safety Checklist

The patient safety consent checklist[55] is another concept gaining popularity in healthcare organizations. As in other areas of healthcare risk management, typically there has been a faulty assumption that caregivers can recall all the information they need in making critical judgments about patient care. When performing many tasks at once or when fatigued, caregivers might forget certain steps or processes in developing a care plan, assessing a patient, or providing treatment. Consent is no different in this regard. Caregivers might forget to ask salient questions that could mean the difference between a patient receiving a prescription for a medication that is an appropriate addition to his or her regime or one that interacts severely with another drug taken routinely. The care provider also might forget to explain the risk of consuming certain types of foods that can have an adverse effect when eaten with certain prescription medications. A checklist that reminds the care provider to ask about over-the-counter preparations, food consumption habits, and related issues can avert needless medication risk exposures.

The Consent Patient Safety Checklist is a tool that helps facilitate the consent process. It promotes patient safety by offering prompts or reminders to caregivers to make certain that key items are addressed in the consent process. These include the following:

- Evaluation of patient or surrogate decision maker to participate in the consent process
- Precise questions on consent (for example, instead of "Do you take medication?", the line of questions in the tool goes further: "Do you use over-the-counter preparations such as aspirin?"; "Do you use any natural or herbal substances or therapies?"; "Have you seen any other doctors or dentists lately who have prescribed medication for you?")
- Follow-up questions to confirm ability of patient or family to adhere to treatment plan
- Follow-up questions to confirm patient's or surrogate decision maker's understanding of test or treatment
- Screening questions for continuing care interventions in end-stage renal dialysis, oncology, or allergy immunization, to ascertain if the underlying circumstances have changed to warrant a review before proceeding with care

The Consent Patient Safety Checklist may be customized to a specific service or healthcare delivery setting. Thus, the tool used in a preoperative workup may be different from the one used in an urgent care center.

The tool may be adapted to serve as evidence of consent. This could be achieved by having the caregiver who uses it sign and date the document. This approach substantiates that the consent process was completed. However, unlike the checklist consent form described previously, this is a patient safety tool designed specifically for caregivers. It is not designed for the patient to sign.

· · · · · · · · ·
CONCLUSION

Consent is double-edged. When completed properly, the consent process is a potent tool for averting liability claims and is the basis for a strong defense to assertions that a patient was not properly informed. However, when the consent process is inadequate or incomplete, it can be used as a weapon against a healthcare facility or professional.

Viewing consent as a loss control mechanism means designing a process that is both practical and used consistently. It means drawing from legal requirements at the state and federal level and from the experience of care providers regarding what will and will not work. Furthermore, as with other aspects of loss control, vigilance is required in terms of monitoring and managing risks that emerge, especially given the vortex of change in the healthcare field, where further modifications can be anticipated that are central to the consent process.

Suggested Readings

Adams, R., and F. A. Rozovsky. *Human Research: A Practical Guide to Regulatory Compliance*. San Francisco: Jossey-Bass, 2003.

Joint Commission on Accreditation of Healthcare Organizations. *Ethical Issues and Patient's Rights Across the Continuum of Care*. Oakbrook Terrace, Ill.: Joint Commission on Accreditation of Healthcare Organizations, 1998.

Rozovsky, F. A. *Consent To Treatment: A Practical Guide*. 3rd ed. Gaithersburg, MD: Aspen Publishing, 2000 (with annual supplements, including December 2004 supplement).

Rozovsky, F. A., and J. R. Woods, eds. *The Handbook of Patient Safety Compliance*. San Francisco: Jossey-Bass, 2005.

Woods, J. R., and F. A. Rozovsky. *What Do I Say? Communicating Intended or Unanticipated Outcomes in Obstetrics*. San Francisco: Jossey-Bass, 2003.

Suggested Web Sites

Agency for Healthcare Research and Quality, www.ahrq.gov.

American Association of Health Plans, www.aahp.org.

American Hospital Association, www.aha.org.

American Academy on Physician and Patient, www.physicianpatient.org.

American Society for Healthcare Risk Management, www.hospitalconnect.com/desktopservlet.

Centers for Medicare & Medicaid Services (CMS), www.cms.gov.

DNV (Det Norske Veritas) National Integrated Accreditation for Healthcare Organizations NIAHO[SM] Accreditation Program, www.dnv.com.

Food and Drug Administration, www.fda.gov.

Health Care Facilities Accreditation Program, www.hfap.org.

Institute for Healthcare Improvement, www.ihi.org.

Institute of Medicine, www.iom.edu.

The Joint Commission, www.jointcommission.org.

National Committee on Quality Assurance, www.ncqa.org.

National Institutes of Health, www.nih.gov.

National Forum for Health Care Quality Measurement and Reporting, www.qualityforum.org.

National Patient Safety Foundation, www.npsf.org.

Partnership for Patient Safety, www.p4ps.org.

Quality Interagency Coordination Task Force (QuIC), www.quic.gov.

The Business Roundtable, www.brt.org.

The Buyers Health Care Action Group, www.choiceplus.com.

U.S. Pharmacopoeia, www.usp.org.

Endnotes

1. Rozovsky, F. A. *Consent to Treatment: A Practical Guide*, 4th ed. Gaithersburg, Md.: Aspen Publishing, 2007. Consent as a process is the same throughout most of the common-law world and in jurisdictions that follow the Napoleonic Code.

2. Note that payment is not necessary for consent to be informed or valid.

3. See *Perspectives on Disclosure of Unanticipated Outcomes of Care*, ASHRM, July 2001; and J. R. Woods and F. A. Rozovsky, *What Do I Say? Communicating Intended or Unanticipated Outcomes in Obstetrics.* San Francisco: Jossey-Bass, 2003.

4. The cases most often described as the benchmarks for the contemporary approach to consent to treatment include *Canterbury v. Spence,* 464 F.2d 772 (D.C. Cir. 1972); *Cobbs v. Grant,* 501 P.2dl (Cal. 1972); and *Wilkinson v. Vesey,* 295 A.2d 676 (RI 1972). These cases marked a watershed in the field of health law, the repercussions of which have been noted in extensive case law and statutory law on the subject of consent to treatment.

5. Department of Health & Human Services. Centers for Medicare & Medicaid Services, *State Operations Manual*, Appendix A-Survey Protocol, Regulations and Interpretive Guidelines for Hospitals, Rev. 47, 06–05-09.

6. *Schloendorff v. Society of New York Hospital*, 105 N.E. 92, 95 (N.Y. 1914), overruled in part, *Bing v. Thunig*, 143 N.E. 2d 9 (N.Y. 1957).

7. See, for example, *Pratt v. Davis,* 79 N. E. 562 (Ill. 1905) and *Mohr v. William* 104 N. W. 12 (Minn. 1905).

8. *Salgo v. Leland Stanford, etc., Board of Trustees,* 317 P.2d 170 (Cal. 1957); *Natanson v. Kline,* 354 P.2d. 670 (Kans. 1960); *Canterbury v. Spence,* 464 F.2d 772 (D.C. Cir. 1972); *Cobbs v. Grant,* 501 P.2dl (Cal. 1972); and *Wilkinson v. Vesey,* 295 A.2d 676 (RI 1972).

9. 21 C.F.R §50.1 through 21 C.F.R §50.56 (2009) (FDA Human Research Requirements) and 45 C.F.R §46.101 through 45 C.F.R §46.409 (2008) (Department of Health and Human Services). Note that several other departments and agencies of the federal government follow the HHS format for regulating human research. This is termed the Common Rule. It is noteworthy that a number of states have legislation on the subject of human research.

10. 42 U.S.C. ß1395dd. The regulations are at 42 C.F.R. ß498.24 (2008).

11. 28 C.F.R. ß42.405 (2008).

12. "National Standards on Culturally and Linguistically Appropriate Services (CLAS) in Health Care." *Federal Register*, Reg. 65(247): pp 80865, et seq., December 22, 2000.

13. 42 U.S.C. §§1395cc(a), et seq., as amended (1990). The law was included in an Omnibus Budget Reconciliation Law.

14. 42 C.F.R. §482.13 (2008).

15. For a more in-depth book on the subject of the clinical research regulations, see, Rozovsky, F. A., and R. A. Adams, *A Practical Guide to Regulatory Compliance*, Human Research. San Francisco: Jossey-Bass, 2003. See also F. A. Rozovsky, "Informed Consent in Federally Regulated Research." In: *Clinical Research Consent Manual: An Administrative Guide*, P. L. Brent and L.W. Vernaglia, editors. New York: Aspen Publishers, 2006; F. A. Rozovsky and J. L. Conley, *Health Care Organizations Risk Management: Forms, Checklists and Guidelines*, 3rd edition. New York: Aspen Publishers, 2009.

16. See, for example, 42 C.F.R. §482.45 (2008) and 42 C.F.R. 482 §§100, 102 and 104 (2008).

17. 42 C.F.R. §483.10 (2008).

18. The HIPAA Privacy Rule was first proposed in the *Federal Register* on November 3, 1999, in 64: 59,918, et seq. The Final Rule, first version, was published on December 28, 2000, in the *Federal Register* 65: 82462, et seq. The Secretary of Health and Human Services opened the Privacy Rule for additional public comment in March 2001, see *Federal Register* 66 12738, and then made it effective on April 14, 2001, see *Federal Register* 65: 12433. On March 27, 2002, the Department of Health and Human Services issued proposed changes to the Privacy Rule, see *Federal Register* 67: 14776. In the August 14, 2002, *Federal Register*, the Department issued the revised Final Rule changes with regard to privacy under HIPAA, see *Federal Register* 67(157): 53182, et seq.

19. See the CDC Vaccine Information Statements www.cdc.gov/vaccines/pubs/vis/default. htm that were developed pursuant to the National Childhood Vaccine Injury Public Law No. 99–660 as amended by Public Law No. 103–183.

20. "Policy Guidance on the Prohibition Against National Origin Discrimination As It Affects Persons with Limited English Proficiency." *Federal Register* 65(169): 52762, et seq., August 30, 2000.

21. "National Standards on Culturally and Linguistically Appropriate Services (CLAS) in Health Care," *Federal Register* 65(247): pp. 80865, et seq., December 22, 2000.

22. Rozovsky, F. A., and J. R. Woods, editors. *The Handbook of Patient Safety Compliance*, Chapter 9. San Francisco: Jossey-Bass, 2005.

23. For a detailed examination of the topic, see Rozovsky, *Consent to Treatment*, Chapter 2.

24. Case law on the topic can be found as early as 1906. See, for example, *Pratt v. Davis*, 79 N.E. 562 (Ill. 1906).

25. See, for example, Ga. Code 31–9–3 (1971).

26. Woods and Rozovsky, *What Do I Say?* See also Rozovsky, *Consent to Treatment*, Chapter 2.

27. Rozovsky, *Consent to Treatment*, 2.4.1.

28. *Ibid.*, 2.5.

29. *Truman v. Thomas*, 611 P.2d. 902 (Cal. 1980).

30. *Ibid.*

31. *Ibid.*

32. *Stamford Hospital v. Vegas*, P 236 Conn. 646 (1996).

33. *Schreiber v. Physicians Insurance Company of Wisconsin*, 588 NW2d 26 (Wis. 1999).

34. See 42 USC sec.12101, et seq. (1990). Title III provides the pertinent legislative requirements on the topic. Although exemptions are provided for certain religious facilities, many have chosen to follow the law.

35. See, for example, 210 ILCS 87/1, et seq. (Smith-Hurd 1994). Language assistance is required if 5 percent of the population served by a healthcare facility on an annual basis do not speak English or are limited in their ability to speak English.

36. For an interesting insight on the topic, see Gostin, L. "Informed Consent, Cultural Sensitivity, and Respect for Persons." *Journal of the American Medical Association* 1995; 274(10): 844–845.

37. *Federal Register* 64: 36070, et seq., July 2, 1999.

38. ASHRM Perspective on Disclosure of Unanticipated Outcome Information, July 2001.

39. [RI.1.2.2] states: "Patients, and when appropriate, their families are informed about the outcomes of care, including unanticipated outcomes." *Comprehensive Manual on Accreditation of Hospitals*, 2002 Standards.

40. Woods and Rozovsky, *What Do I Say?*

41. See, for example, Arizona Revised Statutes 36–3602. (2004); California Business & Professional Code ß 2290.5. (1998) and Vernons Texas Insurance Code Annotates Art. 21.53F. (2001).

42. Interpretive Guidelines §482.24(c)(2)(v), State Operations Manual, Appendix A, Survey Process for Hospitals, (Rev. 47, 06–05–09).

43. *Ibid.*

44. *Federal Register* 64: 36070, et seq., July 2, 1999.

45. For more information on the WHO Surgical Checklist and Consent, see, www.who.int/patientsafety/safesurgery/en/.

46. See *Federal Register*, 72(162): 47130–48175, 47214 (August 22, 2007).

47. CMS, Pub 100–03 Medicare National Coverage Determinations, Transmittal No. 102, July 2, 2009.

48. *Ibid.*

49. *Ibid.*

50. *Ibid.*

51. CMS stated in the NCD that it "… cannot envision a scenario in which HINNs or ABNs could be validly delivered in these NCD cases. However, an ABN or a HINN could be validly delivered prior to furnishing follow-up care for the non-covered surgical error that would not be considered a related as defined in the Pub. 100–02, BPM, Chapter 1, Sections 10 and 120 and Chapter 16, section 180."

52. See Chapter 17 "Consent to Treatment: An ERM Perspective." In: *Enterprise Risk Management Handbook for Healthcare Entities,* E.L. Barton, editor. Washington, D.C.: AHLA, 2009.

53. See, for example, *Lunsford v. Regents, University of California,* No. 837936 (Superior Ct., San Francisco County, California, Apr. 19, 1990).

54. *Medicare Carrier Manual,* CMS-R-131-G.

55. See Rozovsky, *Consent to Treatment*; see also Woods and Rozovsky, *What Do I Say?*

5

Clinical Research: Institutional Review Boards

Sheila Cohen Zimmet

All research subjects really want is to be able to trust the system.

"Jesse's Intent" by Paul Gelsinger
www.circare.org/submit/jintent.pdf

The successful conduct of medical research in a free society depends on trust between the scientific enterprise and the public, trust in the integrity of the discovery process, and especially trust in the safety of patients and healthy volunteers who participate in the process. Maintaining strong safeguards for the safety of human subjects in medical research is a paramount obligation of clinical investigators and their institutions. Institutional review boards (IRBs) are the heart of the protection regime; they are responsible for reviewing all clinical and translational research conducted at their respective institutions and for making ethical determinations that risks to human subjects have been minimized to the greatest extent possible; risks are reasonable in relation to anticipated benefits, if any; and the risks, benefits, and alternative options are clearly communicated to the potential participants in the informed consent process.[1]

J.J. Cohen
Academic Medical Centers and Medical Research

Governmental vigilance regarding research is intensifying, and noncompliance with pertinent regulations can result in significant loss of dollars, organizational reputation, and community trust, as well as an increase in potential for civil liability. This chapter provides an overview of the history, mandated structure, and regulatory authority for IRBs. The complex requirements that accompany IRBs and risk management strategies will also be addressed.

· · · · · · · · ·
ETHICAL PRINCIPLES

The central concept of the modern system of human subject protection in biomedical research is the primacy of the human subject.[2] It has its roots in the ethical principles of respect for persons, beneficence, and justice, the hallmarks of the *Belmont Report* issued in 1979 by the National Commission for the Protection of Human Subjects in Biomedical and Behavioral Research. (The *Belmont Report* is available from the National Institutes of Health at http://ohsr.od.nih.gov/guidelines/belmont.html. See also the Nuremberg Code available from the National Institutes of Health at http://ohsr.od.nih.gov/guidelines/nuremberg.html and the Declaration of Helsinki, which provide, the accepted ethical standards for international human subject research, is available at www.wma.net/en/30publications/10policies/b3/17c.pdf.)

The underlying ethical principles for the current regulations governing human biomedical research, which derive from the *Belmont Report*, are defined in the report as follows:

● Respect for persons means a recognition of the personal dignity and autonomy of individuals, and special protection of those persons with diminished autonomy . . . an affirmative obligation to protect vulnerable populations.

● Beneficence involves an obligation to maximize benefits and minimize risks of harm (nonmaleficence).

● Justice requires a fair distribution of the benefits and burdens of research.

Adherence to these basic ethical concepts ensures that the disadvantaged are not used as research subjects for the benefit of the advantaged and that the goal of social progress resulting from human research does not take precedence over the rights of the individual subject.[3]

The federal research requirements are founded on respect for the autonomy of the research subject, evidenced by stringent informed consent requirements, the protection of vulnerable populations, the absence of coercion, and the reasonable balance of benefits and burdens of the proposed research for the individual subject, not for society at large. An individual's decision not to participate in research may not in any way affect the ability of the individual to receive medical care or other benefits to which the individual otherwise would be entitled. It is the role of the IRB to review and monitor the conduct of research and to educate the research community about the proper conduct of research.

Is It Human Subject Research?

The code of federal regulations for treatment of human subjects (45 C.F.R. Part 46) define research as "a systematic investigation, including research development, testing, and evaluation, designed to develop or contribute to generalizable knowledge" [45 C.F.R. 46.102(d)]. A human subject is "a living individual about whom an investigator (whether professional or student) conducting research obtains (1) data through intervention or interaction with the individual or (2) identifiable private information" [45 C.F.R. 46.102(f)].

Is It Research or Is It Treatment?

The *Belmont Report* distinguishes between research and clinical practice in discussing which activities require special review. Research is defined as an activity designed to test a hypothesis, permit conclusions to be drawn, and thereby to develop or contribute to generalizable knowledge (expressed, for example, in theories, principles, and statements of relationships). Clinical practice includes interventions that are designed to enhance the well-being of a patient through diagnosis or treatment and have a reasonable expectation of success. A departure from standard practice or the institution of a novel or innovative treatment is not viewed as research. This distinction is incorporated into the regulatory definition of human subject research noted above.[4]

The Office of Human Research Protection (OHRP) provides a helpful tool to help determine whether an activity is research involving human subjects. See OHRP's human subjects regulations decision charts at www.hhs.gov/ohrp/humansubjects/guidance/decisioncharts.htm.

Applicable Federal Regulations

Following publication of the *Belmont Report*, both the Department of Health, Education and Welfare (formerly DHEW, now the Department of Health and Human Services [HHS]) and the Food and Drug Administration (FDA) strengthened their human subject protections, increasing but not altering the role of the institutional review boards (IRBs). The HHS human research regulations, including IRB requirements, are codified at C.F.R., Title 45, Part 46. This includes the federal policy known as the Common Rule, which encompasses the human subject protections followed by, and therefore common to, all executive federal agencies that sponsor research. FDA regulations on human research are codified at C.F.R. Title 21, Parts 50 (informed consent), 56 (Institutional Review Boards), 312 (Investigational New Drug Application), 812 (Investigational Device Exemptions), and 860 (Medical Device Classification Procedures).

Each healthcare institution that receives federal funding for human research from a department or agency covered by the federal policy or Common Rule, or that conducts research that is regulated by the FDA, must have one or more IRBs with authority to prospectively review, monitor, require modification of, approve, or disapprove the research. The IRB may be established by the institution or, less often, may be an independent IRB under contract to the institution to provide IRB services.[5] A document assuring compliance with human subject protection regulations must be negotiated between the institution and HHS before HHS-funded research may be conducted. The document, known as an assurance, may be for a single project or, more often, may be a federal-wide assurance (FWA), which applies to the pertinent activities of the institution. Applicable regulations are codified at 45 C.F.R. 46.103. In addition, individual IRBs must register with OHRP, and IRBs that review FDA-regulated research must also, as of September 2009, register with the FDA. IRB registration for both OHRP and the FDA may be accomplished via the OHRP Web site (the IRB electronic registration homepage can be found at http://ohrp.cit.nih.gov/efile/Default.aspx.

HHS and FDA have the authority to conduct compliance inspections of institutions engaged in research, including the activities of IRBs, and to halt or restrict federally funded or FDA-regulated research if institutions are found out of compliance with applicable human subject protections.

Institutional Review Boards

For Dr. Gary B. Ellis, who was director of the former federal Office for Protection from Research Risks (OPRR),[6] the relationship between subject and researcher is one based on trust, and that trust must be respected. Ellis said,

> [i]n the final analysis, research investigators, research institutions, and federal regulators are stewards of a trust agreement with the people who are research subjects. For research subjects who are safeguarded by the federal regulations, we have a system in place that (1) minimizes the potential for harm, (2) enables and protects individual, autonomous choice, and (3) promotes the pursuit of new knowledge. By doing so, we protect the rights and welfare of our fellow citizens who make a remarkable contribution to the common good by participating in research studies. We owe them our best effort.[7]

It is the role of the IRBs to safeguard that trust and to assess research in terms of risks and benefits, the adequacy of informed consent, the adequacy of safeguards to protect the privacy and confidentiality of subjects,[8] and the equitable selection of subjects. Maintaining strong safeguards for the safety of human subjects in medical research is a paramount obligation of clinical investigators and their institutions.

IRB Membership and Quorum

IRBs must be composed of at least five members with diverse backgrounds, including at least one scientific member, one nonscientist, and one nonaffiliated member. IRBs acting under an assurance must be registered with the OHRP. IRB registration requires a listing of members, their affiliations, and whether they serve as scientist or nonscientist members.

No IRB member may participate in any IRB review of a study with which the member has a conflict of interest. It is useful to remind IRB members at the beginning of each meeting of the need to recuse on any matter in which they might have a conflict and to include the following (or similar) reminder on all IRB agendas: No member of the IRB may participate in the review of any project in which the IRB member is an investigator, has a financial conflict of interest, or has any other interest which has an adverse impact on the IRB member's ability to exercise independent judgment. Under such circumstances, the IRB member shall not be present during IRB deliberations, except to provide information requested by the IRB.

To satisfy quorum requirements, a majority of IRB members, including a nonscientist member, must be present and voting. In other words, a nonscientist member must always be present and voting for the IRB to take official action. Many institutions include at least two nonscientist members on their IRBs to ensure that at least one nonscientist is present whenever the IRB convenes. For IRB action to be taken on research involving minors, prisoners, or mentally impaired individuals, an IRB member with expertise in the particular area involved (for example, pediatrician, prisoner activist, mental health professional) must be present and voting.

IRB Review

If an institution subject to the Common Rule is engaged in human subject research, a prospective and ongoing IRB review is required, unless the research qualifies for an exemption under 45 C.F.R. 46.101(b). (See the sample Request for Exemption with listing of eligible categories at www.med.cornell.edu/research/for_pol/forms/IRB_Exemption_Form_rev_2-09.doc. See also the human subject regulations decision charts at www.hhs.gov/ohrp/humansubjects/guidance/decisioncharts.htm.)

IRB review is classified as either full board or expedited review, based on the nature of the proposed research. Research activities that present no more than minimal risk and involve only procedures listed in one or more expedited review categories as specified by the FDA may be reviewed by the IRB through expedited procedures. (See Request for Expedited Review, which lists categories of research eligible for expedited review at www.med.cornell.edu/research/for_pol/forms/IRB_Expedited_Protocol_Form_rev_12-09.doc. See also human subject regulations decision charts cited above.)

IRB review and approval of research must be conducted "at intervals appropriate to the degree of risk, but not less than once per year." (See OHRP Guidance on Continuing Review, www.hhs.gov/ohrp/humansubjects/guidance/contrev2002.html.)

IRB approval lapses after one year, resulting in administrative suspension. Accordingly, unless the IRB schedules an annual continuing review sufficiently in advance of the annual approval date to accommodate delays in IRB meetings and requests additional information, modifications to consent forms, and so on, IRB approval of research may expire, and all research activity must cease. In the event of an administrative suspension, the IRB may determine and inform the investigator that it is in the best interest of enrolled subjects to continue research activities. However, new enrollment must cease. (See OHRP Guidance on Continuing Review cited previously.)

Note that HHS regulations require that the IRB review the actual application or proposal when reviewing proposed HHS-funded human subject research to verify that the application or proposal is consistent with the proposed IRB protocol (45 C.F.R.

46.103[f]). Many IRBs have been required to rereview all previously approved HHS-funded research because of a failure to review the grant application as part of the initial IRB review and approval.

Investigators are also responsible for notifying the IRB of adverse events and unexpected risks to human subjects and for seeking IRB approval for any amendments or modifications to protocols and consent forms before such changes are instituted.

Required IRB Findings

To approve research on human subjects, the IRB must (1) identify risks of the research; (2) determine that the risks will be minimized to the extent possible; (3) identify probable benefits of the research; (4) determine that the risks are reasonable in relation to the benefits to the subject and the knowledge to be gained; (5) ensure that research subjects are provided with an accurate and fair description of the risks, discomforts, and anticipated benefits; (6) ensure that research subjects are offered the opportunity to voluntarily accept or reject participation in the research, or discontinue participation, without coercion or fear of reprisal or deprivation of treatment to which the patient is otherwise entitled;[9] and (7) determine intervals of periodic review and, when necessary, determine the adequacy of mechanisms for monitoring data collection. OHRP not only requires that these findings be made, it also requires that the findings and actions be documented in IRB minutes and that information necessary to support the determinations be included in the records of the IRB. Approval of research involving minors requires specific IRB determinations that must be documented in the minutes of the IRB (see 45 C.F.R. 46.404–46.407). A useful IRB tool is a protocol review form that includes a checklist of required findings that can be incorporated into IRB minutes. (See IRB Protocol Review Form for Reviewers, available at med.cornell.edu/research/for_pol/forms/policies.pdf and Request for Review of Investigation Involving Use of Human Subjects, available at www.med.cornell.edu/research/for_pol/forms/IRB_Protocol_Application_rev_6-1-09.doc.)

Informed Consent

A human being may be included as a subject in research only if the "investigator has obtained the legally effective informed consent of the subject or the subject's legally authorized representative."[10] Required individual elements of informed consent, which must be documented in an informed consent form, and the circumstances under which certain elements or documentation may be waived, are set forth at 45 C.F.R. 46.116 and 45 C.F.R. 46.117. To ensure inclusion of all required information, it is recommended that each IRB have an informed consent template that includes both the required elements and preferred local boilerplates (such as the institution's policy on compensation for research-related injury). For more information see www.med.cornell.edu/research/for_pol/forms/ICF_template_revised_3-16-10.doc. To help develop an informed consent template, refer to the Informed Consent Checklist — Basic and Additional Elements, at www.hhs.gov/ohrp/humansubjects/assurance/consentckls.htm. IRBs also should be alert to research studies that elicit private information about persons other than the subjects who have consented, for instance third parties such as family members whose private information is obtained in the context of the research being reviewed. In those circumstances, the IRB should consider whether consent of the third party is necessary.

Informed Consent in Emergency Settings

The FDA regulations and the Common Rule provide a mechanism to waive informed consent requirements for studies conducted in certain emergency settings. For example, informed consent may be waived for human subjects in need of emergency medical intervention for which available treatments are unproven or unsatisfactory and for which it is not possible to obtain informed consent. (See the relevant FDA information sheet at fda.gov/oc/ohrt/irbs/except.html and OHRP guidance at www.hhs.gov/ohrp/humansubjects/guidance/hsdc97-01.html.)

Exculpatory Language in Consent Forms

Both the Common Rule and FDA regulations preclude use of exculpatory language in consent forms by which the subject is deemed to have waived any right or benefit. This has been interpreted by OHRP and the FDA to preclude often-used consent form provisions related to tissue donation, transfer of ownership of tissue to researcher or sponsor, and right to income from intellectual property developed using research data or tissue. Refer to www.hhs.gov/ohrp/humansubjects/guidance/exculp.htm for examples of impermissible exculpatory language and examples of acceptable language. Courts that have considered related issues have not agreed. See *Washington University v Catalano*, U.S. D Ct E Distr Missouri, Case No.4:03-cv-01065, Mar 3, 2006, aff'd, 8th Cir, No. 06–2286, June 15, 2007, holding that the governing federal regulation relating to research consents (45 C.F.R. 46.116) only prohibits exculpatory language in the form of a waiver or release from liability. Also, agency interpretations in guidance documents that apply the prohibition to the type of language noted above are not legally binding. OHRP subsequently made its disagreement with this judicial interpretation public. OHRP issues assurances and has the authority to revoke assurances.

Clinical Trial Web Sites

Information that is provided to potential human research subjects must be approved by the IRB and must be noncoercive in the manner that it is conveyed, as in content. This requirement for IRB review and approval also applies to recruitment material, including clinical trial Web sites.[11]

Reporting Incidents to OHRP and Other Federal Oversight Bodies

HHS regulations require that institutions have written procedures to ensure reporting to the institutional official, funding department or agency head, and OHRP of (a) unanticipated problems involving risks to subjects or others, (b) any serious or continuing noncompliance with the Common Rule or determinations of the IRB, and (c) any suspension or termination of IRB approval. See the guidance and decision tree at www. hhs.gov/ohrp/policy/incidreport_ohrp.html.

For gene transfer protocols, notification must also be provided to the NIH Office of Biotechnology Activities. For more information, see www.od.nih.gov/oba.

Note that there is an additional reporting requirement for gene transfer protocols conducted in NIH-supported general clinical research centers (GCRC); namely, whenever a gene transfer protocol conducted through the GCRC results in a report to the FDA of a serious unexpected adverse event or a report to the IRB of an unanticipated problem involving risks to subjects or others, a copy of that report should be sent to NCRR's Division of Clinical Research Resources, which funds the GCRC.

These reporting obligations are in addition to the FDA reporting obligations of the investigator who has been authorized to conduct work under an IND (Investigational New Drug) or IDE (Investigational Device Exemption) category.

Compliance

Governmental agency and congressional oversight activities have increased significantly since 1999 and are expected to continue at increased intensity, continuing a pattern of increasing public interest in the ethical and procedural propriety of biomedical research. This intensified oversight is occurring at a time of declining clinical revenue, when there might be increased pressure from principal investigators and administrators to cut corners and speed up the approval process for sponsored research. Such an approach places the welfare of the researcher and the research institution ahead of the welfare of the subject and is inconsistent with the ethical foundation of biomedical research and the derivative regulatory framework. The results of research, whether in terms of scientific recognition or financial reward, must never be allowed to take priority over the research subject. Compliance activities of federal regulatory bodies, public scrutiny of adverse outcomes, and financial interests of investigators, as well as civil actions, have shown that an approach to research that minimizes protection of the subject can ultimately prove very costly, both in revenue and reputation.

OHRP posts its compliance actions on its Web site, including the text of determination. Letters sent to research institutions operating under OHRP assurances are posted at ohrp.osophs.dhhs.gov/detrm_letrs/lindex.htm and provide a good source of information for risk management professionals on OHRP compliance and enforcement priorities.

A review of the OHRP determination letters reveals a pattern of common deficiencies:

1. Consent form deficiencies, such as language that is not understandable to the public, inadequate explanation of potential risks, failure to address all required elements of informed consent, and failure to describe all research procedures

2. IRB procedural and process deficiencies, such as inadequately written policies and procedures; failure to meet regularly as a full board; improper use of expedited review

for research not within permissible categories; inadequate information available to the IRB to support required risk-benefit determinations (particularly with respect to research involving pediatric and other vulnerable subjects, for which specific documented findings are required); substantive changes to protocols and consent forms without full board rereview; failure of documentation of IRB actions, including attendance, specific votes on actions taken, and summary of IRB discussions

3. Lapsed IRB approval (as previously noted, IRB approval is valid for no greater than one year; therefore, study approval expires after one year and the study administratively terminates when the approval expires)

4. Failure to report unanticipated problems involving risks to subjects, serious or continuing noncompliance, and suspensions and terminations to OHRP

5. Inadequate or absent meeting minutes.

The risk management professional should review the OHRP determination letters, informed consent checklist, guidance documents, and decision charts on the OHRP Web site (www.hhs.gov/ohrp/), for a more detailed analysis and useful tools for compliance with the IRB's obligations in each of these areas. Comprehensive, mistake-proof IRB application forms, consent form templates, and IRB reviewer forms that elicit all required information, address all necessary informed consent elements, and contain required IRB findings are important tools in maximizing the safety of human subjects and minimizing institutional liability.

It is the responsibility of each research institution and its IRB to educate investigators, to monitor the conduct of research (for example, through random and for cause audits), and to ensure that the IRB members are adequately and continually trained in human research protection. Ultimately, the expectation is that there will be increasing institutional support for the research compliance infrastructure, including adequate staff resources that incorporate a research compliance officer function for implementation and monitoring of research activities and for management of research funds.

Conflict of Interest

The failure of some IRBs to consider whether the investigator and institution have a potential conflict of interest and to determine how to manage or eliminate that conflict, along with the failure to inform the subject of these potential conflicts of interest, has resulted in significant public condemnation and increased regulatory scrutiny of clinical research efforts. It is essential that each research institution establish its own policies and procedures for reporting and managing investigator and institutional conflicts of interest. Does an investigator, for example, have an impermissible financial conflict of interest because of a paid consultancy or an equity interest in the sponsor? Can the conflict be managed with an independent oversight committee to verify the integrity of the data? Institutions that receive Public Health Service funding for research must have an administrative mechanism to identify significant financial interest of investigators (defined as the principal investigator and any other individual responsible for the design, conduct, or reporting of research), to manage, reduce or eliminate the conflict, and to report to PHS. (For more information, see http://grants.nih.gov/grants/policy/coi/index.htm. For information on recommended individual and institutional conflict policies for academic medical centers, see www.aamc.org/members/coitf/.) The intent of these requirements is to ensure there is no reasonable expectation or appearance that the design, conduct, or reporting of research will be biased by any conflicting financial interest of an investigator.

It is recommended that institutions implement a study-specific disclosure policy for each research study to be used by the grants and contracts office, as well as the IRB, so that the institution acquires the information it needs to meet disclosure and reporting obligations. For a study specific financial disclosure form see http://weill.cornell.edu/research/for_pol/forms/Form_SSD_New.pdf.

Gene or Recombinant DNA Research

Research involving recombinant DNA or gene transfer conducted at institutions that receive any NIH funding for rDNA research requires additional levels of review and approval at the institutional level (institutional biosafety committee) and at the federal level (Recombinant DNA Advisory Committee [RAC] of the Office of Biotechnology Activities [OBA]). Researchers at institutions that receive NIH funding for rDNA research must comply with these requirements even if their individual projects are not NIH funded. The RAC was established to respond to public concerns about the safety of research that involves gene manipulation. See the OBA Web site at http://oba.od.nih.gov, particularly "Frequently Asked Questions" on the OBA Web site at http://oba.od.nih.gov/rdna/rdna_faq_list.html.

· · · · · · · · ·

REGISTRATION OF CLINICAL TRIALS

The requirement that clinical trials register at www.clinicaltrials.gov was implemented in 2005 by the International Committee of Medical Journal Editors (ICMJE) as a prerequisite for publication in journals that adhere to ICMJE standards. This requirement was a precursor to the registration requirements that became law in 2007 (Public Law 110–85, Title VII). Under this law, registration is required prior to enrollment for clinical trials either supported by federal funds or subject to FDA regulations. Results data must also be submitted for public posting. (For more information see www.clinicaltrials.gov and http://grants.nih.gov/grants/guide/notice-files/NOT-OD-08-023.html.)

Additional Areas of Research Interest

Additional information of interest to those overseeing clinical trials is available from the following Web sites.

For *Issues to Consider in the Research Use of Stored Data or Tissues* from the Office for Protection from Research Risk, see http://humansubjects.energy.gov/doe-resources/files/ethframe/appendix_i.pdf.

For information regarding guidance on research involving human embryonic stem cells, germ cells, and stem cell-derived test articles see www.hhs.gov/ohrp/ humansubjects/guidance/stemcell.pdf.

For the most complete information on the National Academies' *Guidelines for Human Embryonic Stem Cell Research*, including all amendments, see www.nap.edu/ catalog.php?record_id=12553.

To familiarize the risk management professional with required research documents several sample protocols, policies, and procedures related to clinical research and IRBs have been included as appendices at the back of this chapter.

· · · · · · · · ·
CONCLUSIONS

Each research institution should review its own policies and procedures and its IRB records for compliance with federal regulations to determine whether it is vulnerable to an adverse action. Does the institution have an internal for cause and random monitoring and audit program to verify that investigators are complying with research protocols? Are signed research consent forms available for all research subjects? Do IRB policies and procedures satisfy federal requirements? Are minutes of IRB meetings maintained, and do they adequately document IRB findings and actions? Does the training of IRB members and investigators address regulatory emphasis on education? Risk managers should assess whether and how they, or research compliance officers or similar officials, can help the institution meet its obligations in the area of human biomedical research. Risk management professionals should also assess coordination of the activities of their research regulatory bodies — the IRB, the institutional biosafety committee for recombinant DNA and biohazards, and the radiation safety committee (which is required by the institution's Nuclear Regulatory Commission license).

If compliance is not adequate, the loss to the institution, in terms of funding and reputation, could be enormous. Institutions must be vigilant in their review and monitoring of the activities of the IRB and investigators and mindful of their own institutional financial conflicts of interest and those of their researchers. If they are not, they can expect that federal oversight and investigative or prosecutorial bodies will be.

Risk management professionals also should be mindful of the potential for costly civil and criminal litigation growing out of regulatory noncompliance. Numerous well-publicized instances of death or serious injury to human subjects in clinical trials have given rise to costly litigation against institutions, investigators, and individual IRB members. In virtually all instances, civil litigants have raised nondisclosure of prior adverse effects experienced by research subjects or nondisclosure of conflicts of interest as bases of their causes of action. It is advised that the risk manager ensure that IRB procedures and audit mechanisms provide for full disclosure to the IRB and research subjects of all potential risks and complications and all conflicts of interest associated with the research. It is further advised that the risk manager investigate whether coverage for personal injury and death arising out of administrative actions, such as actions of IRB chairs and members, is included in its insurance portfolio, whether through its professional and general liability coverage or its directors' and officers' (D&O) insurance. Risk managers should note that D&O policies traditionally do not include coverage for personal injury and death.

An additional area of potential risk arising out of regulatory noncompliance relates to enforcement activities of the HHS Office of the Inspector General (OIG) and the U.S. Department of Justice. The risk manager should be aware that obtaining federal funds in a fraudulent manner, for instance, through billing of the federal government for health-care services provided pursuant to a clinical trial for which service billing is not permitted, failing to disclose conflicting financial interests of investigators, engaging in scientific misconduct (fabrication, falsification, or plagiarism) in a federally funded research proposal, or improper time and effort and cost reporting in federally funded grants, can serve to support both civil and criminal charges under the federal fraud and abuse laws, including the False Claims Act.[12] In the civil context, the government is entitled to treble damages for successful prosecution.

Federal prosecutors have indicated that noncompliance with IRB requirements, such as false information or a failure to provide required information to the IRB regarding adverse events, can serve as a basis for prosecution under the fraud and abuse laws. In a press release announcing civil settlements in an enforcement action relating to the death of a subject in a gene therapy trial at the University of Pennsylvania, the U.S. Department of Justice, Eastern District of Pennsylvania, stated the following:

> Perhaps most significant is the impact that these settlements will have on the way clinical research on human participants is conducted throughout the country . . . This action covers two major research centers which (sic) have instituted important changes in the conduct and monitoring of clinical research on human participants. We hope that these settlements will now serve as a model for similar research nationwide.[13]

The press release goes on to say that

> [t]he government has alleged, among other allegations, that the study had produced toxicities in humans that should have resulted in termination, but the study continued. Reports were submitted to FDA, NIH, and to the Institutional Review Boards (IRBs) charged with oversight of this study that misrepresented the actual clinical findings associated with the study. Additionally, the consent form and process did not disclose all anticipated toxicities.[14]

The Fiscal Year 2009 Work Plan of the HHS Office of the Inspector General lists several research compliance–related areas earmarked for scrutiny, including college and university compliance with cost principles, use of Data Safety Monitoring Boards in clinical trials, FDA oversight of medical device postmarketing surveillance studies, adverse event reporting, and NIH oversight of financial conflicts of interest of extramural grantees.

Federal enforcement of regulatory requirements as they apply to research has been and will continue to be aggressive, whether through agency enforcement activities, application of civil and/or criminal penalties, or congressional mandates. The cost of noncompliance to the institutions and its employees and agents could be high.

The risk management professional plays a key role in ensuring that the institution avoids the considerable risk associated with noncompliance.

Endnotes

1. Cohen, J. J. "Academic Medical Centers and Medical Research," *JAMA*, 2005, 294(11):1367–1372.

2. In discussing the policy of the *New England Journal of Medicine* not to publish the results of unethical research, then Executive Editor Dr. Marcia Angell wrote, "Denying publication even when the ethical violations are minor protects the principle of the primacy of the research subject. . . . [R]efusal to publish unethical work serves notice to society at large that even scientists do not consider science the primary measure of a civilization. Knowledge, although important, may be less important to a decent society than the way it is obtained." Angell, M., "The Nazi Hypothermia Experiments and Unethical Research Today," *NEJM*, 1990, 322:146–164.

3. Jonsen, A. R. "The Ethics of Research with Human Subjects: A Short History." In Jonsen, A. R., R. M. Veatch, and L. Walters, editors, *Source Book in Bioethics*. Washington D.C.: Georgetown University Press, 1998, pp. 5–9.

4. In distinguishing between research, which requires adherence to human subject protection regulations, including prospective IRB review, and innovative therapeutic intervention, which does not, consider whether the primary intent is to develop generalizable knowledge or treat an individual patient. Consider also whether the intent is to publicly present or publish results or whether the activity is for internal quality improvement purposes. See Baruch, A. B., L. B. McCullough, and R. R. Sharp. "Consensus and Controversy in Clinical Research Ethics," *JAMA*, 2005, 294(11):1411–1414.

5. The National Cancer Institute Central IRB (CIRB) initiative is an effort to reduce the administrative burden of multiple local IRB reviews of multisite cancer trials sponsored by the NCI and cooperative groups. Institutions that join the CIRB may rely on the CIRB as the IRB with primary jurisdiction to review these studies and use a local facilitated review mechanism in lieu of local full board review. See www.ncicirb.org/.

6. OPRR is the former federal office with human subject research oversight authority. The office relocated from the National Institutes of Health (NIH) to the Office of Public Health and Science, HHS, and is now called the Office for Human Research Protection (OHRP). The move was generally accepted as a means to increase the visibility of federal oversight of human subject protection and access to the secretary of HHS.

7. Ellis, G. "Protecting the Rights and Welfare of Human Research Subjects." *Acad Med*, 1999, 74(9):1008–1009.

8. There is a mechanism for protection of data for particularly sensitive research, such as genetic research, when there is a concern that the release of information regarding the results of research could lead to discrimination in the workplace or in the ability of individuals who are found to be carriers of genetic diseases to obtain life or health

insurance. The secretary of HHS, or the secretary's designee, may issue a certificate of confidentiality "to protect the privacy of research subjects by withholding their identities from all persons not connected with the research. . . . Persons so authorized to protect the privacy of such individuals may not be compelled in any Federal, State, or local civil, criminal, administrative, legislative, or other proceedings to identify such individuals." 42 U.S.C. 241(d), Section 301(d) of the Public Health Service Act, Protection of Identity, Research Subjects. For further information, call NIH at (301) 402–7221 or see the certificate of confidentiality kiosk at grants1.nih.gov/grants/policy/coc/.

9. For example, is the amount of compensation offered so excessive as to be coercive? Is the subject compensated only at the end of a six-month clinical trial so that the subject cannot withdraw during the trial without loss of all compensation? Or is the compensation prorated for the amount of time the subject participated?

10. 45 C.F.R. 46.116.

11. www.hhs.gov/ohrp/policy/clinicaltrials.html.

12. 31 U.S.C. sec 3729 et seq.

13. Press release by the U.S. Department of Justice, Eastern District of Pennsylvania, "U.S. Settles Case of Gene Therapy Study That Ended With Teen's Death," Sept. 9, 2005.

14. *Ibid.*

6

Patient Safety in Surgery: The Essential Continuum

Marshall Steele, MD
Susan Harris
Craig Westling
Asheesh Gupta

Patient safety is the first priority in the operating room (OR). Keeping a patient safe requires talented professionals; however, the foundation of safety in the OR does not lie in individual capability, but rather is based on *systems* and processes to ensure patient safety. This sometimes flies in the face of a medical culture that is deeply rooted in individual performance. After all, physicians and nurses pride themselves on being independent and self-reliant. However, as Steven Covey wrote in his book, *The Seven Habits of Highly Successful People,* first published in 1989, it is interdependence, not independence, that is the characteristic most likely to lead to success.

Take, for example, a scene that one of the authors witnessed. After working with nurses and physicians to institute a policy that required every surgeon to mark the site of the incision before the patient left the holding area, the OR medical director was confronted by several indignant surgeons who said they knew their patients well and had never performed wrong-site surgery. They felt that marking the site was an unnecessary requirement and an affront to them. The medical director's response was that he was certainly happy that they had never made a mistake, but the goal was that they could say that at the end of their careers. That medical director twice had the wrong extremities prepped, and once had the wrong patient brought into his OR. It was only luck and individual effort that prevented catastrophe in all three cases. Not every surgeon has been so lucky. Well-designed systems, not luck and individual performance, are the pillars of safety. Leaders, particularly physician leaders, are responsible for safety, and they must work with the staff in the trenches to design safety systems.

FIGURE 6.1   Patient Safety Continuum

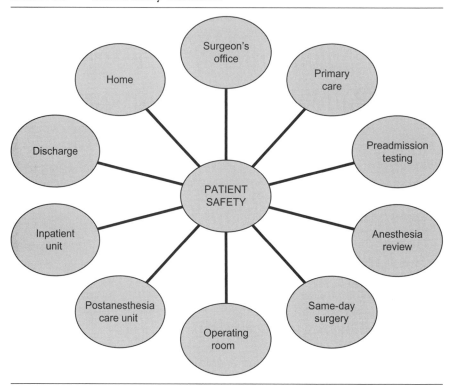

In this chapter, we present a model for patient-centric safety that begins long before the patient arrives at the hospital and ends after they have left (see Figure 6.1).[1]

SAFETY LEADERSHIP

Most hospitals attempt to address safety in a multitude of different ways. For optimal patient safety, it is imperative to break down those silos and understand how each area is affected by the other areas. Talking about safety isn't the same as ensuring it. Leadership must define the metrics of success and failure, and a system must be put in place to measure and manage the information. Accomplishing this infrastructure requires processes that cut across the silos. If safety is really that important, and it is essential to achieving the healthcare organization's mission, put someone in charge of OR safety and extend his or her responsibilities beyond the walls of the OR. Appoint a safety care coordinator to serve as navigator, liaison, and overall safety leader with the following responsibilities:

1. Maintain a roster of medical staff privileges with specific approved procedures.
2. Work with scheduling to validate privileges for every surgeon.

3. Train all staff and physicians on safety systems and protocols.

4. Maintain a roster, privileges, and insurance coverage of all independent contractors, including vendors, perfusionists, and so forth.

5. Develop and ensure the use of checklists, time-outs, and surgical site identification.

6. Ensure electrical safety, anesthesia equipment safety, and laser safety.

7. Ensure there is a system for accomplishing and tracking Surgical Care Improvement Project (SCIP) measures.

8. Develop a dashboard of key measures.

9. Chair the OR safety committee.

10. Conduct root cause analysis of adverse events.

11. Ensure the adequacy of presurgical risk assessments.

12. Ensure that all Centers for Medicare & Medicaid Services (CMS) and The Joint Commission (TJC) guidelines are followed.

To ensure optimum success, the OR safety coordinator should partner with a physician whose role will be one of advisor, champion of the OR patient safety cause with the medical staff and senior leadership and to assist with safe practices implementation. The OR safety coordinator and physician advisor should cochair the OR safety committee, a multidisciplinary team tasked with ensuring OR safety for every patient, every time. The OR itself can be thought of as a hub with many spokes, the spokes being the surgeons, nurses, primary care providers, anesthesia providers, medical subspecialists, registration staff, staff of presurgical holding and preadmission departments, risk management professionals, central sterile processing staff, vendors, postanesthesia care unit (PACU) staff, floor nurses and therapists, and the patients themselves. Taken together, this team will ensure transparency, manage risk, implement safe practices, and develop metrics by which safety efforts will be measured and monitored over time.

· · · · · · · · ·

PATIENT EDUCATION

The entire healthcare team (doctors, surgeons, therapists, nurses, etc.) has a responsibility to set appropriate expectations for patients to ensure safety. One major concern is a lack of communication with patients about these expectations, for example, patient education. Most facilities lack a cohesive system to ensure that patients are asked, and receive, consistent and accurate information regarding their procedure and treatment plan. Patients often ask their surgeon, nurse, or therapist the same question, but they receive different answers. This leads, at minimum, to confusion and frustration. Inconsistent information may also be the precursor to an adverse outcome. Clearly, all caregivers do their best to give the right answers; the problem is not a lack of effort or desire to do better. The problem is the lack of a framework that makes possible coordination and standardization of information so that a consistent message can be delivered, reflecting the fulfillment of proper expectations and facilitating safety along the entire patient continuum of care.

In the Surgeon's Office

We have heard it said many times that it is the surgeon's responsibility to properly prepare the patient. However, the reality is that the vast majority of surgeons must rely on the work of many other professionals to achieve a successful outcome. Therefore, although safety is the responsibility of the surgeon, it is not his or her responsibility alone. Standardized practices must be implemented in every surgeon's office and linked to other caregivers to ensure safety. Often the most basic information is miscommunicated between the surgeon's office and the OR, such as the need for specialized equipment or instrumentation. As a result, the OR staff may not have what the surgeon needs when he or she is ready to begin the procedure, with a resultant increase in surgical and anesthesia times. Simply having preprinted checklists of required equipment for particular surgical procedures can solve this vexing problem. If the equipment and instruments available in the OR do not match the procedural checklist, a misstep has occurred somewhere in the process. This misstep should be evaluated and the process reinforced or changed if necessary. Many surgery centers and OR suites have standardized the equipment and instrumentation that is available for any given procedure to minimize variation and promote cost efficiency. The days of having individual cards for each surgeon's equipment, instrument, and suture preferences based on their specific privileges and list of approved procedures is slowly fading away due to cost of maintaining expensive inventory and the inability to be proficient with all items used.

Previously, we mentioned that surgery should be viewed as a team project. Consider the following scenario. An anemic patient is scheduled for a total hip replacement. According to policy, her hemoglobin is checked preoperatively and is within acceptable limits for surgical clearance at 10 g/dL. However, it has been found by a review of surgical outcomes that postoperative patients whose presurgical hemoglobin was above 10 g/dL, but below 12 g/dL were at greater risk for requiring a postoperative transfusion a day or two after surgery, a fact previously unknown. To support patient-centered care, surgical quality outcomes should be reviewed, and when policy and procedures are periodically evaluated, these outcomes should be considered. Questions to ask include Are preoperative policies and procedures appropriate given the present outcomes? Do they need revision? Who will be responsible for bringing forth this type of outcomes data to the OR safety committee? Who will be responsible for implementing and monitoring change to improve outcomes? Lacking this type of collaboration, risks are reviewed on a separate basis, with no coordination among the other team members outside the OR suite.

Clearance for Surgery

Many primary care physicians (PCPs) are asked by the surgeon to clear the patient for surgery. In other words, the PCPs are to give their opinion as to whether the patient is an appropriate candidate for anesthesia and surgery. To make this determination, they may order tests or additional consultations. PCPs seem like a logical choice to shoulder this responsibility because they know the patient best. However, many PCPs are unfamiliar with specific surgical procedures, and few have contact with anesthesiologists. Many times the PCP is not given procedural information, and anesthesia guidelines are not usually provided to the PCP. As a result, the PCP's assessment and resulting clearance may not take into account clinical ramifications that are important to patient safety. Moreover, because the PCP's assessment may not pick up on key issues, many anesthesiologists admit to relying on the nursing notes instead of the history and physical examination performed by the surgeon or PCP. Either PCPs must be folded into the OR team in some creative way (we have seen hospitalists performing this role for certain surgical procedures), or a system that ensures preoperative collection of the proper data must be devised. A sophisticated, reliable preadmission testing center is one solution to this problem.

The Buck Stops with Anesthesia

The anesthesiologist is a key player in managing risk during surgery. Years ago, all patients were admitted to the hospital the day before their procedure and visited by the anesthesiologist the evening before surgery. This gave the anesthesiologist time to review the patient's medical record and confirm key information in person with the patient prior to surgery. Today, this process varies, and there is no consistent manner in which the anesthesiologist visits or clears the patient for surgery. This is compounded by the high percentage of surgical procedures done in the ambulatory surgery center setting. No consistently implemented information-gathering process has been developed to replace the old model. Based on visits to over one hundred ORs, it was found that very few anesthesia providers review patient information prior to the day of surgery, even for major surgeries and patients with multiple comorbidities.

Obtaining information from patients the day of surgery is fraught with patient safety issues and potential liability risk. Many patients are so frightened that they do not clearly hear or understand questions raised by physicians. Physicians are in a hurry and patients are nervous and fearful. This promotes poor communication, increasing the risk in an area already considered high risk.Improved anesthetic techniques and sophisticated monitoring equipment make anesthesia far safer than ever before. However, the lack of effective patient assessment and communication with the patient before surgery is an area of concern.

Best practice is for the anesthesia providers to review their cases the day before, and if not seeing the patient the day before surgery, to, at a minimum, call their patients the night before surgery to allay any fears. This phone call may also be the anesthesiologist's best opportunity to answer any lingering patient questions and ask any last minute questions he or she may have, and it supports obtaining the patient's informed consent for anesthesia.

· · · · · · · · ·
PREOPERATIVE PREPARATION

After the surgeon's office has scheduled the case, the preadmission testing (PAT) department should begin the process of preparing the patient for surgery. Depending on the facility, this can be accomplished in several ways: either with a phone assessment and/or by having the patient visit the PAT center before surgery. Surgery and anesthesia protocols and orders should be established to determine which patient should visit the PAT. This is a critical process in which the patient's individual medical needs must be considered. Understanding the patient's history, allergies, special needs, and level of psychological preparation allows the staff to incorporate preoperative education that is critical to a successful outcome. In addition, this is an opportunity for the PAT department to obtain documentation of informed consent, the history and physical, and any other required documents such as consultations, advance directives, clearances from other specialists, images, and so forth.

With regard to informed consent, it is essential that patients make an informed decision about whether to have the procedure based on information provided by the treating clinicians, and there must be documentation of this process. Usually, the patient is asked to sign a consent form, verifying that his or her consent is an informed consent and that the patient has decided to proceed. Although the specifics of informed consent can vary from state to state, the basic requirements are the same. The physician explains the following:

1. The diagnosis and procedure

2. The reasons the procedure should be performed

3. The material risks of the proposed procedure

4. The likelihood of success

5. The alternatives to the proposed procedure, including not having the procedure

6. The risks, benefits, and side effects of the procedure and any alternatives, including not having the procedure

7. The risks, benefits, and side effects of subsequent alternatives offered

8. The prognosis, if he or she decides to reject the proposed procedure

The physician is best suited to provide the information which is the basis for an informed consent, and the process should be conducted in the doctor's office, a setting which provides the patient with an opportunity to listen closely and ask questions. Asking the patient to sign the consent form five minutes before surgery is not a good practice. At this point, a patient may not clearly recall the earlier discussion, and asking for a signature at the last minute can increase apprehension. Such an approach is therefore a patient safety issue.

Before the patient is asked to sign the consent form, he or she should be given the opportunity to read the form (or have someone read it to him or her) and ask questions. If the patient indicates that there are questions or that he or she is unclear about the procedure, the physician should respond to those questions and/or provide clarification before the patient signs the form. (Please see Chapter 4 on informed consent in this volume for additional information.)

Patients should also receive preoperative instructions from the surgeon, the department of anesthesia, and nursing. As previously noted, this information should be consistent. For example, patients should be very clear that they are not to drink any liquids or eat any food after the midnight before surgery. If they are to take medications with a sip of water the morning of surgery, they must understand what those medications are. They should also understand exactly what to expect postoperatively, as they may not be able to absorb this information easily immediately after a procedure. Finally, the plan for discharge should be discussed with patients to ensure ample time for transportation arrangements and home care to be established. All these aspects of education are critical to a successful outcome. Encourage patients undergoing surgery to bring a family member, significant other, or neighbor (their choice) to help them remember all these points. Encourage note taking and asking questions, and get them to repeat back critical information such as their understanding of "no liquids and food after midnight" or that they will not be discharged home without having someone present who can drive them.

. . . .
OUTPATIENT SURGERY

Hospital outpatient surgery centers and free-standing ambulatory surgery centers have been established to meet the public and provider demand for surgery on an outpatient basis. Physicians particularly like this setting because they have greater autonomy, flexibility in scheduling, and less operating downtime, allowing them to schedule and perform more surgeries. The goal is to physically and psychologically prepare all patients for surgical intervention. TJC requires that assessment in this setting be performed by a registered nurse. The nurse must understand not only what to ask but also how to ask it. For instance, it is important that the nurse never speak for the patient or prompt the patient with the right answer. For example, the nurse must ask the patient to tell him or her what procedure is being done, instead of telling the patient the procedure and requesting agreement. Wrong-site surgeries have occurred when the patient agrees to ambiguously communicated, incorrect information. The nurse must also make sure that the appropriate identification band has been placed on the patient. This band then becomes one of the ways in which patient identification is verified. TJC's National Safety Patient Goal 01.01.01 requires that two patient identifiers be used before providing treatments or procedures. Therefore, each institution must have policies and procedures that address which two patient identifiers will be used to ensure that the preprocedural patient identification is verified consistently and correctly.

The Day of Surgery

The nursing assessment on the day of surgery is critical to patient safety and liability risk reduction. In addition to identity verification, surgical site confirmation, informed consent corroboration, and other important measures that reduce liability exposure, this is the time when questions to ascertain potentially life-threatening risks such as latex allergies and malignant hyperthermia should be asked. It is important to note that much of this information will have already been addressed preoperatively in the physician offices, so that the nurse will, for the most part, be reinforcing known information.

Hospitalized patients must also be screened closely for preexisting conditions that are considered nonreimbursable events by CMS unless they are present on admission (POA). Conditions such as pressure ulcers, poor glycemic control, and deep vein thrombosis are considered hospital-acquired conditions (HACs) if they are not POA. Even though a physical assessment of the patient is made upon admission to the hospital, it is nevertheless good practice to evaluate the existence of these conditions and to document their existence preoperatively. Should these conditions become manifest during the hospital stay and not noted as POA, CMS will not reimburse for the additional dollars if the presence of one of these hospital-acquired condition would prompt a higher payment.

In addition to the physical aspects of the assessment and preparation, the patient must be screened for psychosocial and special needs. TJC's National Patient Safety Goal (NPSG) 13.01.01 requires that caregivers encourage patients and their families to be actively involved in their care. This goal also requires that the patient be provided with information regarding infection control and measures that will be taken to prevent adverse events in surgery.

Of particular importance is the need to ensure compliance with SCIP measures. For example, beta blockers given perioperatively reduce the risk of cardiovascular complications, so patients who are on beta blockers should receive a dose during the perioperative period. SCIP also requires the administration of specific prophylactic antibiotics to patients undergoing defined procedures to minimize surgical site infections (SSI), and the dose must be received within one hour before the surgical incision. In addition to these important measures, SCIP recognizes that shaving the surgical site with a razor does more harm than good and mandates that, if hair removal is required, it should be removed with clippers.

When the patient leaves the preparation area (sometimes called the holding area) for the OR, an effective transfer must take place. TJC's National Patient Safety Goal 02.05.01 requires that this transfer include "interactive communication that allows for the opportunity for the questioning between the giver and receiver of patient information."

· · · · · · · · ·

IN THE OPERATING ROOM

Risk in the OR can be exaggerated or minimized by the culture and environment, the ability to communicate effectively, and the ability (or inability) of staff to function as a team.

Culture

The culture of the OR plays an important role in safety. It is important for all staff to feel empowered to protect the patient and not defer to the surgeon simply because of his or her leadership role. The hospital setting as a high-risk environment has often been compared to the aviation industry. Small process and systems failures by individuals can have deadly consequences in both industries. The difference is that the aviation industry has taken proactive measures to encourage speaking out, introduced a common language signifying concern, instituted the development of crew resource management, and created a robust nonthreatening adverse event and near-miss reporting system. Compared to the not too distant past, the aviation industry is now considered a safer industry. Healthcare, and in particular the specialty of surgery, is struggling to change the environment and culture of the OR to be more patient focused, with an emphasis on team empowerment.

In many ways, the OR is analogous to the cockpit of an aircraft. From a traditional perspective, the surgeon has always been the captain and the staff are junior officers. The flatter the hierarchy in the OR and the more equal staff members feel, the less likely it is that they will be intimidated and reluctant to speak up when they detect something that could affect patient safety. By fostering a culture that supports critical communication processes, the organization provides staff with the resources to authoritatively deal with potentially unsafe situations.

Teamwork

Even for clinicians who spend their entire careers providing care to surgical patients, the daily complexities and stimulation of the OR environment ensures that the setting rarely becomes commonplace. The OR presents unique challenges involving complex technology and distinct personalities, both of which must be carefully navigated. However, with good leadership and ongoing education that emphasizes safety and risk management, the OR can be an exciting and rewarding place to work.

All members of the OR team must be taught the basic elements of safety. When mistakes do occur, they are often related to poor communication or sensory overload. The second goal of TJC National Patient Safety Goals notes that ineffective communication is the most frequently cited root cause of sentinel events. Supporting this conclusion, Arien Mack, PhD, who has written extensively about inattentional blindness, has postulated that "there is no perception without attention."[2] Consequently, mistakes do occur when communication is ambiguous and not understood by the recipient or when a professional's mind is required to multitask beyond its ability to do so. It is important for the staff to understand this concept. Staff must feel comfortable knowing when to stop the process and ask for clarification to ensure that everything is occurring as planned, for example, by doing a time-out at the beginning of each case. It is also important for the staff to be able to understand and read written orders, progress notes, and so forth. Consequently, hospitals are converting to an electronic medical record (EMR), which enhances clarity of documentation, as well as computerized provider order entry (CPOE), which often incorporates prompts and other safety checks to prevent error in orders.

Roles and Responsibilities of the OR TEAM

A well-functioning operating suite is like a well-scripted play in which every move is deliberate and each role is well-defined. The players include a registered nurse who circulates within the room for each case, a surgical technologist who hands the instruments to the surgeon, an anesthesiologist or certified registered nurse anesthetist (CRNA) who provides anesthesia and sedation, and the surgeon. Depending on the specific procedure to be preformed, there could be additional team members, such as an extra corporeal perfusion technologist for open heart procedures, neonatologist for complex obstetrical cases, and so forth. The surgeon may also have a first assistant who may be another physician, a physician's assistant, a registered nurse first assistant, or a surgical technologist first assistant. CMS and TJC require the circulator to be a qualified registered nurse who is immediately available to respond to emergencies. It is important to note that organizations considering establishing a first assistant role should consult American Association of Operation Room Nurses (AORN) standards and become familiar with any relevant provisions in their state's nurse practice act.

The circulator is responsible for checking the patient into the room; confirming that the documentation of informed consent, histories, and physicals, and so forth are present and properly executed; overseeing the sterile field; securing supplies during the case; assisting the anesthesiologist or CRNA; and ensuring that all safety requirements are met, including a call for the time-out before surgery commences.

All staff members must be properly credentialed and educated. Medical staff privileges must be available to the staff at all times, and student affiliations and guidelines should be clearly delineated and understood by everyone. When residents are present, it is important for everyone to be clear on their limitations and the role that the attending physician should play. Ongoing education for all staff is mandatory in order to stay abreast of new technology and to reiterate basic risk safeguards.

When present for a procedure, vendors also play an important role in the OR. The Association of Operating Room Nurses (AORN) 2005 Position Statement on the Role of the Health Care Industry Representative in the Perioperative/Invasive Procedure Setting states that

- the RN as a team member is accountable for safe patient care;
- vendors may be permitted in the OR to provide technical support in accordance with facility policies, local, state, and federal regulations;
- vendors should never provide direct patient care or be allowed in the sterile field (with specialized training and facility approval, they may perform calibration/synchronization to adjust/program devices under the direction of a physician); and
- the patient has a right to be informed of their presence.

The vendor must not function outside of his or her role in the OR. Because vendor management has grown so complex, many healthcare organizations use vendor credentialing and compliance monitoring strategies similar to those used for the organization's clinical staff to address the hospital's responsibility for ensuring patient safety when vendors are present.

Infection Control

A common misconception about the OR is that the room itself is sterile. This implies that it is free from all living organisms, which is not true. Understanding the boundaries of sterility in the OR is critical to providing safe care. All team members in the OR are required to adhere to facility dress codes, which are designed to protect both the patients and the surgical team members. For example, all must wear eye protection and don gloves anytime contact with the patient occurs or is anticipated. Protective barriers are critical to protecting staff from blood and body fluids that can carry hepatitis, HIV, and other infectious agents, so personal protective equipment (PPE) must be available to the staff at all times. Double-gloving, wearing eye protection, and using blunt sutures, safety scalpels, and safety zones for passing instruments are additional strategies that provide protection from exposure to blood and body fluids. The doors to the OR should remain closed at all times, and traffic in and out of the room should be discouraged. Instrument trays should be checked carefully to ensure that sterilization requirements, such as expiration dates, have been met, and drapes and wrappers must be inspected to ensure that no holes or moisture are present.

It is very important that every OR be terminally cleaned at least once within each twenty-four-hour time period. Terminal cleaning involves more extensive cleaning than that performed between cases, including wet-vacuuming the floors; cleaning all horizontal surfaces, hallways and floors; cleaning the substerile areas; and wiping down the walls. This approach helps to eliminate any dust and debris that may have accumulated during the day.

Labeling Solutions and Medications

Medication safety issues are of great importance in the OR, as in other clinical environments. The following are of particular concern in the surgical environment.

Preassessment by the nurse and a thorough preoperative review of the medical record will assist staff in understanding the patient's medication regime and identify any known allergies prior to the administration of any medication or solution. This information is obtained by direct questioning of the patient before the procedure begins and by referring to the history, physical, and nursing assessment. It is also important to know the medications currently being used by the patient to avoid administration of incompatible medications.

Delivering solutions and medications to the sterile field requires a high level of diligence to avoid potential catastrophic mix-ups. The person delivering the solution or medication to the field is not the person who uses or administers it. Consequently, additional steps must be taken to ensure that the correct medication, in the correct dose, is administered via the correct route to the correct patient at the correct time. This is accomplished in part by requiring that all medications be labeled with the name, strength, and dose, as well as the date, time, and identity of the preparer. The scrub technician uses sterile stickers and a sterile marker to mark all unidentified medication on the field, and both the scrub technician and the circulating nurse verbally and visually confirm the medication containers to ensure accuracy, as required by AORN's 2008 Perioperative Standards and Recommended Practices. When handoffs occur during transitions in care, the medication verification process is repeated for each medication that has been so prepared. Unlabeled medication in any form is never to be on the field during surgery.

Counting Instruments and Surgical Supplies

Every effort must be made to ensure that instruments, sponges, needles, or other supplies are not inadvertently retained in patients postoperatively. Healthcare risk management professionals are thoroughly familiar with the indefensibility of a court case in which an X-ray showing a retained surgical device is shown to a jury. Appropriate efforts to avoid such unfortunate outcomes include counts that take place before the surgery starts, before the closure of a large cavity, anytime staff members are relieved, and when the surgeon is ready to close. Any additions to the sterile field during the surgery must be added to the count and accounted for at pertinent junctures in the procedure. Discrepancies must be reported immediately to the surgeon so that he or she has an opportunity to search for a potentially retained object before closing. In the event that discrepancy in the count cannot be resolved, an X-ray should be ordered to ensure that the item is not in the patient's wound. Although AORN notes that needles 17 mm and smaller may not be consistently visible on an X-ray, this key professional organization does not offer any advice other than (1) to be as diligent as possible as the needles are being used and (2) to make sure the count remains correct instead of waiting until the end. This suggests that an X-ray may be advisable in the event of any missing needle, no matter how small.

The retention of unintended or unplanned foreign objects in surgery is being addressed partially through advances in technology. The use of bar codes and radio frequency identification (RFID) tags are two such technologies that are thought to minimize the potential for retention of foreign objects through tagging and scanning technologies.

Positioning

Failure to appropriately position the patient on the surgical table places the patient at risk and can result in an exacerbation of a preexisting condition(s), neurological and vascular damage, and the development of stasis or pressure ulcers, some of which, depending on the extent of damage, may be designated as a nonreimbursable event by CMS. Improper positioning can also increase employee-related injury due to the use of improper body mechanics when lifting and moving patients into the appropriate position.

For these reasons, proper positioning is one of the first practices OR staff must learn and then methodically execute. Because this is a shared responsibility among team members, consistent delivery of safe care also requires processes that delineate who does what, in general, as well as in a given procedure. For example, for many surgical procedures, the anesthesiologist or CRNA is responsible for ensuring proper positioning of the patient's head, neck, and arms. The surgeon and the circulator are usually responsible for positioning the patient from the neck down. Because the approach to positioning is determined by the procedure to be performed and the patient's individual needs, a thorough knowledge of pressure points and circulatory, respiratory, integumentary, musculoskeletal, and neurological structures is essential for all staff who participate in this aspect of care. Every OR should have access to the 2010 AORN Perioperative Standards and Recommended Practices. These standards and practices are offered in a variety of media formats including, an electronic version, CD-ROM, and hard-copy print version.[3]

Staff involved in positioning must also understand the proper role of positioning-related equipment, because the proper use of such resources can promote both employee and patient safety. For example, the increased bariatric population in all healthcare organizations demands that staff be oriented to the use of lifts, if available, and proper lifting techniques, if lifts are not available. Staff who may care for the obese patient should also receive training to raise awareness of proper techniques and to help them deal with any limitations on the existence of standard OR resources, such as surgical tables. For more information on managing and protecting the obese patient, please see Chapter 18, in this volume, on managing the risks of obese patients.

Fire Safety

A fire in the OR is a critical event by any standard and requires swift action to prevent harm to staff and patient alike. The best efforts should be in prevention. The OR is replete with fuel sources (described loosely as anything that will burn) such as linens, drapes, sponges, dressings, clothing, blankets, and alcohol-based surgical preparations. According to TJC's Sentinel Event Alert 29, having an oxygen-enriched environment was a contributing factor in 74 percent of surgical fires reported. Unless proper precautions are taken, simple occurrences such as leaving the end of a high-intensity light cord on a drape or not properly holstering an electrocautery pencil between uses can ignite the drapes covering the patient. Failure to allow an alcohol-based preparation to dry before using the cautery instrument can also result in a fire. As reported by TJC, 62 percent of all surgical fires involved the airway, head, or face. The Joint Commission for the Accreditation of Healthcare Organizations (now The Joint Commission) issued Sentinel Alert 29, Preventing Surgical Fires, on June 24, 2003. This alert can be found online at www.jointcommission.org/SentinelEvents/SentinelEventAlert/sea_29.htm.

All members of the team must take the threat of fire very seriously, and fire drills specifically oriented to the OR environment should be conducted routinely. (Please see the AORN Guidance Statement, Fire Prevention in the OR, which can be accessed at www .aorn.org/PracticeResources/AORNPositionStatements/Position_FirePrevention/.)

Exposure Prevention

Additional strategies to reduce the opportunity for employee injury are also important. For example, everyone working in the OR must understand the risk of exposure to HIV, hepatitis B and C, tuberculosis, and other infectious diseases. To this end, Occupational Safety and Hazard Administration (OSHA) requires employers to provide PPE and train all employees to properly use such equipment. OSHA also requires hospitals to protect the staff from sharps, for example, by using safety devices to prevent accidental needle or blade sticks. Another primarily employee-related issue is the need to address the presence of noxious fumes in the OR setting. OSHA and AORN require smoke evacuation systems in all ORs to prevent inhalation of electrocautery smoke and laser plume, both of which have been demonstrated to have hazardous properties. Staff should also be trained on measures to avoid the hazards of methyl methacrylate bone cement, certain chemotherapeutic agents, and suction waste disposal.

Preventing Wrong-Site Surgery

Wrong-site surgery (WSS), generally described as surgery performed on the wrong patient, wrong body part, wrong operative site, wrong organ, wrong procedure, or at the wrong level, occurs due to a breakdown in communication. There are a host of issues that contribute to surgical error of WSS, including patients with unusual characteristics, those undergoing multiple surgical procedures, those with multiple surgeons, and time pressure to commence the procedure due to the emergent nature of the patient's condition. Other factors, such as distractions, new or different equipment, understaffing or wrong staffing mix, and lack of access to patient information, also contribute to WSS. TJC and the World Health Organization have both advocated the use of the Universal Protocol to prevent wrong site/patient/procedures. This strategy is similar to the preflight checklist used on an aircraft. Proper use of such check-off lists requires that everyone on the team halt, pay attention, and be aware.

A sample check-off list developed by AORN for the OR may be accessed at www. aorn.org/docs_assets/55B250E0–9779–5C0D-1DDC8177C9B4C8EB/A33D0AE3–17A4– 49A8–8622F379968BC1CF/AORN_Sample_Patient_Records_Introperative.pdf. Another example of such an approach is seen in Box 6.1. You will note that the top portion of this sample form requires that the nurse preparing the patient for surgery ensures certain parameters are met before the patient comes to the OR, including verification of the site. TJC's National Patient Safety Goal Universal Protocol 01.02.01 further specifies that "the site is marked by a licensed independent practitioner or other provider who is permitted by the hospital and qualified through a residency program to perform the procedure. This individual will be involved directly in the procedure and must be present at the time the procedure is performed." The surgeon should involve the patient and/or family and significant others during this process and refer to the patient's history and physical examination findings.

Should a wrong-site procedure occur, it must be reported to TJC as a sentinel event, and in some instances it must be reported to the state office of regulatory services. A root cause analysis must be performed, in which all parties participate in an inquiry to explore causation and develop future prevention.

In 2009, CMS announced three National Coverage Determinations (NCDs) that affect payment by Medicare for serious and reportable errors in medical care. All three of these NCDs are on the list of never events as described by the National Quality Forum. They are (1) surgery on the wrong body part, (2) surgery on the wrong patient, and (3) the wrong surgery performed on a patient. Unlike the hospital-acquired conditions (HACs) provisions, which affect only payments to hospitals for inpatient stays, these NCDs may affect payment to hospitals, physicians, and any other healthcare providers and suppliers

BOX 6.1   Universal Protocol Operating Room Surgical Safety Checklist

Each line is to be checked or, if not applicable, an "N/A" written   Date _____

Pre-procedure, and prior to arrival in the procedure or surgery suite (exception: Minor Treatment Prep Room)

Verification of the correct patient with correct ID band using two identifiers

Patient identification matches schedule (if applicable)

Documentation is completed and, using two identifiers, matches the patient's identification on the following:
- ☐   H & P
- ☐   Nursing Assessment. Allergies are noted
- ☐   Pre-Anesthesia Evaluation Form (if applicable)

Consent forms are accurately completed (signed, witnessed and dated/timed) and, using two identifiers, matches the patient's identification:
- ☐   Hospital consent form
- ☐   Anesthesia consent form (if applicable)
- ☐   Informed consent for Special Procedure, Special Procedure or Diagnostic Test (if applicable). The consent form accurately lists the procedure to be done and notes laterality (if applicable)

Required blood product(s), implant(s), device(s) and/or special equipment is available for the procedure

Correct diagnostic and radiology tests are available and properly labeled

The patient is NPO (if applicable)

Surgical / procedure site (side and surface, if applicable) has been initialed by the physician or LIP performing the procedure

Signature and Title_____

Upon Arrival into the Procedural or Surgical Suite

Prophylactic antibiotics have been given or will be given within the appropriate time frame

All members of the team are introduced to the patient

Time Out   Time Called: _____

#1   #2

Circulating Nurse verbally calls the Time Out and rings the bell indicating the Time Out

All team members stop and actively participate in the Time Out, confirming the following:

Verification of the correct patient with correct ID band using two identifiers

Two identifiers on ID band match chart, consent, schedule

Team agrees on the procedure and position

The consent form accurately lists the procedure to be done

Correct site (and side, surface) has been initialed by the physician or LIP performing the procedure

Images are displayed

Prophylactic antibiotic has been given in the past 60 minutes (120 minutes for aminoglycosides or quinolones), if ordered

Safety precautions based on patient history or medication use have been noted

(Continued)

Anesthesia has completed equipment safety check (if Anesthesiologist or Anesthetist is present)

Pulse oximeter is on the patient and functioning appropriately

Intravenous access is patent and adequate for purposes of procedure

Difficult airway cart is present if needed

Sterility of instrumentation has been confirmed

Equipment issues or concerns have been addressed

Implants are available and sterile

Time Procedure Started: _____ **Participating Team Members:**

Name:	Name:
Name:	Name:
Name:	Name:

End of Case—Nurse verbally confirms with the team:

The name of the procedure recorded

That all counts are correct

How the specimen is labeled

If there are any equipment issues to be addressed

Transfer to Phase I or Phase 2 PACU or post-procedural unit

Key concerns for recovery and management are reviewed by Anesthesia and Nursing; hand-off communication occurs to the next provider

Discrepancy noted

Physician notified at _____ time. Resolution documented in the medical record

Signature and Title _____
_____

Source: Dekalb Regional Healthcare System, Decatur, GA 2003. Reprinted with permission.

involved in the erroneous surgeries. Their effective date was immediate upon announcement. To read the full NCD see the following:

wrong body part, www.cms.hhs.gov/mcd/viewdecisionmemo.asp?id=222;

wrong patient, www.cms.hhs.gov/mcd/viewdecisionmemo.asp?id=221; and wrong surgery performed on a patient, www.cms.hhs.gov/mcd/viewdecisionmemo.asp?id=223.

Management of Specimens in the OR

Patient or specimen identification errors involving the laboratory cause some 160,000 adverse patient events each year in the United States, according to the authors of a 2005 College of American Pathologists Q-Probes study.[4] Consequently, every effort must be made to ensure that a specimen is collected properly in the correct medium and sent to the lab promptly. Incorrect identification or preservation of OR specimens has resulted in unnecessary surgery, surgery on the wrong patient, and the failure to conduct a procedure the patient needed. In the best case scenario, a patient may require a repeat procedure to obtain another specimen. Unfortunately, this occurs every day in hospitals throughout the country, primarily due to problems with communication.

The circulating nurse is ultimately responsible for specimens, and he or she must speak up if there is any question as to the identity or management of the specimen. Mislabeling errors must be avoided by ensuring that the label has the correct patient information as well as brief description of the specimen contained within. The process for transporting the specimens to the lab must be delineated very specifically in a procedure to which all staff who handle specimens are oriented. Both the bearer of the specimen from the OR and the recipient in the laboratory must document compliance with this procedure. After the procedure, the circulating nurse must also ensure that the OR suite has no leftover labels, which might cause confusion for staff managing a subsequent case. (Please see Chapter 10 in this volume on risk management in the laboratory for more information.)

The circulating nurse must also ensure that the proper receptacle containing the appropriate preservative is available before the procedure begins. It should also be noted that another employee-related exposure source is the presence of formalin, a common preservative used in the OR. This substance must be handled with care, and the staff should be educated on its management using the material safety data sheets (MSDS) that all healthcare organizations are required to maintain in each clinical setting, for example, the OR.

Traffic Control

Traffic control (or patient flow) in the OR is very important for patient safety. Proper control of human movement in the OR facilitates infection and drug control, as well as security of staff and patients. Every hospital should have an identification process in place that prevents unauthorized access to restricted areas, including the OR. To achieve this goal, all staff, including physicians, should be required to wear photo identification badges, and anyone attempting to enter a restricted area without one should be stopped and questioned. Exterior doors should be secured and video surveillance should be used in appropriate areas. Emergency exit doors should also be fitted with emergency alert devices, and signage specifying restrictions should be clear and easily interpreted.

An additional related issue that may create patient and employee exposure to risk is construction. When facility modifications are planned, TJC requires performance of an infection control risk assessment to identify any issues that may increase exposure, including those related to traffic patterns. The assessment should culminate in recommendations that are implemented in a timely fashion.

Biomedical Support

In large facilities, the OR is usually supported by on-site biomedical technicians who maintain the complex technology used today. In addition, such staff can help troubleshoot technological issues that arise during procedures. Having this support reduces risk and provides a safety net for the staff. In smaller facilities, biomedical staff may be on call. The risk management professional and OR manager should ensure that availability of biomedical staff resources and equipment replacement capabilities are adequate to meet the needs of the surgical area.

Additionally, all OR staff should be oriented to healthcare organization procedures concerning what to do if a piece of equipment malfunctions. For example, they should remove such equipment from service until it can be repaired and involve the healthcare risk management professional immediately if the malfunction may have harmed or caused the death of a patient. Such circumstances call for leaving the equipment "as is" as much as possible and not returning it to the manufacturer without first discussing the value of a forensic assessment with the healthcare risk management professional. A medical device report (MDR) as mandated by the Safe Medical Device Act (SMDA), is required to be completed within ten working days from the knowledge that the device caused harm or death. (Please see Chapter 3 on biomedical technology in this volume and Chapter 1 in Volume 3 on statutes, standards, and regulations.)

· · · · · · · · ·
POSTANESTHESIA CARE UNIT

The postanesthesia care unit (PACU), also referred to as the recovery room and postanesthesia recovery, is usually contiguous to the OR and is designed to care for patients recovering from regional anesthesia, general anesthesia, and managed anesthesia care. The transfer from the OR team requires that the anesthesiologist and circulating nurse give a handoff report to PACU staff. TJC's National Patient Safety Goal 02.05.01 requires that the handoff include "interactive communication that allows . . . opportunity for questioning between the giver and receiver of patient information."

The American Society of Perianesthesia Nurses (ASPAN) requires PACU nurses to be certified in advanced cardiac life support (ACLS) and certified in pediatric advanced life support (PALS) if pediatric patients are to be in the recovery room. PACU nurses must also have appropriate training for rendering care to the immediate postoperative patient to identify and address any anesthesia-related issues. The primary responsibilities of the PACU nurse are (1) monitoring vital signs, (2) treating symptoms of postoperative nausea and vomiting, and (3) managing postoperative pain. Housewide management of patient flow sometimes calls for interplay between the ICU and the PACU. Patients may recover in the ICU, or the PACU may be called upon to house intensive care patients when the ICU is full. Whichever situation occurs, all nurses must be credentialed to care for the patient population they are assigned to care for, and their competencies in this environment should be evaluated annually in the course of routine performance appraisals. It must also be noted that, if the patient is being cared for in the ICU as an alternative to the PACU, there must be appropriate availability of anesthesia support.

It is important to remember that the PACU is an open ward with patients who cough frequently and staff who may have a great deal of contact with discharge from airways. The staffing ratio in the PACU is generally two patients to one nurse, which poses the challenge of cross-contamination. Careful hand hygiene, as well as other infection control prevention strategies, is critical to prevent the spread of infection. Once discharge criteria have been met, outpatients are discharged accompanied by a competent adult and inpatients are transferred to the appropriate unit in the hospital. Handoff communication takes place once again between the PACU staff and caregivers in the recipient setting.

Transfer to the Outpatient Discharge Unit

Patients leaving the PACU must meet the postanesthesia recovery scoring (PARS) system discharge criteria, which are much more complex than the criteria that must be satisfied before the patient can advance from the second phase of recovery, which enables them to leave the healthcare facility. (Please see Box 6.2.) Second-phase discharge criteria may be as simple as maintaining vital signs and urinating before discharge.

BOX 6.2   Postanesthesia Recovery Scoring (PARS) System

I. CLINICAL POLICIES

A. The Post Anesthesia Recovery Score (PARS) will be used to:
  1. evaluate and determine the recovery progress of the patient post-anesthesia
  2. evaluate and determine the recovery progress of the patient after administration of moderate sedation/analgesia (conscious sedation)
  3. provide objective information on the physical condition of patients arriving in PACU after anesthesia
  4. set criteria for discharge from any recovery area

B. The scoring system is as follows:

Activity—the muscular activity is assessed by observing the ability of the patient to move his/her limbs either spontaneously or on command	
Score = 2	moves all extremities
Score = 1	moves 2 extremities
Score = 0	unable to move

Respiration—respiratory effort is assessed by observation rather than mechanical diagnostics	
Score = 2	able to deep breathe/cough independently
Score = 1	respiratory effort limited/airway management required
Score = 0	mechanical assistance

Circulation—circulatory status is evaluated using arterial blood pressure	
Score = 2	BP+/- 20 points of preanesthetic level
Score = 1	BP+/- 20 to 50 points of preanesthetic level
Score = 0	BP+/- 50 points of preanesthetic level

Consciousness—assessed by the patient's ability to answer simple questions and follow verbal commands	
Score = 2	oriented to time, place, and person
Score = 1	responds to verbal stimuli
Score = 0	no response

Color—patients are to be scored on their color whether their skin/nailbeds/mucosa color was present prior to surgery or not	
Score = 2	normal color
Score = 1	pale, dusky, flushed
Score = 0	cyanotic

(Continued)

C. Standardized discharge criteria, based on the Post Anesthesia Recovery Scoring system, will be approved by the Department of Anesthesia for all patients who have received anesthesia and/or moderate sedation/analgesia.

II. RATIONALE

A formalized scoring system will ensure continuity for all patients who have received moderate sedation/analgesia.

III. DATES

Originally formulated:	as Diagnostic Treatment Center unit-specific policy POST-ANESTHESIA RECOVERY SCORE
Originally approved:	Department of Anesthesia, August 1997
Reviewed/Revised:	Policy and Procedure Committee, July 1997, September 2000, August 2003
Approved:	Operations Directors Team September 15, 2003

Source: Dekalb Regional Healthcare System, Decatur, GA 2003. Reprinted with permission.

Medication reconciliation is particularly important for surgical patients because of the need to ensure that medications that were withheld during a procedure are reinstated. A consistently managed approach to medication reconciliation is an important element of key general strategies to reduce the risk of adverse drug events. TJC's National Patient Safety Goal on medication reconciliation was released in 2005. TJC recognizes the complexity and difficulty of reconciling medication at all transitions of care and announced in March of 2009 that it will evaluate process to reconcile medication at the time of survey, but no requirements for improvement (RFIs) will be generated and comments will not be in the accreditation report. Nevertheless, medication reconciliation should be a goal for all organizations at all transitions in care.

In addition to discussion of the medication regime, postoperative teaching that accompanies discharge instructions should address concerns specific to the procedure performed, for example, dressing changes. It is also important that such education addresses general healthcare needs, such as smoking cessation advice, diabetic teaching, and other disease-specific management information. Discharge instructions should be clear and in writing, and the nurse must make every effort to ensure that the patient understands what is expected of him or her. The family and/or significant others play a key role in the discharge process and should be included whenever possible. Patients are typically not allowed to drive themselves home, and it is often suggested that they have someone with them for the first twenty-four hours.

Transfer to the Inpatient Unit

Just as for outpatients, inpatients may be transferred to the appropriate surgical unit only after PACU discharge criteria have been met. Some units are generalized surgical settings, and others have developed a procedure-specific model of care. One model used for postoperative total joint surgery patients has revolutionized the way in which these patients navigate the first three postoperative days. The plan of care is built on a wellness theme that promotes movement and group participation instead of bed rest and isolation. Such models result in a faster return to the normal activities of daily living and overall patient and family satisfaction.

Other surgical patients may require more intense observation, such as that provided in the intensive care unit. Varying levels of care are usually available throughout the hospital, and the surgeon determines the environment that best meets the individual patient's needs.

In the ambulatory surgery center (ASC) environment, the patient is usually discharged to home to recover because the procedures performed are generally less risky and less invasive than those that require more acute care. Ambulatory surgery centers by their nature do not house patients longer than twenty-four hours, and most are considered day facilities. To ensure patient safety, transfer agreements for facilities that can manage a higher level of care (acute care hospital) and protocols to address when and where patients in crisis are sent should be recorded in writing and known to all staff. In addition, surgeons on staff at the ASC need to be credentialed and have privileges at a local hospital where patients can be sent for care if necessary. Organizations that accredit ambulatory surgery centers have criteria and policies and procedures with which the ASC must comply. Accrediting bodies include American Association for Accreditation of Ambulatory Surgical Facilities (AAAASF), Accreditation Association for Ambulatory Health Care (AAAHC), TJC, and the American Osteopathic Association (AOA).

· · · · · · · · ·
OPERATING ROOM ENVIRONMENT

Physical Structure

The best possible location for the OR is proximate to both the emergency department and the critical care unit(s). This is particularly true in hospitals that function as trauma centers. The surgical suite is considered a restricted area, which means that traffic is closely monitored and a specific dress code is required to minimize infection. Many suites in large hospitals consist of a holding area, control desk, storage rooms, stage one instrument decontamination room, biomed office, substerile areas, and ORs. Some have camera systems that allow the control desk to view the room, and many have tube systems that allow transportation of documents and other items between the OR and the laboratory and the pharmacy. Most large hospitals have a satellite pharmacy located in the OR to issue and control the drugs ordered by the surgeons and anesthesiologists. Some of the larger, more complex operating suites, in addition to using RFID technology to prevent the unintended retention of surgical objects, also use this or similar technology to track patients and manage patient flow.

Outbreaks of infections have been traced to airborne contamination; consequently, it is important to remove contaminants from the air and control airflow patterns. This is one major reason that ORs have heating, ventilating, and air-conditioning (HVAC) systems that have been specifically designed for this environment. AORN states that the quality of air entering the OR should be carefully controlled and filtered. The period of time required for the ventilation system to achieve a 99.9 percent air exchange is twenty-eight minutes for a cycle of fifteen air exchanges per hour.[5] The relative humidity should be maintained between 30 percent and 60 percent, and the temperature should be maintained between 68 and 73 degrees Fahrenheit. The pressure gradient in the rooms should be positive, and the doors should remain closed whenever possible. AORN standards also require alternate sources of lighting and electrical power, and this source should begin operating within ten seconds after the interruption.

The increased role of technology in surgical procedures over the past twenty years has necessitated larger ORs, with rooms expanding from a norm of 400 square feet to 800 square feet or more. Most ORs also have ceiling-mounted booms to house equipment and keep electrical cords and other clutter off the floor. Computers and picture archiving and communication systems (PACS) that allow access to radiological images take up room, and if applicable, a remote console for robotic surgery requires even more space. Also, endovascular labs are often located in the surgical suite, and most have additional space for imaging equipment. Overall, the less invasive procedures become, the more room is required to house the technology responsible for this quality of care improvement.

Gas cylinders that are stored in the surgical suite should be kept in a secure area separate from industrial gases (AORN Perioperative Standards and Recommended Practices). Empty cylinders must never be kept in the same area as the full ones. Specific guidelines for storage areas must be followed, and the cylinders must be kept in a holder designed to prevent tipping.

Surgical lights must be bright but produce a minimum of radiant heat to reduce damage to exposed tissues and prevent discomfort to the surgical team. Lights should also be equipped with an automatic switch that initiates emergency power should an interruption occur.

Surgical Instrument Processing

All surgical suites require a surgical processing department to provide supplies, sterilize individual instruments, and provide sterilized instrument trays for the procedures. Most large hospitals use a case cart system to transport case-specific supplies to the OR. Many surgical processing departments also serve as the sterilization center for the entire facility, providing services to labor and delivery, the emergency department, and other procedure areas. Both AAMI (Association for the Advancement of Medical Instrumentation) and AORN provide very complex standards of operation for sterilization and instrument processing, recognizing that if sterilization is compromised in any way, patient risk increases exponentially. Proper sterilization, handling of trays, storage of trays, and maintaining quarantine parameters are an essential aspect of this department's role in patient care.

In most surgical processing departments today, the primary means of sterilization are steam, peracetic acid, and hydrogen peroxide. All related processes require instrument technicians who receive ongoing education and constant updates on sterilization methods, as well as the instrument and equipment manufacturers' recommended guidelines. This department is the foundation for the successful use of surgical equipment in the OR.

Flash Sterilization

Flash sterilization, a shortcut for processing instruments, is associated with increased patient infection risks. Flashing occurs when (1) an instrument(s) is cleaned by someone other than the central instrument processing department, using abbreviated decontamination methods; (2) a gravity displacement steam sterilization is used for an abbreviated amount of sterilizing time; or (3) the instrument(s) is autoclaved and transported in an open pan. AORN suggests that flash sterilization should not be used routinely, and it should not be used in lieu of purchasing additional instrumentation. However, TJC surveyors note that many hospitals employ flash sterilization routinely. If flash sterilization is used, it should be limited to specific equipment with clearly delineated guidelines for use. The compliance of staff with such restrictions and the effectiveness of any flash sterilization function must be continually assessed.

· · · · · · · · ·

ORGANIZATIONAL STRUCTURE

Medical Director

In most hospitals, a medical director or chief of surgery serves as the primary medical administrative officer for the department of surgery. Department chiefs or medical directors are responsible for all medical activities occurring within their departments and must account for departmental performance. They are expected to help coordinate activities within the department, including the overall operation and budgeting process. Although many medical directors are paid employees, more physicians who serve as chief of the service are voted into this position by their colleagues. Nursing and administration rely heavily on this role, and thus the individual with this responsibility must demonstrate a high level of competence and strong negotiating skills. In short, this is a leadership role, and as TJC noted in a sentinel event alert (which can be accessed at www.jointcommission.org/SentinelEvents/SentinelEventAlert/sea_43.htm), leadership is absolutely essential to safety.

Anesthesia Director

Anesthesia plays a key role in the daily operations of any surgical suite, and a successful outcome is dependent on the clear direction established by the anesthesia director or chief. In many ORs, the department of anesthesia actually runs the daily schedule, including determinations about add-on cases, blocks, and future schedules. The ability to start cases on time and have a quick turnover is clearly contingent on the anesthesia department's commitment to its business metrics. Anesthesia is also essential in ensuring the department's ability to meet regulatory and quality requirements. The attitude required to achieve these goals is determined by the director or chief.

Nursing Director

AORN Standard II of Standards of Perioperative Administrative Practice states that a registered nurse qualified by advanced education and management experience shall have administrative responsibility for perioperative nursing services. The director, working in collaboration with the chiefs of surgery and anesthesia, is responsible for articulating the mission of the area, as well as strategic planning, meeting regulatory and quality requirements, fiscal oversight, risk management, staffing, and clinical applications. This position requires someone who embraces change and can function as a change agent by motivating staff to understand and accept it.

Team Leaders

Many ORs have team leaders who multitask throughout the department. Often they are head nurses of the different surgical area service lines, and as such, they are responsible for ensuring that each patient on their service is supported with appropriate equipment and supplies. They also serve as resource nurses and participate in the orientation of new employees. Their role in this regard is key to patient safety and risk management, because patients' risks increase when a new staff member comes on board. The department must have well-designed programs to orient the new staff member and help ensure his or her contribution to safe care.

Performance Improvement Teams

Clinical processes and systems define our ability to be successful and safe. Both are a sequence of steps directed at achieving a goal or outcome. These steps should be subject to constant scrutiny for opportunities that may result in refinement or change. And, because surgery has so many far-reaching ramifications for the patient, the pursuit of performance improvement is an ongoing endeavor. Many perioperative services have a dedicated quality coordinator who coordinates the assessment, reassessment and improvement activities of the performance improvement (PI) teams. In addition, the coordinator oversees the collection of data that support participation in SCIP and other surgery-related quality improvement initiatives. Perioperative morbidity and mortality rates should be evaluated concurrent with these efforts.

· · · · · · · · ·
PERIOPERATIVE SCORECARD

ORs are a hospital's biggest revenue generator, as well as its largest expense. Therefore, although our primary goal is patient safety, we must also be efficient and productive. That's why it's important to measure all the dimensions that contribute to a safe patient environment, including revenues and costs.

The goal is quality care for the best possible price. It is important that clinicians understand how these two forces interact. For instance, we have often heard surgeons complain that they don't have enough of the right tools in the OR. It is important to make clear that the money to acquire the needed tools could be available if, for instance, procedures weren't as frequently delayed, causing overtime costs, or cancelled. The surgeon can help the OR run more efficiently and safely by telling the patient to go to PAT and preoperative class. Although the interrelatedness of all these processes makes measuring just one of them a challenge, it is essential that all aspects of care continually be assessed. Results must then be shared with clinicians to facilitate quality improvement and efficiency.

A balanced scorecard is the foundation for the alignment of processes because what gets measured is what gets done.[6] See Table 6.1, Balanced Scorecard Project.

TABLE 6.1   **Balanced Scorecard Project**

Summarize Objectives, Measurements, Targets & Initiatives/Programs

	Strategic Objectives	*Measurements*	*Targets*			*Initiatives/Programs*
			Period 1	*Period 2*	*Period 3*	
Financial	*Insert financial objective*	*Insert financial measurement*	*Target*	*Target*	*Target*	*Since financial is the final outcome, there may not be any formal programs directly related to the Financial Perspective.*
Customer	*Insert customer objective*	*Insert customer measurement*	*Target*	*Target*	*Target*	*Briefly describe the programs that will address your customer-related objectives.*
Internal Processes	*Insert internal process objective*	*Insert internal process measurement*	*Target*	*Target*	*Target*	*Briefly describe the programs that will address your internal process–related objectives.*
Learning	*Insert learning & growth objective*	*Insert learning & growth measurement*	*Target*	*Target*	*Target*	*Briefly describe the programs that will address your learning- & growth-related objectives.*

Source: Reprinted with the permission of Marshall / Steele

Sample Measures

The template in Table 6.1 is the basis for a balanced scorecard for perioperative services, using a sample set of measures. The final scorecard should allow the review of both current levels and trends in key measures or indicators of organizational performance. These may include productivity, turnaround times, use rates, cost reduction, waste reduction, clinical quality, partner performance, and other appropriate measures of effectiveness and efficiency.[7] Table 6.2 identifies some sample measures.

TABLE 6.2   Sample Measures

Perspective and Measures	*Frequency*	*Segment*[i]	*Additional Comment*
Financial: To succeed financially, how should we appear to our stakeholders?			
OR cases and OR hours	Weekly	Physician, group	Assessment of weekly budget vs. actual volumes
Variable cost per case	Monthly	CPT code	
Total cost per case	Monthly	CPT code	
Cost per minute	Monthly	Top 10 procedures	
Paid hours per OR hour	Biweekly	—	
Days to final bill for OR cases	Monthly	By payer	
Overtime hours per day	Biweekly	—	
Net margin per OR minute	Monthly	Top 10 procedures	
Customer: To achieve our vision, how should we appear to our patients?			
Patient satisfaction	Monthly	Physician, anesthesiologist, inpatient, same-day surgery	Covers preadmission testing, patient intake, and PACU. Questions include five standard dimensions of service quality measurement[ii] (empathy, assurance, reliability, responsiveness, and tangibles).
Case cancellations on day of surgery	Weekly	Reason code	
Patient wait on day of surgery (minutes)	Weekly	Reason code	Determine the root cause of delays.
Number of patients requiring day of surgery testing	Weekly	Reason code	
Internal Processes: To satisfy our stakeholders and patients, at what key processes must we excel?			
Average minutes in PACU after recovery	Monthly	Anesthesia type	
Census days in PACU	Monthly	—	
% of first cases on-time patient in-room	Weekly	Physician, anesthesiologist	
% of cases with room turnover in less than *x* minutes	Weekly	Physician, nursing team	

(Continued)

TABLE 6.2   Sample Measures (*Continued*)

Perspective and Measures	*Frequency*	*Segment*[i]	*Additional Comment*
% of cases with incomplete instrumentation	Weekly	Physician	To identify opportunities for preference card updates and request for additional instrumentation.
% of cases with incomplete supplies	Weekly	Physician	
OR block utilization	Daily	Physician, group	
% of OR days with more than *y* cases	Weekly	—	
Infection rates	Monthly	Physician, CPT code	
Patient safety measures (antibiotics selection, started, stopped, intraoperative temperature, shaving, time-outs)	Monthly	Physician, anesthesiologist	
Booked vs. actual case duration variance	Monthly	Physician	
Average case duration		Physician	
Average days between case scheduling and surgery	Monthly	Physician	
Number of repeat diagnostic tests	Monthly	PA, anesthesiologist	

Learning and Growth: To achieve our vision, how will we sustain our ability to change and improve?

Staff satisfaction	Quarterly	Staff type	
Physician satisfaction	Quarterly	—	
Training hours per FTE per year	Annual	Staff type	
Staff turnover	Quarterly	Staff type	

[i]Segment refers to the logical grouping used to disaggregate data in a way that allows for meaningful analysis of performance.

[ii]Parasuraman, A., Berry, L.L., and Zeithaml, V.A. (1988) "SERVQUAL: A multiple-item scale for measuring customer perceptions of service quality."*Journal of Retailing* 64 (1) Spring:12–40.

Source: Reprinted with the permission of Marshall / Steele

• • • • • • • • •

CONCLUSION

OR safety is the responsibility of leadership. Although efficiency is extremely important, it must always take a backseat to safety. The most critical component of safety in the OR is the culture of safety that the surgeons, anesthesiologists, and staff create together for the patient. This culture is supported by the checklists, tasks, metrics, and systems that are implemented. ORs must be SAFE.

S — Superior systems

A — Absolute accountability

F — First priority

E — Enthusiastic engagement

Endnotes

1. Marshall, S. "Managing for Metrics." In: *Orthopedics and Spine: Strategies for Superior Service Line Performance*. Marblehead, Mass.: *HealthLeaders Media*, 2009. Available at: www.healthleadersmedia.com/print/PHY-239886/Managing-from-Metrics. Accessed March 31, 2010.

2. Mack A., Rock I. "Inattentional Blindness: An Overview" *PSYCHE*, 1999, 5(3).

3. More information on the Standards and Practices and ordering information can be found at: www.aorn.org/PracticeResources/AORNStandardsAndRecommendedPractices/. Accessed April 8, 2010.

4. Valenstein, PN, Raab SS, and Walsh MK. "Identification errors involving clinical laboratories: A College of American Pathologists Q-Probes study of patient and specimen identification errors at 120 institutions." *Archives of Pathology and Laboratory Medicine* 2006, 130(8):1106–1113.

5. AORN Recommended Practices Committee. *Recommended Practices Environmental Cleaning in the Surgical Practice Setting*, VII.d.1, pp 13–14. Available at: www.aorn. org/docs/assets/EEE0D99B-DC58–58BD-EEC88C83DD6AA9CB/RPEnviron_Clean_ pub%20com_10–29–07.pdf. Accessed April 8, 2020.

6. Aplan, R. S. and D. P. Norton. "Using the balanced scorecard as a strategic management system." *Harvard Business Review* 1996, 74(1):75–85.

7. The term *effective* refers to how well a process or measure addresses its intended purpose.

7

Managing Risks and Improving Safety in the Intensive Care Unit

Cynthia Wallace
Linda Wallace

Intensive care units (ICUs) account for 10 percent of all inpatient acute care beds in the United States, collectively making up one of the largest and most costly components of the nation's healthcare system.[1] ICUs provide care to more than five million acutely ill patients per year at an annual cost of $180 billion, accounting for 30 percent of U.S. hospital costs.[2] In addition to being high volume and high cost, ICUs are also very high risk. Despite the dedication and competency of ICU caregivers, patient mortality rates in ICUs approximate 10 to 20 percent, and some studies suggest that medical errors and adverse events affect nearly all ICU patients.[3]

The combination of high-risk patients and an error-prone environment makes ICUs high-risk settings, exposing healthcare organizations to potentially high medical malpractice losses and to operational and other losses. Consider the following figures. The associated annual costs of managing adverse events in two 10-bed ICUs is nearly $1.5 million for one 720-bed hospital.[4] Additionally, one medical malpractice insurer reports that the average indemnity payment (for closed ICU claims resulting in a payment) in its insured hospitals between 2000 and 2008 was $319,000, and the average cost to defend the claims was $62,300.[5]

Note: The authors gratefully acknowledge the work of Peter J. Pronovost, MD, PhD, and Kathleen Shostek, RN, ARM, BBA, FASHRM, coauthors of this chapter when it first appeared in the fifth edition of ASHRM's *Risk Management Handbook for Health Care Organizations.*

Modern error theory suggests that ICUs are error prone due to the complexity of the environment, the presence of multiple caregivers, and the high number of interactions among them. Contributing to the intricate nature of the ICU is the high acuity of patient illnesses, the use of complex medical technologies, the performance of invasive procedures, and the need to continuously monitor patients who are medically unstable. In addition, the devices and technology used to perform procedures or monitor patients all carry the potential for failure or misuse if not operated or maintained properly.

Principles of human factors analysis also indicate that the high stress, high complexity, and staff diversity typically found in ICU environments make them fertile ground for distractions, miscommunications, and fatigue that lead to mistakes, errors, and adverse events.[6] Time pressures, space limitations, and budgetary constraints also affect patient safety in ICUs by restricting the availability of direct care providers at the bedside, limiting the ability of family members to remain with (and advocate for) patients, and reducing staff access to critical equipment and supplies.

Common occurrences that contribute to adverse events and poor outcomes, which lead to increased lengths of stay and potential liability claims in ICUs, include medication and intravenous (IV) errors, events during physical transport outside the ICU or transfer of responsibility for care (handoffs), injuries associated with airways or ventilator use, central catheter–related complications, infections such as catheter-related bloodstream infections (BSIs) and ventilator-associated pneumonias (VAPs), and failures to rescue or intervene in a timely or appropriate manner when a patient's condition worsens. Studies of human errors in ICUs indicate that communication breakdowns and the failure to convey important information from one caregiver to another contribute significantly to these types of occurrences.[7] This is consistent with the finding that communication issues are the most frequent root cause of all categories of sentinel events reported to The Joint Commission.[8]

The aging of the nursing workforce and a shortage of critical care–trained nurses also affects the ability of ICUs to provide high-quality bedside care. Provision of medical care to ICU patients by resident physicians in various levels of training is common in facilities in which teaching programs exist. The quality of supervision provided by senior physicians who oversee critical care in teaching facilities varies, as does compliance with limitations on residents' work hours, and inexperience and fatigue inevitably have a major effect on patient safety. Also, the use of intensivists in ICUs, physicians with specialized training in critical care medicine, is low,[9] even though evidence suggests that the use of intensivists in ICUs is associated with lower hospital mortality and reduced hospital and ICU stays.[10]

The quality of hospital support services also affects ICU care. Hospital information systems vary in their ability to support clinicians in communicating the information necessary for critical decision making. Pharmacy, laboratory, and imaging services may or may not provide an optimal level of therapeutic and diagnostic support for the care of critical patients. Inefficient and incomplete systems and services may negatively impact the timeliness, accuracy, and quality of care provided in this setting.

Risk management professionals and patient safety officers can address these and other challenges by collaborating with senior leaders, physicians, ICU managers, and the critical care staff to transform critical care units into safer, more patient-friendly units with lower liability risk exposure. They can also help the hospital and community capitalize on the value of critical care services. With proper support and commitment, critical care units can embody the elements of high-reliability organizations (HROs), organizations that perform extremely well with few errors or adverse events over the long term even though they face high intrinsic hazards and risks.[11] In this chapter, current approaches to improving quality, enhancing safety, and managing risks in ICUs are reviewed, and examples of advances and successes in critical care safety are highlighted.

· · · · · · · · ·
ICU CULTURE AND PATIENT SAFETY

An integral part of improving reliability and quality of services provided is the creation of a culture of safety across the healthcare organization. Patient safety initiatives focused on the ICU have a much greater chance of success if they are preceded by such a culture.[12] In fact, safety culture can be thought of as the lubrication that allows system redesign. Organizations with a culture of safety, either in healthcare or in other industries such as aviation and nuclear energy, approach safety systematically; indeed, system safety is the number one priority. A safety culture supports openness about errors and problems so that the organization can learn from these events and focus on improving performance within the organization.

Characteristics of a culture of safety in ICU include a commitment to speak up and raise concerns about behaviors and processes of care that have the potential to compromise safety. Equally important, an ICU culture of safety also fosters a willingness to listen when others express concerns, especially when those concerns involve risk to patients that may be rooted in "the way we do things around here." The organization with a culture of safety strives to identify system flaws and process errors, and when system defects are identified, the organization makes changes to eliminate or minimize the defects. The degree to which communication and teamwork failures contribute to The Joint Commission's sentinel events highlights the impact of safety culture on patients. Indeed, The Joint Commission's leadership standards for many of its accreditation programs, including its program for hospitals, require a culture of safety and a systems approach to quality improvement focused on responsibilities and accountabilities of leadership.

Crucial to a safety culture is enduring support from key leadership of the organization's administration and medical staff. Hospital administrative support is vital to obtaining the financial, staff, and moral support necessary for organizational change and care unit improvement. Physician champions are particularly vital to critical care patient safety programs because they facilitate the support of other clinicians and promote motivation of the frontline staff. Fundamental to the success of a culture of safety is involving all critical care staff in the initiative. Staff must understand that they are the backbone of a team that fosters the unit's safety culture.

Safety culture is both measurable and improvable. Several safety culture survey instruments that evaluate communication, teamwork, management support, and other aspects of a safety culture are available. The Hospital Survey on Patient Safety Culture, performed by the Agency for Healthcare Research and Quality (AHRQ) and available at www.ahrq.gov/qual/patientsafetyculture/hospsurvindex.htm, measures safety culture in specific work areas, such as the ICU. Data collected from more than twelve thousand individuals working in ICUs in four hundred hospitals show that ICUs, like most other hospital units, score highest in facilitating teamwork within the ICU and lowest in non-punitive approaches to error reporting.[13]

A safety attitudes questionnaire (SAQ), developed by the University of Texas-Memorial Hermann Center for Healthcare Quality and Safety, provides another valid and reliable way to measure safety culture.[14] A SAQ designed specifically for the ICU is available at www.utpatientsafety.org. The SAQ was incorporated as part of a comprehensive unit-based safety program (CUSP) for improving safety culture and other safety outcomes in the ICU settings at Johns Hopkins Hospital (JHH), Baltimore, Maryland. The improvement of safety culture was validated in the hospital's two ICUs,[15] and it was then expanded to nearly one hundred ICUs in a statewide ICU improvement project in Michigan. A federally funded project, known as On the CUSP: Stop BSI, will implement a slightly modified version of a CUSP in more than one hundred hospitals in ten states to improve ICU safety, particularly with regard to central line–associated BSIs.

The CUSP model used for the JHH and Michigan projects is based on the following six steps:[16]

1. Assess the culture of safety: A starting point for the achievement of an improved culture of safety is an assessment of the current culture (or climate), using tools such as the SAQ and/or AHRQ's safety culture survey, to determine whether and how that culture affects the provision of safe patient care.

2. Provide education on the science of safety: Physicians and staff need to understand system safety concepts to apply them to patient care processes. Resources for developing safety science education programs are provided at the end of this chapter.

3. Identify system safety concerns: Safety teams seek to identify system safety concerns. There are multiple ways to accomplish this, including walking rounds by leadership, patient safety reporting systems, morbidity and mortality conferences, review of the facts underlying liability claims, and perhaps most important, asking staff how the next patient might be harmed and what they could do to prevent it.

4. Develop senior leader partnerships with units: Successful system safety programs assign responsibility to senior executives for specific care units and make them accountable to follow through on culture of safety improvement initiatives. With this approach, senior leaders become part of the unit-based teams, meeting with them regularly and seeking to mitigate system safety error-prone process concerns.

5. Learn from one defect per month: Staff are asked to learn from one defect (safety concern) per month. Patient safety issues are prioritized and improvements are implemented. To achieve a better understanding, employees are provided with a structured tool with which to learn from defects in care. Specific questions include the following: What happened? Why did it happen (that is, what contributed to it)? What could you do to reduce the probability that it will happen again? Results are summarized as a one-page document for sharing in the organization. Employees are

also asked to implement tools to improve teamwork and communication and to reduce system safety hazards. These tools include, among others, a daily goals sheet, shadowing another professional, observing rounds, and briefings and debriefings. Refer to the resource list at the end of this chapter for information on accessing these tools online.

6. Reassess the safety culture: The successful organization periodically reassesses its system safety culture.

The success of CUSP at JHH has been demonstrated in several ways, including improved safety climate, reduced ICU patient lengths of stay, fewer medication errors, and decreased nurse turnover rates.[17] In Michigan, the safety program was also used successfully to improve the system safety climate of nearly one hundred ICUs and eliminate catheter-related BSIs.[18] In addition to improving patient care, these efforts aimed at transforming ICU care demonstrate the value of patient safety efforts from a business perspective.

The Patient Safety Group, a Massachusetts-based patient organization whose mission is to promote a safety culture in healthcare, provides the electronic version of the comprehensive unit-based safety program (eCUSP) to healthcare organizations. The eCUSP greatly aids in project management by keeping a database of safety concerns and active and completed projects. It also summarizes what was learned in a shared story that can be broadly disseminated. Information about eCUSP is available online at www.patientsafetygroup.org.

· · · · · · · · ·
COMMUNICATION AND TEAMWORK

To effectively manage the complex work involved in providing care to critically ill patients, staff need a clear understanding of what tasks and treatments are to be performed and when, what observations and interventions need to be made, as well as how to prevent, detect, and manage complications and pain. But, most important, the entire care team must know what the goals of treatment are: what needs to be done today to help a patient progress to the next level of care. The whole team must also be aware of any changes in the patient's condition that require treatment or enhanced monitoring. Clear, concise, and complete communication is a crucial component of critical care. Errors attributed to communication failures are recognized as a significant issue in the ICU and in malpractice litigation.[19]

The AHRQ safety culture survey assesses teamwork and communication throughout the hospital and within the ICU. The 2009 results include responses from twelve thousand individuals working in the critical care setting. Although these individuals indicated that their units foster an environment of teamwork, there was room for improvement in communication and openness (see Table 7.1, Critical Care Settings Rate Unit's Patient Safety Culture).

Communication breakdowns in the critical care setting are frequent and may occur in a variety of ways. A 2006 report by Pronovost and colleagues found that, of 2,075 incidents from twenty-three ICUs over a period of twenty-seven months, a wide range of

TABLE 7.1   Critical Care Settings Rate Unit's Patient Safety Culture

Survey Item	Percent Positive Response
Teamwork within units	
People support one another in this unit.	88%
When a lot of work needs to be done quickly, we work together as a team to get the work done.	88
In this unit, people treat each other with respect.	80
When one area in this unit gets really busy, others help out.	74
Average composite-level response	83
Organizational learning/continuous improvement	
We are actively doing things to improve patient safety.	83
Mistakes have led to positive changes here.	57
After we make changes to improve patient safety, we evaluate their effectiveness.	67
Average composite-level response	69
Communication openness	
Staff will freely speak up if they see something that may negatively affect patient care.	75
Staff feel free to question the decisions or actions of those with more authority.	44
Staff are afraid to ask questions when something does not seem right.	63
Average composite-level response	61
Teamwork across units	
Hospital units do not coordinate well with each other.	39
There is good cooperation among hospital units that need to work together.	52
It is often unpleasant to work with staff from other hospital units.	60
Hospital units work well together to provide the best care for patients.	60
Average composite-level response	53

Source: Agency for Healthcare Research and Quality. "Hospital Survey on Patient Safety Culture: 2009 Comparative Database Report." Available at www.ahrq.gov/qual/hospsurvey09/hosp09tabb2.htm and www.ahrq.gov/qual/hospsurvey09/hosp09tabb1.htm. (Accessed August 6, 2009).

Note: The "Hospital Survey on Patient Safety Culture" includes responses by work areas or units. The findings for critical care units are based on 12,040 responses at 401 hospitals. The percent positive response is based on those who responded "Strongly disagree" or "Disagree," or "Never" or "Rarely" (depending on the response category used for the item).

factors related to communication were found to underlie critical incidents.[20] For example, team factors contributed to 32 percent of errors. These errors consisted of problems with verbal/written communication during routine care (19 percent of incidents) and problems with verbal/written communication during handoffs (12 percent of errors).

Risk management professionals should work with the critical care team to develop strategies to improve communications during routine care, handoffs, and crises. For example, consideration may be given to providing critical care staff members with training in communication and teamwork, including techniques that have proven successful in other high-intensity organizations such as aviation, which uses a teamwork tool called crew resource management.

Examples of ICU handoff situations include staff shift changes, transfer of treating physicians in or out of units and to or from on-call responsibility, and patient transfers into and out of the critical care unit. It is clear that a taped change of shift report that does not allow for real-time interaction between caregivers is no longer acceptable.

Recognizing the importance of communication during transitions in care to patient safety, The Joint Commission requires specific approaches to improve the effectiveness of communication among caregivers. The Joint Commission's National Patient Safety Goal on improving communication among caregivers, has included strategies to improve handoff communications by encouraging staff to ask and respond to questions. For example, the handoff communication between the giver and receiver of patient information should include up-to-date information regarding the patient's condition, care, treatment, medications, services, and any recent or anticipated changes. These provisions were incorporated into The Joint Commission's accreditation standards as of 2010.

Another provision of The Joint Commission's goal to improve the effectiveness of communication among caregivers addresses communication of critical test results, an important issue in critical care because many therapies are predicated on the results of laboratory and radiology tests and on consultations with specialists. For example, when an individual receives critical test results by telephone, The Joint Commission requires that the individual giving the test result verify that the correct information has been communicated by having the person receiving the information record and read-back the complete test result.

Risk management professionals must monitor the effectiveness and timeliness of communication between physicians. The use of newer communication technologies (e.g., wireless communication devices) may facilitate communication between physicians; however, if the organization encourages the use of cellular technology, it is recommended that consideration be given to the possibility of electromagnetic interference that can disrupt the operation of critical medical equipment (e.g., by causing malfunction of mechanical ventilators) and create a safety hazard.[21]

The use of prompts, such as communication checklists, may also help to improve critical care communication. One organization developed a handoff protocol checklist that was combined with simulation training for nursing staff in a step-down ventilator unit.[22] The checklist addresses important information to discuss with the next caregiver, such as medications, events during the last shift, laboratory and radiology test results, and tasks expected to be done in the next shift. Communication at change of shift was improved, although certain aspects of care, such as checking the monitor alarms and ventilator at handoff, were not improved. A similar handoff tool for critical care nursing staff to use during multidisciplinary rounds was developed by the Virginia Mason Medical Center in Seattle, Washington, and is available for download from the Web site of the

Institute for Healthcare Improvement (IHI), a patient safety and healthcare quality improvement group in Cambridge, Massachusetts, at www.ihi.org/IHI/Topics/CriticalCare/IntensiveCare/Tools/MultidiscplinaryRoundsCCUNurseHandoffTool.htm. (Free registration is required.)

An innovative means of verbal communication now being used to enhance exchanges of information among caregivers can be applied in the ICU. It follows the acronym SBAR, which stands for[23]

- situation (define the problem);
- background (keep information brief, related, and to the point);
- assessment (summarize what you found or think)
- recommendation (describe what you want).

When all members of the care team understand how to communicate in a consistent way, such as by using SBAR, authority gradient issues are reduced, differences in communication styles are less problematic, and patient safety is enhanced. This has huge implications for the ICU setting for which the quality of collaborative communication is a key factor in patient outcomes.[24]

One healthcare organization, Kaiser Permanente, adopted a multifaceted approach to improving patient safety through improving teamwork and using human factors applications designed to improve patient safety and strategies to enhance interpersonal relationships, as well as a common understanding of how best to communicate important patient information. In implementing this approach, Kaiser used many tools and techniques to educate physicians and other clinical staff in human factors science and empower them to practice safely. Assertiveness training, briefings and debriefings, and situational awareness are among the communication and teamwork training programs that Kaiser continues to provide today.[25] Assertiveness empowers staff to speak up and "stop the line" if necessary when they have a safety concern. Briefings are communications between team members that allow concerns to be raised, the plan of care to be clarified, and important information to be relayed, for example, before a procedure begins. Situational awareness is just that, being aware of what is going on around you to decrease the risk of errors. In addition, because it is important for teams to practice their skills and rehearse the handling of high-risk or emergency situations, lifelike simulators are used at Kaiser in conjunction with human factors education and communication training to enhance teamwork. Simulation allows the team to develop critical thinking skills while rehearsing the procedures to be implemented when certain situations arise. It also helps team members learn how to work together.

Generally, critical care patients who must be transferred to another department for examination or treatment are accompanied by critical care staff. Handoff communication in these instances should be face to face. Critical care staff should bring the medical record and other important documentation with them to the off-unit department for reference. Less critical patients who are transferred may have a "ticket to ride," which lists important information about the patient to be communicated to a receiving department.

When patients are transferred from the ICU to other units for continued care, critical care staff need to ensure that information about patients is carefully communicated to the receiving staff. One hospital developed a discharge record to accompany patients who were transferred from the ICU to other units in the hospital.[26] The authors concluded that the discharge plan positively affected patient transfers from critical care to other units.

Improving quality and creating a culture of safety in the ICU necessarily involves training in patient safety and risk management. All levels of medical, nursing, and ICU support staff should receive education in safety science and be oriented to institutional and unit-specific risk and safety procedures. Ideally, a staff that works as a team should train as a team. In addition to providing education and training for staff members to develop the capacity to successfully function as team members, the organization should strive to provide an environment that promotes teamwork.

ICU staff should also be trained in how to report events, errors, and near misses through easily accessible reporting systems and should receive regular feedback on causes and trends identified through reported events, as well as actions taken to prevent or reduce them. See additional information on this topic later in this chapter.

· · · · · · · · ·
ICU STRUCTURE, STAFFING, AND TRAINING

The makeup of the medical, nursing, and support staff varies greatly in ICUs, as do their organizational structures. Even the terminology for ICU staffing models varies.[27] The terms *open*, *closed*, and *hybrid* have been used to describe critical care organizational models. The open ICU model, the predominant approach in the United States, allows for patient care and management by a diverse medical staff (not all of whom have specific training in critical care medicine), with no single physician responsible for overall management of the ICU. The closed model assigns an intensivist, specially trained in critical care medicine, to the management of patients. The hybrid model incorporates aspects of both open and closed units.

Recent studies of critical care staffing have grouped ICU physician staffing into high intensity, a closed model or an open model with mandatory intensivist consultation, and low intensity, with elective intensivist consultation or no intensivist available.[28] An estimated 73 percent of ICUs in the United States have low-intensity coverage (20 percent with some intensivist coverage and 53 percent with none), and 26 percent have high-intensity coverage.[29]

There is extensive evidence that staffing ICUs with physicians who are specifically trained in critical care medicine improves patient outcomes. Studies of ICU attending physician staffing strategies and outcomes of hospital and ICU mortality and length of stay have consistently shown that hospitals using specially trained intensivists in their ICUs had lower hospital and ICU mortality rates as well as lower hospital lengths of stay.[30] One exception to this support was a recent study of nearly 125 ICUs, published in 2008. This research raised questions about the earlier findings by determining that mortality rates were higher for patients managed by critical care physicians than those who were not.[31]

Although this study may prompt further evaluation of the effectiveness of intensivist-staffed ICUs, professional groups and healthcare purchasers continue to press for use of intensivist-based staffing. The Society of Critical Care Medicine (SCCM) has advocated an intensivist-led, multiprofessional ICU team as a model for ICU staffing.[32] Indeed, support for the use of ICU-certified physicians to staff ICUs has been echoed by AHRQ and included in the 30 Safe Practices endorsed by the National Quality Forum.[33,34] Both organizations cite evidence that, through the use of intensivists, adverse events and errors in ICUs can be reduced or prevented. Likewise, the Leapfrog Group, a coalition of employers and other purchasers of healthcare services, has required use of intensivists among the standards it uses for rating patient safety in healthcare organizations.

Of the 1,282 hospitals that responded to the Leapfrog Group Hospital Quality and Safety Survey in 2008, 31 percent said they had physicians who are intensive care specialists (intensivists) on their ICU staff, and another 7 percent indicated that they planned to implement the use of intensivists by 2009.[35] Compliance with this particular Leapfrog standard is up from 10 percent in 2002. Nevertheless, intensivist staffing in the United States still trails behind that used in Europe and Australia, where closed ICUs are the norm and the majority of care (80 percent) is initiated by intensivists. The reasons for the underuse of intensivists in the United States are varied and may include perceived costs of implementing intensivist-staffed ICUs, a shortage of critical care–certified physicians, and resistance to a major change in how critical care is provided.

The above-noted shortage of critical care physicians is a concern. Most of the facilities with high intensivist-use ICUs are teaching hospitals. Outside the academic medical setting, smaller hospitals may be unable to support full-time intensivists, making it necessary for them to explore options that can help them achieve optimal ICU physician coverage. Such strategies include using specialists, such as pulmonologists and anesthesiologists, who can demonstrate appropriate training and extensive ICU experience; hiring hospitalists to work in the ICU; increasing the number of physician extenders, such as nurse practitioners, working in the ICU setting; implementing telemedicine to enable an off-site intensivist to oversee care remotely; and regionalizing critical care services so that facilities without critical care units can transfer critically ill patients to facilities with the capability to provide critical care.[36]

Physicians who provide care to patients in the ICU should continuously seek to improve and maintain skills in the management of the critically ill. SCCM recommends that non-ICU specialists improve their skills by taking critical care courses and continuing education programs geared toward the management of critically ill or injured patients in the first 24 hours and in the handling of the sudden deterioration of a patient.[37]

Proper credentialing of critical care physicians and midlevel providers is fundamental to managing provider-related risk. One aspect of credentialing that is particularly important to the safety of ICU patients is the granting of privileges according to validated training and skill level, which is crucial to patient safety. Guidelines for granting privileges for the performance of high-risk, high-volume, and problem-prone procedures such as central venous catheterization, pulmonary artery catheterization, airway intubation, mechanical ventilation, and cardioversion and defibrillation have been published by SCCM. Nevertheless, there is wide variation in training, certification, and supervision of these procedures, and related failures commonly contribute to patient harm. It is also important for the ICU staff to have ready access to information about who can perform specific procedures and what degree of supervision is required, especially in teaching facilities.

Staffing a sufficient number of properly trained critical care nurses is also essential for safe and effective ICU care. In fact, researchers have demonstrated the important role of critical care nurses in intercepting medical errors in the ICU before they reach the patient.[38] Further research is warranted, however, to determine the most cost effective nurse staffing ratios for achieving optimal patient outcomes. Many hospitals report an average ICU nurse-to-patient ratio of $1:2$.

Annual validation of critical care competencies for ICU nurses is also recommended. It is especially important to evaluate and document the skills of agency or temporary nursing staff before the start of an assigned shift in the ICU. Certification in critical care nursing provides a specialty credential that also enhances ICU nurse competencies.

As previously noted, SCCM advocates an intensivist-led ICU multidisciplinary team model to optimize the delivery of critical care. In addition to physicians and nurses, pharmacists, respiratory therapists, and other ICU support staff play important roles in promoting optimal outcomes and preventing errors and adverse events. Team staffing plans for ICUs should identify all members of the team and delineate their roles and responsibilities.[39] Additionally, all staff members should receive education that emphasizes patient safety and the importance of event reporting to identify system flaws and prevent future events.

· · · · · · · · ·
INITIATIVES REQUIRE INTEGRATED SYSTEMS

ICUs operate as subparts of larger healthcare facilities; they are subsystems within larger systems, namely, hospitals. When transforming critical care, it is important that the rest of the hospital organization recognize and support the efforts of the ICU because of the interdependency of the ICU and various other hospital departments, personnel, and processes. For example, a successful statewide initiative in Michigan, called the Michigan Keystone ICU Project, identified a goal to reduce potentially lethal catheter-related BSIs, a major contributor to ICU morbidity and mortality. The project involved the coordinated efforts of hospital leaders, ICU doctors and nurses, and ICU staff. For example, as part of the initiative, central catheter insertion kits were redesigned to include a 2 percent chlorhexidine-based solution for skin disinfection to reduce the risk of catheter-related BSIs. This redesign required not only the input of the ICU staff, but also the commitment and cooperation of personnel and departments outside the ICUs.[40]

Although these steps sound easy to accomplish, in many organizations they constitute major purchasing adjustments that require product changes, renegotiation of applicable supply-related contracts, solicitation of alternate distributors, and reevaluation of inventories. Therefore, the subsystem (the ICU) is dependent upon the larger system (the hospital) having an administrative system capable of minimizing system defects. As illustrated by this example, a potential defect is an inability to make changes in products and supplies deemed necessary for improved patient safety. By working together to make change, the combined efforts of the ICUs and hospitals resulted in a 66 percent reduction in BSIs throughout Michigan during the eighteen-month study, thousands of lives were saved, and there were significant cost savings because the hospitals were treating fewer infections.[41]

The emergence of numerous initiatives, whereby payers will no longer reimburse poor-quality care, requires extensive collaboration among multiple stakeholders within hospitals. For example, under an initiative started in 2008, the Centers for Medicare & Medicaid Services (CMS) no longer pays for treatment of certain preventable conditions that develop during a beneficiary's hospital stay because these hospital-acquired conditions (HACs) could have been avoided if caregivers had adhered to accepted guidelines. Of the ten HACs no longer paid for by CMS, several (including catheter-associated urinary tract infection, pressure ulcers, vascular catheter–associated infection, poor glycemic control, and deep vein thrombosis/pulmonary embolism following hip and knee replacement surgery) involve care provided throughout the hospital, including care given in the ICU. Other conditions that can develop in the ICU, such as VAP, are also being considered by CMS for inclusion on the list. Although the bulk of attention has focused on the CMS initiative, other payers in the public and private sector have put similar provisions in place, freeing them from responsibility to pay for certain HACs.

CMS and other payers have also initiated pay-for-performance measures offering physicians financial incentives to achieve performance benchmarks. CMS's Physician Quality Reporting Initiative (PQRI) has several performance goals, for example, a central venous catheter insertion protocol and a directive for head-of-bed elevation to prevent VAP, that are relevant to ICU physicians, who should integrate these measures into their practice.[42]

In addition to designing payment systems that focus on quality, CMS is providing the public with greater access to quality of care information about healthcare providers. CMS's Hospital Compare Web site provides hospital-specific information about their care processes for some conditions, heart attack, heart failure, and pneumonia, for example, that may be managed in the critical care setting.

Enterprise Risk Management

Payment initiatives that target quality of care and public access of information about hospital quality expose facilities to risk across multiple departments, finance, legal, clinical, public relations, information systems, performance improvement, compliance, and utilization departments, to name a few. As discussed elsewhere in this text, organizations can use enterprise risk management (ERM) to address these multiple risks. ERM stresses the value of managing and capitalizing on available resources to address a broad range of risks faced by the healthcare organization, rather than concentrating on narrowly focused issues through risk avoidance alone. This approach goes far beyond the traditional issue of clinical error that increases professional liability exposure or of environmental safety issues that create general liability or property exposures.

The quality and safety of ICU care affects many ERM risk domains, for example, operational, human capital, and strategic. It is important to note that applying this approach in the ICU reinforces the ERM principle that risks can be managed for positive gain. Strategies aimed at reducing the complications of ICU care (central line infections, ventilator injuries, errors of omission, and so on), improving patient outcomes, and reducing lengths of stay clearly create opportunities for operational gain. In addition to the cost reductions associated with fewer complications, benefits include improved patient and family satisfaction, increased availability and turnover of ICU beds, reduced length of stay, and better scores on patient safety indicators and quality/outcome data reports. Such results can clearly help the hospital realize gains in reputation, improved ICU usage, and increased patient volume. Once thought of merely as risks to be managed, the activities associated with ICU operations (providing medical care to high-risk, acutely ill patients) can instead be considered sources of capital to help the hospital gain advantage in the healthcare marketplace.

· · · · · · · · ·
EVENT, ERROR, AND NEAR-MISS REPORTING

Event reports (often called incident reports) were originally designed to serve as risk-identification tools for the risk management professional and notices of potential claims for liability insurance companies. The patient safety movement, stimulated by the Institute of Medicine's 1999 report, *To Err is Human*, increased the importance and expanded the purpose of event reports and highlighted the potential value of examining near misses or close calls, errors that could have harmed the patient but were intercepted before reaching the patient, to understand the causes of errors. The value of reporting events, learning what factors contribute to their occurrence, and taking action to reduce or eliminate those factors is now recognized as key to improving patient safety. However, protection of event reports under peer review and other quality improvement statutes is largely a state-specific and jurisdictional matter with wide variation among states. A voluntary federal initiative, described in more detail below, may help to address some of the variation in state peer review by extending federal protections to organizations that report to patient safety organizations (PSOs).

Because of the high incidence of close calls, errors, and adverse events in ICUs, the internal reporting and collection of ICU events for analysis and trending promotes the identification of system problems that contribute to the events.[43] Therefore, an easily accessible, low-burden system for reporting will enhance the staff's willingness and ability to report errors, events, and near misses. To be successful, however, the culture of the ICU (and the hospital) must be a nonpunitive one in which event reporting is supported and the staff does not fear reprisal for reporting. Hospital leadership must demonstrate their support for the reporting program. For example, by personally thanking staff that report and identify hazardous conditions, leaders show their commitment to safety culture. Also, to encourage continued compliance with event reporting, the staff needs meaningful feedback on how the information in the reports was used and whether any changes were made as a result.

Despite some limitations, the value of external event reporting in identifying trends and common causes of adverse events has been demonstrated through national and state event reporting programs and by The Joint Commission's sentinel event database.[44-46]

FIGURE 7.1   ICU Adverse Events and Near Misses Reported to Pennsylvania Patient Safety Authority, 2008

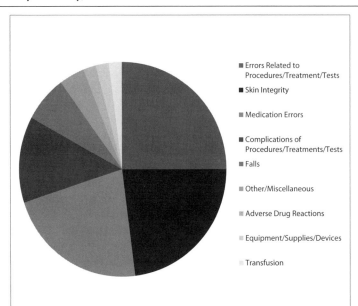

Legend:
- Errors Related to Procedures/Treatment/Tests
- Skin Integrity
- Medication Errors
- Complications of Procedures/Treatments/Tests
- Falls
- Other/Miscellaneous
- Adverse Drug Reactions
- Equipment/Supplies/Devices
- Transfusion

Source: Pennsylvania Patient Safety Authority, Harrisburg, Penn. Unpublished data. June 29, 2009

One state-mandated adverse event and near-miss reporting program is the Pennsylvania Patient Safety Authority. In 2008, the authority received 23,040 reports of adverse events and near misses from ICUs, representing 10.5 percent of all hospital reports received. Reports of medication errors, adverse drug reactions, and complications of procedures, treatments, and tests involving the ICU were more likely to be categorized as serious events than reports not involving the ICU (10.2 percent of all serious event reports from hospitals involved the ICU). Refer to Figure 12.1.

Critical care patients are at greater risk of adverse events and errors than are patients in general care settings. A recent study of the incidence and nature of adverse events in intensive care at an academic, tertiary care urban hospital in the United States revealed additional insights into the risk of iatrogenic injury for critically ill patients.[47] The AHRQ-sponsored critical care safety study was conducted from July 2002 to June 2003 in two critical care units, using direct continuous observation, review of incident reports, information from a computerized adverse drug event detection system, and chart extraction. Among the systems factors associated with the serious medical errors identified in the study, treatment and procedure errors, including those involving medications, accounted for nearly 75 percent of the errors. Sterility hazards occurred in over half of central intravascular catheter insertion procedures when interns failed to wash their hands. Also, a significant number of errors in reporting or communicating clinical information were the result of system failures. Other study findings with important patient safety and risk management implications for ICUs include the following:[48]

- More than 20 percent of patients admitted to the ICUs experienced an adverse event.
- Almost half (45 percent) of the ICU events were preventable.
- More than 90 percent of incidents occurred during routine care, not at admission or during an emergency.

Further analysis of the data confirmed that the cost of adverse events in ICUs is substantial. Adverse events added an additional day to a patient's hospital stay and cost nearly $4,000 to treat.[49] The researchers calculated that the nation's annual cost for adverse events involving critical care provided at nonfederal hospitals is between $5.8 and $7.2 billion. Efforts to improve event reporting in ICUs will not only improve patient care but also cut costs of care.

To benefit from reporting of ICU events and near misses, hospitals must understand the root causes of these events. They can then take steps to eliminate or prevent the situations that contribute to errors. An external ICU-specific event reporting system was implemented to detect systemic patient safety issues common to many ICUs and to improve the identification of errors and events that occur too infrequently for individual ICUs to easily trend based solely on their own data.[50] Although no longer in operation, the ICU Safety Reporting System (ICUSRS) was a voluntary Web-based reporting system that collected reports of adverse events and near misses. Funded for four years by AHRQ, ICUSRS involved twenty-three participating ICUs. Based on an analysis of 2,075 incidents submitted during a two-year period, the researchers found that 42 percent of the incidents resulted in some degree of harm to the patient. The majority of events involved medications and therapeutics (42 percent), followed by incorrect or incomplete care delivery (20 percent), equipment and medical devices (15 percent), and lines, tubes, and drains (13 percent).[51]

The program helped identify systemic patient safety issues common to many ICUs as follows (the percentages exceed 100 percent because more than one contributing factor may have been involved with each event):

- Training and education issues (e.g., knowledge or skill deficiencies, failure to follow protocol) contributed in 49 percent of events.
- Team factors (e.g., communication) contributed in 32 percent of events.
- Patient factors (e.g., acuity) contributed in 32 percent of events.
- ICU environmental factors (e.g., workload) contributed in 22 percent of events.
- Provider factors (e.g., fatigue) contributed in 20 percent of events.
- Institutional environmental factors (e.g., time pressures) contributed in 16 percent of events.
- Information technology/computerized provider order-entry system factors (e.g., user or software errors) contributed in 12 percent of events.
- Task factors (e.g., unavailability of test results) contributed in 10 percent of events.

Based on their analyses of the factors that contribute to adverse events, the ICUSRS facilities developed strategies to eliminate or prevent these contributing factors from occurring. For example, data from the ICUSRS reports helped one site recognize the need for a pharmacist to make daily rounds of the ICU to help in the prevention of medication errors.

In a report to AHRQ summarizing the benefits and limitations of ICUSRS, the researchers said that the reporting system provided a means to identify and mitigate hazards; however, to truly benefit from the information, hospitals must be able to assign priority and focus their limited resources on the improvement efforts likely to have the biggest impact on patient safety.[52] A federal initiative, established by the Patient Safety and Quality Improvement Act of 2005 (PSQIA), created the first national system for providers to voluntarily report medical errors, near misses, and other patient safety events to designated organizations while having assurance that the information will be protected from legal discovery and kept confidential. The voluntary reporting program allows organizations that collect the data, called patient safety organizations (PSOs), to aggregate and analyze it and share findings and lessons learned. By collecting data from many providers, PSOs can spot problems and trends that an individual hospital, with its limited pool of data, may be unable to detect. Critical care units that participate in the reporting program may benefit by better targeting their patient safety improvement efforts. (Please see Volume 1, Chapter 10, for more information on PSOs.)

In addition to event reporting systems, other methods are available to identify and prevent ICU adverse events. IHI has developed a trigger tool to use during a random review of medical records to identify adverse events and possible clues underlying the events. The tool has twenty-four triggers, such as readmission to the ICU or development of pneumonia during the ICU stay, to identify adverse events during the chart review. Designed as an adjunct to adverse event reporting, the adverse event trigger tool can be used to evaluate adverse events and target improvement efforts.[53] IHI's resource for ICUs is available for download from its Web site at www.ihi.org.

Data from medical malpractice claims and lawsuits involving critical care also provide insights into the need for improved safety in ICUs. The Doctors Company/OHIC Insurance, the largest national insurer of physician and surgeon medical liability, conducted a 2009 study of closed claims arising in ICU locations (surgical ICUs, medical ICUs, and coronary care units) for claims that were closed between 2000 and 2008.[54] Although just 219 (approximately 2.2 percent) of the company's claims and lawsuits from 2000 to 2008 were coded to an ICU location, more than two-thirds (69 percent) of these ICU claims involved the death of the patient. Thirty-eight of the 219 claims (17 percent) resulted in payments to patients or their families. Some of the findings from the 219 claims and lawsuits coded to an ICU location provide information about common allegations and risk management implications.

Allegations

The most common allegation for ICU claims, failure to diagnose, occurred in approximately 33 percent of all ICU claims. Improper management of treatment course was the

TABLE 7.2   The Doctors Company/OHIC Insurance Top 10 Allegations in ICU Claims, 2000 to 2008

Allegation	Claim Count	Percent of Total
Failure to diagnose	71	32.7%
Improper management of treatment course	23	10.6
Delay in diagnosis	16	7.4
Delay in treatment/procedure	14	6.5
Improper performance of treatment/procedure	14	6.5
Failure to treat	13	6.0
Improper management of surgical patient	10	4.6
Failure to monitor patient's physiological status	9	4.1
Administration—wrong dose	7	3.2
Treatment—other	6	2.8

Source: Darrell Ranum. *Study on Closed ICU Claims.* Columbus, Ohio: The Doctors Company/OHIC Insurance.

second most common allegation, accounting for approximately 11 percent of ICU claims. Delay in diagnosis was the third most common allegation, representing 7 percent of ICU claims. The diagnosis-related allegations failure to diagnose and delay in diagnosis, combined, accounted for more than 40 percent of ICU claims. See Table 7.2 for a further breakdown of allegations.

Risk Management Issues

When reviewing and analyzing cases, The Doctors Company/OHIC Insurance identified risk management issues that may have contributed to allegations, injuries, or initiation of the claims. The insurer considers these issues during the development of strategies for prevention and mitigation of future cases. A review of risk management issues in the company's ICU claims indicates that "communication among providers regarding the patient's condition" and "lack of or inadequate assessment with a failure to note clinical information" were the most common problems. Both issues were identified in more than 22 percent of cases.

"Communication among providers regarding the patient's condition" reflects inadequate sharing of information among healthcare providers that is important to the care and treatment of patients. The "lack of or inadequate assessment—failure to note clinical information" risk management issue is indicative of a failure to attend to relevant findings (laboratory values, diagnostic tests, symptoms, and so on) for all pertinent information that has been received. Allegations such as failure to diagnose and delay in diagnosis can result. Notably, these are among the most common allegations.

The next most common risk management issue identified through Doctors Company/OHIC Insurance review of ICU cases is "failure or delay in ordering diagnostic test." This

TABLE 7.3   The Doctors Company/OHIC Insurance Top 11 Risk Management Issues in ICU Claims, 2000 to 2008

Risk Management Issue	Claim Count	Percent of Total
Communication among providers regarding the patient's condition	49	22%
Lack of or inadequate assessment—failure to note clinical information	49	22
Failure or delay in ordering diagnostic test	47	21
Failure to rule out abnormal finding	45	21
Failure to establish differential diagnosis	44	20
Patient monitoring—physiological	32	15
Staff training/education	30	14
Failure/delay to obtain consult/referral	24	11
Patient assessment issues—other	22	10
Selection/management of therapy—medical	22	10
Policy/protocol not followed	20	9

Source: Darrell Ranum. *2009 Study of Closed ICU Claims*. Columbus, Ohio: The Doctors Company/OHIC Insurance.

Note: This table includes the top 11 risk management issues and the percentage of claims identifying these risk management issues. There were a total of 89 risk management issues that were identified 737 times in these 219 ICU cases.

issue was seen in approximately 21 percent of the cases. These cases include situations in which patient symptoms were not adequately explored, according to reviewing experts. In their opinions, specific tests were warranted in light of these patients' clinical pictures.

The fourth most common risk management issue, "failure to rule out abnormal finding," is related to the other patient assessment issues. It represents situations in which patients have abnormal test results or symptoms that are not investigated. Later findings reflected bone fractures, internal hemorrhaging, incorrect drug levels, and so forth, that should have been identified and addressed, according to the reviewers. See Table 7.3 for a further breakdown of risk management issues.

· · · · · · · · ·

TECHNOLOGY AND SAFETY IN THE ICU

The critical care environment requires an array of equipment and technology to monitor patients and deliver care. ICU caregivers must ensure the safe operation of critical care equipment such as infusion pumps, physiological monitoring systems, and ventilators. Additionally, they must adopt measures to prevent equipment-related safety issues such as clinical alarm–related incidents and tubing disconnections and misconnections.

Infusion Pumps

IV infusions in critical care areas are most often delivered via infusion pumps to more carefully regulate the flow of infusate. However, because of the dangers associated with IV pump free flow (an unregulated flow of infusate into a patient through an intravascular line), the frequency with which such hazards occur when unprotected sets are used, and the availability of set-based mechanisms that effectively prevent this condition, facilities seldom use IV pumps with unprotected administration sets.

In response to recommendations from ECRI Institute (an independent nonprofit research institute that researches the best approaches for improving patient care), The Joint Commission, and other organizations, healthcare facilities have switched over to the exclusive use of infusion pumps with set-based free-flow protection.[55]

Medication errors typically occur with infusion pumps either because an operator fails to correctly program an order into the pump or because a provider issues an incorrect order. Such errors can be reduced by establishing clear protocols for the ordering of infusions and by using pumps with dose-calculation capabilities. Several infusion pump suppliers now offer pumps that incorporate a dose error reduction system, or DERS. Such systems, sometimes referred to as *smart pumps*, alert clinicians if programmed doses exceed preset limits for a specific drug, clinical location, or application. Organizations must take necessary steps to deter caregivers from overriding the safety features on this equipment. Risky workarounds sometimes occur in response to delays caused by issues generated by the system itself, such as a requirement that numerous steps be taken to properly program appropriate settings. Clinicians and risk managers must work with the manufacturer, biomedical professionals, and others to circumvent these and other barriers to the pumps' efficient operation.

ECRI Institute recommends that healthcare facilities adopt smart pump technology as they replace older-generation pumps.[56] Because DERSs vary greatly in their features and functionality, evaluating these systems is a critical part of the pump selection process. Also, effective use of a DERS depends heavily on implementation, education, and ongoing system support. The key to using any new technology to improve patient safety is educating physicians and staff in its use and appropriately redesigning the processes in which the equipment is used to ensure adoption of the safety features.

Physiological Monitoring Systems

Physiological monitoring systems help clinicians assess vital parameters, such as ECG, temperature, blood pressure, and cardiac output, so they can track changes in the patient's condition and intervene appropriately. In the ICU, where patients typically require the highest level of monitoring, every patient has a bedside monitor, and patient information is usually displayed at a central station. An ICU monitor should be capable of displaying at least six waveforms and monitoring a wide variety of parameters, such as cardiac output, ECG, pulse oximetry, invasive blood pressure, noninvasive blood pressure, respiratory rate, and temperature.[57]

A variety of patient safety concerns accompany the use of physiological monitors, and the following measures are particularly important for monitoring systems in the ICU:[58]

- Improvements in the flexibility and networking capability of monitoring systems now allow facilities to provide continuum of care monitoring wherever the patient may be in the healthcare facility. This is an essential feature for physiological monitoring systems in the ICU, particularly if critically ill patients must be transported to areas outside the ICU. Professional organizations recommend that critically ill patients receive the same level of physiological monitoring during intrahospital transport as they received in the ICU.[59]

- Staff must be educated to recognize, understand, and properly respond to electro-cardiogram arrhythmia waveforms and other abnormal physiological monitoring parameters wherever the patient is in the facility, including areas outside the ICU where patients must sometimes be transferred for testing or procedures.

- Alarm coverage protocols should be established and compliance assessed, to ensure that alarms are addressed promptly and appropriately. Please see the section in this chapter on clinical alarms for more information.

- Facilities with multiple critical care service settings must determine the staffing levels required to meet the clinical and monitoring needs of the patients in each ICU. Any use of alternative notification approaches, such as the use of full-time, dedicated personnel who are dedicated to observing monitors 24 hours a day or remote ICU monitoring, must be carefully considered, with patient safety being the paramount factor in the choice of appropriate staffing and alarm notification models.

- How physiological monitoring equipment will interface with other clinical devices such as ventilators and IV pumps, as well as with the hospital's information systems, must be considered when evaluating the capabilities of each vendor's monitoring system. Such integration of clinical and demographic data within department and enterprise-wide systems has become an integral part of hospital equipment planning.

Ventilators

Intensive care ventilators provide temporary support to patients who cannot breathe on their own or require assistance to maintain adequate ventilation. In a 2002 Sentinel Event Alert on ventilator-related injuries, The Joint Commission identified ventilator-related alarms problems and tubing disconnections as the leading safety issues associated with ventilator deaths and injuries.[60] The Joint Commission published recommendations for enhancing ventilator safety in that alert, and ECRI Institute reiterated and expanded on those recommendations as follows:[61]

- Include job-specific ventilator safety content in staff competency assessments.
- Ensure effective staffing for ventilator patients at all times.
- Implement regular preventive maintenance and testing of alarm systems and ensure that alarms are sufficiently audible.

- Provide interdisciplinary training for staff that care for ventilator patients.
- Recognize that alarms do not replace direct observation of ventilator-dependent patients.
- Confirm that the respiratory care group follows an accepted and documented method for calculating ventilator alarm settings.
- Require staff to confirm, during regular ventilator checks, that all alarms are active and that the alarm volume is loud enough to be heard outside the room.
- Identify staff authorized to operate ventilators, and do not allow other staff to make changes to settings.

A common risk associated with intensive care ventilators is VAP. Refer to the section "Clinical Care Bundles" for more information on preventing VAP.

Clinical Alarms

ECRI Institute has identified clinical alarm hazards as the top medical device hazard in hospitals.[62] Alarm-related issues are among the problems most frequently reported to ECRI Institute, which maintains a voluntary and confidential reporting program for hospitals and others to report medical device–related incidents and deficiencies. Alarm issues are of particular concern when they affect ICU equipment such as ventilators and physiological monitoring systems. The Joint Commission also called attention to this problem by making clinical alarm safety a National Patient Safety Goal in 2003. Although the goal was retired in 2005, concerns remain about ineffective alarm coverage, inappropriate alarm use, and failure to hear alarms. To reduce the frequency of alarm-related adverse incidents, ECRI Institute recommends the following:[63]

- When evaluating a device for purchase, ask whether the device alarms are designed in a way that is logical, safe, and consistent with the facility's practice. Look for designs that limit nuisance alarms (that is, false or excessive alarms), which can desensitize staff, possibly leading them to ignore true hazards.
- Make sure that staff members understand the purpose and significance of alarms. Are personnel aware of the types of hazards about which each alarm is supposed to warn? Do they know how to set alarm limits to appropriate, physiologically meaningful values? ECRI Institute continues to learn of incidents in which staff unintentionally disable critical alarms by setting them far outside reasonable parameters. Low-saturation alarms on pulse oximetry monitors and low minute volume or high peak-pressure alarms on ventilators are regular subjects of this sort of misuse.
- Ensure that alarm conditions are consistently conveyed to staff on the floor in as efficient a manner as possible. Make sure that factors such as speaker volume, floor layout, and physical distance from the device do not prevent staff from hearing audible alarms. If such factors can't be controlled, consider implementing an alarm-enhancement system, which can increase alarm volume or convey alarms remotely, for example, via pagers, mobile phones, or the nurse-call system. Visual alarm indicators should be positioned so that they can be easily seen.

Tubing Disconnections and Misconnections

Critical care patients may be attached to numerous devices, such as IV pumps for several critical infusions, central line catheters, and ventilators, which pose the risk of tubing misconnections or disconnections. In a 2006 Sentinel Event Alert, The Joint Commission warned of the dangers associated with tubing and catheter connection errors.[64] For example, invasive lines may disconnect accidentally, resulting in blood loss, and feeding tubes may mistakenly be connected to IV tubes. When recommending strategies to reduce tubing misconnection errors, The Joint Commission cited ECRI Institute's recommendations. ECRI Institute reiterated those recommendations in a 2009 report[65] as follows:

● Purchase devices that are designed to prevent misconnections.

● Provide periodic training about misconnection prevention and risks specific to the ICU. Remind staff of safe work practices and the consequences of misconnections.

● Discourage the use of adapters unless they are clearly appropriate for the application. For example, using adapters to force two female Luer connectors to join or using a similar approach to force two different-sized breathing device components together, when these pieces of equipment are not normally partners, could cause an incorrect connection.

● Instruct staff to trace all lines back to their origin before making connections. Doing so helps to ensure that the correct lines will be joined.

● Ensure that staff recheck connections and trace all patient tubes and catheters to their sources upon the patient's arrival in the ICU from another setting as part of the handoff process.

● Prohibit staff from forcing connections. If a connection requires a lot of effort, chances are that it is not the right connection. If a connection is not secure or leaking, staff should check to see that the right components have been connected.

● Require staff to label certain high-risk catheters, such as epidural, intrathecal, and arterial lines.

· · · · · · · · ·

MEDICATION ERRORS IN THE ICU

Medication errors, including errors that involve IV infusions, are common in healthcare organizations, and the problem is of major concern in the ICU setting, where many high-alert medications are administered. In one study of medical errors in an ICU, medication errors accounted for slightly more than 20 percent of all reported events.[66] A Jury Verdict Research® (JVR) analysis of medical negligence plaintiff awards from 2001 to 2007 found that the jury award median for medication errors was $1.25 million.[67] As of June 2009, medication errors were the fourth most frequent type of sentinel event reported to The Joint Commission and accounted for 8.3 percent of all events in The Joint Commission sentinel event database.[68] To reduce medication errors, a healthcare organization should evaluate its strengths and weaknesses in medication-use safety by completing a medication self-analysis. Assessment tools are available from organizations such as the Institute for Safe Medication Practices (ISMP) www.ismp.org, Horsham, Pennsylvania, and ECRI Institute www.ecri.org, Plymouth Meeting, Pennsylvania. In addition, risk management professionals should be familiar with the 2006 Institute of Medicine report, *Preventing Medication Errors,* which provides information that can be used throughout the hospital to prevent medication errors.[69]

Medication event and error reporting, along with near-miss reporting, is crucial to identifying the factors and systems that contribute to the occurrence of errors. For example, ISMP operates the Medication Errors Reporting Program, a confidential, national voluntary reporting program for medication errors that is used to analyze the system causes of medication errors and identify recommendations for prevention. Another national adverse drug event reporting system, MedMarx®, operated by Quantros Inc. in alliance with the U.S. Pharmacopoeia, is used by client hospitals as a comparative database of medication-related errors and adverse drug reactions. Although reports from external medication error databases can be extremely useful for collecting and analyzing aggregate data, they are also limited because they cannot support real-time event reporting for internal, ICU-specific purposes, including follow-up and root cause analysis.

In general, a medication error reporting system should meet the needs of the organization as a whole. Therefore, ICUs should have hospital-specific internal medication error-reporting processes in place. How to make the best use of external reporting resources such as MedMarx® and patient safety organizations (as discussed in the Event, Error, and Near-Miss Reporting" section of this chapter) may be a suitable topic for discussion by ICU unit leaders in conjunction with risk management and quality improvement representatives. When possible, incident reporting systems should include those errors and potential errors (near misses) that are captured by automated prescribing or administration systems.

In addition to medication error reporting systems, automated pharmacy or medical record–based triggers have been useful in monitoring adverse drug events caused by many high-alert drugs used in the ICU. One example includes triggers that indicate when a patient received a medication used to reverse the effect of a drug, such as when naloxone is given for opiate overdose, prompting an investigation of the reason for the use of the reversal agent. In particular, IHI's adverse event trigger tool for ICUs captures medication and other inadvertent events that may occur in critical care. For more information on adverse event reporting systems see Chapter 6 in Volume 1 on early warning systems for the identification for organizational risk.

Medication safety experts have expounded on the value of pharmacists on the patient care team and recommended that they be available on patient care units, particularly when medication orders are written. One study found that the availability of pharmacists in one hospital's ICU helped identify potential errors with medication orders.[70] Also, according to ISMP, medication errors are reduced by two-thirds when a senior pharmacist accompanies physicians on rounds in an ICU.

·········

HIGH-ALERT MEDICATIONS IN THE ICU

ISMP defines *high-alert medications* as drugs that bear a heightened risk of causing significant harm when they are used in error.[71] This does not imply that errors with these medications occur more frequently, but rather that the consequences of errors involving their use can be devastating. According to ISMP, common high-alert medications include insulin, opiates and narcotics, injectable potassium chloride (or phosphate) concentrate, anticoagulants, thrombolytics, and chemotherapeutic agents, many of which are commonly administered in ICUs. Special precautions must be taken when prescribing, dispensing, and administering high-alert medications. These precautions are especially applicable to the ICU. They include the following:[72]

- Eliminating high-alert drugs from floor stock wherever feasible
- Requiring independent checks (a double-check by a second clinician) of doses and preparations of high-alert medications
- Using premixed infusion products
- Having a pharmacist review all high-alert medication orders
- Using safety checklists that prompt clinicians to review important safety considerations for high-alert medications and delivery systems

Compounding the risk of administering high-alert medications in the ICU, the parenteral routes of administration (that is, IV, intramuscular, subcutaneous, and epidural) are frequently used to administer ICU medications. These routes provide a more direct means of delivering medication for faster and more effective results and are beneficial to patient care. However, high-alert drugs administered rapidly by direct routes can be especially dangerous if given erroneously because there is little time to reverse their immediate effects. Furthermore, when a high-alert drug is administered with an infusion device capable of rapid IV delivery, a mistake in dosing or rate programming can have grave consequences. A 2007 survey by the American Nurses Association (ANA) reported that nurses attributed being too busy or working in a rushed environment as the top factors contributing to medication errors, particularly those involving injectable medications, somewhat common conditions in the ICU.[73]

Following the deaths of three infants in a Midwestern neonatal intensive care unit (NICU) that were attributed to accidental overdoses of heparin, ISMP issued new recommendations to ensure that systems are established to safeguard against administration of inappropriate doses of high-alert drugs. In this instance, six NICU patients received 1,000 times the appropriate dosage of heparin when heparin solution of 10,000 unit/mL was given instead of the 10 unit/mL heparin flush solution. ISMP's recommendations included the following:[74]

- Sequester 10,000 unit/mL vials and store them away from vials of all other concentrations.
- Store doses greater than 100 units/mL in areas separate from concentrations normally used as flushing solutions.

- Dispense flushing solutions not normally available in the required concentration only from the pharmacy.

- Independently validate products that are pulled for stocking in automated dispensing cabinets before sending them to the unit.

- Purchase different concentrations of a product from different vendors to avoid having labels that look similar.

- Use bar-code technology for stocking and administering drugs.

- Review any dispensing unit stock and remove potentially unsafe medications, allowing only the pharmacy to dispense such medications.

Despite the attention surrounding this incident and the recommendations that followed, other, similar mistakes continue to occur. For example, incidents involving different concentrations of nitroglycerine for IV administration have occurred in ICU settings. As well, there are documented errors in which insulin has been mistakenly given for heparin. ISMP provided additional recommendations to prevent confusion of the two drugs as follows:[75]

- Always compare the indication for heparin or insulin with the patient's diagnosis/conditions to ensure they match before dispensing or administering insulin or heparin.

- Write verbal orders directly on order forms and read back the orders to verify understanding and accuracy.

- Require an independent double-check of IV insulin and IV heparin before administration.

Independent checks are recommended to help prevent errors that involve high-alert medications. An independent check must involve independent verification of a drug or dose by a second clinician. In practice, the checks are often not independent, and as such, the preventive effects are negated. For example, nurses standing next to one another commonly check insulin, narcotics, and other high-risk medications and dosing computations, potentially encoding each other's errors, rather than independently checking them. Physicians often cosign chemotherapy orders rather than independently calculating the required dose. These misuses of the concept suggest that broad education about the meaning and benefits of independent checks might be helpful to the ICU staff.

The lesson for risk management professionals is to be ever vigilant when near misses occur and to learn from these incidents because they may herald medication accidents waiting to occur. Analysis of near misses and close calls can be used to identify strategies to prevent these types of errors from harming patients. Additionally, during walking rounds they must also investigate whether look-alike/sound-alike medications are stored together in cabinets, on medication carts, or on pharmacy shelves and ensure that measures are in place to prevent errors from potential mix-ups of these drugs.

As noted previously, ICU care involves multiple transfers and transitions in care, transitions that present opportunities for medication errors and adverse events to occur. The Joint Commission includes the improvement of medication safety in its National Patient Safety Goals, with reconciliation of medications across the continuum of care being one specific goal. To decrease medication errors that occur during patient transfer from an ICU to other healthcare settings, organizations should ensure that measures are in place to reconcile the patient's medications, including those taken before the patient's admission to the ICU and those ordered during the patient's stay in the ICU. In a 2004 report, researchers at Johns Hopkins Hospital reported on a computerized tool developed to reconcile patient medications before a patient's transfer out of the surgical ICU. ICU nurses used the tool to record all preoperative and ICU-ordered medications. Before transfer out of the surgical ICU, a nurse reviewed the form for any discrepancies in orders or medication allergies. The tool was effective in detecting medication errors in transfer orders in the surgical ICU and prevented potentially harmful errors in 21 percent of patients.[76] The success of this electronic tool has been attributed to making medication reconciliation a system process, rather than leaving it solely to the discretion of individual physicians and nurses.[77]

INFECTIONS IN THE ICU

The incidence of healthcare-acquired infections, a major health issue and a serious patient safety concern, has become a focus for the Centers for Disease Control and Prevention (CDC), CMS, and The Joint Commission. ICU patients, in particular, are at increased risk of infection because of their critical illnesses, possible comorbidities, and compromised immunity. Additionally, they tend to have many invasive devices that can increase the risk of infection. Device-related infections of particular concern for ICUs are central catheter (or central line) associated BSIs, infections related to indwelling urinary catheters, and VAP.

CMS will no longer pay for two of these three conditions, infections from urinary catheters and BSIs associated with central catheters, if they develop during a Medicare beneficiary's stay in the hospital as a result of caregivers' failure to follow established guidelines to prevent these hospital-acquired conditions. VAP is on the agency's radar screen as a preventable condition that may also be identified as a hospital-acquired condition for which there will be no payment. Infection control strategies, such as vigilant attention to hand hygiene, in place throughout the hospital are essential in the ICU.

CDC tracks device-related infections occurring in adult, pediatric, and neonatal ICUs through its National Healthcare Safety Network, a surveillance system for hospitals to voluntarily report healthcare-associated infection data. The surveillance system was modified in 2007 to open participation to all hospitals. As a result, recent year-to-year comparisons of ICU infections are difficult to make because of the change in facilities reporting to the network. Nevertheless, in its 2004 National Healthcare Quality Report, AHRQ summarized data on nosocomial infections in ICU patients from 1998 through 2002 using CDC data and showed a gradual overall decline in some types of ICU infections.[78]

CDC has issued several guidelines to help healthcare facilities reduce infection. They include guidelines for hand hygiene, for prevention of healthcare-associated pneumonia, and for prevention of intravascular catheter-related infections. The Joint Commission's focus on reducing the risk of healthcare-associated infections includes National Patient Safety Goals centered on compliance with CDC's hand hygiene guidelines and on measures to prevent central line–associated BSIs. Public reporting of healthcare-associated infections is now required by the majority of states. Additionally, there has been renewed interest in bringing lawsuits against healthcare facilities, alleging acquisition of infections in hospitals due to substandard care and negligence, and this could prove a harbinger of future litigation. Previously, because of the difficulty in proving the causes and sources of infection, liability cases involving infections centered mainly on prompt diagnosis and treatment and not on whether they were hospital-acquired infections.

The potential for operational losses due to increased lengths of stay for critical care patients experiencing infection complications is high. When this is coupled with the threat of liability losses from infection-related suits, it becomes clear that risk management and patient safety efforts should concentrate on prevention and reduction of infections in the ICU. Some specific strategies aimed at preventing infections are discussed next.

· · · · · · · · ·
CLINICAL CARE BUNDLES

Bundling is the grouping of evidence-based interventions to improve patient safety. One bundling initiative, which originated in the ICU, focuses on reducing catheter-related (central line) BSIs. This initiative is known as the *central line bundle*, and it includes the following five components:[79]

1. Hand hygiene: compliance with strict hand hygiene practices before insertion and use of central lines

2. Maximal barrier precautions: use of sterile gloves, gown, mask, and large enough drapes to prevent contamination of the catheter on insertion

3. Chlorhexidine skin antisepsis: use of faster-drying disinfectant to reduce remaining bacteria on the skin

4. Optimal catheter site selection: insertion site individualized to patient's needs, for example, avoiding the femoral vein for central venous access in adults, and standardized, meticulous care of the line once placed

5. Daily review of line necessity with prompt removal of unnecessary lines: ongoing assessment of need for central lines and removal as soon as possible

Organizations that have successfully implemented the central line bundle have reduced their rates of central line infections (and death rates) significantly.[80] An estimated 80,000 central line–associated BSIs occur annually in the United States in ICUs leading to 28,000 deaths.[81] At an estimated cost of $45,000 per case to treat these infections, the nation spends an estimated $2.3 billion annually to treat ICU patients who have central line infections.

Following on the success of several single-hospital studies, the Michigan Keystone ICU project, using a systems approach, eliminated catheter-related BSIs through multifaceted interventions in nearly 100 ICUs within the state. The overall median rate of central line–associated BSIs dropped to 0 from 2.7 per 1,000 catheter-days within three months of the start of the eighteen-month project.[82] This systems approach consisted of the following five interventions developed at Johns Hopkins Hospital to reduce central line infections:[83]

1. Educating providers about practices to control infection and harm from catheter-related BSIs

2. Creation of a catheter line insertion cart containing all necessary supplies to avoid staff skipping essential steps due to lack of equipment

3. Asking providers during daily rounds whether catheters could be removed to reduce exposure to central lines

4. Implementing a checklist to be completed by the bedside ICU nurse to ensure adherence to evidence-based guidelines for preventing catheter-related BSIs

5. Empowering nurses to stop the catheter insertion procedure if a violation of the guidelines was observed, and notify the attending physician if a violation was not corrected

The interventions required significant support by the clinical leaders of the ICU and by hospital executives and a focus on the creation of a culture of safety in the unit whereby interpersonal communications and teamwork prevailed. Staff received feedback about their efforts from monthly and quarterly reports on the number and rates of catheter-related BSIs. Tools developed at Johns Hopkins Hospital to promote the use of this systems approach are available online. (Please refer to the resource list at the end of this chapter for information on accessing these tools and others.)

Another set of evidence-based interventions originating in the ICU, the ventilator bundle, is being used to prevent and reduce the incidence of VAP, the leading cause of death among hospital-acquired infections with a mortality rate of 46 percent. VAP is also associated with longer time spent on a ventilator, an increased length of stay, and an increase in hospital costs estimated at $40,000.[84] The ventilator bundle has four key components:

1. Elevation of the head of the bed to between thirty and forty-five degrees

2. Daily "sedation vacation" and daily assessment of readiness to extubate

3. Peptic ulcer disease (PUD) prophylaxis

4. Deep venous thrombosis (DVT) prophylaxis (unless contraindicated)

Many hospitals are using the VAP bundle developed by IHI to reduce the incidence of VAP. Two Pennsylvania hospitals report success in implementing the ventilator bundle to reduce their VAP rates and maintain very low or zero rates by consistent application of risk reduction strategies. The combined use of the ventilator bundle, professional infection control guidelines, ongoing monitoring, education, and feedback resulted in a reduction of VAP. Also contributing to the drop in VAP was the pride and ownership by staff members regarding their ongoing success in targeting zero infections.[85]

A third set of care bundles focuses on sepsis, an infectious process that is life-threatening if treatment is delayed and that is frequently encountered in, but not limited to, the ICU. With mortality rates of up to 50 percent for septic shock, the most severe form of sepsis, sepsis treatment has gained worldwide attention. SCCM, in partnership with other international groups, formed a coalition to improve sepsis care through adoption of evidence-based guidelines for the care of critically ill patients with sepsis. The initiative, which concluded at the end of 2008, developed two bundles for severe sepsis: the sepsis resuscitation bundle, to begin within six hours of identifying patients with severe sepsis or septic shock, and the sepsis management bundle, to begin within 24 hours of the diagnosis.[86] The tasks for each bundle are as follows:

- Sepsis resuscitation bundle

  - Measure serum lactate

  - Obtain blood cultures prior to antibiotic administration

  - Administer broad-spectrum antibiotics within three hours for emergency department admissions and within one hour for ICU admissions

  - Treat hypotension and/or elevated lactate with fluids

  - Maintain adequate central venous pressure and central venous oxygen saturation

- Sepsis management bundle

  - Administer low-dose steroids for septic shock in accordance with standardized ICU policy

  - Administer recombinant human activated protein C in accordance with standardized ICU policy.

  - Maintain glucose control greater than 70, but less than 150 mg/dL

  - Maintain a median inspiratory plateau pressure (<30 cm H_2O) for mechanically ventilated patients

With the sepsis care bundles now available, the IHI is promoting widespread adoption of the bundles by clinicians to reduce deaths from sepsis by 25 percent. Additional information about this Surviving Sepsis Campaign, including a Web-based suite of information and tools for hospitals and caregivers to use in implementing sepsis care bundles, is available online at www.ihi.org/IHI/Topics/CriticalCare/Sepsis.

Although not an official care bundle, another intervention aimed at improving patient outcomes in the ICU involves the management of blood glucose levels in critically ill patients. Based on the premise that critically ill patients experience hyperglycemia, or high blood sugar levels, due to the release of certain hormones, which occurs under stress even in the absence of a history of diabetes, clinicians have recommended insulin infusion for critical care patients. Studies to date have been inconclusive. One of the largest multinational studies compared intensive and conventional glucose control and found that tight glucose control, contrary to a growing consensus, was more harmful because it led to more cases of severe hypoglycemia, or low blood sugar levels.[87] Until investigators sort out the findings from the multinational study, critical care clinicians are focusing on managing extremes of hyperglycemia and hypoglycemia in their ICU patients. An editorial accompanying the published results of the multinational study noted that many hospitals have implemented refined insulin-infusion protocols to achieve glucose control and that this strategy has improved outcomes for their ICU patients.[88] Another intervention aimed at reducing possible exposure to microorganisms that cause urinary tract infections (UTIs) from indwelling urinary catheters is a simple reminder system for physicians to evaluate the need for patients to continue having the indwelling catheters after 48 hours. Researchers at the University of Michigan Health System found that the use of a urinary catheter reminder can reduce the incidence of indwelling urethral catheterizations and thereby decrease the number of hospitalized patients who develop nosocomial UTIs.[89]

Although not yet available as of mid-2009, CDC's updated guidelines for the prevention of catheter-associated UTI will likely promote protocols for the appropriate use of urinary catheters, increased awareness among caregivers of patients who have indwelling catheters, and measures to ensure that the catheter is removed promptly when appropriate. CDC's draft of the guideline, issued in 2008, did recommend such approaches.[90] Some facilities with electronic medical records use programmed reminders and alerts to prompt clinicians to evaluate removal of the catheter in patients who have received them. In addition, documentation in the patient's medical record that the catheter was ordered and inserted also reminds clinicians to consider whether the catheter is still needed. All too often, clinicians forget that a catheter is in place and allow it to remain longer than needed. Urinary catheters should only be used when needed for clinical care; they should never be used for staff convenience.

A risk management issue that arises when care bundles are used is that of compliance. The question of whether instances of noncompliance with care bundles can result in liability claims alleging deviations from the standard of care has not been directly answered, although it can be reasonably assumed that if care bundles become the recognized standard of care, then noncompliance with the care bundle can be considered substandard care when a patient is injured and causation is linked to the noncompliance. Indeed, components of the ventilator bundle have been included in national quality measures. Additionally, hospitals are encouraged to adopt evidence-based guidelines to prevent instances of central line–associated BSIs and catheter-associated UTIs that could trigger CMS's no-payment initiative. However, whether the delivery of medical care is thought of in terms of standards or care bundles, the overriding precedence should be to do the right things right, in the interest of improving quality and safety, while seeking protection of compliance monitoring data under whatever peer review, quality improvement, or PSO protective statutes are available. Documentation in committee minutes of clinical rationale supporting the choice or modification of care bundles can help the organization track progress and prove that a reasonable approach was used if "protected" minutes are ever successfully subpoenaed.

· · · · · · · · ·

INFORMATION TECHNOLOGY AND THE ICU

Information technology (IT) holds the promise of improving safety and efficiency in the critical care unit as well as throughout the healthcare system. An electronic medical record (EMR) enables the critical care provider to access all the necessary information (laboratory and other test results, medications provided, medical records, and so forth) about a critical care patient at the point of care. Although hospitals have been slow to implement a fully integrated EMR, financial incentives from the federal government for facilities to adopt an EMR could spur the effort, provided facilities comply with the provisions for receiving the bonus payments.

Critical care physicians whose organizations have adopted EMRs have shared their recommendations regarding features on an EMR used in the ICU as well as tips for successful implementation.[91] Among features they felt were desirable for EMR are the following:

- Access to all vital signs, vascular monitoring, pulse oximetry, and waveforms
- Immediate access to laboratory, pathology, and microbiology reports as well as radiology images and reports
- Immediate access to electrocardiograms and rhythm strips
- Medication administration record with documentation of changes and explanations
- Input and output records with intravenous drip documentation and cumulative shift totals
- Computerized provider order entry
- Progress and nursing notes
- Access to online medical reference information
- Clinical decision support
- E-mail capability for all system users
- Access to face sheet information such as insurance, next of kin, and contact phone numbers

To ensure successful implementation of EMR in the critical care setting, organizations must involve a critical care physician in the planning process.[92] The critical care physician champion can ensure that the system meets the needs of critical care caregivers and that the ICU EMR is sending and receiving necessary information to and from various hospital departments such as pharmacy, laboratory, radiology, medical records, billing, and central supply. Additionally, the physician champion can help support the system's adoption in the ICU and its acceptance by physicians and staff.

As listed above, one desirable component of the EMR system is a computerized provider order entry (CPOE) system to help prescribers order medications, treatments, and tests more safely. CPOE systems are networked computer systems used to electronically document the full range of orders found in a paper-based environment, including patient-specific diagnostic orders (such as laboratory tests and radiology exams) and medication orders. Characteristics that may make CPOE systems safer than paper-based systems include the fact that orders are input electronically in typewritten format so that there is no handwriting to be misread. Similarly, the use of CPOE means no dictated orders to be misheard. Most notably, CPOE systems offer safety alerts and clinical decision support to help guide caregivers. For example, orders entered in the system are automatically analyzed for appropriateness, and improper orders (such as for a contra-indicated treatment or a test that has already been performed) will cause the system to display an alert. Additionally, some CPOE systems are able to perform drug dose calculations based on a patient's condition or physical characteristics.[93]

CPOE systems were originally developed for general areas of the hospital and not the complex environment of the ICU. Therefore, computerized systems must be adapted to meet the needs of a critical care environment. As with EMR, adoption of CPOE in the ICU has been slow, and planning for this technology can be challenging. Much of the current experience with ICU CPOE systems is based on homegrown systems, although newer commercial ICU systems have built-in CPOE, which may facilitate its adoption.[94]

Although additional research is needed, studies of CPOE in the ICU have shown that the technology can help reduce the number of medication errors, including adverse drug events.[95] Nevertheless, as with any technology, CPOE systems may have unintended consequences because they introduce the potential for new types of errors. For example, the technology may induce a false sense of security, prompting a provider to accept the system's proposed suggestion for a drug dose without question.[96] In some cases, an override of the system's suggested course of action may be needed.

With both EMR and CPOE systems, risk management professionals should ensure that staff are encouraged to report near misses and errors associated with implementing the technology, that such reported data is analyzed, and that necessary fixes are accomplished to prevent similar errors. Feedback on identified issues and their resolution should also be provided to staff and appropriate committees involved in the technology's implementation.

SCCM has set forth essential elements required for a functional ICU CPOE in its *CPOE System Requirements for Intensive Care Use* available online at www.sccm.org/corporate_resources/coalition_for_critical_care_excellence/Documents/cpoe.pdf.

· · · · · · · · ·
QUALITY IMPROVEMENT IN THE ICU

In the years since the Institute of Medicine's seminal reports *To Err Is Human* and *Crossing the Quality Chasm* called attention to systems approaches that can enhance safety and prevent error, hospital activity to improve quality has increased, including in the ICU. Within the ICU, some professional groups have suggested quality measures that can be used to monitor care provided and identify areas for improvement. A SCCM task force defined a good quality measure as one that is "important, valid, reliable, responsive, interpretable, and feasible."[97]

In the same vein, The Joint Commission has introduced the concept of using performance measures to complement its accreditation process and allow healthcare organizations to monitor internal quality. The Joint Commission recommendations pertaining to the ICU include four ICU quality measures and two additional measures that are proposed as test measures. Although these measures have not been adopted on a full-scale national basis, The Joint Commission says its ICU measure set is an excellent, fully tested set for monitoring quality in the critical care setting.[98] The four quality measures that are recommended target VAP, stress ulcer disease, deep venous thrombosis, and central catheter–associated BSIs. The two test measures monitor ICU length of stay and mortality for ICU patients. Other highly recommended ICU quality measures address patients with vancomycin-resistant enterococcus, patient complications, gastrointestinal bleeding, and patient satisfaction.[99] Effective quality monitoring requires rigorous data collection aimed at answering the question, How do we know we are safer?

With similar goals, several large collaborative projects in ICU quality improvement have proven effective in facilitating improvement among individual institutions.[100] In addition to the Michigan Keystone ICU Project, other ICU quality initiatives have been adopted by hospitals belonging to VHA Inc., as well as hospitals in New Jersey and Rhode Island.[101] Largely because of Michigan's success in reducing central line infections, AHRQ is funding a ten-state project to reduce central line infections in ICUs by 75 percent by 2012.[102]

As described elsewhere in this chapter, the Keystone ICU Project, a partnership between the Michigan Health & Hospital Association Keystone Center for Patient Safety & Quality and Johns Hopkins University established goals to improve quality of care, enhance safety culture and staff satisfaction, and eliminate unnecessary and additional costs through best-practice and evidence-based interventions.[103] In addition to a 66 percent reduction in catheter-associated BSIs, the hospitals tracked declining VAP rates, a strengthened sense of teamwork between executives and clinicians, improved communication between caregivers, and an enhanced culture of safety.[104]

The Michigan Health & Hospital Association's Keystone Center, Johns Hopkins University, and the American Hospital Association's Health Research and Educational Trust are continuing the work of the Keystone ICU project with an AHRQ-funded project to reduce central line BSIs in ICUs in ten states. The project, On the CUSP: Stop BSI, will implement many of the same tools and strategies used by the Michigan hospitals such as a comprehensive unit-based safety program for ICUs, including checklists to ensure compliance with safety practices, staff education on evidence-based practices to reduce BSIs, staff education on team training, regular feedback on infection rates to hospitals and hospital units, and monthly team meetings to assess progress.[105] The tools for the project are available at www.hret.org/hret/programs/cusp.html.

· · · · · · · · ·
ICU TELEMEDICINE

The electronic ICU (eICU) is steadily gaining acceptance as a viable means of providing intensivist care, demonstrating enhanced patient outcomes in spite of a shortage of physicians and nurses trained in critical care medicine. Having a centralized medical intensivist monitor critically ill patients in multiple ICUs by way of an intricate system of cameras, monitors, and communication links powered by specialized software provides an extra set of eyes on each patient in each ICU. On-site physicians and nurses still conduct regular rounds for each patient in the ICUs; however, a real-time video of each patient, vital signs data, X-ray and laboratory data, and medical records are also transmitted to a centralized ICU command center that monitors the patients remotely.[106]

The full extent of the advantages and disadvantages of telemedicine for delivering critical care is not yet completely understood, although data are starting to emerge that demonstrates the eICU's positive impact on mortality, length of stay, patient outcomes, and clinician satisfaction.[107] Much of these data have been reported in published abstracts; however, clinicians still await the publication of data in peer-reviewed journals to substantiate claims from vendors and users of eICUs.[108] To date, most eICUs are in larger healthcare organizations, which may be better able than smaller operations to address integration of the eICU with other pertinent information technology systems and to finance the significant upfront costs of the eICU.[109] Third-party reimbursement for telemedicine visits is minimal.

Risk management professionals should be involved in organizational planning for the eICU. For example, they will need to ensure that the same credentialing procedures that are in place for on-site physicians are also in place for physicians staffing the remote site. All off-site physicians providing care by telemedicine should be credentialed at each hospital in which the ICU is monitored. Additionally, risk management professionals will need to ensure that the eICU complies with the organization's privacy and security policies for information technology and that on site staff have sufficient means for contacting the off-site physician as needed.

The eICU may also face barriers to its adoption, such as resistance from clinicians opposed to its use. To minimize resistance, one physician with experience in the eICU recommends the following steps:[110]

- Require that all physicians in the eICU be board-certified in critical care.
- Ensure that physicians and nurses in the eICU also provide bedside care and are well respected.
- Request that ICU medical directors take regular shifts in the eICU so they can appreciate how remote monitoring can benefit bedside clinicians.

· · · · · · · · ·

TRANSPARENCY, DISCLOSURE, AND THE PATIENT-CENTERED ICU

In its report, *Crossing the Quality Chasm*, the Institute of Medicine called for transparency as one of the six aims to improve healthcare. Steps have been taken toward this goal in the hospital quality reporting for full reimbursement initiatives sponsored by CMS, which makes the quality data reported to them available to consumers and purchasers alike. Similarly, The Joint Commission has posted quality reports on accredited organizations at its Web site, and several other quality and safety organizations and coalitions are publishing reports on performance of healthcare providers and organizations. ICUs have a vested interest in continuously striving to improve and maintain positive patient outcomes because much of the care provided to patients whose outcomes are monitored for quality and safety reporting is provided in the ICU. The ICU safety and quality programs and projects described in this chapter and in the literature present opportunities for critical care providers and ICUs to move forward in achieving improvements that will reflect positively when viewed by patients and payers alike.

In keeping with honest and open communication among physicians, administrators, and healthcare staffs as a means of promoting patient safety, open communication with patients and their families is also considered characteristic of a culture of safety. Numerous regulatory, accrediting, and professional organizations, including The Joint Commission, ASHRM, and the National Patient Safety Foundation (NPSF), have published standards, monographs, and guidelines that support informing patients and families about outcomes of care, including unanticipated outcomes, errors, and adverse events. Also, several state-mandated laws on disclosure and reporting of serious or sentinel events have been enacted. Concerns initially expressed about increased liability claims resulting from the disclosure of medical errors persist today, but to a lesser degree. In fact, some studies suggest that although the frequency of healthcare liability claims may increase (with disclosure), the severity (costs of monetary payments) of those claims will not.[111] At the same time, other analyses support the other side of the argument. For example, a 2007 study found that full disclosure of adverse events is unlikely to result in a decrease in medical malpractice claims and may actually lead to increases in claim frequency and cost.[112]

Given that the evidence about disclosure's impact on litigation remains inconclusive, additional research is needed. Obviously, there will be some lawsuits filed after a medical mistake has been disclosed to the patient or the patient's family. Often, without a disclosure policy in place, the patient or family may have been completely unaware that a mistake occurred. But there may be many instances in which a lawsuit was prevented because of open and honest communication between provider and patient throughout the patient's medical experience, not just after an unanticipated outcome.

Taking this concept further, apologizing when an error occurs and has been determined to cause injury, and offering to compensate the patient up front, might eventually become standard practice. Disclosure with apology is increasingly common because it is being accepted as the right thing to do and because it is a viable liability claim avoidance strategy. ICU leaders, physicians, and staffs should understand and promote the communication and disclosure policies of their institutions and strive to incorporate improved patient and family involvement in care, treatment, and decision making. Achieving such partnership might require training, education, and skill building.

A partial list of resources on communication and disclosure includes the following:

- National Patient Safety Forum, at www.npsf.org, has a video, "Let's Talk: Disclosure After An Adverse Medical Event," available for $45.

- University of Michigan Hospitals and Health Centers' guidelines for disclosing medical errors are available online at www.med.umich.edu/patientsafetytoolkit/disclosure/howto.doc.

- The Institute for Healthcare Improvement Web site, at www.ihi.org, has numerous shared tools for policies and training.

- The Sorry Works! Coalition, at www.sorryworks.net, was established in 2005 to promotes disclosure, apology (when appropriate), and upfront compensation (when necessary) after adverse medical events.

The concept of patient-centered care is not new. However, the patient safety movement has increased its visibility and importance to healthcare organizations. In addition to open communication and active involvement in care, environmental modifications and nontraditional interventions are being embraced by organizations desiring to become patient centered. There is a growing belief that patient and family involvement improves outcomes and decreases the incidence of errors and mishaps, and this is exemplified nowhere in the healthcare organization more readily than in the ICU, where great strides have been already been made in actively involving patients (and families) in their own care.

To further the implementation of such patient safety strategies, the SCCM and American College of Critical Care Medicine assembled a multidisciplinary task force of experts in critical care practice to review the published literature relative to clinical practice guidelines for support of the family in the patient-centered ICU. The task force issued its guidelines for support of the family in the patient-centered ICU with some of the following recommendations:[113]

- Endorsement of a shared decision-making model
- Early and repeated care conferencing to reduce family stress and improve consistency in communication
- Honoring culturally appropriate requests for truth-telling and informed refusal
- Spiritual support
- Staff education and debriefing to minimize the impact of family interactions on staff health
- Family presence at both rounds and resuscitation
- Open, flexible visitation
- Way-finding and family-friendly signage in the unit
- Family support before, during, and after a death

. . . .

END-OF-LIFE CARE IN THE ICU

The critical care setting is a common place to die; an estimated 22 percent of all deaths in the United States occur in or after admission to the ICU.[114] As the population ages and requires more critical care, more end-of-life decision making will be made in the critical care setting. Risk management professionals can assist their ICU physicians and nurses with guidance in this area.

It is clearly established in the United States that patients who are legally competent and who have the mental capacity to make decisions about their healthcare have the right to refuse treatment, even when such refusal is likely to result in death. The majority of critical care patients may not be able to make decisions for themselves because of their illness or sedation. When patients lack the capacity to make healthcare decisions, their rights can be exercised by a family member or an appointed surrogate. The Patient Self

Determination Act of 1990 gives competent individuals the right to designate a surrogate to make their healthcare and treatment decisions for them in the event that they lose the capacity to make decisions for themselves.[115]

SCCM's 2008 guidelines on end-of-life care emphasize the importance of family-centered care and decision making as the ideal for end-of-life care.[116] The cornerstone to a successful process, says SCCM, is good communication among patients, their surrogates, and clinicians. Nevertheless, conflicts may occur. Families may insist on interventions that the patient's physician considers inadvisable. To resolve these conflicts, patients and families must understand the goals for care and clinicians must provide clear information about the patient's prognosis and what can be accomplished with specific interventions. Clinicians must be prepared to discuss the practical and ethical aspects of withdrawing different modalities of life-sustaining treatment and approaches to easing the dying process. In addition, they should be prepared to answer patients' and families' questions about death. How, for example, is death clinically determined and how can this be explained in terminology that can be easily understood and absorbed by family members?

A good risk management practice is to require accurate documentation of end-of-life discussions and decisions in the patient's medical record. Documentation should include the following:[117]

- Materials documenting the conclusion of a licensed physician concerning the patient's ability or inability to make informed medical decisions on his or her own behalf

- A full description of the patient's medical condition

- Documentation describing efforts that satisfy conditions of state laws

- If the patient is incompetent, notes of all relevant discussions with the family, including discussions about the patient's beliefs and wishes concerning death and termination of life support

- A copy of any written advance directives

- Written informed consent (if the patient is competent) or the family's or designated proxy's written informed consent for withdrawing or withholding a specific treatment

- Orders for sedatives and analgesics for palliative care, as well as documentation of drugs used.

· · · · · · · · ·
CONCLUSION

Critical care is an integral part of the healthcare system, providing complex care to the sickest of patients. ICUs of today and tomorrow must balance increased demand for critical care services from an aging population and increased need for properly trained caregivers for safe and effective intensive care. Providers best able to address these challenges are those that create a culture of safety whereby caregivers work in teams that communicate effectively and understand the goals of medical treatment, that focus on improved care and outcomes, that embrace a systems safety approach to diminish errors, and that partner with patients and their families in providing care. These units will also capitalize on the efficiencies that information technology can bring to medical care and will explore the use of telemedicine to bring critical care capabilities to underserved populations.

The high risks inherent in the ICU can be managed so that patients, caregivers, and healthcare institutions benefit from safer environments, better clinical outcomes, and improved reputations in the communities served. A culture of safety in the ICU is characterized by people and processes aimed at identifying and correcting system defects that affect patient safety and quality of care. All levels of critical care providers, managers, and staff should receive education in the science of systems safety. Medical error reporting must be supported and rewarded through continuous feedback on how learning takes place through the analysis of individual errors and aggregate event data. Because the potential for human and financial loss is arguably the highest when medication errors occur and infections result, these should be a priority for prevention and reduction in the ICU. System and process improvements must be measured to determine the effectiveness of strategies and interventions undertaken to enhance safety and improve outcomes. Technology should be employed to improve safety and decrease errors whenever possible, but with the understanding that new equipment and devices present their own potential for failure that can be exacerbated by human factors and workflow issues.

With the support of risk management professionals and patient safety officers and the commitment of leaders, physicians, and staff; the execution of a clear plan of action; and the verification of effectiveness through measurement of improvements, ICUs can be units in which caregivers work as teams to implement best practices, prevent complications, identify errors, potential errors, and adverse events and strive to reduce and prevent them.[118]

ICU Risk and Safety Resource List

In addition to the references listed in the endnotes to the chapter, the following resources are provided to assist with risk management and patient safety efforts in critical care.

Agency for Healthcare Research and Quality, www.ahrq.gov

Hospital Survey on Patient Safety Culture, http://www.ahrq.gov/qual/patientsafetyculture/

Making Health Care Safer: A Critical Analysis of Patient Safety Practices; Evidence Report/ Technology Assessment, "'Closed' Intensive Care Units and Other Models of Care for Critically Ill Patients," Jeffrey M. Rothschild, M.D., M.P.H., www.ahrq.gov/clinic/ptsafety/chap38.htm

Medical Errors and Patient Safety, www.ahrq.gov/qual/errorsix.htm

Patient Safety Network, www.psnet.ahrq.gov/

Patient Safety Organizations, www.pso.ahrq.gov/

TeamSTEPPS Curriculum Tools and Materials, http://teamstepps.ahrq.gov/abouttoolsmaterials.htm

Web M&M Morbidity and Mortality Rounds, www.webmm.ahrq.gov/

American Association of Critical-Care Nurses, www.aacn.org

Education, Certification, Publications

Centers for Disease Control and Prevention, www.cdc.gov

Hand Hygiene in Healthcare Settings

Prevention of Catheter-Associated Urinary Tract Infections

Prevention of Intravascular Device–Related Infections

Preventing Healthcare-Associated Pneumonia

National Healthcare Safety Network

ECRI Institute, www.ecri.org

Critical Care Safety: Essentials for ICU Patient Care and Technology

Health Devices System, www.ecri.org/Products/Pages/Health_Devices_System.aspx?sub=Device Safety

> Evaluations of infusion pumps, physiological monitoring systems, and ventilators; guidance articles on clinical alarms and tubing disconnections and misconnections

Healthcare Risk Control System, www.ecri.org/hrc

> Risk analyses: clinical alarms, invasive lines, physiological monitoring systems, risk management and patient safety in the ICU, ventilator safety; Self-assessment questionnaires: Critical Care patient safety, infusion therapy, medication

Medical Device Safety Reports, www.mdsr.ecri.org

Patient Safety Organization, ECRI Institute PSO, pso.ecri.org

Top 10 Health Technology Hazards

Health Research & Educational Trust, www.hret.org/hret/programs/cusp.html

Toolkit for National Implementation of the Comprehensive Unit-Based Safety Program (CUSP) to Reduce Central Line Associated Blood Stream Infections (CLABSI) in the Intensive Care Unit

Institute for Healthcare Improvement, www.ihi.org

Topics in Critical Care

Central Line Bundle

ICU Adverse Event Trigger Tool

Multidisciplinary Rounds: Critical Care Unit Nurse Handoff Tool

Severe Sepsis Bundles

Ventilator Bundle

Institute for Safe Medication Practices, www.ismp.org

Error-Prone Abbreviation List

High-Alert Medication List

ISMP Medication Safety Alert! newsletter

Medication Safety Self-Assessment For Hospitals

Johns Hopkins Medicine, www.hopkinsmedicine.org

Science of Safety Educational Program, http://mediasite.jhu.edu/JHU/Viewer/Viewers/Viewer240TR.aspx?mode=Default&peid=386cadcd-66aa-45a8–8e86-df8c86ed3642&playerType=WM7&mode=Default&shouldResize=true&pid=a01d436a-3e82–4027-b07a-07e881540053&playerType=WM7#

Johns Hopkins University Quality and Safety Research Group, http://www.safetyresearch.jhu.edu/QSR/Safety/toolbox/index.asp

Blood Stream Infection (BSI) Checklist

Daily Goals Checklist

How to Investigate a Defect

Morning Briefing

Ventilator Bundle

Shadowing Another Professional

Michigan Health and Safety Coalition, www.mihealthandsafety.org/icu/1.htm

A Toolkit for Intensive Care Units to Improve the Safety and Quality of Patient Care

Patient Safety Group, www.patientsafetygroup.org

eCUSP: Electronic Comprehensive Unit-based Safety Program

Society of Hospital Medicine, www.hospitalmedicine.org

Online Education: Core Competencies and CME Courses: Society of Critical Care Medicine, www.sccm.org

Professional Resources, Online Guidelines

Clinical Practice Guidelines for Support of the Family in the Patient-Centered Intensive Care Unit

CPOE System Requirements for Intensive Care Use

Critical Care Delivery: Defining Clinical Roles and the Best Practice Model

Guidelines for Granting Privileges for the Performance of Procedures in Critically Ill Patients

Guidelines for the Inter- and Intrahospital Transport of Critically Ill Patients

Improving Your ICU: Tips for Better Care

Recommendations for End-of-Life Care in the Intensive Care Unit

Surviving Sepsis Campaign: International Guidelines for Management of Severe Sepsis and Septic Shock

Surviving Sepsis Campaign, www.survivingsepsis.org

Guidelines, Severe Sepsis Bundles

The Joint Commission, www.jointcommission.org

National Patient Safety Goals

Sentinel Event Alerts

National Hospital Quality Measures — ICU

University of Texas-Memorial Hermann Center for Healthcare Quality and Safety, www.utpatientsafety.org

Safety Attitudes Questionnaire (ICU Version)

> Resource listings are representative of information and tools available at selected Web sites and were current as of October 2009.

Endnotes

1. Society of Critical Care Medicine. "Critical Care Statistics in the United States." 2006. Available at: http://sccmwww.sccm.org/Documents/WebStatisticsPamphletFinalJune06. pdf. (Accessed on 8/3/2009.)

2. *Ibid.*

3. Donchin, Y., D. Gopher, M. Olin et al. "A Look into the Nature and Causes of Human Errors in the Intensive Care Unit." *Critical Care Medicine* 1995; 23(2):294–300.

4. Kaushal, R., D. W. Bates, C. Franz et al. "Costs of Adverse Events in Intensive Care Units." *Critical Care Medicine* 2007; 35(11):2479–2483.

5. Ranum, D. "2009 Study on Closed ICU Claims." Columbus, Ohio: The Doctors Company/OHIC Insurance.

6. Human factors is the study of the interrelationships between humans, the tools they use, and the environment in which they live and work. This type of analysis can be applied to the complex systems and processes for delivering healthcare. Source: National Patient Safety Definitions. Available at: www.npsf.org/rc/mp/definitions.php. (Accessed on 7/20/2009.)

7. Donchin, Y., supra note 3.

8. "Root Causes of Sentinel Events (1995–2004)." In: *Sentinel Events and National Patient Safety Goals*. Available at: http://healthpolicy.stanford.edu/PtSafety/ OnlineDocuments/Meetings/2006/Croteau_JointCommission.ppt. (Accessed on 8/5/2009.)

9. Gajic, O., and B. Afessa. "Physician Staffing Models and Patient Safety in the ICU." *Chest* 2009; 135(4):1038–1044.

10. Pronovost, P. J., D. C. Angus, T. Dorman et al. "Physician Staffing Patterns and Clinical Outcomes in Critically Ill Patients: A Systematic Review." *Journal of the American Medical Association* 2002; 288(17):2151–2162.

11. ECRI Institute. "Healthcare Embracing Concept of the High-Reliability Organization." *Risk Management Reporter* 2005; 24(1):8.

12. Perspectives on Safety. "In Conversation With … Peter Pronovost, MD, PhD." Morbidity & Mortality Rounds on the Web, June 2005. Available at: http://www. webmm.ahrq.gov/perspective.aspx?perspectiveID=6. (Accessed on 8/3/2009.)

13. Agency for Healthcare Research and Quality. "Item-Level Average Percent Positive Response by Work Area/Unit." 2009. Available at: www.ahrq.gov/qual/hospsurvey09/ hosp09tabb2.htm. (Accessed on 8/3/2009.)

14. Sexton, J. M., R. L. Helmreich, T. B. Neilands et al. "The Safety Attitudes Questionnaire: Psychometric Properties, Benchmarking Data, and Emerging Research." *BMC Health Services Research* 2006; 6:4. Available at: www.biomedcentral.com/content/pdf/1472–6963–6–44.pdf. (Accessed 3/31/2010.)

15. Pronovost, P., B. Weast, B. Rosenstein et al. "Implementing and Validating a Comprehensive Unit-Based Safety Program." *Journal of Patient Safety* 2005; 1(1):33–40.

16. *Ibid.*

17. *Ibid.*

18. Pronovost, P. J., S. M. Berenholtz, C. A. Goeschel et al. "Creating High Reliability in Health Care Organizations." *Health Services Research* 2006; 41(4 Pt 2):1599–1617.

19. Reader, T. W., R. Flin, and B. H. Cuthbertson. "Communication Skills and Error in the Intensive Care Unit." *Current Opinion in Critical Care* 2007; 13(6):732–736.

20. Pronovost P.J., D. A. Thompson, C. G. Holzmueller et al. "Toward Learning from Patient Safety Reporting Systems." *Journal of Critical Care*, 2006; 21(4):305–15.

21. ECRI Institute. "Cell Phones and Electromagnetic Interference." *Healthcare Risk Control* 2009; Jan. 3 Medical Technology 12.

22. Berkenstadt, H., Y. Haviv, A. Tuval et al. "Improving Handoff Communications in Critical Care." *Chest* 2008; 134(1):158–162.

23. ECRI Institute. "Teamwork Takes Hold to Improve Patient Safety." *Risk Management Reporter* 2005; 24(2):4.

24. Baggs, J. G., M. H. Schmitt, A. I. Mushlin et al. "Association Between Nurse-Physician Collaboration and Patient Outcomes in Three Intensive Care Units." *Critical Care Medicine* 1999; 27(9):1991–1998.

25. ECRI Institute, supra note 23.

26. Williams, T. A., G. D. Leslie, N. Elliott et al. "Introduction of Discharge Plan to Reduce Adverse Events Within 72 Hours of Discharge From the ICU." *Journal of Nursing Care Quality* 2010; 25(1):73–79.

27. Rubenfeld, G. D., and D. C. Angus. "Are Intensivists Safe?" *Annals of Internal Medicine* 2008; 148(11):877–879.

28. Pronovost, Angus, Dorman, supra note 10.

29. Angus, D. C., A. F. Shorr, A. White et al. "Critical Care Delivery in the United States: Distribution of Services and Compliance with Leapfrog Recommendations." *Critical Care Medicine* 2006; 34(4):1016–1024.

30. Pronovost, Angus, Dorman, supra note 10.

31. Levy, M. M., J. Rapoport, S. Lemeshow et al. "Association Between Critical Care Physician Management and Patient Mortality in the Intensive Care Unit." *Annals of Internal Medicine* 2008; 148(11):801–809.

32. Brilli, R. J., A. Spevetz, R. D. Branson et al. "Critical Care Delivery in the Intensive Care Unit: Defining Clinical Roles and the Best Practice Model." *Critical Care Medicine* 2001; 29(10):2001–2019.

33. Agency for Healthcare Research and Quality. "30 Safe Practices for Better Health Care." 2005. Available at: www.ahrq.gov/qual/30safe.htm. (Accessed on 8/3/2009.)

34. National Quality Forum. "Safe Practices for Better Health Care 2010 Update," Available at: www.qualityforum.org/Projects/Safe_Practices_2010.aspx. (Accessed on March 31, 2010.)

35. The Leapfrog Group. "Leapfrog Hospital Survey Results." 2008. Available at: www.leapfroggroup.org/media/file/leapfrogreportfinal.pdf. (Accessed on 8/3/2009.)

36. Joint Commission Resources. *Improving Care in the ICU.* Oakbrook Terrace, Ill.: Joint Commission Resources, 2004; pp. 61–63.

37. Society of Critical Care Medicine. "Improving Your ICU: Tips for Better Care." 2004. Available at: http://sccmwww.sccm.org/tips/Documents/ccLite_brochure.pdf. (Accessed on 8/5/2009.)

38. Rothschild, J. M., A. C. Hurley, C. P. Landrigan, et al. "Recovery from Medical Errors: The Critical Care Nursing Safety Net." *Joint Commission Journal on Quality and Patient Safety* 2006; 32(2):63–72.

39. Brilli, R. J., A. Spevetz, R. D. Branson et al., supra note 32.

40. Pronovost, P., and C. Goeschel. "Improving ICU Care: It Takes a Team." *Healthcare Executive* 2005; 20(2):14–22.

41. Pronovost, P., D. Needham, S. Berenholtz et al. "An Intervention to Decrease Catheter-related Bloodstream Infections in the ICU." *New England Journal of Medicine* 2006; 355(26):2725–2732.

42. Raoff, N. D., and N. A. Halpern. "Pay for Performance in Critical Care: Like It or Not, Here It Comes!" *Critical Care Medicine* 2009; 37(3):1132–1133.

43. Rothschild, J. M., C, P. Landrigan, J. W. Cronin et al. "The Critical Care Safety Study: The Incidence and Nature of Adverse Events and Serious Medical Errors in Intensive Care." *Critical Care Medicine* 2005; 33(8):1694–1700.

44. National Healthcare Safety Network (NHSN). Centers for Disease Control and Prevention. Available at: www.cdc.gov/nhsn/. (Accessed on 3/31/2010.)

45. Pennsylvania Patient Safety Authority. Available at: http://patientsafetyauthority.org/Pages/Default.aspx. (Acccessed 3/31/2010.)

46. The Joint Commission. "Preventing Ventilator-Related Deaths and Injuries." *Sentinel Event Alert* 2002; 25(2). Available at: www.jointcommission.org/SentinelEvents/SentinelEventAlert/sea_25.htm. (Accessed on 8/5/2009.)

47. Rothschild, Landrigan, Cronin et al., supra note 43.

48. *Ibid.*

49. Kaushal, supra note 4.

50. Pronovost, Thompson, Holzmueller et al., supra note 20.

51. *Ibid.*

52. Pronovost, P. J., L. L. Morlock, J. B. Sexton et al. "Improving the Value of Patient Safety Reporting Systems." Available at: www.ahrq.gov/downloads/pub/advances2/vol1/Advances-Pronovost_95.pdf. (Accessed on 8/5/2009.)

53. Resar, R. K., R. D. Rozich, T. Simmonds et al. "A Trigger Tool to Identify Adverse Events in the Intensive Care Unit." *Joint Commission Journal on Quality and Patient Safety* 2006; 32(10):585–590.

54. Ranum, D., supra note 5.

55. The Joint Commission. "Infusion Pumps: Preventing Future Adverse Events." *Sentinel Event Alert* 2000; 15(11). Available at: www.jointcommission.org/SentinelEvents/ SentinelEventAlert/sea_15.htm. (Accessed on 8/5/2009.)

56. ECRI Institute. "General-Purpose Infusion Pumps." *Health Devices* 2007: 36(10):309–336.

57. ECRI Institute. "Physiologic Monitoring Systems." *Health Devices* 2005; 34(1):5–45.

58. ECRI Institute. *Critical Care Safety: Essentials for ICU Patient Care and Technology*. Plymouth Meeting, Pa.: ECRI Institute, 2007.

59. Society of Critical Care Medicine. "Guidelines for the Inter- and Intrahospital Transport of Critically Ill Patients." *Critical Care Medicine* 2004; 32(1):256–262.

60. The Joint Commission, supra note 46.

61. ECRI Institute. "JCAHO, ECRI Offer Advice to Prevent Ventilator-Related Deaths, Injuries." *Risk Management Reporter* 2002; 21(3):9–10.

62. ECRI Institute. "Top 10 Health Technology Hazards." *Health Devices* 2008; 37(11):343–350.

63. *Ibid.*

64. The Joint Commission. "Tubing Misconnections—A Persistent and Potentially Deadly Occurrence." *Sentinel Event Alert* 2006; 36(4). Available at: www.jointcommission. org/SentinelEvents/SentinelEventAlert/sea_36.htm. (Accessed on 8/5/2009.)

65. ECRI Institute. "Fixing Bad Links: Preventing Misconnections in Your Hospital." *Health Devices* 2009; 38(7):220–227.

66. Osmon, S., C. B. Harris, and W. C. Dunagan. "Reporting of Medical Errors: An Intensive Care Unit Experience." *Critical Care Medicine* 2004; 32(3):727–733.

67. Jury Verdict Research. *Current Award Trends in Personal Injury*, 48th edition. Horsham, Pa.: LRP Publications, 2009.

68. The Joint Commission. "Sentinel Event Statistics—Updated through June 30, 2009." Available at: www.jointcommission.org/SentinelEvents/Statistics/. (Accessed on 8/17/2009.)

69. Aspden, P., editor. *Preventing Medication Errors*. Institute of Medicine Committee on Identifying and Preventing Medication Errors, Washington, D.C.: National Academies Press, 2006.

70. Leape, L. L., D. J. Cullen, M. D. Clapp et al. "Pharmacist Participation on Physician Rounds and Adverse Drug Events in the Intensive Care Unit." *JAMA* 1999; 282(3):267–270.

71. Institute for Safe Medication Practices. "Survey on High-Alert Medications. Differences between Nursing and Pharmacy Perspectives Revealed." *ISMP Medication Safety Alert* 2003; 8(21):1–2.

72. ECRI Institute. "High-Alert Medications." *Healthcare Risk Control* 2004; Mar, 4 Pharmacy and Medications 1.4

73. ECRI Institute. "Medication Safety." *Healthcare Risk Control* 2007; Nov, 4 Pharmacy and Medications 1.

74. Institute for Safe Medication Practices (ISMP). "Three Neonates Die from Heparin Overdoses: How Will Your Organization Respond?" *ISMP Medication Safety Alert Nurse Advise-ERR* 2006; 4(10):1–2.

75. Institute for Safe Medication Practices (ISMP). "Action Needed to Prevent Dangerous Heparin-Insulin Confusion." *ISMP Medication Safety Alert, 2007*; May 3. Available at: www.ismp.org/Newsletters/acutecare/articles/20070503.asp. (Accessed on 8/17/2009.)

76. Pronovost, P., D. B. Hobson, K. Earsing et al. "A Practical Tool to Reduce Medication Errors During Patient Transfer from an Intensive Care Unit." *Journal of Clinical Outcomes Management* 2004; 11(1):26–33.

77. *Ibid.*

78. Agency for Healthcare Research and Quality. *National Healthcare Quality Report Dec. 2004*; AHRQ Publication No. 05–0013. Available at: www.ahrq.gov/qual/nhqr04/fullreport/Index.htm. (Accessed on 8/5/2009.)

79. Mermel, L. A. "Prevention of Intravascular Catheter-Related Infections." *Annals of Internal Medicine* 2000; 132(5):391–402.

80. Institute for Healthcare Improvement. Implementing the central line bundle. Available at: www.ihi.org/IHI/Topics/CriticalCare/IntensiveCare/Changes/ImplementtheCentralLineBundle.htm. (Accessed on 7/30/2009.)

81. Pronovost, P., supra note 41.

82. *Ibid.*

83. Berenholtz, S. M., P. J. Pronovost, P. A. Lipsett et al. "Eliminating Catheter-Related Bloodstream Infections in the Intensive Care Unit." *Critical Care Medicine* 2004; 32(10):2014–2020.

84. Institute for Healthcare Improvement. "Implement the Ventilator Bundle." Available at: www.ihi.org/IHI/Topics/CriticalCare/IntensiveCare/Changes/ImplementtheVentilatorBundle.htm. (Accessed on 7/31/2009.)

85. Pennsylvania Patient Safety Authority. "Successful Reduction of Ventilator-Associated Pneumonia." *Pennsylvania Patient Safety Advisory* 2009; 6(2):63–68.

86. Dellinger, R. P., M. M. Levy, J. M. Carlet et al. "Surviving Sepsis Campaign: International Guidelines for Management of Severe Sepsis and Septic Shock: 2008." *Critical Care Medicine* 2008; 36(1):296–327.

87. The NICE-SUGAR Investigators. "Intensive versus Conventional Glucose Control in Critically Ill Patients." *New England Journal of Medicine* 2009; 360(13):1283–1297.

88. Inzucchi, S. E., and M. D. Siegel. "Glucose Control in the ICU—How Tight Is Too Tight?" *New England Journal of Medicine* 2009; 360(13):1346–1349.

89. Saint, S., S. R. Kaufman, M. Thompson et al. "A Reminder Reduces Urinary Catheterization in Hospitalized Patients." *Joint Commission Journal on Quality and Patient Safety* 2005; 31(8):455–462.

90. ECRI Institute. "Urinary Catheter-Associated Infections Drop with Focus on Indications." *Risk Management Reporter* 2009; 28(5):18–19.

91. Friedman, L. N., N. A. Halpern, and J. C. Fackler. "Implementing an Electronic Medical Record." *Critical Care Clinics* 2007; 23(3):347–381.

92. *Ibid.*

93. ECRI Institute. "Computerized Provider Order-Entry Systems." *Healthcare Risk Control* 2002; May(Supp A) Pharmacy and Medications 6.

94. Colpaert, K., and J. Decruyenaere. "Computerized Physician Order Entry in Critical Care." *Best Practice & Research Clinical Anesthesiology* 2009; 23(1):27–38.

95. *Ibid.*

96. *Ibid.*

97. Curtis, J. R., D. J. Cook, R. J. Wall et al. "Intensive Care Unit Quality Improvement: A "How-To" Guide for the Interdisciplinary Team." *Critical Care Medicine* 2006; 34(1):211–218.

98. The Joint Commission. National Hospital Quality Measures — ICU. Available at: www .jointcommission.org/PerformanceMeasurement/MeasureReserveLibrary/ Spec+Manual+-+ICU.htm. (Accessed on 8/5/2009.)

99. McMillan, T. R., and R. C. Hyzy. "Bringing Quality Improvement into the Intensive Care Unit." *Critical Care Medicine* 2007; 35(2 Suppl):S59–65.

100. *Ibid.*

101. *Ibid.*

102. Department of Health and Human Services. "Secretary Sebelius Releases Inaugural Health Care 'Success Story' Report." 2009. Available at: www.hhs.gov/news/ press/2009pres/07/20090713a.html. (Accessed on 8/3/2009.)

103. ECRI Institute. "Michigan's Focus on ICU Patient Safety Achieves Success." *Risk Management Reporter* 2008; 27(1):1–8.

104. *Ibid.*

105. Agency for Healthcare Research and Quality. "10-State Project to Study Methods to Reduce Central Line-Associated Bloodstream Infections in Hospital ICUs." 2009. Available at: www.ahrq.gov/news/press/pr2009/clabsipr.htm. (Accessed on 8/3/2009).

106. National Coalition on Health Care and Institute for Healthcare Improvement. "Imagining the ICU of the Future." In: *Care in the ICU: Teaming Up to Improve Quality*. September, 2002. Available at: www.nchc.org/documents/CareintheICU2.pdf. (Accessed on 8/18/2009.)

107. Ries, M. "Tele-ICU: A New Paradigm in Critical Care." *International Anesthesiology Clinics* 2009; 47(1):153–170.

108. Sapirstein, A., N. Lone, A. Latif et al. "Tele-ICU: Paradox or Panacea?" *Best Practice & Research Clinical Anaesthesiology* 2009; 23(1):115–126.

109. Ries, M., supra note 107; A. Sapirstein, N. Lone, A. Latif et al, supra note 108.

110. Ries, M., supra note 107.

111. Popp P. "How Will Disclosure Protect Future Litigation?" *Journal of Healthcare Risk Management* 2003; 23(1):5–9.

112. Studdert, D. M., M. M. Mello, A. A. Gawande et al. "Disclosure of Medical Injury to Patients: An Improbable Risk Management Strategy." *Health Affairs* 2007; 26(1):215–226.

113. Davidson, J. E., K. Powers, K. M. Hedayat et al. "Clinical Practice Guidelines for Support of the Family in the Patient-Centered Intensive Care Unit: American College of Critical Care Medicine Task Force 2004–2005." *Critical Care Medicine* 2007; 35(2):605–622.

114. Truog, R. D., M. L. Campbell, J. R. Curtis et al. "Recommendations for End-of-Life Care in the Intensive Care Unit: A Consensus Statement by the American College of Critical Care Medicine." *Critical Care Medicine* 2008; 36(3):953–963.

115. ECRI Institute. "Termination of Life-Sustaining Treatment." *Healthcare Risk Control* 2006; Nov; Ethics 2.

116. Truog, R. D., supra note 114.

117. ECRI Institute, supra note 115.

118. Perspectives on Safety. In: Conversation With … Peter Pronovost, MD, PhD. Morbidity & Mortality Rounds on the Web, June 2005. Available at: www.webmm.ahrq.gov/perspective.aspx?perspectiveID=6. (Accessed on 8/3/2009.)

8

Management of Risk: Promoting Perinatal Patient Safety

G. Eric Knox, MD
Kathleen Rice Simpson

SCOPE OF PROBLEM

The personal, professional, and financial cost of perinatal liability remains significant and problematic. For more than twenty years, obstetrics has led or been close to the top of severity (dollars paid) for professional liability claims.[1] The 2006 American College of Obstetricians and Gynecologist (ACOG) Survey on Professional Liability reflects little change since the last survey (2003).[2] During a sixteen-year career, the average obstetrician can expect 2.62 professional liability claims. A total of 89.2 percent of the respondents indicated they had at least one professional liability claim filed against them during their professional careers and 5 percent of ACOG fellows surveyed reported three or more claims. In response to affordability and availability issues with professional liability insurance, 65 percent to 70 percent of ob-gyn survey respondents significantly decreased the number of high-risk obstetric patients cared for, increased the number of C-sections in routine practice, and refused to perform or offer vaginal birth after caesareans (VBACs). Between 7 and 8 percent of respondents stopped practicing obstetrics altogether (average age forty-eight years old). Twenty-three "red alert" states now exist with a medical liability insurance crisis. Factors that contribute to designation as a red alert state are a lack of available professional liability coverage for obstetricians because only a few carriers are currently writing policies in the state; the number of carriers leaving the medical liability insurance market; and the cost and rate of increase of annual premiums based on reports from industry monitors.

ACOG also found in their 2006 survey that the primary clinical issue in an obstetric claim was a neurologically impaired baby (34.3 percent) followed by stillbirth or neonatal death (15.3 percent). Hospital-based treatment such as fetal monitoring (47.7 percent for a neurologically impaired baby; 21.9 percent for a stillbirth or neonatal death) and oxytocin administration (43.4 percent for a neurologically impaired baby; 14.7 percent for a stillbirth or neonatal death) were significant factors in both types of claims.[3] The mean length of time from filing of an obstetric claim involving neonatal harm to resolution is four years, with 13.4 percent requiring seven years or longer to resolve.[4] The average payment for claims involving a neurologically impaired infant was $1,150,687. Other average payments for obstetric claims include "other infant injury–major," $477,504, and "stillbirth/neonatal death," $259,017. Healthcare organizations face similar liability/financial risk. The average settlement for a claim against a hospital is just over $1.5 million, and the average jury verdict exceeds $7 million.[5]

The devastation of families that occurs when a labor and birth result in a brain-damaged baby is enormous and long-standing, particularly when the adverse outcome is determined to have been preventable. The psychological and emotional impact on the healthcare clinicians who are involved cannot be minimized. They often suffer a wide range of distressing emotions (shock, outrage, denial, anxiety, guilt, shame, and despair) and increased stress, which can disrupt their personal lives and the lives of their families; sometimes the clinician gives up his or her clinical practice entirely.[6] Coping with medical professional liability litigation is an ongoing, complex process in which physicians and nurses often struggle to regain a sense of personal identity and professional mastery as well as control of their clinical practices.

· · · · · · · · ·

AN EMERGING SOLUTION?

Despite the somewhat static and discouraging picture painted by the 2006 ACOG survey and related claims data, recent information suggests an emerging consensus on broad principles capable of successfully managing perinatal risk and increasing obstetrical patient safety. Obstetrical patient safety initiatives with the goals of decreasing the financial loss associated with claims and promoting safer care for mothers and babies during labor and birth are reporting impressive results (see below).[7,8] Essential basic principles of the successful initiatives include the following:

- Standardization of key clinical protocols and physician orders based on professional standards, guidelines, and the latest evidence

- Accountability for creating a culture of safety based on trust, transparency, and teamwork as opposed to provider autonomy, hierarchy, and unprofessional behavior

- Respecting oxytocin as a high-alert medication as designated by Institute for Safe Medication Practices (ISMP) and providing accountability for all aspects of appropriate administration

This chapter will discuss the evolution of loss prevention practices that have culminated in these principles and will suggest strategies for implementation.

·········

ATTEMPTS TO MANAGE OBSTETRICAL RISK

Until recently, the following traditional approaches to managing obstetrical risk have been employed by a majority of healthcare organizations:

- Blaming and training
- Documentation
- Technology
- Credentialing
- Outcome screening
- Causation defenses

However, as pointed out in the introduction, none of these techniques, either alone or in combination, have been able to stop the increasing dollar amounts of plaintiff settlements, jury awards, or the percentage of cases decided against hospitals or physicians.[9] However, within these discouraging overall trends, there exists an important dichotomy not readily explained by legal jurisdiction; that is, some perinatal units have encountered a disproportionate number of obstetrical claims whereas others have had very few or only minor nuisance-type liability claims brought against them.[10] This dichotomy mirrors that of the physicians' professional liability experience; that is, a minority of physicians account for a majority of claims filed and dollars paid.[11,12] Understanding the differences between high liability and lower risk OB units and provider practice has been crucial in understanding the principles underlying a systematic and successful approach to managing obstetric risk.

Units at High Risk for Patient Injury and Harm

Perinatal units that experience an unacceptably high amount of patient harm or professional liability have the following organizational features:[13]

- Patient safety is not explicitly stated as a primary and important goal or value.
- Production and financial considerations have a higher priority than patient safety in operational decision making.
- Clinical practice is not based on evidence and professional standards. Instead, clinical action and decision making are determined by "the way we've always done it." Wide variation in clinical practice persists in spite of existing clearly articulated professional standards and guidelines. Autonomy routinely trumps standardization.
- Nurses and physicians cannot articulate or agree to the mission, vision, or goals of the clinical team.
- Provider convenience takes precedence over patient safety.
- Effective peer review and interdisciplinary case analysis are nonexistent.
- Reporting of near misses or good catches is not done or valued.

- Systems or unit operations are not evaluated as potential sources of error. Rather, individuals are blamed when errors occur.

- Accidents are often attributed to "circumstances beyond our control."

- Physician–patient relationships are patriarchal, with little effective patient-centered decision making.

- Women are not fully informed of risks and benefits of procedures prospectively, as applicable.

- Labor and birth are routinely viewed as medical procedures to be managed and controlled rather than a natural, predominantly low-risk phenomenon made riskier by unnecessary iatrogenic (induced inadvertently by a physician or surgeon or by medical treatment or diagnostic procedures)[14] intervention.

- Hierarchical deference in nurse–physician relationships is the expected behavioral norm.

- Nurse–physician relationships are characterized by ongoing conflict, overt or covert. Professionals uneasily coexist or barely tolerate one another's presence.

- Hostility and inappropriate workplace behavior are tolerated or taken for granted.

- A formal chain of command is frequently used to modify behavior instead of informal group norms and open, direct communication.

- Conflict is downplayed or avoided rather than used as an opportunity for learning.

In sum, organizational and individual behavior in high-liability, high-risk perinatal units is dysfunctional at best and destructive at worst.[15] The atmosphere is one of hierarchy, blame, and retribution, with professionals in constant conflict. Clearly, this is the antithesis of teamwork, high reliability, and patient safety as defined in other high-risk domains.[16]

Low-Risk Units Are Different

In contrast to obstetrical units at high risk for professional liability, in the authors' experience low-risk units, regardless of size or level of care, operate with a markedly different set of general principles. For example, administrative leadership, though recognizing the importance of fiscal stewardship, ultimately believes that the mission of preventing fetal and neonatal injury creates the margin and makes safety first a day-to-day reality. The tension between production and safety is balanced rather than shifted in a hazardous way toward production. The resulting clinical environment fosters a much more objective and transparent appreciation of risk for all stakeholders. Low-risk units have invested in an administrative medical director of obstetrics who works in tandem and in partnership with the nursing leader of perinatal services to ensure high reliability and quality. Education is viewed as an essential component of clinical work with adequate educational support provided. The unit is routinely staffed according to American Academy of Pediatrics[17] and Association of Women's Health, Obstetric and Neonatal Nurses (AWHONN)[18] recommendations. Administrators recognize that their organization holds the majority of perinatal risk and are willing to hold providers accountable for standards-based practice and, most important, professional workplace behavior.

Complementing the administrative infrastructure, low-risk units also feature a supportive clinical infrastructure. There is a commitment to creating and sustaining a culture of safety[19] for mothers, babies, and healthcare professionals. Strong interdisciplinary clinical leadership and an interdisciplinary perinatal practice committee[20] define unit policy and hold all providers accountable for standards-based practice.[21] The interdisciplinary practice committee has a standing agenda item each month to review the most recently published science, standards, and guidelines from professional organizations such as AWHONN, ACOG, AAP, and The Joint Commission on Accreditation of Healthcare Organizations (JCAHO, or TJC). When new standards and guidelines are published, the discussion should focus on how and when (rather than if) such professional guidance will be incorporated into unit operations and daily practice. Obstetric department membership requires a commitment to clinical practice based on good science, the latest evidence, and published national professional standards of care. Standardization and simplification of clinical protocols and unit operations is accepted and routine. In rare cases, where there might be a need to practice outside unit policy, interdisciplinary discussion occurs, medical record documentation objectively details clinical rationale, and the case is evaluated through the quality review process.[22]

Professional attitude, behavior, and unit culture are recognized as major determinants of degree of perinatal risk. Collegial professional relationships and superb communication predominate, rather than a more traditional hierarchical way of doing business. There is the expectation that all professionals will act professionally all of the time. There is meaningful direct, real-time follow-up when behavior is inappropriate. Teamwork is promoted and practiced. For example, the different but equal contribution of nurses to patient care and clinical outcomes is recognized, acknowledged, and valued by physicians and administrators. Constant communication by everyone is encouraged. Briefing and debriefing to enhance communication is used extensively. Creating and maintaining a safety net is part of unit mindset. The "one thing that could go wrong" and "what ifs?" are routinely and openly discussed, and change of shift reports emphasize the questions what if?" and "are we prepared?" Emergency protocols are rehearsed.[23] As specified by unit policy, physicians come to the unit and personally evaluate a patient at any time they are requested to do so by a nurse. Clinical disagreements are managed directly on the unit; chain of command is viewed as a failure or sentinel event that requires root cause analysis (RCA) to determine the factors that produced it. In sum, there is universal agreement to use professional standards and professional behavior as the basis for clinical practice, all within the context of a culture of safety.

· · · · · · · · ·
STEPWISE STRATEGY FOR MANAGING PERINATAL RISK

Creating a safe clinical environment during labor and birth requires effective leadership, a clearly articulated and shared philosophy, professional workplace behavior, and excellence in key clinical practices. Without effective administrative and clinical leaders, staff members are challenged to implement essential criteria for safe care. Leaders must be fully committed and must have the will to do the right thing for mothers and babies, caregivers, and the institution, even as they are faced with the very real pressures of economics, production, and perceived provider convenience.[24]

Several organizations have recently published the results whereby they have increased the safety of their perinatal environments by employing the basic set of principles outlined in this chapter. It should be noted that although broad principles are identical, specific strategies, tactics, and approaches to managing perinatal risk are based on organizational structure, history, and administrative strengths:

- Yale University, a representative member of MCIC Vermont (university teaching hospitals representing academic leadership) demonstrated significant improvement in a broad range of obstetrical safety outcomes (i.e., AOI).[25]

- Catholic Healthcare Partners, a community faith-based institution with systemwide risk analysis and collaboration has demonstrated improved systemwide infrastructure and process together with a reduction in number and cost of OB professional liability claims.[26] HCA, a data-driven and protocol/check list-driven for-profit hospital company recently published data indicating a decrease both in claims and C-section rates.[27]

- Swedish Healthsystem, a large nonprofit community hospital in Seattle, has shown improved safety by limiting elective inductions.[28]

Although the methodological emphasis or tactics differ slightly from organization to organization, there is an emerging consensus among successful organizations that executive leadership needs to be absolute in its support of the perinatal safety initiative. Clinical consensus grounded in standardization based on national standards, a culture of safety emphasizing multidisciplinary learning, and correct administration of oxytocin are prerequisites for decreasing perinatal harm and liability.[29]

Policy and Protocol Development

Organizations that have enhanced obstetric safety apply national and professional standards to all unit policies. They give priority to induction and augmentation of labor; timely, accurate fetal assessment and response to nonreassuring fetal status; and second-stage labor management (see also specific clinical issues discussed below).

The following are steps by which organizations can achieve this objective include the following:

- Use an interdisciplinary perinatal practice committee to review and revise policies and procedures to be consistent with current national standards of all pertinent professional organizations.

- Develop a uniform set of standing orders that reflect unit policy based on national professional standards. With the exception of rare clinical situations, variation of practice that is outside good science (the latest evidence and national professional standards) should be prohibited.

- Educate all providers together as an interdisciplinary team on national professional standards and standing orders.

- Review perinatal practice for compliance with national professional standards through direct observation and medical record audits.

- Identify, update, and implement practice as new standards are published.

Conduct a Baseline Perinatal Safety Attitude Survey   The previously mentioned organizations have found it helpful to anticipate perinatal safety enhancement by measuring effectiveness of unit teamwork, patient safety, and provider attitude, that is, the sum and substance of a perinatal culture of safety.

- The perinatal safety attitude questionnaire (SAQ) provides information on teamwork climate, safety climate, job satisfaction, perceptions of management, working conditions, and individual stress recognition.[30]

- Professional attitude and organizational culture help explain other forms of healthcare performance data such as absenteeism, turnover, case delays, length of stay, and readmission rates, in addition to safety performance in other high-risk domains.

- The SAQ is designed to be a preintervention and postintervention measurement tool and should be initiated with this capability in mind.

Initiate Teamwork and Patient Safety Education

Once the SAQ is completed, effective perinatal organizations address issues of dysfunctional communication, collaboration, and teamwork that have been identified. They also encourage the value of including principles of human factors and the role of systems in creating harm in all unit orientation and ongoing work.[31, 32]

The following are related insights and suggested approaches:

- Poor teamwork and communication (miscommunication or lack of communication) are often significant factors in mishaps that occur in nonmedical high-risk domains, medical accidents, and perinatal malpractice claims.[33]

- Initial education should emphasize assertive communication, situational awareness, and conflict management.

- It is important to routinely conduct drills for common high-risk clinical situations such as shoulder dystocia, emergent cesarean birth, and postpartum hemorrhage.[34]

- Use role-playing to simulate clinical situations with potential for conflict between team members.

- Routinely observe handoffs and use opportunities for improvement that are identified to improve the handoff process.[35]

Begin Daily Interdisciplinary Unit Reviews and Debriefings

Daily interdisciplinary unit reviews and debriefings of select medical records can help improve team performance and educate all care providers to the system issues involved when a near miss or harm occurs. The following points are to be considered:

- Standardize and select patient safety indicators specific to risk or potential liability for medical record review every twenty-four hours (for example, unanticipated maternal return to the operating room (OR), admission to the intensive care unit (ICU), intrapartum fetal death, and neonatal pH of less than 7.20).

- Focus on process of care rather than adverse outcomes. Such adverse outcomes occur rarely and are difficult to assess with statistically stable data, even in large samples. For example, a "failure to rescue" indicator can be a useful way to measure fetal safety because it captures gaps and limitations in unit processes.[36]

- Monitor medical records for adherence to unit policies and protocols (care processes).

- Include fetal monitor strips with the medical record as part of each case review.

- Transmit lessons learned to all unit providers.

Use Neonatal Injuries for Credentialing and Peer Review

Include and emphasize defined neonatal injuries as an integral component of obstetrical peer review, credentialing, and privileging activities.

- Conduct peer review of the maternal medical records leading to the neonatal injuries (for example, intrapartum fetal death, neonatal asphyxia, brachial plexus injury, meconium aspiration, forceps or vacuum extraction injury).

- Include fetal monitoring strips with the medical record as part of each case review. Process and outcome should be assessed and emphasized.

Institute Interdisciplinary Education and Certification in Electronic Fetal Monitoring

Successful perinatal programs emphasize the importance of interdisciplinary education to increase team communication and proficiency through adoption of a common electronic fetal monitoring (EFM) language and demonstration of competence. This initiative should be both individual and team based.

Physicians and nurses in these settings should obtain certification in EFM from a nationally recognized certifying organization that provides psychometrically valid and reliable examinations. Privileging and credentialing should require documentation of such certification. It is important to continue EFM team review and learning through regular interdisciplinary forums.

Create the Position of Perinatal Patient Safety Nurse

The perinatal patient safety nurse works in collaboration with perinatal physicians and nursing leaders.[37] The role is designed to do the following:

- Actively advocate safety first, ask the tough questions, and stop the line when reevaluation of risk is indicated.
- Be a clinical link to and support organizational risk management professionals.
- Ensure that all care providers in the unit, and unit practices, adhere to national professional standards and the principles and practice of a culture of safety.
- Coordinate safety culture survey process and team training.
- Coordinate analysis of medical records to objectively measure process and improvement.
- Coordinate electronic fetal monitoring certification.
- Provide interdisciplinary education in the principles of patient safety.
- Serve as a constant reminder of the organization's commitment to safe care for mothers and babies.

· · · · · · · · ·
CLINICAL PRACTICES THAT INCREASE RISK OF INJURY AND HARM

A discussion of key clinical practices known to increase risk of prenatal injury and harm and the solutions for specific obstetric issues follows in this section.[38]

Fetal Assessment

As previously discussed, safety during fetal assessment is based on a common language for fetal heart rate (FHR) patterns, common knowledge and understanding of fetal physiology, and common expectations for interventions when the FHR pattern suggests fetal compromise. The terminology to describe FHR patterns recommended by the National Institute of Child Health and Human Development is used in all professional communication concerning fetal assessment.[39–41] The written and electronic medical records provide cues to the appropriate terminology. There is ongoing interdisciplinary fetal monitoring education. Knowledge and skills in fetal assessment are not assumed to be discipline specific. All members of the team participate in case reviews and offer suggestions for future care improvement. Communication among team members about nonreassuring FHR patterns should include baseline rate, variability, presence or absence of accelerations and decelerations, the clinical context, and pattern evolution.[42]

Intrauterine Resuscitation

There should be common expectations for intrauterine resuscitation with documentation in real time as interventions occur, including the following:

- Promotion of fetal oxygenation
- Placement in lateral position (either left or right)
- Administration of oxygen at 10 L per minute via non-rebreather facemask
- Administration of intravenous fluid bolus of at least 500 mL of lactated Ringer's solution
- Discontinuation of pushing temporarily or pushing with every other or every third contraction (during second stage labor)
- Reduction of uterine activity (discontinue Cytotec or Cervidil and oxytocin)
- Correction of maternal hypotension[43,44]
- Agreement among team members concerning which type of FHR patterns require bedside evaluation by the primary care provider and within an identified time frame[45]
- Intervention for nonreassuring fetal status, including emergent cesarean birth, in a timely and appropriate time frame
- Neonatal resuscitation based on the Neonatal Resuscitation Program (NRP)[46]
- Completion of the NRP course by all team members

Labor Induction

Labor induction should be carried out on suitable candidates, with proper timing, pharmacological agents, dosing protocols, and recognition and treatment of complications as recommended by ACOG[47,48] and AWHONN.[49] Elective births should not be performed for women who are less than thirty-nine completed weeks of gestation. Miscalculations in gestational age and estimated dates of birth are common and can result in the birth of a late preterm baby if labor is induced prematurely. In addition to risk of iatrogenic prematurity, elective birth before thirty-nine completed weeks of gestation poses a professional liability risk. If care during labor induction and/or cesarean section of a woman having elective birth before thirty-nine completed weeks of gestation leads to an adverse outcome and subsequent litigation, the plaintiffs have readily available evidence that there was a breach of the standard of care before any other aspects of the clinical situation are reviewed.

There is a cumulative body of evidence that late preterm babies compared to term babies have higher incidence of prematurity-related medical and surgical conditions, such as respiratory distress syndrome, transient tachypnea, patent ductus arteriosus, hypothermia, apnea, infection, feeding difficulty, necrotizing enterocolitis, hyperbilirubinemia and kernicterus, seizures, and intracranial hemorrhage.[50] Late preterm babies have higher mortality rates than term babies throughout infancy[51] and need closer monitoring than term babies, often requiring special care or Newborn Intensive Care Unit (NICU) admissions or readmissions after initial hospital discharge, resulting in significantly more hospital costs.[52]

Every week matters for fetal growth and development. Babies born even one to two weeks before thirty-nine completed weeks of gestation are also at significant risk for neonatal morbidity.[53] Rates of adverse respiratory outcomes, mechanical ventilation, newborn sepsis, hypoglycemia, admission to the NICU, and hospitalization for five days or more are increased 1.8 to 4.2 times for births at thirty-seven weeks and 1.3 to 2.1 times for births at thirty-eight weeks.[54]

Iatrogenic neonatal morbidity from elective birth before thirty-nine completed weeks of gestation is unacceptable in contemporary perinatal practice.

There are standard unit policies and corresponding order sets for each pharmacological agent. There is an expectation that all providers will practice based on these established unit policies. There are ample data that a standard oxytocin protocol (start at 1 mU/min and increase by 1 to 2 mU/min no more frequently than every thirty minutes based on the maternal-fetal response) has numerous benefits to mothers and babies (decreased risk of oxytocin-induced tachysystole, fetal hypoxemia and acidemia, maternal pain, placental abruption, uterine rupture, unnecessary cesarean birth for indeterminate/abnormal FHR patterns, postpartum hemorrhage and infection[55]) and should be used as routine clinical practice. Patient injury from drug therapy is the single most common type of adverse event that occurs in the inpatient setting.[56] Patient harm resulting from use of a drug is defined as an *adverse drug event* (ADE). Other terms used include *potential adverse drug event*, circumstances that could result in patient harm by the use of the drug, but did not harm the patient, and *medication error*, inappropriate use of a drug that may or may not cause patient harm. Oxytocin-induced uterine tachysystole can be classified as one or more of these conditions.

In 2007, ISMP added intravenous (IV) oxytocin to their list of high-alert medications.[57] High-alert medications are drugs that have a heightened risk of causing significant patient harm when they are used in error. Errors with high-alert medications may or may not be more common than with other drugs; however, patient injury and consequences of associated errors may be more devastating, thus special considerations and precautions are required prior to and during its administration. As with other high-alert medications, the lowest dose of oxytocin possible to achieve the desired clinical effect should be used. Tachysystole is a major feature in successful obstetrical malpractice cases[58] and makes it challenging to find a credible defense expert.

Nurses must never be pressured by physician colleagues to "push the pit" or "pit to distress." Labor induction should be initiated only when there are enough qualified nurses to safely monitor the mother and fetus. Consider using a checklist before initiating oxytocin[59]:

- A minimum of thirty minutes of fetal monitoring is required.

- At least two accelerations (15 bpm × 15 sec) in thirty minutes are present, or a biophysical profile of 8 out of 10 is present within the past four hours, or moderate variability is present.

- There have been no late decelerations within the last thirty minutes.

- No more than two variable decelerations exceeding sixty seconds and decreasing greater than sixty beats per minute from baseline within the previous thirty minutes.

Consider use of a checklist every thirty minutes while oxytocin is being administered, before increasing the dose, and before restarting oxytocin if it has been discontinued for tachysystole and/or an indeterminate/abnormal FHR pattern.[60]

Fetal Assessment

- At least one acceleration of fifteen beats per minute for fifteen seconds in thirty minutes or moderate variability for ten of the last thirty minutes
- No more than one late deceleration within the previous thirty minutes
- No more than two variable decelerations exceeding sixty seconds in duration and decreasing greater than sixty beats per minute from the baseline within the previous thirty minutes

Uterine Contractions

- No more than five uterine contractions in ten minutes for any twenty-minute period
- No more than two contractions longer than 120 seconds in duration
- Uterus palpates soft between contractions

Labor Progress

- Labor has not progressed 0.5 to 1 cm per hour for nulliparous women or 1 cm per hour for multiparous women

Second-Stage Labor Care

It is recognized that the second stage of labor is a period of stress for the fetus, and efforts are made to minimize that stress by shortening the active pushing phase and using applicable pushing techniques. There should be common expectations among team members concerning when to begin pushing and how to encourage women to push. Women with epidural anesthesia who do not feel the urge to push at 10-cm cervical dilation should be allowed to rest until the fetus has descended enough to stimulate the urge to push (up to two hours for nulliparous women and up to one hour for multiparous women).[61] When the urge to push is noted, women are encouraged to bear down as long as they can at the peak of the contraction, no more than three times per contraction.[62] Women are no longer told to take a deep breath and hold it while the nurse or physician counts to ten.[63] Breath-holding longer than six to eight seconds per pushing effort is discouraged.[64]

Women are assisted to suitable positions for pushing, such as upright, semi-Fowlers, lateral, and squatting.[65] The supine lithotomy position and stirrups are not used during pushing efforts. The woman's knees are not forcibly pushed back against her abdomen in positions that stretch the perineum or risk joint or nerve injury; rather, she is allowed to position herself for comfort or keep her feet flat on the bed as desired.[66] Repetitive pushing efforts are not encouraged if the FHR is nonreassuring. Instead, women are coached to push with every other or every third contraction to maintain a stable baseline FHR and allow the fetus to recover between pushes. Uterine tachysystole is avoided during the second stage, and the same intrauterine resuscitation techniques used during first stage of labor are used during the second stage.

Vaginal Birth After Cesarean Section

In the early 1990s, organizations such as ACOG and the National Institutes of Health (NIH) endorsed trials of labor by women who had had cesarean delivery who met specific criteria with a goal to reduce a national cesarean rate of approximately 25 percent.[67] Subsequently, whereas many mothers successfully attempted a vaginal birth after cesarean (VBAC) delivery, a small number (just under 1 percent) experienced uterine rupture that occurred with little or no warning. In 1999, ACOG issued a Practice Bulletin that cautioned that, although trial of labor is "appropriate for most women who have had a previous low transverse cesarean delivery, increased experience with VBAC indicates that there are potential problems."[68]

In July 2004, ACOG reiterated that selection criteria for VBAC included "one previous low transverse cesarean; clinically adequate pelvis; no other uterine scars or previous rupture; physician immediately available throughout active labor capable of monitoring labor and performing an emergency cesarean delivery; availability of anesthesia and personnel for emergency cesarean section." In addition, the July 2004 ACOG Practice Bulletin on VBAC went further, discouraging physicians from using prostaglandins for these patients.[69]

The 2004 ACOG statement has been interpreted by many organizations to require in-house support immediately capable of performing a cesarean section. In the case of VBAC, the earlier ACOG position requiring that the team take no longer than thirty minutes from the time the decision is made to perform an emergent cesarean procedure to the procedure itself is arguably inapplicable.[70] Many hospitals have ceased to offer VBAC opportunities to mothers because they cannot provide the requisite support.

Clinicians and organizations providing VBACs should provide a thorough informed-consent process for the woman who elects VBAC over a cesarean section. The practitioner must also remember that maternal consent to try VBAC can mean VBAC consent can be withdrawn at any time. Refer to Chapter 4 in this volume for more information on informed consent.

Another important risk management strategy for those electing to have VBAC or for other high-risk patients, as well as the general population, is the importance of making certain that the maternal medical records are transferred from the practitioner's office to the hospital setting at least a month before the expected date of confinement.

Shoulder Dystocia

Shoulder dystocia is a condition that creates delivery difficulty because of the mother's inability to deliver vaginally due to the size and position of the infant's shoulders. In essence, the upper body of the infant becomes wedged behind the maternal pubic bone, the umbilical cord becomes compressed, reducing the amount of oxygen to the baby, and delivery is impeded. More than 30,000[71] babies are born in the United States each year with shoulder dystocia, making it another source of litigation. Allegations include the failure to predict the adverse outcome and the lack of communicating risk. Once shoulder dystocia becomes evident, the physician is faced with limited options, all of which are risky at best and can lead to further damage to the brachial plexus due to stretching or injury. Erb's palsy is injury to the upper part of the brachial plexus, and injury to the lower part of the brachial plexus is called Klumpke palsy. Both can have lifelong devastating effects upon the baby, mother, and family.

Most babies born with a diagnosis of shoulder dystocia and brachial plexus injury will recover in time, with no long-lasting injury. However, for those who do not fully recover, injuries can be severe. They include fractured clavicle and injury to the brachial plexus, both leading to and contributing to long-term disability. If the physician's efforts to deliver the baby are not successful and timely, the resulting damages can also include brain damage and death. Avoidance is facilitated to some degree by screening patients with the potential for the condition, for example, diabetic mothers who are prone to have infants with large upper bodies and heads. However, most shoulder dystocia events have not been predictable, and if the circumstance arises suddenly, emergency management is required. Strategies to address shoulder dystocia include McRoberts' maneuver, which involves sharply flexing the legs above the mother's abdomen, and suprapubic pressure, in which an attendant makes a fist and pushes the infant's shoulder to the right or left.[72] A well-researched and clear resource on shoulder dystocia can be found at the Web site of Dr. Henry Lerner, clinical instructor in obstetrics and gynecology at Harvard Medical School, at www .shoulderdystociainfo.com.

One issue that historically has been problematic in defending shoulder dystocia-related malpractice suits is the substitution by staff of fundal pressure for suprapubic pressure. Fundal pressure is applied much higher than suprapubic pressure and can result in a ruptured uterus. Nursing staff and others who might assist in addressing shoulder dystocia in the delivery room must be educated regarding the difference between these two approaches. It is also critical that all interventions be objectively documented.

Shoulder dystocia is an excellent example of a clinical situation that arises infrequently, yet requires rapid and correct execution of a team approach. Steps to manage shoulder dystocia should be formalized in a protocol, and staff members should then participate in shoulder dystocia drills as often as necessary to maintain their proficiency. An excellent resource for planning and critiquing shoulder dystocia drills is an ACOG video on this topic, which can be obtained at www.acog.com.

With the proliferation of advances in medical technology, the risk inherent in conditions such as shoulder dystocia may be reduced by the application of advanced technology. The evolution of computer-generated predictive modeling will expand the treatment options for practitioners, allowing them to evaluate the potential for dystocia prior to delivery and to facilitate a planned strategy with full disclosure to and informed consent from the mother.[73] For further discussion on the use of advanced technology, see Dr. Henry Lerner's Web site mentioned previously.

Drills for Obstetric Emergencies

Safety is enhanced when all team members know what to do during other common obstetric emergencies such as nonreassuring FHR patterns, emergent cesarean birth, postpartum hemorrhage, and neonatal resuscitation. Routine drills for these emergent clinical situations have been recommended by TJC.[74] Although there are no specific recommendations for how to conduct drills, these basic suggestions may be useful.

- Develop pocket cue cards with clinical algorithms for intrauterine resuscitation, shoulder dystocia, emergent cesarean birth, and postpartum hemorrhage.

- Use the clinical algorithm for neonatal resuscitation as outlined.[75]

- Use a scribe or video to record what happens during each drill so that team member roles and organization can be reviewed retrospectively as a basis for planning for improvement.

- Debrief after actual emergencies, comparing care provided with the clinical algorithms.

- Pay particular attention to team communication and timely response.

- Develop a list of everything that went well and things that could have been done better.

- Use the list as a basis for interdisciplinary discussion concerning what the perinatal team needs to do should a similar clinical situation occur in the future.

· · · · · · · · ·

CONCLUSION

The risk management professional is encouraged to facilitate implementation of principles that will enhance perinatal safety. The specific approaches discussed in this chapter can both improve safety and reduce liability for obstetric providers and organizations.

Endnotes

1. Jury Verdict Research. *Current awards trends in personal injury*. Horsham, Pa.: Author. 2004.

2. American College of Obstetricians and Gynecologists (ACOG), 2007. *2006 ACOG survey of professional liability*. Washington, D.C.: Author.

3. *Ibid.*

4. *Ibid.*

5. Jury Verdict Research, 2004, *op. cit.*

6. Wu, A. W. "Medical error: The second victim." *British Medical Journal* 2000; 320(7237):726–727.

7. Knox, G. E., K. R. Simpson, and K. E. Townsend. "High reliability perinatal units: Further observations and a suggested plan for action." *Journal of Healthcare Risk Management* 2003; 23(4):17–21.

8. McFerran, S., J. Nunes, D. Pucci, and A. Zuniga. "Perinatal patient safety project: A multicenter approach to improve performance reliability at Kaiser Permanente." *Journal of Perinatal & Neonatal Nursing* 2005; 19(1):37–45.

9. Jury Verdict Research, 2004, *op. cit.*

10. Knox, G. E. and K. R. Simpson. "Teamwork: The fundamental building block of high reliability organizations and patient safety." In: B. Youngberg and M. J. Hatlie (eds). *The Patient Safety Handbook*. Chicago, Ill.: American Hospital Association, 2003.

11. Rolph, J. E. "Merit rating for physicians malpractice premiums: Only a modest deterrent." A Rand Note (N-3426-MT/RWJ/RC). Santa Monica, Calif.: Rand Corporation, 1991. Available at: www.rand.org/pubs/notes/2009/N3426.pdf. (Accessed March 31, 2010.)

12. Sloan, F. A., P. M. Mergenhagen, W. B. Burfield et al. "Medical malpractice experience of physicians." *Journal of the American Medical Association* 1989; 262(23):3291–3297.

13. Knox, Simpson, Townsend, *op. cit.*

14. *Merriam-Webster Online Dictionary*. Available at: www.merriam-webster.com/. (Accessed January 26, 2006.)

15. Knox, Simpson, Townsend, *op. cit.*

16. Knox, G. E., K. R. Simpson, and T. J. Garite. "High reliability perinatal units: An approach to the prevention of patient injury and medical malpractice claims." *Journal of Healthcare Risk Management* 1999; 19(2):24–32.

17. American Academy of Pediatrics & American College of Obstetricians and Gynecologists. *Guidelines for Perinatal Care*, 5th ed. Elk Grove Village, Ill.: Author. 2002.

18. Schofield, L. M. *"Perinatal Staffing and the Nursing Shortage: Challenges and Principles-based Strategies."* Washington, D.C.: Association of Women's Health, Obstetric and Neonatal Nurses. 2003.

19. Reason, J. T. "Understanding adverse events: The human factor." In: C. Vincent (ed). *Clinical Risk Management*. London: BMJ Books, 2001.

20. Simpson, K. R. and G. E. Knox. "Strategies for developing an evidence-based approach to perinatal care." *The American Journal of Maternal Child Nursing* 1999; 24(3):122–132.

21. Simpson, K. R. and G. E. Knox. "Common areas of litigation related to care during labor and birth: Recommendations to promote patient safety and decrease risk exposure." *Journal of Perinatal and Neonatal Nursing* 2003; 17(1):94–109.

22. Simpson, K. R. and G. E. Knox. "Essential criteria to promote safe care during labor and birth." *AWHONN Lifelines* 2005; 9(6).

23. The Joint Commission on Accreditation of Healthcare Organizations. Preventing infant death and injury during delivery. Sentinel Event Alert No. 30. Oak Brook, Ill.: Author. 2004.

24. Simpson, Knox. "Essential criteria to promote safe care."

25. Pettker, C. M., S. F. Thung, E. R. Norwitz et al. "Impact of a comprehensive patient safety strategy on obstetric adverse events." *American Journal of Obstetrics and Gynecology* 2009; 200:492.e1–492.e8.

26. Simpson, K. R., C. C. Kortz, and G. E. Knox. "A comprehensive perinatal patient safety program to reduce preventable adverse outcomes and costs of liability claims." *Joint Commission Journal on Quality and Patient Safety* 2009; (Nov) 35(11):565–574.

27. Clark S., M. Belfort, G. Saade et al. "Implementation of a conservative checklist-based protocol for oxytocin administration: Maternal and newborn outcomes." *American Journal of Obstetrics and Gynecology* 2007; 197:480.e1–480.e5.

28. Reisner D. P., T. K. Wallin, R. W. Zingheim et al. "Reduction of elective inductions in a large community hospital." *American Journal of Obstetrics and Gynecology* 2009; 200:674.e1–674.e7.

29. Knox et al. "High reliability perinatal units," *op. cit.*

30. Sexton, J. B., E. J. Thomas, R. L. Helmreich et al. "Frontline assessments of healthcare culture: Safety attitudes questionnaire norms and psychometric properties," Technical Report 04–01, 2001. The University of Texas Center of Excellence for Patient Safety Research and Practice AHRQ Grant # 1PO1HS1154401.

31. Reason. "Understanding adverse events," *op. cit.*

32. *Ibid.*

33. JCAHO. "Preventing infant death," *op. cit.*

34. *Ibid.*

35. Simpson, K. R. "Handling handoffs safely." *MCN The American Journal of Maternal Child Nursing* 2005; 30(2):152.

36. Simpson, K. R. "Failure to rescue: Implications for evaluating quality of care during labor and birth." *Journal of Perinatal & Neonatal Nursing* 2005; 19(1):23–33.

37. Will, S. B., K. Hennicke, L. Jacobs et al. "The perinatal patient safety nurse: A new role to promote safe care for mothers and babies." *Journal of Obstetric, Gynecologic, and Neonatal Nursing* 2006; (May-Jun) 35(3):417–423.

38. Simpson, K. "Essential criteria to promote safe care," *op. cit.*

39. "Electronic Fetal Heart Rate Monitoring Research Guidelines for Interpretation" from The National Institute of Child Health and Human Development Research Planning Workshop published in the *Journal of Obstetric, Gynecologic and Neonatal Nursing*, 1997; (Nov.-Dec.) 26(6):635–640, and in the *American Journal of Obstetrics and Gynecology* 1997; (Dec.) 177(6):1385–1390.

40. American College of Obstetricians and Gynecologists. *Intrapartum fetal heart rate monitoring*. Practice Bulletin No. 62. Washington, D.C.: Author. 2005.

41. Association of Women's Health, Obstetric and Neonatal Nurses. "Fetal heart monitoring principles and practices." Washington, D.C.: Author. 2005.

42. Fox, M., S. Kilpatrick, T. King, and J. T. Parer. "Fetal heart rate monitoring: Interpretation and collaborative management." *Journal of Midwifery and Women's Health* 2000; 45(6):498–507.

43. ACOG, "Intrapartum fetal heart rate monitoring," *op. cit.*

44. Simpson, K. R. and D. C. James. "Effects of immediate versus delayed pushing during second-stage labor on fetal well-being: A randomized clinical trial." *Nursing Research* 2005; 54(3):149–157.

45. Fox. "Fetal heart rate monitoring," *op. cit.*

46. American Academy of Pediatrics & American Heart Association. *Textbook of Neonatal Resuscitation*. Chicago, Ill.: Author. 2002.

47. American College of Obstetricians and Gynecologists. *Induction of Labor*. Practice Bulletin No. 10. Washington, D.C.: Author. 1999.

48. American College of Obstetricians and Gynecologists. *Dystocia and Augmentation of Labor*, Practice Bulletin No. 49. Washington, D.C.: Author. 2003.

49. Simpson, K. R. *Cervical ripening and induction and augmentation of labor*, Practice Monograph. Washington, D.C.: Association of Women's Health, Obstetric and Neonatal Nurses. 2002.

50. *Ibid.*

51. *Ibid.*

52. *Ibid.*

53. Clark, S. L., D. D. Miller, M. A. Belfort et al. "Neonatal and maternal outcomes associated with elective term delivery." *American Journal of Obstetrics and Gynecology* 2009; 200:156.e1–156.e4.

54. Tita, A. N., M. B. Landon, C. Y. Spong et al. "Timing of elective repeat cesarean delivery at term and neonatal outcomes." *New England Journal of Medicine* 2009; 360:111–120.

55. Clark, S. L., K. R. Simpson, G. E. Knox et al. "Oxytocin: New perspectives on an old drug." *American Journal of Obstetrics and Gynecology* 2009; 200:35.e1–35.e6.

56. Simpson K. R., and G. E. Knox. "Oxytocin as a high-alert medication: Implications for perinatal patient safety." *The American Journal of Maternal Child Nursing* 2009; (Jan-Feb) 34(1):8–15; quiz 16–17.

57. "ISMP 2007 survey on HIGH-ALERT medications: Differences between nursing and pharmacy perspectives still prevalent." May 17, 2007. Available at: www.ismp.org/newsletters/acutecare/articles/20070517.asp. (Accessed March 31, 2010.)

58. ACOG Practice Bulletin No. 54

59. Clark et al., 2007, *op. cit.*

60. Clark et al., 2007, *op. cit.*

61. Hansen, S. L., S. L. Clark, and J. C. Foster. "Active pushing versus passive fetal descent in the second stage of labor: A randomized controlled trial." *Obstetrics and Gynecology* 2002; 99(1):29–34.

62. Roberts, J. E. "The push for evidence: Management of the second stage." *Journal of Midwifery and Women's Health* 2002; 47(1):2–15.

63. Simpson, K. R. and D. C. James. "Efficacy of intrauterine resuscitation techniques in improving fetal oxygen status during labor." *Obstetrics and Gynecology* 2005; 105(6):1362–1368.

64. Roberts, "The push for evidence," *op. cit.*

65. Association of Women's Health, Obstetric and Neonatal Nurses. "Nursing management of the second stage of labor." Washington, D.C., 2000.

66. *Ibid.*

67. ACOG Practice Bulletin No. 54, July 2004.

68. ACOG Practice Bulletin No. 5, July 1999.

69. ACOG, 2004, *op. cit.*

70. American Academy of Pediatrics, American College of Obstetricians and Gynecologists, *Guidelines for Perinatal Care*, 4th ed., 1997, p. 112.

71. LMS Medical Systems, Inc. Press release, LMS Announces Clinical Breakthrough in Predicting Key Obstetrical Challenge, June 21, 2005, Montreal, Quebec. Available at: www.lmsmedical.com/4105/pdf/PR_June%2021_Dystocia.pdf or www.lmsmedical. com. (Accessed March 31, 2010.)

72. Lerner, H. "Shoulder Dystocia Information." Available at: www.shoulderdystociainfo. com/index.htm. (Accessed March 31, 2010.)

73. LMS Medical Systems, Inc. Press release, *op. cit.*

74. *Ibid.*

75. Simpson, J. "Efficacy of intrauterine resuscitation," *op. cit.*

9

Pediatric Risk Management

David Stallings
Jeff Sconyers

P ediatric patients are one of the most vulnerable populations cared for by the health care professional. This chapter will identify and analyze key risks that pertain to this "at risk" class of patients. It will also suggest strategies to enhance safety and reduce liability.

CLINICAL ISSUES

Although pediatric patients are often small people, they are not also little adults. There is significant risk associated with inappropriate modification of adult treatment approaches for pediatric patients. Also, providers must have age-specific training in their specialties.

Age and Size-Specific Clinical Needs

Highly skilled adult cardiologists usually know very little about congenital malformations of the heart seen in infants or children. Even within the ranks of pediatric specialists, there is a broad range of expertise. Some are highly skilled in conditions affecting the neonate, while others specialize in adolescent medicine, and so on.

The granting of pediatric medical staff privileges must require that the provider's skill level qualify them for the care they will deliver. Any need for supplemental training and practice should be identified and addressed immediately. The same principle applies to nurses and other allied health care professionals who care for children.

It is also potentially desirable, in pediatrics more than any other specialty, to delineate circumstances under which consultation is required for specific diagnoses and procedures. Similarly, if a facility lacks practitioners skilled in managing the particular condition of a given patient, it is potentially wise to transfer the patient to a pediatric facility that can manage that condition (referral center) rather than to attempt care without needed expertise. The common sense exception is emergency care, which is necessary to save the patient's life. However, once a complex critical pediatric patient in a non-tertiary setting is stabilized, transfer should be considered.

One of the most obvious differences between adult and pediatric patients is simple: it is size. Healthcare providers and organizations entrusted to care for children must ensure that they have on hand and use the right supplies and equipment to provide needed care. Beds, ventilators, endotracheal tubes, thermometers, surgical instruments, infusion pumps, and casting supplies are just some of the many products that must be sized to the patient receiving care. And of course, within the pediatric population, there is also great variation, from the 500-gram neonate to the 200-pound adolescent. These special size issues make it more complicated to protect the pediatric patient from equipment-related injury than it is to protect adult patients. However, this issue must be addressed to promote safety and avoid medical malpractice cases with the potential for substantial damages.

Communication with Pediatric Patients

Age-specific competencies are required of providers by The Joint Commission (TJC) and other regulators. Arguably, pediatric communication skills should be considered an age-specific competency. The ability to communicate with pediatric patients and to facilitate their participation in their own care is an important therapeutic measure that also reduces risk. Effective communication enhances the quality and substance of the pediatric provider's physical assessment. It also enables the practitioner to present information in a way that helps children understand what to expect and prepare themselves for their treatment.

The amount of information that can be shared, and the time required to accomplish this, varies by age level. For example, techniques involving storytelling and playtime provide the best possible comfort level for some young patients, while still imparting significant information. Simply developing rapport with children can help make them more amenable to the things that need to be done to treat their illness.

Particular challenges are presented by infants and toddlers, two groups with limited ability to communicate. Providers must find ways to elicit the information they need. Infants might exhibit auditory and visual clues when they are experiencing painful stimuli; however, the clues may be nonspecific. For toddlers who have not yet developed significant language skills or are hard to understand, providers must rely on parents to help them assess what a child may be trying to express. This puts pediatric practitioners at a significant disadvantage, when compared with providers who deal with adolescent and adult patients.

The child's parents can provide important assistance to the provider trying to assess the patient's communication, and they can provide additional information about particular behaviors and vocalizations. However, cases often arise in which the parents are not sure what is wrong and cannot provide more information. In situations with limited information, the provider must rely on a thorough clinical assessment, and age-specific communication skills become invaluable. Particularly important are skills that facilitate assessment of pain, and implementation of the correct interventions to address the pain, of pediatric patients. In general, many facilities are finding that the assistance of child life specialists who routinely see pediatric patients can also help in assessing communication.

Communication with Parents, Guardians, and Families

Pediatric facilities often employ the concept of family-centered care, which recognizes that the family is an integral part of the patient's life and a critical factor in helping the patient manage illness. Parents or guardians who are present should be woven into the ongoing activities that surround the patient's care once providers determine how involved these individuals want to be. Most parents are anxious when their child is hospitalized. Informing and assisting them to participate in a satisfactory level of care is helpful from several perspectives. For example, helping parents or guardians understand treatment plans and giving them an opportunity to ask questions promotes dialogue that can enhance the quality of care. Knowledgeable parents might, for example, detect deviations from the expected course of recovery or the care plan and raise good questions. Keeping the parents informed on an ongoing basis also naturally keeps expectations realistic and reduces the chances of misunderstanding the course of treatment. Finally, teaching the parent or guardian about treatments the child might require at home is an important step in effective discharge planning.

The parent or guardian who is with the patient all the time during the hospitalization can play a significant role in patient safety. Here are some ways that properly informed parents or guardians can help maintain a safe environment of care. Parents or guardians should

- keep crib or bed rails up when they are not actively interacting with the patient;
- notify the assigned nurse when they will be leaving the patient unattended;
- know the importance of hand hygiene and avoid visiting when they are sick;
- know and follow whatever isolation restrictions are in effect and make sure that care providers do the same; and
- speak up and ask questions when a care provider is doing something that differs from the discussed plan or when something just doesn't seem right.

It is particularly important that staff members let parents and guardians know that they are expected to speak up and help them overcome any hesitation they might have about questioning providers.

There are several points pertaining to security and accountability that the staff should explain to parents:

- Parents must wear facility-approved or sponsored identification tags and abide by the facility's security policies.

- Parents are expected to respect the needs of other patients and families and therefore must respect quiet hours and avoid disruptive behavior.

- Parents must not bring in weapons, liquor, or illicit drugs.

- Parents must support facility policies designed to protect patients and staff.

- Parents who stay overnight must be aware that the nursing staff is responsible for checking on the patient at all hours.

It might help to develop an outline of these principles as a basis for teaching parents about their role.

One challenge associated with involving parents in care may be maintaining the necessary privacy for the patient. Pediatric patients often have many family members and friends visiting, so providers need to be cognizant of the effect of large groups on the child's well-being and on the expectations of parents or guardians regarding privacy. Privacy can be particularly challenging when there are two (or more) patients to a room. Providers must work through such issues on a case-by-case basis. Keeping the parents informed of their efforts may ease any tension about a semiprivate room.

. . . .
SLEEPING POSITION

The sleeping position of an infant is a very important safety factor.[1] It is general knowledge that infants sleeping prone, or on their stomachs, are at risk for sudden infant death syndrome (SIDS). In 1992, the American Academy of Pediatrics (AAP) recommended that infants sleep in the supine position to reduce of the risk of SIDS. Since that time, epidemiological evidence and infant mortality statistics show that the U.S. SIDS rate has fallen markedly. The possible cause of SIDS has to do with the fact that prone patients may rebreathe exhaled air, a phenomenon has been shown to cause ventilatory compromise and death. Sleeping in the prone position has also been linked to changes in cardiovascular and arousal responses in infants. Another unrelated potential cause of SIDS is hyperthermia due to excess bedclothes or room temperature.

The supine position should be used during sleep until the infant is developmentally able to independently roll out of supine. At that point, the infant should be placed for sleep in the supine position and be allowed to assume a preferred sleep position. Although the supine position is the recommended position for healthy infants, there are certain exceptions to this rule, including the following:

- Any preterm infant with signs of respiratory distress, such as increased work in order to breathe, apnea, or tachypnea, may benefit from the prone position.

- Prone positioning provides a respiratory and developmental advantage for asymptomatic, very low birth weight preterm infants (less than 1,250 grams).

- Infants with known or suspected airway obstruction may benefit from prone positioning.

- Infants on assisted ventilation may benefit from prone positioning.

- Children with birth defects in which supine sleep would be contraindicated, such as neural tube defects and Pierre Robin malformation sequence, clearly benefit from sleeping prone.

- Infants receiving phototherapy also benefit from being in the prone position.

- Infants with severe gastroesophageal reflux may also respond positively to prone positioning.

Parents of infants fitting any of the above categories need to be educated regarding the rationale for positioning their child and how to help the child maintain the most clinically desirable position.

Also, whereas the supine position may be generally recommended for sleeping, prone and side-lying positioning for infants during supervised awake periods helps to promote development of symmetrical head control and age-appropriate motor skills. It may also reduce the risk of skull deformity (positional brachycephaly or plagiocephaly).

In addition to the sleeping position of the infant, suitable bedding materials are another important safety factor. Infants should be dressed warmly but avoid overheating. Blankets or other bedding materials might provide warmth, but they should not cover the infant above the chest or shoulders. This prevents any accidental pulling of the covers over an infant's face during movement, which is dangerous because the covers might trap air that the infant will be forced to rebreathe.

Use of Restraints

As is required by TJC and Centers for Medicare & Medicaid Services (CMS), all facilities must minimize the use of restraints and maximize the patient's health and safety when restraints must be used. Restraints should be used only in behavioral emergencies when there is an imminent risk of physical harm to the patient or others (including staff members). They may also be judiciously used to protect a patient from injury. Any use of restraints requires clear indications, considered in the light of reasonable alternatives, and a frequently reviewed physician's order specifying the type of restraint to be used.

According to AAP, there should also be an explanation given to the child as to the rationale for the restraint. If the restraint is to help the child control his or her emotions, there should be consideration of an alternative approach known as *therapeutic holding*. If used, the restraint should be applied correctly, the patient's skin condition and other parameters routinely monitored, and the need for continuation of the restraint frequently evaluated.[2] Of note, a 2004 study of emergency department (ED) clinician practice regarding pediatric restraints found that resident physicians were not often educated on their use.[3]

· · · · · · · · ·

MEDICATION MANAGEMENT

Pediatric medication errors can be devastating. They can result in harm that affects patients for many years or even death. In the 2008 Sentinel Event Alert on Preventing Pediatric Medication Errors, TJC cited a study identifying an "11.1 percent rate of adverse drug events in pediatric patients . . . This is far more than described in previous studies. The researchers also found that 22 percent of those adverse drug events were preventable, 17.8 percent could have been identified earlier, and 16.8 percent could have been mitigated more effectively."[4]

Exacerbating concerns about the high number of medication-related pediatric adverse events is the concern that children are often less able to tolerate medication errors due to still developing renal, immune, and hepatic functions. Young children are also less likely to be able to communicate about negative effects of medication, including misadministration of a medicine.

Causes of pediatric medication errors in the adult-focused general hospital often include a lack of trained staff oriented to pediatric care, pediatric care protocols and safeguards, and up-to-date and easily accessible pediatric reference materials, especially with regard to medications. The need for such reference material is made more urgent by the fact that many medications simply do not come in pediatric dosages. This is, in part, because certain pediatric illnesses occur rarely in comparison to the incidence affecting the adult population, and therefore there is a smaller market for manufacturers to serve. Despite urging by TJC,[5] it is expected that pharmaceutical development will continue to focus on the adult, rather than on the pediatric patient. Regardless of the reasons, the care provider faced with administering an adult strength medication to a child may be forced to manipulate the adult pharmaceutical, for example, cut tablets in half or crush pills so that pediatric patients can ingest them. Pediatric dosage determination is yet another risk issue. For example, dosage must be based on parameters such as age, weight, and body surface area.

Of particular importance, weight of a child, especially a small child, can change rapidly, so it is essential that medication dosage be based on a recent weight and that the patient's weight is routinely assessed and documented. A single system of measurement should be used to assess pediatric weight, preferably metric. Grave errors may occur when English units are confused with metric or vice versa.

More light is shed on causes of pediatric medication errors by the MedMarx® study discussed by TJC in their previously referenced Sentinel Event Alert.

> During calendar years 2006–2007, USP's MedMarx database shows nearly 2.5 percent of pediatric medication errors led to patient harm. The most common types of harmful pediatric medication errors were: improper dose/quantity (37.5 percent), omission error (19.9 percent), unauthorized/wrong drug (13.7 percent), and prescribing error (9.4 percent), followed by wrong administration technique, wrong time, drug prepared incorrectly, wrong dosage form, and wrong route. Medication errors involving pediatric patients were most often caused by performance deficit (43.0 percent), knowledge deficit (29.9 percent), procedure/protocol not followed

(20.7 percent), and miscommunication (16.8 percent), followed by calculation error, computer entry error, inadequate or lack of monitoring, improper use of pumps, and documentation errors . . ."[6]

The MedMarx Data Report A Chartbook of Medication Error Findings from the Perioperative Settings from 1998–2005 reveals that approximately 32.4 percent of pediatric errors in the operating room involve an improper dose/quantity compared with 14.6 percent in the adult population and 15.4 percent in the geriatric population.[7] A recent study indicates that children are particularly at risk for chemotherapy medication errors, they often reached the patient and were potentially harmful.[8]

TJC's Sentinel Event Alert goes on to recommend specific risk reduction strategies to promote safe pediatric medication administration:

- Standardize and identify medications effectively, as well as the processes for drug administration.

- Establish and maintain a functional pediatric formulary system with policies for drug evaluation, selection, and therapeutic use.

- To prevent timing errors in medication administration, standardize how days are counted in all protocols by deciding upon a protocol start date (e.g., day 0 or day 1).

- Limit the number of concentrations and dose strengths of high-alert medications to the minimum needed to provide safe care.

- For pediatric patients who are receiving compounded oral medications and total parenteral nutrition at home, ensure that the doses are equivalent to those prepared in the hospital (i.e., the volume of the home dose should be the same as the volume of the hospital-prepared products).

- Use oral syringes to administer oral medications. The pharmacy should use oral syringes when preparing oral liquid medications. Make oral syringes available on patient care units when as-needed medications are prepared. Educate staff about the benefits of oral syringes in preventing inadvertent intravenous administration of oral medications.

- Ensure full pharmacy oversight, as well as the involvement of other appropriate staff, in the verifying, dispensing, and administering of both neonatal and pediatric medications.

- Assign a practitioner trained in pediatrics to any committee that is responsible for the oversight of medication management.

- Provide ready access, including Web site access, to up-to-date pediatric-specific information for all hospital staff. This information should include pediatric research study data, pediatric growth charts, normal vital sign ranges for children, emergency dosage calculations, and drug reference materials with information about minimum effective doses and maximum dose limits.

- Orient all pharmacy staff to specialized neonatal/pediatric pharmacy services in your organization.

- Provide a dosage calculation sheet for each pediatric critical care patient, including both emergency and commonly used medications.

- Develop preprinted medication order forms and clinical pathways or protocols to reflect a standardized approach to care. Include reminders and information about monitoring parameters.

- Create pediatric satellite pharmacies or assign pharmacists and technicians with pediatric expertise to areas or services such as neonatal/pediatric critical care units and pediatric oncology units. At a minimum, pediatric medications should be stored and prepared in areas separate from those where adult medications are stored and prepared.

- Use technology judiciously.

- Use methods to ensure the accuracy of technology that measures and delivers additives for intravenous solutions, such as for total parenteral nutrition.

- If dose and dose-range checking software programs are available in hospital or pharmacy information systems, enable them to provide alerts for potentially incorrect doses.

- Medications in automated dispensing cabinets that do not undergo appropriate pharmacist review should be limited to those needed for emergency use and to those medications under the control of a licensed independent prescriber, as specified in TJC standard MM 4.10.

- Recognize that the use of infusion pumps, or smart pumps, is not a guarantee against medication errors. Appropriate education for nurses, pharmacists, and other caregivers regarding these technologies is important for all institutions caring for pediatric patients.

- To prevent adverse outcomes or oversedation, use consistent physiological monitoring, particularly pulse oximetry, while children are under sedation during office-based procedures. Use age- and size-appropriate monitoring equipment and follow uniform procedures under the guidance of staff appropriately trained in sedation, monitoring, and resuscitation.

- Providers are encouraged to develop bar coding technology with pediatric capability. Potential errors should be carefully considered when adapting this technology to pediatric processes and systems. For example, a pediatric bar coding solution must be able to provide readable code for small-volume, patient-specific dose labels.

Still other practical suggestions in TJC's Sentinel Alert include the following:

1. Because patient weight is used to calculate most dosing (either as weight-based dosing, body surface area calculation, or other age-appropriate dose determination), all pediatric patients should be weighed in kilograms at the time of admission (including outpatient and ambulatory clinics) or within four hours of admission in an emergency situation. Kilograms should be the standard nomenclature for weight on prescriptions, medical records and staff communications.

2. No high-risk drug should be dispensed or administered if the pediatric patient has not been weighed, unless it is an emergency.

3. On inpatient medication orders and outpatient prescriptions, require prescribers to include the calculated dose and the dosing determination, such as the dose per weight (e.g., milligrams per kilogram) or body surface area, to facilitate an independent double-check of the calculation by a pharmacist, nurse, or both. Exceptions to this are medications that do not lend themselves to weight-based dosing, such as topicals, ophthalmics, and vitamins.

4. Whenever possible, use commercially available pediatric-specific formulations and concentrations. When this is not possible, prepare and dispense all pediatric medications in patient-specific unit dose or unit of use containers, rather than in commercially available *adult* unit doses. For oral liquid preparation medications, use oral syringes to ensure correct dosage.

5. Clearly differentiate from adult formulations all products that have been repackaged for use in pediatric populations. *Use clear, highly visible warning labels*. To prevent overdoses, keep concentrated adult medications away from pediatric care units. Avoid storing adult and pediatric concentrations in the same automated dispensing machine or cabinet drawer.

6. Ensure comprehensive specialty training for all practitioners involved in the care of infants and children, as well as continuing education programs on pediatric medications for all healthcare providers. Training and education should include information on how adverse effects should be reported.

7. Communicate verbally and in writing information about the child's medication to the child, caregivers, and parents/guardians, including information about potential side effects. Ask the caregiver/parent/guardian to repeat back their understanding of the drug and how it is to be administered. Encourage the asking of questions about medications.

8. Have a pharmacist with pediatric expertise available or on-call at all times.

9. Establish and implement medication procedures that include pediatric prescribing and administration practices.[9]

Without doubt, medication administration is one of the highest risk care processes in the pediatric setting. Risk management professionals are encouraged to monitor resources such as related TJC publications and the Institute of Safe Medication Practice (ISMP) Web site to stay current with identified issues and best practices in this area of concern.

·········
OFF-LABEL USE OF MEDICATIONS

The previously noted lack of pharmaceutical industry focus on the pediatric patient sometimes leaves pediatricians without resources to address their patients' unique needs. In the absence of other alternatives, they may turn to use of a medication in an unapproved, or off-label, manner, or even to medications that are approved in other countries but not in the United States. Clinicians considering such applications must work with pharmacy, administration, and their peers to evaluate the risks and benefits of the potential use; determine appropriate safeguards; and develop appropriate written and verbal information. The patient and parent guardian should also be engaged in a true informed consent process so that he or she may understand both risks and benefits of any unconventional approach, and all elements of that discussion, including their decision to proceed, should be documented. (For more information on informed consent, please see Chapter 4 in this volume.)

Patient or Family Role in Medication Administration

Medications From Home   Two issues related to medication administration often present in the pediatric facility. The first issue is that patients or parents may request that medications from home be administered rather than medications from the hospital's pharmacy. Some facilities allow this when the medication is not on their formulary and an alternative cannot be arranged in a timely manner. Other facilities prohibit it under any circumstances.

If such medications are to be administered, the organization should have a protocol requiring that the pharmacist inspect the medication and approve its use during an inpatient stay. Such approved use should be supported by a current written physician order. Addressing such a request would be just one result of the medication reconciliation process that TJC now requires be carried out on admission, transfer to another care area, and at discharge.

Generally, only medications that can be positively identified by the pharmacist are permitted. This means that tablets and capsules with an imprint code and manufacturer's name or emblem must be identifiable. Liquid medications must be contained in a properly sealed, original manufacturer's container. The pharmacist will inspect the prescription label and the container. The medication will not be used if there is any concern about cleanliness, storage, or contents of the medications. Once a product is identified, it should be labeled by the hospital pharmacist as approved.

It must be noted that there are limited exceptions to the requirement of identifiability. For example, the facility may allow research patients on investigational drugs to supply their own medications because investigational drugs might not have identifying imprints, thus not identifiable to a pharmacist. The research drug may be used if, in a pharmacist's judgment, it meets requirements for cleanliness, storage, and content.

Another potential exception may apply to drugs available in other countries but not in the United States. Both exceptions require that a physician write an authorizing order.

Self-Administration   The second issue involving pediatric medication is the patient or family member may ask to self-administer medications while the child is an inpatient, rather than rely on the hospital staff. The clinical care team should determine whether the request is acceptable. If so, the nurse or pharmacist should instruct the patient or non-staff caregiver about the indication for the medication, dosage form, administration route, frequency, side effects, and objective ways to monitor the effectiveness of the medication. This instruction should be documented in the medical record. The caregiver's technique should also be assessed through observation. When the non-staff member administers the medication, he or she should advise the nursing staff, who will document that the medication was administered by this individual.

Psychiatric Patients

Facilities that serve pediatric psychiatric patients and hospital emergency rooms that potentially manage such patients must evaluate their physical and clinical environment(s) and implement any interventions needed to reasonably ensure safe care while protecting other patients, staffs, and property. Depending on age and specific diagnosis, pediatric psychiatric patients may be both strong and volatile. Emotional outbursts can therefore result in harm to other patients, the patients themselves, or staff members. Property is also at risk because these patients might be capable of damaging walls, furnishings, and equipment.

Additional clinical staffing might be needed to manage this population. Some facilities use a sitter who is trained to work with psychiatric patients to keep the patient safe and free other clinical personnel to care for other patients. Some emergency settings that are seeing an influx of acute pediatric psychiatric patients have also implemented seclusion areas for these patients. Although seclusion might benefit the patient therapeutically, it does not reduce the need for monitoring. Also, any seclusion area must allow such monitoring and be routinely screened for risk, such as projections from the ceiling that patients might use to hang themselves. Training in de-escalation techniques is beneficial for all staff who manage these patients.

In general, all patient care areas that see pediatric psychiatric patients must be made as safe as possible by eliminating objects that the patients might use to harm themselves and by constructing the area with materials that are hard to destroy.

· · · · · · · · ·

ENVIRONMENTAL SAFETY

Obstetric and neonatal facility personnel work hard to establish precautions that will prevent infant abduction. Pediatric facilities face a broader range of potential scenarios because pediatric patients are vulnerable to abduction at any age. In general, abductors are more likely to be noncustodial parents or other family members known to the staff than a stranger. Therefore, protection of pediatric patients is complicated by the need to be alert to potentially deceptive intent on the part of the child's family.

Infant and Child Abduction and Patient Elopement

The possibility of abduction varies with the type of facility. To some degree, the level of risk depends on whether the facility is a dedicated pediatric operation or simply a healthcare setting with a maternity ward and newborn nursery or small pediatric unit.

Risk management professionals must work with safety and security and the clinical staff to determine where their vulnerabilities are and how to minimize or alleviate them. Basic issues that should be examined include (1) access to and from the facility; (2) methods to control and secure entrances such as the use of proximity card readers; (3) video surveillance; (4) staff, parent, and visitor identification; and (5) patient identification band products that alert the staff if the patient leaves a designated area.

In addition, facilities may require infants and toddlers to be transported only in transport devices rather than by carrying them. If such an approach is implemented, staff members and family must be educated accordingly. Routine mock abduction drills for pediatric staff are important to help them maintain ability to manage this frightening situation. It is also very important that the staff knows what to do if a patient is actually taken. Mock drills related to abduction follow-up are also worthy of consideration.

Another potential risk that is more likely to pertain to the older pediatric patients is patient elopement, for example, leaving the facility without parental supervision or against medical advice. Adolescents are particularly vulnerable because they might long to get a break from treatment. Younger children may run or simply get separated from their parents in clinic areas, lobbies, elevators, cafeterias, and other public areas. Facilities need mechanisms to alert staff to a lost child situation and to mobilize a timely search for the child. The same response mechanism should be used consistently for all events because it is not often immediately clear whether the child has run away, gotten lost, or been abducted. In the worst case scenario, a child or abductor can leave the facility grounds quickly, necessitating an immediate and satisfactory response.

Patients and Parents Who Are Sexual Offenders

In a facility that works with a large pediatric population, it is possible that the risk management professional and staff may occasionally see a pediatric patient who is a registered sex offender. Some of these patients may be identified at the outset because they are being admitted from a juvenile detention facility, and the detention facility should clearly share such information with the healthcare organization to ensure that pertinent safety issues are addressed. However, for those patients admitted from home, it is unlikely that the healthcare facility will receive any warning about the patient's status. Because it is important to know about sex offender status, and any other propensity that the patient has for violence, it is important for clinicians who perform the admitting assessment to ask the patient and parent or guardian whether there are any security issues that might create safety or security problems for the patients themselves or anyone else at the facility. Documentation that this question has been raised may later help to refute any allegation that the facility did not exercise due diligence concerning protection of other patients or staff.

Once a patient is confirmed to be a registered sex offender, reasonable precautions may include placing the patient in a private room. Although a bracelet monitoring device that tracks the patients when they leave their rooms may be used, this does not prevent undesirable behavior. The use of a trained sitter may more effectively ensure that other patients and staff are not affected by the patient's presence.

A similar situation arises when a patient's parent or relative is a sexual offender. Information about the status of these individuals usually comes from one of the parents through the admission or psychosocial assessment. These situations are sometimes addressed preemptively because the offender may be judicially limited by restraining orders, probation-related provisions, and so on, from being near children. In this case, security must be notified of the identity of such individuals, and they should be barred from the institution. Where the parent is a sexual offender, but their presence might be therapeutically valuable to the child, clinicians, the security staff and the risk management professional may devise an approach that allows supervised visitation. Clinical providers should be trained on how to identify and manage such situations, and they should understand how to access resources who can help determine a rational approach that is beneficial and safe for patients and the organization.

Another concern for the safety of the pediatric patient is the admitted adult patient who is a sexual offender or sexual pedophile. Every precaution must be taken to ensure that these patients have no access to the pediatric population of patients. The use of private rooms, monitoring devices, sitters, and limited access to pediatric areas are all ways to minimize the potential for contact. The pediatric staff needs to be made aware of the admission of such people and their potential whereabouts. They should be accompanied when off their assigned floor for any reason and not be left to wander or have free access to the hospital.

Infection Control

Infection control is both important and challenging for the pediatric staff. Special considerations include the need to educate parents, who are sometimes with their children continually, and visitors,who might want to hold or feed a child, about infection control. In particular, staff should educate all family and visitors about the importance of hand washing and the frequency and technique with which hands should be cleaned. If parents are ill, they need to be informed about the risks of transmitting infectious disease to the patient. Staff should be alert to the potential of infection from sick family members or visitors and should be prepared to ask them not to visit the child if they may be contagious. Finally, the staff should educate parents as to what to do if they come in contact with the child's infectious waste.

Balloons, Flowers, and Plants

Friends and family often want to bring flowers, plants, and particularly balloons, to cheer a child. Flowers and plants could spread infection, thus many facilities limit their presence. They are typically not allowed in intensive care units, on hematology or oncology units, in clinics, or in any room occupied by an immunocompromised patient. Parents and other visitors should be advised to check with the staff before they purchase flowers or plants.

Latex balloons in particular can create several problems for the pediatric patient. Latex balloons affect those who have latex allergies, and they also present a potential choking hazard for children when deflated or popped. Children who chew or suck on deflated balloons can aspirate them, choke, and even die. Balloons and other soft objects that potentially conform to the shape of a child's airway are especially dangerous because they cannot be removed by the Heimlich maneuver. Children therefore should not be allowed to continue playing with a balloon that has popped or deflated.

According to the American College of Allergy, Asthma and Immunology,[10] at least 1 percent of the American population is allergic to latex. About 10–15 percent of healthcare workers may be allergic to latex, from their frequent exposure to latex gloves. Because latex balloons pose risk of exposure through touch, or by releasing rubber particles into the air, many healthcare facilities have banned them.

Mylar balloons are a safer alternative to latex balloons because they eliminate both the risk of latex allergy and aspiration. Many hospitals have chosen to stock only Mylar balloons in their gift shops. The staff must still be vigilant, however, to the possibility that latex balloons will be brought into the facility by visitors or family members. The security staff and others based at the entrance should be trained to intercept anyone who brings latex balloons into the facility and explain the policy to them. Facilities can also proactively contact local flower and balloon vendors with information about their policy. However, this approach can be difficult because of the large number of potential vendors, so the most important strategy is for the staff to be vigilant about such items.

Pets in the Hospital

Many facilities have policies that allow visits from service animals (an animal that is trained to do work or perform tasks for the benefit of a person with a disability) and animal-assisted activities such as pet therapy. All such policies must address infection control issues such as the need for hand hygiene, and so on. Reasonable expectations and limitations must be established and monitored. Facility environmental services should also be prepared to manage animal urination, defecation, and vomiting.

In addition to hygiene requirements, it is essential that the behavior of a service or pet therapy animal be the responsibility of the owner or handler. The animal must be trained and controlled to permit the staff to care for the patient and work in the room. The facility should establish reasonable limits on where the animal can go within the premises; for example, pet therapy animals may visit only certain units. If the animal is disruptive or presents a risk to other patients, hospital staff, or property, the animal should be removed immediately.

It is generally a good practice to obtain the consent of the physician and the bedside nurse before a pet therapy animal's visit to make sure that the child's condition will allow him or her to participate, to validate that the child is not afraid of the animal, to ensure the child is not allergic to pet dander, and so on. In addition, the hospital staff should accompany the handler to make sure that the visit goes as planned and that each patient or family member performs hand hygiene at the end of the visit.

If the family asks to bring the patient's pet in for a visit, the same criteria should apply as to service animals and pet therapy animals. Additional points to consider include common sense issues such as size, and consideration of other patients.

Allowable Toys and Cleaning Toys

The toys that parents, relatives, and friends may bring to the child in a pediatric setting introduce additional risk issues.[11] For example, some toys create a choking or digestive hazard for small children. Toys not suitable for children under age three include small cars and planes, minianimals, wind-up toys, bubbles, and games with small pieces. Such items might create a choking hazard for children this age, who often put things in their mouths. If plush or stuffed toys have buttons or eyes that can be chewed off, they might create similar problems. Most plush toys are marked by the manufacturer as to age appropriateness. Staff must be vigilant about the type of toys brought in to cheer the child up and educate family members and visitors as necessary about pertinent safety concerns.

Another toy-related concern involves devices with portable radio transmitters (for example, radio-controlled or remote-controlled toys) that can cause electromagnetic interference. Such interference might cause biomedical equipment malfunction, and restrictions similar to those that pertain to cell phones should apply.

Yet another toy-related issue is infection control. Playrooms in hospital waiting areas, in pediatric units, and in physicians' offices are particularly high-risk environments in this regard. To make these toys safe for patients, facilities need to have adequate procedures for checking the serviceability of all toys, proper storage for unused toys, and cleaning and maintenance of all toys.

With regard to infection control, it is important that toys that contain fabric or cloth (material) such as chenille, velvet, and fur not be shared between patients and that they should be discarded after the patient leaves the facility, or if suitable, given to the patient to take home. Shared toys should be made of materials that are easy to clean, such as hard plastic, vinyl, metal, finished wood, and so on.

Before buying toys, games, and so on, facilities should work with their infection control practitioners to determine whether the materials they are made of can be cleaned once they have been contaminated with moist body substances, such as saliva, respiratory secretions, urine, stool, blood, and so on. If they can be cleaned, it is also important to know what cleaning agent and method should be used. Procedures should be developed and distributed to the areas controlling the toys. Any items being evaluated for purchase should also be checked to ensure that they do not represent a choking or digestive risk, as noted previously regarding concerns about toys for small children.

Crib Tops, Canopy Beds, and Side Rails

Parents of toddlers know that sometimes it can be hard to keep their children in the bed. When a child is in the hospital, adequate sleeping arrangements need to be made to keep the child safe. One solution is to use crib tops or canopy beds that will not allow the child to get out of bed unassisted. These beds help protect the patient from falls and also prevent wandering, thus helping the staff avoid using restraints.

If a facility does not have beds to prevent falling and wandering, it might be necessary to engage a sitter to protect the patient. If a family member who is staying with the patient around the clock is expected to prevent them from falling or getting out of bed unassisted, the staff must communicate this expectation and document the discussion with the parent, including their agreement. Parents or guardians in such circumstances should be specifically instructed to alert the facility staff whenever they will be leaving the child alone, even for a short period of time.

Side rails are important safety features for both the younger and older pediatric patient. Side rails can help prevent patients from falling or rolling out of bed. It is critical that side rails be kept up. Leaving them down, even for a short time, can lead to a fall. The hospital staff, including volunteers who may interact and play with the patient, must be aware that it is their responsibility to put the rail back up any time they are not with the child. In addition, the staff should advise the parent or guardian about maintaining this safety feature when they are interacting with the child. All such instructions to the parent must be documented in the medical record.

Other Environmental Hazards

Just as in the child's home, a pediatric facility needs to be childproofed to protect the patient and others from any negative effects that might result from the child's natural curiosity. Items that are important to include in such a childproofing inventory are discussed next.

Electrical Outlets   Children are fascinated with electrical outlets. Some think that this is because outlets are near their eye level, drawing the child's attention to them. Although the chance of electrocution is very small, such a result clearly would be devastating. Any related litigation would be indefensible because there are simple ways to make outlets safe. The facility's bioengineering resources should be knowledgeable about, and facilitate, implementation of child tamper-resistant outlets. It might also be possible simply to reposition the outlets out of reach.

Plastic Bags   As is noted on most products such as dry cleaning and other plastic bags, they create the risk that a child might suffocate if the bag adheres to the patient's nose and mouth. This hazard has been so well publicized that parents should be familiar with it. However, the staff should still be alert to those who might not recognize the risk of bringing toys or clothing for the patient into the facility in a plastic bag and then leaving it in the patient's room. Staff should remind such individuals about the hazard, and direct them to place any such bags out of reach of the child. They should also be told to remove the bag when they leave. If they do not, the staff should dispose of it.

Needle Boxes, Sharps Containers, and Hazardous Waste   Needles and other sharps used in medical care must be disposed of properly, using an approved disposal container. Pediatric patients create a particular safety issue regarding sharps receptacles because these containers provide a tempting target if they are within reach of young hands. Sharps containers must thus be mounted at a proper height, and providers in the pediatric setting must be especially cautious to avoid overfilling them. Other hazardous waste should also be placed in suitable containers for pickup and proper disposal. Such containers should be placed in areas that are not accessible to curious children or their parents.

Doors and Stairs   Doors and stairs might also be tempting to a child. Some pediatric facilities place door handles and other opening mechanisms higher than usual to keep them out of reach of young hands. Others increase staffing to provide for close monitoring of external exits. Doors that lead to stairs are associated with particular risk because stairs are a potential fall hazard for young children. Stairs also might allow patients access to other parts of the facility and even allow them to leave the building. Facilities that work with older children and teens who might want to investigate the floor below, or brain-injured or psychiatric patients who might not understand that they are exiting the building, may consider tracking devices like the identification bands used to keep elderly patients from wandering in nursing homes.

Medication Storage   There are many potential locations for medication storage besides the pharmacy. These locations include medication rooms, medication carts, treatment room medication cabinets, code carts, and transport boxes, among others. The pharmacy should be responsible for maintaining a list of sanctioned medication storage locations and items for which drug storage outside the pharmacy is allowed. Medication may also be stored in a patient room either by use of an in-room medication cabinet or within a childproof bedside box. The nursing staff should be responsible for documenting the medications given on the medication administration record. When the patient is discharged, the box should be cleared of the medications, and the medications should be credited to the patient or labeled and sent home as required.

· · · · · · · · ·

PERSONNEL ISSUES

The pediatric provider must undergo an annual competency review, like other healthcare providers, to ensure that they have the knowledge and skills to provide competent, safe care to patients. Competency requirements should be assessed at least annually for any necessary revisions related to changes in the diagnoses and ages cared for and procedures performed.

Competency Assessment

There are seven pediatric age ranges that may be appropriate for specific competency delineation, including newborns, infants, toddlers, preschoolers, school age, adolescents, and adults, because many pediatric facilities continue to see patients through the age of twenty-one or beyond for certain conditions.

Lifting Patients

As mentioned earlier, pediatric patients come in all shapes, sizes, and weights. Although the infant or small toddler is easy to lift, staff may also be faced with a six-foot, 250-pound high school football player or a bariatric patient struggling with obesity issues. Staff risk injury to themselves if they take on the task of moving such patients alone.

The staff should be trained in lifting techniques and related procedures that are in place to minimize injury and should follow them. Particularly important are the following:

- Staff must be trained to assess the task, determine the resources needed, and request those resources.

- Two or more staff members should be used when transporting patients in full-size beds or beds that are difficult to maneuver. Use of additional personnel should also be considered when moving or positioning a patient with the following risk factors: limited cognitive abilities and difficulty following verbal directions, history of violence and unpredictable behavior, and recent sedation, including those awakening from anesthesia.

- Facilities should consider obtaining assistive devices such as slider boards and ceiling lift systems.

- Staff should apply ergonomic principles when moving patients, for example, adjusting the bed or other surface to waist height when working with patients who are lying down.

Background Checks

Healthcare organizations owe patients a duty to ensure adequately screened individuals are staffing their facilities. To protect the pediatric population, in particular, the organization must avoid having staff with criminal backgrounds caring for patients, especially if the charges against them involve violence or abuse of a child. During the preemployment process, the facility should perform a criminal background check on all applicants. In addition to checking the local database, the facility should also use a background check service that identifies charges and convictions from other jurisdictions.

To reduce the risk of liability due to inadequately conducted hiring processes, the employment application form must clearly identify those items that prospective employees must disclose to be considered for employment. Applicants who fail to disclose requested background information should automatically be ineligible for hire. Note that convictions do not necessarily bar an applicant from employment. The facility should consider the relationship between the conviction and the duties of the job for which the applicant is applying.

Professional Relationships with Patients and Families

Staff who work with pediatric patients often encounter very compelling and emotional stories. To ensure proper therapeutic relationships, organizations must have policies or guidelines in place to help the staff identify acceptable professional boundaries and set proper limits on relationships between patients and families. Some guiding principles include the following:

- Provide care only within the scope of your practice.
- Provide care only within regularly scheduled work hours.
- Provide care and support to patients and families consistently, without preferential treatment.
- Refrain from accepting gifts of significant monetary value from patients and families.
- Do not offer gifts of money or significant financial value to patients or family.
- Refrain from sharing personal information with patients or families, including home phone numbers, addresses, e-mail addresses, and fax numbers.
- Do not engage in romantic, sexual, or intimate physical relationships with any patient, any members of a current patient's family, or any former patients under the age of eighteen.
- Do not provide foster care or initiate adoption proceedings for patients encountered in the role as employee.
- Never transport patients or patients' family members in your personal vehicle.

Staff should understand that the reason some of these acts are not sanctioned is because they might result in liability for them and for the organization. Supportive supervisors should help staff identify resources that can help the patient and family once the limits of their professional relationship have been reached.

Chaperones

The use of chaperones can reduce the risk for both patient and clinician. Chaperones should be considered when the patient care will involve an examination or procedure involving a sensitive area such as the breast, genital/gynecological, or rectal areas. With a young patient, the parent or guardian may be an appropriate individual to witness the care. Older patients, including adolescents, may be too embarrassed to have a relative present for a sensitive examination or procedure. The facility and clinician should determine when to offer a facility-provided chaperone rather than rely on a parent/guardian.

A chaperone will provide a witness that an exam was performed within appropriate clinical bounds. Another way to decrease the risk of such encounters is by using one of the risk management core skills: communication. Clinicians can help minimize the patient's apprehension and embarrassment by sharing information with the patient about what will be done as well as the purpose for the examination. Clinicians may also find it useful to communicate during the examination to describe what they are looking for and reinforce the clinical need for the specific actions. Showing respect, and possibly empathy, to the patient can lessen the patient's and parent's concerns and any lingering questions about whether the clinician's actions were appropriate.

· · · · · · · · ·

SPECIAL ISSUES

Risk management professionals in pediatric healthcare face the same range of issues, and responses to those issues, as do risk management professionals in adult healthcare. But these issues deserve special mention regarding their application in the pediatric context.

Informed Consent

Informed consent, although important for patients of all ages, is an extremely important and potentially complex process for a practitioner providing pediatric care. In most adult cases, practitioners can obtain consent directly from the patient. The reverse is true for pediatric patient situations, where, with a few exceptions, such as those that apply to emancipated or mature minors, the provider is usually obtaining consent from a third party. Clearly, practitioners must be diligent in identifying and involving the correct authorized parent or guardian. (Refer to Chapter 4 on informed consent for more information.)

Obtaining Consent in a Variety of Family and Social Situations   The pediatric practitioner works with many family situations in which it is challenging to determine the individual who is authorized to give an informed consent. These situations include, but are not limited to (1) parents who disagree on treatment options, (2) divorced parents, (3) putative fathers, (4) court-appointed custodians or guardians, (5) patients undergoing adoption, and (6) parents who are no more than adolescents themselves. In addition, practitioners might be faced with family members who are caring for the child in the parents' absence and therefore believe that they have the authority to make healthcare decisions. Laws regarding who may consent for a child can vary from state to state, so it is essential that practitioners be familiar with the regulations in their jurisdictions.

Such challenging scenarios also make it necessary for the practitioner, office, or hospital staff to address the topic of legal custody when the patient enters the practice or is admitted to the hospital. A copy of any pertinent legal documents should be placed in the medical record. It may also be necessary to provide a resource to help interpret legal documents for staff so that staff know who can provide consent. Questioning the existence or level of consent authority can be challenging when it involves interacting with potentially sensitive parties such as adoptive parents, same sex partnerships, foster parents, etc. Custody documents, court orders, parenting plans and other legal documents can range in size from a single page to a large document (10–20 pages). It is expecting too much to have individual staff members try to interpret documents in which consent authority is complicated and confusing. Staff should have a resource such as the risk manager who can help define the scope of legal authority so that staff involve the correct individual in the consent process.

Emancipated and Mature Minors   Many states allow an adolescent to pursue full legal rights, including the right to make care decisions, when they can show that they are emancipated from their parents or guardians. Minors can demonstrate in several ways that they live, or can live, independent of a parent or guardian. Rules on emancipation vary state by state. For example, depending on the state, a minor can make a case for emancipation through circumstances such as being married, being the parent of a child, serving in the military, or living independently. To obtain an official determination of emancipation, the minor must go through the legal system and receive that determination from the court. Therefore, when patients identify themselves as emancipated minors, the facility staff should request a copy of the court documents to confirm the status. A copy should also be placed in the medical record so the process will not have to be repeated in the future. If no determination exists, the practitioner should consult the risk management professional or hospital counsel to determine whether the minor can be treated as emancipated.

Mature minor is a designation that physicians in some states bestow upon a minor if it is determined that the patient has a level of judgment and reasoning that is sufficient for medical decision making. The courts in many states have elevated the rights of minors by ruling that minors who are age fourteen and older can consent to certain types of healthcare treatments. These include treatments for drug and alcohol abuse, pregnancy, sexually transmitted diseases, and mental health. Given this legal precedent, it might be desirable to allow minors to consent to other care, if they can show the required maturity level. Practitioners should make sure that they are familiar with the regulations of their particular jurisdiction. If mature minor statutes exist, the clinician should be diligent in assessing minors' ability to understand the treatment options and assessing their decision-making abilities. This should be followed up with explicit documentation regarding specific observations that the practitioner relied upon to determine maturity.

In general, the right to obtain treatment is associated with the right to have the organization maintain confidentiality of the medical record. Practitioners should be careful to maintain the confidentiality of records of mature minors and should not disclose them to others, including parents, without the minor's consent or as otherwise permitted or required by law.

Preparing Patients for Adulthood and Decision Making   Pediatric practitioners can greatly benefit their adolescent patients by involving them in decision making, along with their parents or guardians. Their involvement will build confidence and prepare them for adult decision making. Without preparation, patients are generally no more ready to make decisions on their eighteenth birthday than they were the day before, when they were still a minor. Also, as adolescent patients with chronic conditions often continue to be seen in a pediatric system between the ages of eighteen and twenty-one, preparing such patients to make their own decisions assists the entire care team. Involving adolescents in decision-making discussions also helps the parents or guardians and the patients better understand the other's point of view. This leads to more collaborative decision making and increases the accountability of the adolescent patient.

End-of-Life Decision Making
End-of-life care creates special issues with pediatric patients. State law will determine whether a minor, of any age, can execute a valid directive to physicians. Such a directive is also known as a living will or durable power of attorney. There is certainly a trend toward allowing older minors to express their wishes about withholding or withdrawing life-sustaining treatment when they are in a terminal condition. Whether the provider can, should, or must follow these wishes varies by state. In addition, it is a matter of state law whether the parents may make their own decision to withhold or withdraw care when a child is in a terminal condition or permanent vegetative state. Some states allow the parents or guardians, acting with the care team, to reach and implement this decision, whereas others require a court hearing, sometimes including appointment of a guardian *ad litem*. In addition to learning the laws of their state, practitioners might want to consult with their institutional ethics committee for advice in these very difficult situations.

Pediatric Clinical Research and Consent
Pediatric patients and their families have benefited from research over the years. Research led to development of vaccines to combat measles, polio, and other deadly or debilitating diseases that used to strike children. Continued clinical research and development of equipment and pharmaceuticals has led to a marked decrease in pediatric morbidity and mortality.

Despite the significant advances in pediatric care that have come from research, children have not benefited as much as they might have, for several reasons. One reason is that the numbers of studies involving children have decreased. Another is the difficulty in conducting research on rare diseases, which by definition have few patients to participate. In some cases, clinicians must treat pediatric patients with drugs that were developed through adult studies, without specific and substantive information about pediatric dosages or effects. Community awareness of this lack of pediatric research–based information has recently led to increased funding, as academic medical centers focus more on this patient population.

Because pediatric patients cannot consent to medical care until they are teenagers, and then only in limited circumstances, informed consent for pediatric research raises important ethical questions. It is of interest that federal regulations governing research create an exception to the common law's general requirement that individuals must achieve the age of majority before they may consent. Specifically, these regulations require assent from children involved in research to the extent that they are capable of understanding and providing it.

Assent is considered to be a child's agreement to participate in research. Assent is a nebulous concept, and the age at which a child can give assent is also vague, as federal regulations do not specify a particular age at which assent should be obtained. Researchers should consider a child's age, maturity, and psychological state. Children six years of age can give assent to participate in research. For children, then, agreement to participate in research is a two-step process. First, the child's parents or guardians must consent to have their child involved in research. Only if this occurs can researchers then discuss the research protocol with the child to determine if the child also wants (assents) to participate. Although this process is more cumbersome than informed consent issues associated with other research, it provides a framework for making sure that researchers deal with children ethically. (Refer to Chapter 5, "Clinical Research, Institutional Review Boards," for more information.)

Pediatric Implications of HIPAA   The Health Insurance Portability and Accountability Act (HIPAA) and its related regulations established federal privacy standards for individually identifiable health information. HIPAA affects all patients, including pediatric patients. Disclosing a child's health information might be necessary for multiple reasons, including the request of a parent or guardian, qualification for services from community resources, program assistance from educational institutions, and so on. Requests for information on pediatric patients should be evaluated to see whether the request is for a purpose for which HIPAA permits disclosure and whether state privacy and medical record confidentiality regulations apply. When a request for information requires an authorization, the provider, in consultation with the risk management professional or counsel, must determine who may provide a valid authorization for the pediatric patient. This is particularly important because HIPAA has been modified by the HITECH Act, an aspect of the recovery legislation that was signed into law in 2009. Among many other provisions, HITECH creates accountability for individual employees of healthcare organizations and makes them potentially responsible for fines ranging from $100 to $50,000, with maximum total fines of $1.5 million annually for repeated egregious offenses. (Please see Chapter 16, Volume 3, on HIPAA/HITECH for more information.)

Often, the pediatric patient's parent or guardian will be the proper individual to authorize release of information. However, depending on state laws and regulations, situations might arise in which the patient must provide authorization. Emancipated or mature minors are likely to be included in this group because it is a general rule that a minor may consent to the release of information pertaining to care that the minor authorized. Such situations might include treatment related to mental health, HIV, sexually transmitted diseases, and so on. Relevant state laws and regulations must be reviewed to clarify the scope of information that may be authorized for release by the minor patient.

Immunizations and the National Childhood Vaccine Injury Compensation Act   Immunizing children is an important part of childhood disease prevention. Diseases such as smallpox, measles, and polio have been greatly reduced or eliminated through vaccine development and administration. The degree to which immunization has become a part of our culture is illustrated by general requirements that children must be immunized before they may attend school. Allegations that adverse outcomes resulted from vaccine administration, however, have created liability-related concerns.

In the 1970s and 1980s, in particular, patients and families were concerned about adverse effects of vaccines and practitioners and manufacturers were concerned about being sued for the adverse events. In some cases, companies ceased to manufacture the vaccines and shortages resulted. In 1986, Congress, spurred on by these events, enacted the NCVIA (U.S. Code 42 U.S.C. 300), which established the National Vaccine Injury Compensation Program (VICP).

Any patient, or parent or guardian on behalf of the patient, may file a VICP claim if particular adverse events are experienced related to several commonly administered vaccines in a specified time frame. A claimant must file a claim under this program before suing a manufacturer or practitioner. If the claimant accepts a settlement from the VICP, then a secondary claim against a manufacturer or practitioner cannot be filed. Risk management professionals and practitioners should be aware of this program so that they can direct patients to applicable resources. Practitioners must also understand their obligations under the program, such as recording certain information in the medical record when a patient receives a vaccine (manufacturer, vaccine, lot number, practitioner who administered the vaccine, and date of administration). In addition, practitioners need to know what adverse events they need to report to the program. The program is a reasonable approach that protects practitioners from lawsuits and ensures that patients get the immunizations they need.

· · · · · · · · ·

CHILD ABUSE AND NEGLECT

Child abuse and neglect reporting laws have been enacted in every state to deal with the large number of children that are physically, emotionally, and sexually abused each year. Healthcare providers are mandatory reporters of child abuse, or suspected child abuse, under these laws.

Abuse Reporting

Authorities to whom such reports must be made may include, depending on the state and the circumstances, a child protective services or law enforcement agency, or both. Many professionals are specifically designated as mandated reporters, for example, audiologists, counselors, coaches, dentists, nurses, pharmacists, phlebotomists, physician assistants, physicians, podiatrists, psychiatrists, psychologists, occupational or physical therapists, optometrists, respiratory therapists, social workers, speech therapists, and so on. Thus the risk management professionals and clinical managers in a healthcare facility or private practice must be aware of local law and which providers must report. All pertinent staff must then be educated as to their responsibilities.

Healthcare providers are generally immune from civil or criminal liability when they report or provide testimony in good faith. If they do not report, however, there might be serious professional consequences, including litigation for failure to act and potential loss of licensure. Although it is less likely, failure to report child abuse could also lead to criminal charges against a provider.

Abuse Identification   Pediatric patients who present with abuse or neglect-related injuries might have been admitted for other conditions as seen by the provider or health-care facility. It is important for the provider to have a clear set of screening criteria to help determine when additional medical care or review is needed and when a potential case of child abuse or neglect should be reported. A provider should consider assessing for child abuse or neglect when any of the following conditions are present. Circumstantial criteria include the following:

- An attending physician or other medical consultant has determined that an injury is not due to an accident.
- The case has been recently referred to child protective services by another community agent, such as another medical center, paramedics, or the police department.
- A parent or caregiver(s) admits to abuse or neglect.
- A witness reports abuse or neglect of the child.
- The child has been exposed to violence of any kind in a living situation.
- There has been delay in seeking medical treatment.
- The pattern of family interaction or involvement does not seem consistent with the child's needs.
- The history related to the injury or condition is dubious.

    Clinical criteria include

- an infant who fails to thrive;
- fracture(s) in patients under the age of two, without sufficient explanation of injury;
- unexplainable bruises, cuts, burns, and so on;
- intracranial or intra-abdominal injury(ies) without sufficient history of accident;
- rectal or vaginal injury with no clear accidental causes; and
- drug or toxic injections (prescription drugs, illegal drugs, gasoline) and so on.

    As these examples illustrate, abuse, neglect, or sexual abuse can look like another condition entirely. The Children's Protection Program at Children's Hospital and Regional Medical Center in Seattle, Washington, has developed a specific list of indicators that identify when an abuse evaluation is warranted. These indicators also specify patient-specific characteristics and parental or caretaker characteristics that might raise questions about the presenting problem and trigger a more in-depth assessment by the provider. (Refer to Box 9.1 and Tables 9.1 to 9.12 for indications for further investigation.)

    When in doubt about whether a situation warrants reporting to the local child protective agency, a provider should consider consulting with the particular agency, which should have staff members designated to assist them on such issues. Remember that agency personnel are not obligated to share information, as their first obligation is to solicit potential abuse reporting. However, agency representatives should be able to respond to any of the following concerns:

- Whether to make a referral to child protective services or law enforcement
- Whether a family has a child protective services history
- Whether there are differences of opinion regarding the handling of a case
- What the protocol is for making complaints to an agency
- What are the general questions regarding the policy or philosophy of child protective services
- Where to turn for more specific answers
- Whether there are cases from other child protective services offices outside the local area

This external resource can help the healthcare team determine how to proceed when they are unsure whether the patient situation involves reportable abuse or neglect. By documenting the attempt at and result of consultation, the provider also minimizes potential liability, because turning to the authorities on questions of reportability is a reasonable approach.

BOX 9.1   Physical Abuse — General Indicators

FACTORS, INDIVIDUAL OR IN COMBINATION, THAT SUGGEST THAT AN INJURY/SITUATION MAY BE THE RESULT OF ABUSE

- **Child's level of development:** It takes a certain stage of development to injure oneself. Judgment should be based on child's own developmental abilities, e.g., any traumatic injury or poisoning of pretoddlers is considered suspicious.

- **Shape of injury:** Assaults may be inflicted by identifiable objects, e.g., shape of some immersion burns may suggest intentional dunking.

- **Location of injury:** Injuries to thighs, upper arms, genital and rectal areas, buttocks, and back of legs or torso are frequently inflicted.

- **Force to produce injury:** It takes substantial force to cause a bruise that remains visible for more than a few hours. Even more force is needed to break a bone.

- **Type of injury:** It is almost impossible for some injuries to be self-inflicted. Metaphyseal fractures or choke marks on a child's neck are two examples.

- **Number of old and new injuries:** Multiple injuries on various parts of body unlikely to occur in accidents and/or multiple injuries in various stages of healing are indicative of a continuing pattern of assaults. Severe injuries that are untreated or signs of delay in seeking treatment are very concerning.

Source: Reprinted with the Permission of Children's Hospital & Regional Medical Center, Seattle, WA.

TABLE 9.1   Specific Indicators that Warrant an Abuse Evaluation

Specific Indicators that Warrant an Abuse Evaluation	SCAN ASSESSMENTS ✓ = recommended		
	Medical*	Psycho Social	SCAN Attending
Intracranial bleeding (especially SDH and SAH) in absence of major documented trauma (such as MVAs) or preexisting bleeding disorders in children 3 years old & under	✓	✓	✓
Altered consciousness plus retinal hemorrhages in children 3 years old & under	✓	✓	✓
All skull fractures in children 3 years old & under not explained by significant trauma	✓	✓	✓
Fractures in preambulatory and preverbal children not explained by significant trauma	✓	✓	✓
Intra-abdominal trauma (bowel perforations, injuries to liver, pancreas or intestines) in absence of documented major trauma such as MVAs in children of all ages	✓	✓	✓
Burn injuries, particularly distinctly shaped burns suggesting an object was used to inflict them; cigarette burns; immersion burns suggesting intentional dipping in hot water in children of all ages	✓	✓	✓
Rib fractures in children 3 years old & under (without abnormal bones or documented major trauma)	✓	✓	✓
Bruises, particularly any bruise on a child under 9 months or not cruising, without documented bleeding disorder	✓	✓	✓
Any bruise with a recognizable pattern; adult bite marks; unusual location; clustered injuries; multiple, apparently inflicted injuries in different stages of healing; injuries on several different body planes in children of all ages	✓	✓	✓
Munchausen syndrome by proxy Any concern for fictitious illness in a child of any age requires a consultation with CA/N attending and children's protection team	✓	✓	Required
Any disclosure by child and/or caretaker; statements by witnesses indicating child maltreatment has occurred.	✓	✓	
Tying, binding, and other forms of tortuous confinement	✓	✓	

*Consider differential diagnosis.
Reprinted with the permission of Children's Hospital & Regional Medical Center. Seattle, WA.

TABLE 9.2   Characteristics of Abuse — Child

The following conditions may have any one of a number of organic or environmental causes besides maltreatment and should be evaluated within the context of a comprehensive assessment, which includes the developmental level of the child and parent's response to the child's problems.

	SCAN ASSESSMENTS ✓ = recommended		
Child Characteristics	*Medical**	*Psycho Social*	*SCAN Attending*
Developmental lags (physical, mental or emotional)	✓	✓	
Extremes of behavior (excessive compliance and passivity or overly aggressive, demanding, negative, hyperactive)		✓	
Wary of physical contact with parents or other adults; fears going home		✓	
Displays hypervigilance		✓	
Is clingy and indiscriminate in her/his attachments		✓	
Overly adaptive behavior (inappropriately adult or inappropriately infantile)		✓	
Shows no expectation of being comforted; extreme sense of hopelessness		✓	
Children who have complications with prenatal exposure to drugs may be at higher risk for maltreatment because of their physical and neurological impairments		✓	
Children with chronic illnesses and/or disabilities, particularly those that lead to difficult child behavior, may be at higher risk for maltreatment.		✓	

*Consider differential diagnosis.
Reprinted with the Permission of Children's Hospital & Regional Medical Center. Seattle, WA.

TABLE 9.3   Characteristics of Abuse — Parental or Caretaker

Parental or Caretaker Characteristics	SCAN ASSESSMENTS ✓ = recommended		
	Medical*	Psycho Social	SCAN Attending
Inappropriate response to seriousness of child's condition	✓	✓	✓
No explanation for injury	✓	✓	✓
Explanations that are at variance with clinical findings	✓	✓	✓
Changing explanations/histories	✓	✓	
Concealment of past injuries	✓	✓	
Delay in seeking medical help; continuing or gross parental inattentiveness to child's need for safety; indifference to repeated accidents	✓	✓	
Hospital and/or physician shopping	✓	✓	
Parental limitations (lack of basic parenting and problem-solving skills); inappropriate discipline; inflexible and controlling behaviors; frequent crises/chaotic lifestyles, homelessness; lack of consistency to family members and peers; cognitive, developmental or physical limitations	✓	✓	
Domestic violence	✓	✓	
Substance abuse	✓	✓	
Severe mental health problems (major depression, psychosis)	✓	✓	
An extended family history of abuse or neglect	✓	✓	
Open Child Protective Services case	✓	✓	

*Consider differential diagnosis.
Reprinted with the Permission of Children's Hospital & Regional Medical Center. Seattle, WA.

TABLE 9.4   Neglect—Specific Indicators

Factors, individual or in combination, that suggest an injury/situation is suspicious

Specific Indicators that Warrant an Evaluation for Neglect	SCAN ASSESSMENTS ✓ = recommended		
	Medical*	Psycho Social	SCAN Attending
Ingestions	✓	✓	
Near drownings	✓	✓	
Failure to thrive in absence of causative major medical problems or if family support issues complicate major illnesses	✓	✓	
Medical neglect, parent's failure to provide medical, dental, or psychiatric care needed to prevent or treat serious physical or psychological injuries or illnesses. It includes failure to provide, consent to, or follow through with: preventative care, such as immunizations; diagnostic care, such as medical exams and hospitalizations; remedial care, such as surgery or regular medication; or prosthetic care, such as eyeglasses or an artificial limb. Apparently untreated injuries, illnesses, or impairments that suggest medical neglect and failure to make court-ordered appointments require medical and psychosocial CA/N assessments. Other missed appointments, treatments, inappropriate medication applications are dependent on acuteness of situation. For some children, a single missed treatment could be fatal.	Assess with social worker. Determine seriousness of consequences for health/safety of child		
Burn injuries of children 3 years old & under. Medical provider consults with social work regarding child's development and history of injury to decide if SCAN psychosocial interview should take place.	Consult with social worker	Consult with PMD	
Any disclosure by child and/or caretaker; statements by witnesses indicating child **maltreatment** has occurred.	✓	✓	
Abandonment of child or child left in physically dangerous situation (consider child's age and maturity as well as actual conditions)	✓	✓	

*Consider differential diagnosis.
SCAN, suspected child abuse and neglect; CA/N, child abuse/neglect; PMD, primary medical doctor.
Reprinted with the permission of Children's Hospital & Regional Medical Center. Seattle, WA.

TABLE 9.5   Characteristics for Neglect — Child

The following conditions may have any one of a number of organic or environmental causes besides neglect and should be evaluated within the context of a comprehensive assessment, which includes the developmental level of the child and parent's response to the child's problems.

	SCAN ASSESSMENTS ✓ = recommended		
Child Characteristics	*Medical**	*Psycho Social*	*SCAN Attending*
Developmental lags (physical, mental or emotional)	✓	✓	
Failure to thrive or less severe deficits in growth or development	✓	✓	
Sudden and severe drops in child's school performance, emotional appearance or general functioning		✓	
Delinquency (e.g. thefts)		✓	
Exploitation, excessive responsibilities placed on child to care for home and other younger children		✓	

*Consider differential diagnosis.
Reprinted with the permission of Children's Hospital & Regional Medical Center. Seattle, WA.

TABLE 9.6   Characteristics for Neglect — Parental or Caretaker

The following conditions may have any one of a number of organic or environmental causes besides neglect and should be evaluated within the context of a comprehensive assessment, which includes the developmental level of the child and parent's response to the child's problems.

	SCAN ASSESSMENTS ✓ = recommended		
Parental or Caretaker Characteristics	*Medical**	*Psycho Social*	*SCAN Attending*
Delay in seeking medical help; continuing or gross parental inattentiveness to child's need for safety; indifference to repeated accidents		✓	
Hospital and/or physician shopping		✓	
Parental limitations (lack of basic parenting and problem solving skills); inappropriate discipline; inflexible and controlling behaviors; frequent crises/ chaotic lifestyles, homelessness; lack of consistency to family members and peers; cognitive, developmental, or physical limitations		✓	
Domestic violence		✓	
Substance abuse		✓	
Severe mental health problems (major depression, psychosis)		✓	
An extended family history of abuse or neglect		✓	
Open Child Protective Services case		✓	

*Consider differential diagnosis.
Reprinted with the permission of Children's Hospital & Regional Medical Center. Seattle, WA.

TABLE 9.7   Characteristics for Emotional Maltreatment—Child

Factors, individual or in combination, that suggest an injury/situation may be the result of abuse

The following conditions may have any one of a number of organic or environmental causes besides emotional maltreatment and should be evaluated within the context of a comprehensive assessment, which includes the developmental level of the child and parent's response to the child's problems.

	SCAN ASSESSMENTS ✓ = recommended		
Child Characteristics	*Medical**	*Psycho Social*	*SCAN Attending*
Developmental lags (physical, mental or emotional)	✓	✓	
Failure to thrive or less severe deficits in growth or development	✓	✓	
Enuresis and/or encopresis	✓	✓	
Habit disorders (head banging, sucking, rocking, biting)	✓	✓	
Conduct disorders (antisocial or destructive behaviors)	✓	✓	
Neurotic traits (sleep disorders, speech disorders, and inhibition of play)	✓	✓	
Psychoneurotic reactions (hysteria, obsession, compulsion, phobias, hypochondria)		✓	
Extremes of behavior (excessive compliance and passivity or overly aggressive, demanding, negative, hyperactive)		✓	
Wary of physical contact with parents or other adults; fears going home		✓	
Displays hypervigilance		✓	
Is clingy and indiscriminate in her/his attachments		✓	
Overly adaptive behavior (inappropriately adult or inappropriately infantile)		✓	
Sudden and severe drops in child's school performance, emotional appearance or general functioning		✓	
Attempted suicide	✓	✓	
Any disclosure by child and/or caretaker; statements by witnesses indicating child maltreatment has occurred.	✓	✓	
Abandonment of child or child left in physically dangerous situation (consider child's age and maturity as well as actual conditions)	✓	✓	

*Consider differential diagnosis.
Reprinted with the permission of Children's Hospital & Regional Medical Center. Seattle, WA.

TABLE 9.8   Characteristics for Emotional Maltreatment—Parental or Caretaker

Parental or Caretaker Characteristics	*SCAN ASSESSMENTS ✓ = recommended*		
	*Medical**	*Psycho Social*	*SCAN Attending*
Inappropriate response to seriousness of child's condition	✓	✓	
No explanation for injury	✓	✓	
Explanations that are at variance with clinical findings	✓	✓	
Changing explanations/ histories	✓	✓	
Concealment of past injuries	✓	✓	
Delay in seeking medical help; continuing or gross parental inattentiveness to child's need for safety; indifference to repeated accidents	✓	✓	
Hospital and/or physician shopping		✓	
Parental limitations (lack of basic parenting and problem-solving skills); inappropriate discipline; inflexible and controlling behaviors; frequent crises/chaotic lifestyles, homelessness; lack of consistency to family members and peers; cognitive, developmental or physical limitations		✓	
Domestic violence		✓	
Substance abuse/drug dealing		✓	
Severe mental health problems (major depression, psychosis)		✓	
Caretaker exhibits psychically destructive behaviors towards child, e.g., extreme rejection, isolation, terrorizing, ignoring or corrupting		✓	
Open Child Protective Services case		✓	

*Consider differential diagnosis.
Reprinted with the permission of Children's Hospital & Regional Medical Center. Seattle, WA.

TABLE 9.9   Sexual Abuse — General Indicators

Factors, individual or in combination, that suggest an injury/situation is suspicious

Signs of sexual activity cannot be automatically interpreted as signs of sexual abuse, but should be further assessed. Even without a disclosure, a report to CPS may be necessary. (Refer to Recommended Guidelines for Sexual Assault Emergency Medical Evaluation, Child 12 years and under; Recommended Guidelines for Sexual Assault Emergency Medical Evaluation, Adult and Adolescent)

| | *SCAN ASSESSMENTS ✓ = recommended* | | |
General Indicators	*Medical**	*Psycho Social*	*SCAN Attending*
Exam indicative of acute penetrating injury, vaginal bleeding, genital trauma, anal injury	✓	✓	✓
STD, including GC, CT HPV, herpes, syphilis, HIV, which are recognized beyond the normal age for appearance of perinatally acquired disease; other in nonsexually active patient. When STDs are found in the consensually sexually active patient, consider age and power difference between the two partners to determine whether consent is legitimate.	✓	✓	✓
Exam concerning for sexual abuse, e.g., trauma to breast, lower abdomen, thighs, genital/rectal areas	✓	✓	✓
Presence of semen	✓	✓	✓
Pregnancy	✓	✓	✓
History of sexual assault/abuse and/or any disclosure by child and/or caretaker; statements by witnesses indicating child maltreatment has occurred.	✓	✓	

*Consider differential diagnosis.
Reprinted with the permission of Children's Hospital & Regional Medical Center. Seattle, WA.

Factitious Disorder, or Munchausen Syndrome by Proxy   According to the *Diagnostic and Statistical Manual of Mental Disorders*, Fourth Edition (*DSM-IV*), "factitious disorders are characterized by physical or psychological symptoms that are intentionally produced or feigned in order to assume the sick role."[12] It is hard to believe that someone would feign illness, but affected individuals apparently have such a great need to gain attention that they subject themselves to unnecessary medical care. Although the condition is more commonly seen in adults than in children or adolescents, and even then affects only a small percentage of the population, practitioners should be aware of the potential that they could have a pediatric patient with factitious disorder.

Factitious disorders are difficult to diagnose. When patients are confronted regarding factitious disorders, they often cease seeing that practitioner and find another practitioner who will provide the attention that they seek. Practitioners may help some of the patients

TABLE 9.10   Characteristics of Sexual Abuse — Child

The following conditions may have any one of a number of organic or environmental causes besides sexual abuse and should be evaluated within the context of a comprehensive assessment, which includes the developmental level of the child and parent's response to the child's problems.

Child Characteristics	SCAN ASSESSMENTS ✓ = recommended		
	Medical*	Psycho Social	SCAN Attending
Insecurity; lack of trust; behavioral problems; denial of painful feelings or perceptions; excessive fears; overwhelming desire to please others; shame; compulsive or obsessive behavior problems; regressive or aggressive behaviors		✓	
Sexualized behavior toward adults, other children; promiscuity or prostitution; expressed unusual curiosity toward sexual parts of the body; has specific knowledge of sex beyond developmental age; inappropriately exposed genitals to others or extreme discomfort with own body		✓	
Nonspecific behavior changes, e.g. fear of being alone with any male, or particular person; sudden refusal to sleep in regular bed; poor peer relationships; unusual ownership of money or gifts		✓	

*Consider differential diagnosis.
SCAN, suspected child abuse and neglect.
Reprinted with the permission of Children's Hospital & Regional Medical Center. Seattle, WA.

afflicted with this condition if they are able to honestly but empathically confront the patient.

Another form of factitious disorder exists in which an adult, usually a parent, exaggerates or feigns illness of a child or deliberately causes or exacerbates actual medical problems that the child is experiencing. This disorder is called *factitious syndrome by proxy* (sometimes called *Munchausen syndrome by proxy*).[13] Sometimes the effects of the feigned illness are minor, but some cases can have tragic outcomes. One example is a parent who smothers a child to the point that the child stops breathing in an effort to pretend that the child has an apnea problem.

Factitious disorder by proxy can be very difficult to prove unless the provider actually observes the perpetrator in the act. Determining the causes of suspicious results or behaviors is a time-consuming and stressful process. It can be particularly difficult in

TABLE 9.11   **Characteristics of Sexual Abuse—Parental or Caretaker**

The following conditions may have any one of a number of organic or environmental causes besides sexual abuse and should be evaluated within the context of a comprehensive assessment, which includes the developmental level of the child and parent's response to the child's problems.

	SCAN ASSESSMENTS ✓ = Recommended		
Parental or Caretaker Characteristics	*Medical**	*Psycho Social*	*SCAN Attending*
Domestic violence		✓	
Substance abuse		✓	
Parental limitations (lack of basic parenting and problem-solving skills); inappropriate discipline; inflexible and controlling behaviors; frequent crises/chaotic lifestyles, homelessness; lack of consistency to family members and peers; cognitive, developmental or physical limitations		✓	
Severe mental health problems (major depression, psychosis)		✓	
Parental concern for sexual abuse: refer to PMD or GYN Specialty Clinic	✓	✓	
An extended family history of abuse or neglect		✓	
Open Child Protective Services case		✓	

*Consider differential diagnosis.
SCAN, Suspected Child Abuse and Neglect; GYN, gynecology; PMD, primary medical doctor.
Reprinted with the permission of Children's Hospital & Regional Medical Center. Seattle, WA.

TABLE 9.12   **Nonspecific Physical Complaints**

The great majority of sexual abuse cases do not involve violent or forced physical assaults. In these nonviolent cases, physical evidence is often ambiguous or nonexistent.

Anorexia (if anorexia nervosa)	If physiological causes are evaluated by a physician and found to be noncontributory to the symptoms, a psychosocial assessment should occur.
Abdominal pain	
Enuresis and/or encopresis	
Dysuria	
Genital or rectal pain, itching, discharge, bleeding, bruising	
Urethral discharge	
Painful defecation	

Reprinted with the permission of Children's Hospital & Regional Medical Center. Seattle, WA.

cases where the child actually does have a physical or medical problem and the perpetrator is simply exacerbating the condition. Practitioners and facilities treating children should have resources available to investigate suspected child abuse with this etiology. The use of video surveillance may be helpful in some cases, although the most helpful tool may be a multidisciplinary team that can help assess whether the factitious disorder by proxy exists. A multidisciplinary assessment can validate that a single practitioner is not overreading or underreading a situation. It can also promote defensibility of the provider if litigation ensues.

Understandably, parents who are reported for child abuse due to factitious syndrome by proxy may be very upset. They may be even more upset if child protection services subsequently determines that the report is unfounded. Furthermore, if the child is returned to the parent after removal, the parent may feel vindicated. In either circumstance, there is high potential for a volatile malpractice suit. It is therefore essential that practitioners be diligent in their investigation of possible abuse. In addition, it is extremely important that they accurately document their assessment, actions, and rationale so that it can subsequently be established that any report was made in good faith.

. . . .

CONCLUSION

By helping pediatric clinicians manage the complex and thorny regulatory, ethical, and safety-related issues that are unique to their fragile population, the risk management professional can address significant liability concerns, minimize risk, and contribute to an enhanced quality of care. Particularly valuable strategies include development of tools and mechanisms that facilitate partnership with patients and their families.

Endnotes

1. Children's Hospital & Regional Medical Center. Seattle, Wash. "Infant Sleep Position and Bedding Recommendations." Policy statement. March, 2005.

2. "The Use of Physical Restraint Interventions for Children and Adolescents in the Acute Care Setting." In: *Pediatrics* 1997; 99(3):497–498. Available at: http://aappolicy. aappublications.org/cgi/content/full/pediatrics;99/3/497. (Accessed November 28, 2009.)

3. Dorfman, D. H. and B. Kastner. "The Use of Restraint for Pediatric Psychiatric Patients in Emergency Departments." *Pediatric Emergency Care* 2004. 20(3):151–156.

4. Takata, G. S., et al. "Development, Testing, and Findings of a Pediatric-Focused Trigger Tool to Identify Medication-Related Harm in US Children's Hospitals." *Pediatrics* 2008; 121:e927–e935. Available at: www.pediatrics.org/cgi/content/full/121/4/e927. (Accessed March 30, 2010.)

5. "Preventing Pediatric Medication Errors" *The Joint Commission Sentinel Event Report* 2008; 39(4).

6. *Ibid.*

7.   Hicks, R.W., S.C. Becker, and D. D. Cousins. *MEDMARX® Data Report: A Chartbook of Medication Error Findings from the Perioperative Settings from 1998–2005*. Rockville, MD: USP Center for the Advancement of Patient Safety, 2006.

8.   Rinke, M.L., A.D. Shore, L. Morlock et al. "Characteristics of pediatric chemotherapy medication errors in a national error reporting database." *Cancer* 2007. 110(1):186–195.

9.   *op. cit.* "Preventing Pediatric Medication Errors."

10. American College of Allergy, Asthma & Immunology, 85 West Algonquin Road, Suite 550, Arlington Heights, Ill. 60005. Telephone: 847–427–1200.

11. Children's Hospital & Regional Medical Center. Seattle, Wash. "Toy Cleaning and Disinfection." *Infection Control Policies and Procedures*. September, 2004.

12. The American Psychiatric Association, *Diagnostic and Statistical Manual of Mental Disorders*, 4th ed. p. 513.

13. Terminology in this area is in some flux. Generally speaking, the term *Munchausen syndrome by proxy* is a diagnosis of the adult who is fabricating the illness. The term *factitious disorder* describes a condition caused by deliberate acts and is sometimes used as a diagnosis of the perpetrator and sometimes (when speaking of factitious disorder by proxy) of the victim. The term *pediatric falsification*, though not yet in wide use, can be expected to become the preferred term for diagnosing the child victim of a falsification disorder because it merely identifies the child as suffering from a falsified condition without attempting a psychiatric diagnosis of the adult perpetrator.

10

Risk Management in the Laboratory

Christine Clark
Laurence Sherman

Risk management in the laboratory requires understanding the structure and background of a highly regulated, information-generating, multiprocess operation. The majority of clinical diagnoses and therapeutic decisions are based, at least partly, on laboratory data. All processes producing this information, whether a blood count, a pap smear, or a throat culture, are subject to error at each of three stages:

1. **Preanalytic** — This phase includes ordering the correct test, which is then obtained in the correct manner, at the correct time, from the correct patient, yielding a correctly obtained and labeled specimen that is then transported safely to a testing facility.

2. **Analytic** — This laboratory-based phase includes accurate specimen identification, verification of order entry, properly executed specimen processing, reliable test performance, accurate result entry, and retention of the specimen in a manner that preserves its integrity.

3. **Postanalytic** — This phase includes the transmission of accurate results to the caregiver who is authorized to act on those results.

For each of these phases there are multiple layers of accreditation organization standards and governmental regulations, which arguably constitute the standard of care. Failure to comply with such regulatory parameters can jeopardize care, subject the healthcare site and workers to possible fines and closure, and potentially weaken any professional liability defense. Other significant influences on the standard of care include formal opinions from organizations such as the FDA; opinions, guidelines, and recommendations from professional organizations; and regulations promulgated by individual states.

Each phase is also fraught with liability issues associated with the potential for error. Paradoxically, although the analytic phase has the most complex regulatory structure, the other two phases can be more challenging to risk management professionals because the preanalytic and postanalytic phases involve many more hospital staff members, in addition to medical staff members and their employees. Most laboratory processes also involve several interfaces and handoffs between departments, often with separate lines of reporting. The result is substantial complexity and thus increased risk.

This chapter will point out key regulatory issues of which the risk management professional should be aware. It will also identify specific risks associated with each of the three phases described previously and offer strategies to reduce exposures.

Although this chapter focuses on laboratory area-specific solutions, it is also important to recognize the many ways that the laboratory supports the quality improvement program of the organization. For example, the pharmacy needs microbiology data to monitor changing antibiotic resistance patterns of infectious organisms, and an effective tissue committee must evaluate surgical pathology data. Similarly, blood bank and hematology reports should be reviewed by the transfusion committee. All of these interactions illustrate the central role that the laboratory plays in reducing exposure and improving quality throughout the healthcare operation. It is of interest that this interactive role is increasingly recognized by regulatory agencies. For example, The Joint Commission (TJC) now reviews laboratory data when they survey hospitals, regardless of whether the laboratory's Clinical Laboratory Improvement Amendments (CLIA) certification was attained through another agency.

· · · · · · · · ·
REGULATORY ENVIRONMENT

Federal Regulations

The primary source of regulations pertaining to the laboratory is the federal legislation known as the Clinical Laboratory Improvement Amendments (CLIA), originally passed in 1967 and updated in 1988. A set of final regulations was issued in 1992, although refinements are routinely published in the *Federal Register*. The purpose of the law is to "ensure the accuracy, reliability, and timeliness of patient test results regardless of where the test was performed."[1] Under CLIA, laboratories are required to be licensed, and they must renew licensure every two years.

The Impact of Other Regulations

Before considering specific CLIA mandates, it is important to note that these regulations often intertwine with those of other organizations whose requirements sometimes exceed

CLIA's.[2] From a risk management perspective, it is key that the standards of these private organizations may establish the standard of care in a related case. For example, many organizations apply for a Certificate of Accreditation (COA) under CLIA.[3] This certificate is awarded when they pass an inspection by a private organization with standards equal to or higher than those set out in the law, such as the College of American Pathologists (CAP) or TJC. As long as the organization holds a COA, it is not subject to routine inspections by employees of the Centers for Medicare & Medicaid Services (CMS), which is the agency responsible for enforcing CLIA. Similarly, facilities that pass an inspection in states whose programs are CLIA exempt, such as New York, are not routinely subject to CMS inspection.[4]

Although compliance with more stringent standards might raise comfort levels about ability to pass a CMS inspection, it is important that accreditation, and exempt status conferred by state program compliance, do not entirely free a laboratory from the specter of federal oversight. The federal government performs random, follow-up inspections to ensure that private and state agencies are conducting inspections equivalent to the federal government's inspections. Also, when there has been a credible complaint or apparent violation of pertinent regulations, federal, state, or nongovernmental inspectors may appear unannounced. The more recent approach by TJC and other accrediting organizations, to routinely survey facilities on an unannounced basis, reinforces the concept that compliance is a twenty-four-hour-a-day, year-round endeavor.

CLIA Is Facility Specific

Risk management professionals should be aware that CLIA defines a laboratory as "any facility [that] performs laboratory testing on specimens derived from humans for the purpose of providing information for the diagnosis, prevention, treatment of disease, or impairment of, or assessment of health."[5] This facility-based approach means that CLIA is generally site specific, and there may be several licenses within one healthcare organization. For example, if respiratory therapists perform blood gas analysis in their department in a large teaching hospital, they may have a separate CLIA license. Remote physicians' offices with labs may have their own licenses, as may medical schools that perform genetic analysis or drug monitoring partially in the context of research. Another important factor that may play a role in licensure is the reporting relationship of the laboratory. For example, satellite labs or special laboratories that report to the central hospital laboratory will usually be inspected under the hospital laboratory's license, even though they are geographically separate within a hospital complex.

The risk management professional should understand the status of laboratory licensure in various settings throughout the organization. One resource may be the laboratory manager of the main laboratory in a large facility, who is likely to be knowledgeable about licenses in other departments or may be able to collect such information. It is also desirable to ask CMS for a list of the laboratories that have your hospital's or healthcare organization's name. Laboratory managers should update the risk management professional about upcoming inspections by any organization and about any negative findings, including any required corrective action or follow-up.

Testing Complexity

The final CLIA regulations, published February 28, 1992, were based on the complexity of the test method. The more complicated the test, the more stringent the requirements. Three categories of tests were established: waived complexity, moderate complexity, and high complexity. Some factors considered in determining complexity include

1. degree of knowledge needed to perform the test;
2. training and experience required;
3. complexity of reagent and materials preparation;
4. characteristics of operational steps;
5. characteristics and availability of calibration, quality control, and proficiency testing materials;
6. troubleshooting and maintenance required; and
7. degree of interpretation and judgment required in the testing process.[6]

For moderate-complexity and high-complexity tests, CLIA specifies quality standards for proficiency testing (PT), in which the laboratory tests samples sent by independent third parties to see if their results are the same as those of peers who have tested the same material,[7] patient test management, quality control, personnel qualifications, and quality assurance for laboratories that perform moderate-complexity or high-complexity tests.[8]

The criteria that define *waived testing* are set out under Sec. 493.15 (b) as follows.

(b)   **Criteria.**

Test systems are simple laboratory examinations and procedures that

- are cleared by FDA for home use;
- employ methodologies that are so simple and accurate as to render the likelihood of erroneous results negligible; and
- pose no reasonable risk of harm to the patient if the test is performed incorrectly.

Although the processes pertaining to waived tests are not subject to routine CMS inspection, in those facilities that have a waived testing certificate the laboratory must follow manufacturer specifications for the testing. Waived test processes are also subject to inspection by surveyors of TJC and CAP, whose standards are more stringent.

Also note that waived tests may generate liability exposure if they are incorrectly performed. For example, some rapid HIV antibody tests are waived tests, as are some rapid streptococcus A tests. Also, if it is inconsistently performed, a fingerstick glucose test, which is another waived test, may yield variable results that could affect insulin dosing.

The second category of testing complexity under CLIA encompasses moderate-complexity tests, which include provider-performed microscopic interpretation (PPMI). The third category, high-complexity tests, includes surgical pathology specimens.

Point-of-Care Testing

Increasingly, testing may be done outside the laboratory, with kits designed for this purpose. These resources have expanded testing capability at the bedside, as well as in clinics. Although many of these tests are waived, as described above, others are moderately complex and subject to all of the requirements of proficiency testing, including more stringent quality control. Adding confusion is the fact that some kit-based tests are waived, for example, for streptococcus A testing. However, other manufacturers' kit-based testing is moderately complex. Institutions should be clear as to which regulatory category applies to the product(s) they are considering.

Regardless of the level of complexity of the point-of-care (POCT) test, it is critical, from a risk management standpoint, that staff follow instructions carefully and that results are integrated in the health record.

State Regulations and Staff Training

State-based regulation of laboratory procedures varies widely. As previously noted, states such as New York have achieved CLIA exempt status because they have comprehensive licensure and inspection programs. At the other end of the spectrum, some states require federal CLIA licensure and compliance.

Staff training requirements in individual state programs are highly variable. For example, some require that medical technologists have state licenses to work in a laboratory, analogous to licensure for registered nurses. This is a step beyond a common requirement that medical technologists earn a bachelor's degree and be tested, certified, and registered by the American Society for Clinical Pathology (ASCP) or a comparable agency.

Also acceptable in some locales are training programs that require less stringent prerequisites for certification, for example, two years of post-high school education or training. Because there are many approaches, human resources departments should be familiar with the requirements of each type of certification presented by job applicants. The significant level of variation in state requirements also makes it critical that each laboratory be familiar with their state(s) requirements and communicate changes to risk management on an ongoing basis. Position descriptions should be based on state and CLIA requirements and the tasks of the individual laboratory. Independent verification of licensure, educational degrees, and special certifications should be carried out routinely, similar to the approach taken with registered nurses. It is of particular note that some clinical staff only perform tests periodically, for example, respiratory therapists may perform blood gas tests and nurses may perform waived tests. Risk management professionals should work with clinical managers to ensure that such tests are addressed in the job descriptions, training, and annual competency reviews of these individuals.

State requirements also vary as to who may order laboratory tests, for example, whether ordering tests is exclusively the responsibility of physicians, or whether other healthcare providers, such as nurse practitioners, may also order tests. State legislative endeavors by nonphysician health professionals to gain this prerogative are ongoing. Risk managers should be aware of current local requirements and whether third-party payers will reimburse for laboratory tests ordered by nonphysicians. Similarly, states may vary with regard to whether patients can directly receive test results from the laboratory, instead of from the ordering physician.

Unless state requirements are more stringent, federal CLIA guidance concerning laboratory personnel must be followed. Current information can be found on the CLIA Web site at www.cms.hhs.gov/clia. Pertinent specific information about training will be provided later in this chapter.

Medical Staff and Outside Laboratories

The pathologist's relationship with the hospital may be that of an independent staff member, a hospital employee, or as an aspect of a contractual relationship with the pathologist's laboratory. Regardless of the basis of the relationship, all pathologists should go through the same credentialing process as the rest of the organization's medical staff. In the course of that process, the healthcare organization should also determine whether pathologists will function exclusively on-site or whether they may occasionally perform testing in an outside, independent laboratory. When such an outside laboratory is used, it is the duty of the hospital to verify the bona fides of that laboratory, including state and CLIA licensure. The same criteria should apply to referral laboratories, and formal contracts with all such laboratories should specify that the outside laboratory is responsible for taking steps to ensure reliable testing. The outside laboratory should also be required to notify the hospital of any change in licensure status or pending investigations that might result in a negative determination about the quality of patient testing.

Safety of Laboratory Conditions

Occupational Health and Safety Administration (OSHA), state, and municipal regulations, as well as those of private organizations, such as TJC, address the safety of environmental conditions under which testing is performed. All specimens are potentially infectious, and information on biosafety issues particular to the laboratory is available at www.cdc.gov/od/ohs/biosfty/bmbl4/bmbl4s2.htm. Certain reagents and controls may also be infectious or contain hazardous materials. Information about chemical safety in the laboratory is available at the OSHA Web site www.osha.gov/SLTC/laboratories/index.html. Laboratory personnel should be familiar with and document compliance with all pertinent OSHA and TJC mandates, as well as state-specific requirements that pertain to laboratory safety.

Federal Oversight of Blood Transfusion and Laboratory Instruments

Blood products are licensed biologics and thus are subject to Food and Drug Administration (FDA) oversight.[9] Hospital transfusion services that perform only minimal processing of blood products are required to register with the FDA, but they are not under the same level of scrutiny as hospitals performing more complex processing. Blood centers and other facilities that collect blood from donors must be licensed[10] and must have periodic unscheduled inspections by the FDA. Unlike CMS, which has delegated certain inspection responsibilities to CAP and TJC, the FDA retains responsibility for blood services and conducts all inspections.

Therefore, an FDA-licensed hospital transfusion service often will be inspected when a state, CAP, or TJC inspects the laboratory or when the American Association of Blood Banks (AABB) performs an accreditation survey. However, no determination of compliance by another organization exempts the transfusion service from unannounced inspections by the FDA. Transfusion services that are registered, but not licensed, may not be visited by the FDA as frequently as those that are licensed. Any transfusion service that has had a serious procedural violation is also likely to be inspected. Additionally, both transfusion-related deaths and serious procedure violations resulting in actual injury, or with potential to endanger a patient, must be reported to the FDA.

Many smaller blood transfusion services are not AABB members. For these services, it is prudent to have policies and procedures consistent with the current edition of the AABB's standards because these standards are sometimes cited as standards of care. (See the AABB Web site at www.aabb.org, for more information on the AABB standards and other related matters.)

The FDA also has jurisdiction over all laboratory instruments and tests that are in any way related to blood collection or testing. A representative list of equipment affected can be found on the FDA Web site under the Center for Biologics Evaluation and Research (CBER).[11]

Although, in general, the requirements of inspecting organizations are similar, some differences do occur. When there is conflict, it is prudent to follow the most stringent set of rules and to always be in compliance with the regulations, recommendations, or advisory publications of the FDA.

· · · · · · · · ·

KEY INFRASTRUCTURE

Policies and Procedures

All laboratory processes should follow current procedures, and these procedures must be in writing. Formalizing the laboratory's interactions with other areas of the hospital is particularly important and challenging. Risk increases exponentially when areas such as the operating room or emergency department have their own individual procedures for processes such as patient identification, obtaining and labeling blood and tissue specimens, and blood administration. Therefore, it is essential that representatives from each area participate in development of common procedures. Once created, there should be no changes to such multidisciplinary procedures without the input of the risk management professional and approval of the laboratory's manager and clinical director.

Procedures should also be routinely reviewed by representatives from applicable clinical areas, and updates must be distributed to all affected staff. All new employees should also be oriented to pertinent procedures. This orientation should include the rationale for procedures and be documented. For example, phlebotomists and the nursing staff must understand why certain specimens must be collected at a certain time, and they should be educated as to the causes of hemolysis and contamination. Phlebotomists and the nursing staff should also be taught to inform other clinical staff, such as the ordering physician, of any difficulty in obtaining specimens. The personnel who develop procedures for the laboratory should be guided by applicable accreditation and licensure requirements. They must also remember that equipment and laboratory test-related procedures should be consistent with the applicable instrument manufacturer's recommendations. Many sample procedures are available from the Clinical and Laboratory Standards Institute. Contact information for the Institute is provided at the conclusion of this chapter.[12]

Laboratory Information System and Data Management

Information systems can facilitate many aspects of the laboratory's work, from ordering tests to printing tube labels with bar codes identifying the patient and the test that has been ordered for him or her. Certain systems now also generate bar-coded wristbands, which help the phlebotomist identify the patient before drawing blood. Such systems should be rigorously tested because they are not always proof against work-arounds. Other systems assist in performing the test, conducting quality-control checks, and reporting results, and may even facilitate billing. The extent to which these features are in use varies among systems and from site to site. The laboratory information system (LIS) may be separate from the hospital information system (HIS) and connected by an interface for ordering, reporting and billing, or the LIS may be part of an integrated system offered by the HIS vendor. Additionally, many individual instruments have complex computer systems that may perform some of these functions on a stand-alone basis. For example, chemistry instrument systems may document specimen identification and processing. Other information technology (IT) resources, located within instruments, perform and document preventive maintenance tests. All this information can then be directly transmitted to the LIS or an HIS.

The chapter will only briefly touch on the practical and regulatory issues associated with information system selection. One major issue involves security of information in the system. Preceding implementation, there must be rigorous analysis as to what information is needed by each healthcare provider with access. For example, a phlebotomist needs to know the types of blood tests to be drawn on a given patient, but often does not need to know the results. In contrast, a nurse performing a fingerstick blood glucose test for immediate blood sugar results must know the result in order to administer insulin according to the attending physician's orders. Attending physicians only need access to the clinical information of patients they are seeing on a primary or consultative basis, not the information of all patients in the hospital. HIPAA (Health Insurance Portability and Accountability Act)[13] and local state laws should be consulted regarding such access issues. This is particularly important because HIPAA has been modified by the HITECH Act, an aspect of the recovery legislation that was signed into law in 2009. Among many other provisions, HITECH creates accountability for individual employees of healthcare organizations and makes them potentially responsible for fines ranging from $100 to

$50,000, with maximum total fines of $1.5 million annually for repeated egregious offenses. (Please see Chapter 16, Volume 3, on HIPAA/HITECH for more information.)

Where management of test results is concerned, information systems should be programmed to meet the standards of various regulatory agencies as well as laboratory-specific requirements. The system must be screened routinely to be certain that it is compliant, and data must be backed up with electronic copies maintained off-site.

Depending on the laboratory test, automated access to previous results (delta checks) can help prevent errors. For example, routine comparison of blood type results with those previously obtained on a patient is a requirement of many private accrediting organizations.

Important steps to take before implementing an LIS include the following:

- The hospital should contact other healthcare organizations to get feedback on the systems under consideration.

- The hospital must also determine how well the candidate system can handle the volume of tests that is generated by the laboratory.

- If the LIS is to be separate from the main HIS, the question of the systems' interface must be addressed early on.

- Because healthcare providers should consult only one source for all patient information, one objective of the interface should be automatic transfer of laboratory reports into the HIS's patient record. Another objective is efficient movement of information into the billing database.

- If possible, the interface should be tested before the system is purchased. High-volume validating test runs are an important part of pretesting, and the staff must plan for potential system malfunctions or crashes during this process.

- Yet another important consideration is training for all staff who will use the system. This comprehensive orientation should be documented.

Design of Data Reports

The laboratory data report, whether electronic or manual, should be formatted with input from the medical staff. Formatting should make it easy to identify abnormal results and to report such results, in keeping with the healthcare organization's critical value reporting system. Reports should facilitate communication of critical results, as well as those results that are noncritical but still outside normal parameters. As discussed later in this chapter, abnormal results that are not timely reported should be monitored through the quality improvement program and followed up as required. It is important that the LIS be able to facilitate data collection for this process. Special attention should also be paid to data report–related processes, including LIS system functions, that may facilitate critical value reporting in the outpatient environment. Because outpatients are remote, and presumably less acute than hospitalized patients, physicians may not be as attuned to the potential for aberrant values. For example, although markedly abnormal results are usually identified and addressed in physicians' offices, sizeable numbers of mildly abnormal radiology and laboratory results of testing on outpatients may be missed or ignored.[14,15]

New laboratory IT initiatives that may help to address critical value reporting include rules-based event engines that automatically route laboratory results to providers, for example, text messaging a physician's pager with critical values. These programs may also include template letters to patients notifying them of aberrant results, and some will even schedule reminders for follow-up testing.

Revised or Amended Reports

On occasion, a laboratory will issue a follow-up report, revising either clinical or anatomic pathology results that were issued previously. In some instances, such reports correct an earlier administrative misstatement. In others, the revision is warranted by new clinical information, for example, results of special studies on a surgical pathology specimen. Regardless of the cause, the information must be communicated to the primary clinician and documented in the health record.

Management of revised or updated reports should be consistently handled throughout the organization. If the revision is the result of an administrative issue, it might be called an *amended report*. If it is the result of new clinical information, it might be called an *updated report*. At no time should later reports of a particular test be described as *corrected*, a term that implies that a clinical error may have occurred.

· · · · · · · · ·
RISK REDUCTION STRATEGIES IN THE PREANALYTICAL PHASE

Specific written procedures on specimen collection should be available to all providers who collect specimens in the facility. These procedures should address test ordering, patient identification, specimen collection, labeling, and transporting. Procedures should also detail preparation, type and amount of specimen to be collected, special timing of collection if applicable, type of container to use, special handling requirements (such as refrigeration), proper labeling, and test requisition completion. Access to current procedures can be facilitated through use of a properly programmed HIS.

Other issues that should be procedurally addressed include the need for all specimen collection processes to be supported by a specific requisition, as well as access to the original order. For a telephone STAT order, or a telephone-added test, it is important to document the telephone order and the identity of the person who orders it. As will be detailed in the postanalytic section that follows, it is now a TJC requirement that orders be read back and verification documented.[16] Any telephone order should also be documented in the medical record and then signed by the ordering practitioner within forty-eight hours of ordering, or as required by state law.

Certain accepted practices, which are reimbursable, allow laboratory personnel to add tests at their discretion. For example, the use of special stains on surgical specimens in anatomic pathology does not require a specific order. Additional discretionary tests are less common in clinical pathology. An example is performing a definitive HIV test after a positive screening test. To ensure consistent performance of such discretionary tests, it is desirable to have specific algorithms reviewed and approved by a medical staff committee.

The highest risk step in obtaining patient samples is the identification of the patient. Most laboratories print specimen labels within the laboratory, based on test orders, and then distribute them to phlebotomists. It is incumbent upon the phlebotomist to properly identify the patient and label the specimen at the time of collection. TJC standards now require the use of two unique identifiers, such as name and medical record number (MRN). Use of the latter assumes that there is a wristband, because patients are unlikely to know the MRN. Date of birth (DOB) is sometimes used instead of the MRN. Although some cultures deemphasize the significance of the DOB, it is a useful alternative when the MRN is not available. Use of inpatient room numbers as a second identifier is unwise and also unacceptable to TJC.[17]

Some facilities use bar-coded labels that can be matched to the bar code on the patient's identification bracelet at the point of collection. Wristband bar coding can reduce error, but it is not error-proof. It must be supplemented by other common sense measures, such as communicating effectively with the patient. Conscious and alert patients should be asked to state their name, rather than being asked if they are "Mrs. Jones." The latter approach is fraught with error potential, particularly when hearing or language barriers are present. When anatomic pathology specimens are obtained, the patient is frequently unconscious, and, in these situations, the patient's identity should be confirmed by wristband. It is also critical that the specimen be labeled before it leaves the procedure area. Similarly, clinical pathology specimens should be labeled at the bedside. Specimen tubes for multiple patients should not be labeled in advance. Some institutions generate multiple specimen labels for a single patient undergoing a long procedure or when several tubes are needed. However, to avoid specimen misidentification, it is essential to destroy any unused labels immediately after the procedure or collection process. This issue is of particular concern in areas such as operating rooms and invasive radiology suites, where several patients go through an individual room in a day.

In general, many erroneous laboratory tests result from mislabeling of tubes or drawing the specimen from the wrong patient. Even if it does not cause delayed or wrong care, misidentification can have a serious impact on the hospital's reputation. For example, some prestigious hospitals are now also known for transfusion-related or transplant-related patient and specimen identification errors. When collecting specimens related to transfusion and tissue transplantation, it is therefore important to implement as many safeguards as are practical. For example, once the phlebotomist has collected and labeled a blood bank specimen, a second person often verifies that the patient identification and specimen labels match. Use of specially numbered transfusion arm bands, with corresponding bands on the blood products, are another identification verification mechanism, which can be used by a single person drawing blood.

Mislabeled or inadequately labeled biopsy or surgery specimens are particularly important issues. Blood samples can usually be redrawn, but intraoperatively obtained surgical biopsy tissue is ordinarily not replaceable.

Another common source of specimen collection error is using the wrong container. For example, the stronger anticoagulants designed to preserve a blood gas specimen (in a green-top tube) or a blood count specimen (in a purple-top tube) may significantly skew the results of a prothrombin test, which measures clotting time and should be collected in a blue-top tube. Most such errors are recognized in the laboratory, after the sample has been improperly collected. Usually, it is then necessary to draw another sample from the patient, which results in delayed communication of test results to the treating provider, as well as patient inconvenience. Depending on the circumstances, such delay may also have a negative effect on the clinical outcome. On the other hand, if the specimen collection error is not recognized, an incorrect test result can bring dire consequences. For example, when a heparinized syringe is used to draw a blood gas sample from a patient in the operating room, and the remaining blood in the syringe is injected into a blue top tube for coagulation tests, the coagulation test results will be quite abnormal. The surgeon may conclude that STAT plasma transfusions are needed, even though the patient is not bleeding excessively.

When the wrong type of container is used for a surgical biopsy tissue sample, it might not be possible to obtain a second specimen. Operating room and other authorized staff should be trained to consult the laboratory, whenever feasible, as to the container and preservative they will need before they collect unusual specimens or specimens for tests with which they are unfamiliar. The operating room staff (and staff in other areas where specimens are collected) should also routinely check the availability of suitable collection containers before the procedure begins.

All specimens must be accompanied by a complete and accurate requisition that documents the date and time that the specimen was collected, the name of the person who collected the specimen, the type and source of the specimen, test(s) requested, and, as relevant, clinical history and differential diagnosis. It is also essential that the source and type of specimen be specific and accurate because these factors often determine how testing will be carried out. For example, in microbiology, growth culture material (media) is selected based on the site of collection and type of specimen. This is partly due to differences in pH among specimen sources. For example, urine has a very different pH from spinal or thoracentesis fluid and must be cultured in a different medium. Even in simple waived tests for the presence of blood in body fluids, the test kit used to assess the presence of blood in gastric contents is different from the one used to check for blood in stool.

Similarly, the history and potential diagnoses are critical to the laboratory's management of tissue specimens for surgical pathology, hematopathology, and cytopathology. This information must be specifically documented by the individual collecting the specimen, and the laboratory should also correlate the test order with the differential diagnosis.

Sample storage and transport might require specific approaches, depending on the test, particularly if a sample is sent to a distant central or reference laboratory. Also, before using a pneumatic tube system for specimen or blood product transport, the laboratory should validate that use of the tube system does not adversely affect the sample or blood product.

· · · · · · · · ·

RISK MANAGEMENT STRATEGIES IN THE ANALYTIC PHASE

To maintain specimen identity, it is essential for laboratory personnel who receive the specimen to check specimens and labels against requisitions for discrepancies. Specimens should be submitted in sufficient quantity in the proper, labeled container with the required preservative, and they should arrive in the laboratory undamaged. If the specimen is unacceptable, the collection location should be notified as soon as possible and another specimen requested.

Written criteria should guide rejection of specimens, and, under certain circumstances, the lab could be forced to test a specimen that otherwise would be rejected. For example, the laboratory might accept difficult-to-replace specimens that are mislabeled, such as timed blood draws, biopsies, or cerebrospinal fluid. In these cases, the laboratory can require clinical staff to label the specimen again, or sign a voucher, affidavit, or confirmation attesting to the identity of the patient from whom the specimen was collected. Please see Exhibit 10.1.

The policy for acceptance of mislabeled specimens should be written with the input of the risk management professional or legal counsel. It should include safeguards such as the following. The specimen should be reasonably identifiable. The person signing the voucher should also receive authorization from the facility's chief medical officer, chief nursing officer, or the medical director of quality or patient safety. A laboratory representative should document objectively on the test report regarding the original error, such as, "This specimen was relabeled prior to testing—see voucher on file." The voucher should then be retained by the laboratory. Some laboratories have resorted to DNA testing, at the expense of the healthcare organization, to match irreplaceable specimens to patients.

When irreplaceable specimens must be relabeled, or their labels must be modified, the laboratory should complete an occurrence report. Mislabeled specimens should be monitored through the healthcare organization's quality improvement program. Failure Mode and Effects Analysis (FMEA) can be also be used to reduce labeling and collection errors.

One general safeguard against the loss of specimen integrity is that, during the analytical phase, a part, or aliquot, of a sample is commonly transferred to another container before the actual testing. All aliquots and dilutions must be readily identifiable, and the identity and integrity of samples must be maintained throughout the entire testing phase.

· · · · · · · · ·

RISK MANAGEMENT STRATEGIES IN THE POSTANALYTIC PHASE

A *critical value* is defined as a laboratory result that indicates that adequate and timely intervention is needed to correct a potentially life-threatening condition. Critical values, formerly known as *panic values*, are those that fall outside high and low limits defined by the laboratory. CLIA, TJC, and CAP require that each laboratory establish a list of

EXHIBIT 10.1   Confirmation of Specimen Identification

SuperDuper Hospital
Anywhere, USA
Irreplaceable Specimen
THIS ENTIRE FORM MUST BE COMPLETED.

Name on Specimen Label _____

Name on Requisition _____

Collection/Patient Location _____

Provider/Physician Notified _____

Notification Date/Time/By _____

Physician's Statement

Use of Confirmation of Specimen Identification Form
This form is completed to verify the accuracy of information for irreplaceable specimens. This form will be used only for the following limited purposes (please check one or more of the following):

___ The test is critical and delay for a new specimen could compromise care.

___ Clinical reasons for not obtaining a second specimen exist—explain:
_____

___ The patient is unavailable for a second collection.

___ Other—explain:
_____

Correct Specimen Information: _____

I affirm the accuracy of the corrected information provided and request that the specimen be analyzed. The process of obtaining a new specimen could have a negative impact on the condition of the patient and is not possible at this time.

Print Physician's Name: _____ Date: _____ Time: _____

Physician's Signature: _____

Collector's Statement (if not the physician above)

I affirm the accuracy of the corrected information provided.

Print Collector's Name: _____ Date: _____ Time: _____

Collector's Signature: _____

Laboratory Medical Director

Print Name: _____ Date: _____ Time: _____

Medical Director Signature: _____

critical values, which may be individualized to reflect the facility's patient population. Turnaround time for critical value reporting must also be established by the facility and monitored for compliance on an ongoing basis.

Reporting Critical Values and Critical Test Results

For some time, hospital laboratories have identified markedly abnormal test results that are or might be an immediate threat to life. When a test result falls outside the parameters on the critical value list, a caregiver must be notified immediately. To accomplish this, laboratory personnel usually place a telephone call to the clinical staff caring for the patient. However, common pitfalls in this process include failure of the laboratory staff to make the telephone call; the failure of the clinical staff, such as nurses on the floor, to communicate the result to the physician or other ordering healthcare provider; and the provider's failure to act on the results in a timely manner. Such communication gaps often lead to allegations of delay in diagnosis or delay in treatment in a related malpractice suit.

To ensure that the critical value reporting process is effective, the values selected should be logical and meaningful and the list of critical values that can be reported should be short and manageable. Critical values should be developed by a team of healthcare providers, and it must be recognized that patient variables such as age, weight, and comorbidities play a role in determining the criticality of a test result. For example, a renal specialist does not want to be continually bothered about a creatinine result of 6.2, which is abnormal for most patients, but normal for an end-stage renal disease patient. One concept that might be helpful, in consultation with the treating physician, is a "first time alert." In this approach, the first time the patient has a creatinine above 4.0, the physician is immediately notified. After that, delta check values (significant changes from shift to shift or day to day or week to week) may be more useful to the physician. Policies must be detailed and then applied to individual patients based on specific physician orders. A general physician order directing the staff not to call should not be acceptable. If orders are not specific, or there is doubt about the meaning of an order, laboratory staff or nurses should call the physician. Guidance in developing critical values is provided by CAP. Another resource is the Massachusetts Coalition for the Prevention of Medical Errors, which has developed a comprehensive "starter set" of critical values for laboratories. This resource, which includes implementation and monitoring guidance can be found at www.macoalition.org/initiatives.shtml#7. The final list of critical values should also include expected turnaround time from ordering to reporting for each test and result. As previously noted, this turnaround time should be monitored for compliance on an ongoing basis.

As previously suggested in this chapter's section on LIS, computer alert programs have proved invaluable in reducing erroneous or omitted reporting of critical values. Several laboratory computer systems detect critical values and notify the laboratory staff through the use of pop-up or colored notice screens. Technologists are not permitted to proceed further in the computer system without acknowledging the result. Laboratory technologists then initiate the critical value reporting process. Some computer systems even page the physician automatically with critical value results, thus reducing delays in necessary treatment.

Because reporting time frames are such an essential part of critical value and test reporting, they should be established in collaboration with the medical staff. Risk managers can assist the laboratory by providing education on key risk management principles, including the use of a back-up strategy, such as access to an alternative provider to receive critical results, and how to access the chain of command if designated caregiver(s) are unavailable or unresponsive.

The chain of command policy should be consistent with other such approaches in the healthcare organization. It should be triggered by written criteria and contain no more than three steps. For example, the chain may be initiated if the laboratory pages the ordering physician three times within forty-five minutes with no response. The next step may be to notify applicable house staff, the hospitalist, or the applicable department chairman with the critical test results to ensure that the patient receives the necessary timely treatment. When the chain of command or back-up system is implemented, the laboratory should subsequently work with the medical staff to learn what can be done to improve the process.

Critical value reporting documentation should include the name of the person reporting the test result, the name and title of the person receiving the results, the test name, the value and interpretation, and the date and time. It is also essential, in keeping with TJC's requirement, that there be documentation that the recipient of the results has confirmed is or her understanding of those results by reading them back to laboratory personnel. Read-backs can be encouraged by using simple dialogue such as, "I want to be sure that you have the correct information, could you please repeat the patient's name, test, and result that I just gave you?" Several facilities have the nursing staff document receipt of critical values results on a special label, which is then placed on the patient's chart. The label also documents action taken, such as implementation of orders received.

The laboratory manager and the risk management professional should educate all healthcare providers regarding the importance of the critical value test-reporting process. For example, ordering physicians should be educated as to their responsibility for tracking the test results of their patients. The laboratory can facilitate this process by providing checklists or other tools to help physicians remember key points in critical value reporting. Physicians should also understand the importance of ensuring their availability, or a covering provider's availability, for receipt of critical test values on a twenty-four-hour basis. For settings such as outpatient, long-term care, and home health, a list of personnel who are to be contacted with critical values results should be provided to the laboratory.

Laboratory personnel must also be educated that communication of critical values does not necessarily stop with the first provider to whom the information is conveyed. For example, if the laboratory calls the nurse caring for the patient, the nurse might assume that the physician already knows about the critical test result. Many organizations, such as the Massachusetts Coalition for the Prevention of Medical Errors, strongly recommend that critical test values be communicated directly by the lab to the physician. Some institutions prefer that, for inpatients, the nurse notify the physician, which makes it possible for the results to be communicated and new orders given in one phone call. Whichever notification system is used, it should be well understood by all involved.

Critical values reporting is an excellent example of a multidisciplinary process, and variances, including excessive turnaround time, should be monitored through the facility-wide quality improvement program. Laboratory managers should also monitor the frequency and effectiveness of the process's use, on a daily basis. The risk management professional can be a valuable resource to assist in resolving any issues.

A more recent concept concerns critical tests.[18] These are tests whose results must be known as soon as possible, regardless of whether they are normal or abnormal.

Laboratory examples might include cardiac markers for an elderly emergency room patient with chest pain or a blood hemoglobin and chest X-rays for a patient with acute blunt chest trauma. Just as with critical values, TJC requires that such tests and their turnaround times be defined and monitored by the hospital. However, the requirements for the two processes differ in that critical results reporting must be measured from the point that the physician orders the test, until the results are received by an individual who is legally authorized to act on them, usually the physician. Thus the measured time frame encompasses the entire system, preanalytical, analytical, and postanalytical, in contrast to critical values, which is only postanalytical, that is, from result to physician notification. Clearly, addressing the turnaround of critical results is potentially more complex than critical values reporting. Such evolving accreditation requirements also illustrate that it is more important than ever to monitor CAP and TJC publications for new information on an ongoing basis.

Specimen Retention

State and private accrediting organizations require that specimens be retained for specific periods of time. For example, CAP has established a set of minimum standards in this regard that may be accessed at www.cap.org/apps/docs/laboratory_accreditation/ retention_1101.pdf.

Specimen retention protocols should reflect compliance with retention requirements and with any specific clinical requirements concerning storage of particular specimens, for example, refrigeration.

. . . .

RISK MANAGEMENT STRATEGIES IN LAB SPECIALTIES

The risk management professional, together with laboratory managers, must address specific risk management implications of each laboratory specialty. These include, but are not limited to, clinical pathology, anatomic pathology, cytopathology, and blood transfusion services.

Clinical Pathology

Clinical pathology includes clinical chemistry, microbiology, virology, urinalysis, blood banking, and parts of hematology. Each of these disciplines performs manual or automated tests on various kinds of blood, body fluids, and tissue samples from patients. The choice of a particular test method can be difficult. For example, counting the number of blood platelets in a sample can be done manually, although more often it is accomplished by one of several indirect methods that uses hematology instruments. Recently, a flow cytometry technique has been advocated as more accurate and reproducible. Approaches vary from laboratory to laboratory, yet procedures should be clearly written and kept current in all cases. All reagents and instruments should be federally licensed, although for some testing, licensed reagents are not available. Flow cytometry is one example of a test for which there may not be licensed reagents, and test reports should clearly indicate when unlicensed reagents are used. These results should be considered less credible than results of tests performed with licensed reagents. Instrument manufacturers should also approve the source of the reagents used in their products. Attempts to cut costs by using reagents that might not work with the organization's instrumentation may result in testing delays, erroneous results, and more costs later.

Proficiency testing is an important CLIA regulatory requirement for many tests. This generally involves the laboratory's receipt of a five-sample set for tests such as blood glucose, hemoglobin, microbiological culture, and so on, from a third party that is also licensed under CLIA. The laboratory usually performs the test and submits the results on sets of samples three times per year. The laboratory's results are then compared to the correct answers and to those of peer settings. Unsatisfactory results on two of three successive sets may result in loss of the ability to do such testing. For most tests, it is possible to fail on one sample of the five and still pass overall (80 percent is the pass rate). For blood typing, a 100 percent passing rate is required. All failed individual samples should be reviewed when they occur, and a written corrective action plan should be developed and implemented.

Blood Transfusion Services

As previously noted, blood transfusion services have additional unique regulatory requirements because blood products are FDA-licensed pharmaceuticals. They also have unique handling requirements because blood products are biologicals with strict temperature and expiration-related monitoring requirements. The reagents used for testing are in large part also biologicals, with similar restrictions. Unlike most other pharmaceuticals, each bag of red cells or plasma is from an individual source (donor) and is considered an individual lot, meant only for patients with that particular blood type. A permanent record must be retained concerning the source of the blood, the testing (including retesting of ABO and Rh of the blood), reagent lot numbers, storage, transfusion process, and name of the recipient.

There are many reasons for the increased focus on the handling of blood products. Blood is a biological with potential for immediate lethal risk if it is given to the wrong patient or incorrectly tested. As compared to drugs, blood has stricter storage needs and a shorter shelf life. It is also important that the complications of a transfusion might not manifest for decades after the transfusion. All staff involved in any aspect of blood transfusion, including collecting recipient blood specimens, and prescribing, cross-matching, administering, and monitoring the transfusion, must realize that they are responsible for creating a record that verifies that each step in a potentially high-risk process was followed.

Logically, adverse reactions to transfusions should be reported immediately to the supplier of blood products so that any related concerns may be identified and addressed. FDA-reporting requirements change frequently, and so laboratory personnel should routinely update themselves regarding events and standards deviations that are reportable.

Transfusion-related deaths must be reported to the FDA,[19] as must any deviation from transfusion-related standards that results in patient injury or the potential for patient injury.[20] For example, a transfusion reaction involving hemolysis of the red blood cell bag warrants reporting, even without severe patient injury, whereas a mild febrile reaction without injury, where there is no evidence of improper processing, storage, testing, or transfusion of the blood, may not be reported. The febrile reaction would, however, be noted in the medical record, as an observation made in the course of a customary transfusion reaction workup.

Requirements for blood bank record retention have steadily increased. In some cases, transfusion services have been asked to identify recipients of transfusions more than ten years previous. One reason for this involves an important regulatory aspect of transfusion known as *lookback*. This term defines the mandatory process that ensues when a blood donor tests positive for HIV, hepatitis, and other bloodborne diseases. Briefly, the blood collection organization must identify previous donations that were transfused from the particular donor that previously tested negative. The recipient patients are identified, contacted, and retested. There are specific federal requirements concerning how far back to review records, time limits for completing the process, and so forth.

It is important for laboratory staff and risk management professionals to stay current with newsletters from CAP, AABB, TJC, FDA, and state agencies for changes in record retention requirements and other regulatory or accreditation changes that pertain to lookback and other blood transfusion-related issues.

Anatomic Pathology

The number of autopsies has steadily decreased over the last forty years. However, a significant number of "missed diagnoses" continue to be identified during autopsies, and sometimes the unsuspected diagnosis was important in the patient's demise. Some physicians avoid requesting autopsies, for fear of such findings and potentially related lawsuits. Others seek autopsy results to help them avoid the same problem in a subsequent patient. The hospital and the pathologist might be concerned that there will be no reimbursement for an autopsy. There is no clear resolution to this multifaceted dispute. However, discouraging the family's request for an autopsy can create suspicion of the physician and the hospital. When an autopsy is performed, it should be done with sufficient care, and attention to the presumed cause of death. When implants such as pacemakers or replaced joints are present, they should be examined for defects. They should be carefully removed and preserved, and pertinent Safe Medical Device Act reporting requirements should be followed if they potentially contributed to morbidity and mortality.

Cytopathology

Cytopathology has risk management ramifications in all its aspects, including, but not limited to, training and proficiency testing and practice requirements, and the special area of cervicovaginal cytology.

Training and Proficiency Testing Requirements

CLIA and private accrediting organization requirements vary for training of laboratory staff who perform cytology testing. The laboratory director of a cytology lab can be a pathologist, other MD, or DO with experience and training, or a Ph.D. with required experience and training. The technical supervisor must be an MD or DO, certified in anatomic pathology. The cytology general supervisor may be qualified as a technical supervisor in cytology or a cytotechnologist with three years of full time experience as a cytotechnologist in the preceding ten years.

Of particular note, CLIA 1988 discussed the importance of proficiency testing for any individual who examines gynecologic preparations. This is in contrast to proficiency testing in the rest of the laboratory, where the proficiency tested is of the laboratory, not the individual. After many years of internal debate, CMS finally approved two national gynecologic cytology proficiency testing programs in December 2004. CAP and others have raised concerns that the programs are based on outdated standards and have recommended their suspension until they can be updated to reflect technological advances. The CAP position articulated first in June 2005 and subsequently can be reviewed on the CAP Web site at www.cap.org/apps/docs/advocacy/advocacy_issues/cytology_proficiency_testing.htm. Risk management professionals should follow this issue carefully. Despite the controversy over the quality of specific proficiency testing approaches, compliance dates were set in 2005, and laboratories must ensure that individuals who examine gynecological preparations are enrolled in one of these programs. All such professionals had to be tested at least once before April 2006 and had to achieve a passing score. If the laboratory fails to ensure that individuals are tested, or fails to take remedial action when an individual fails gynecologic cytology proficiency testing, sanctions will be imposed. On several occasions bills have been unsuccessfully introduced in Congress to suspend or modify this program. More information on resources to assist providers in achieving compliance can be found on the CAP Web site at www.cap.org/apps/docs/news_service/0503/0503_Resources.html, or in the CAP newsletter.[21]

Practice Requirements for Cytopathology

The laboratory must ensure that diagnostic interpretations are not based on unsatisfactory smears and that all cytology slide preparations are evaluated on the premises or referred to a laboratory certified to conduct testing in cytology. All gynecologic smears are to be stained using a Papanicolaou or modified Papanicolaou method. Workload limitations are also imposed by CLIA 1988. Each individual who evaluates cytology preparations by nonautomated microscopic technique must examine no more than one hundred slides (gynecological and nongynecological or both) in a twenty-four-hour period. The total number of slides examined by each individual during each such period must be documented. The maximum workload of one hundred slides can be completed in no less than an eight-hour workday, and this number includes all slides that an individual reads during employment in another setting.[22] The hospital should consider requiring that those who are employed elsewhere report the total number of slides read daily, for the protection of the laboratory, the individual technologists, and the patients whose results are being interpreted.

Overreading requirements for slides are based on criteria that prioritize certain pathological conditions. All gynecological smears interpreted to show reactive or reparative changes, atypical squamous or glandular cells of undetermined significance, or to be premalignant or in a malignant category are to be confirmed by a technical supervisor in cytology. A technical supervisor in cytology must review all nongynecological preparations.

The laboratory must establish and follow a program designed to detect errors in the performance of cytological examinations and the reporting of results. A 10 percent rescreen of negatives must occur from random patients and from high-risk patients, based on available patient information. The review must be completed before reporting patient results on those selected cases. The laboratory must also compare all malignant and premalignant gynecological reports with the histopathology report, if available in the laboratory, and determine the causes of any discrepancies. For each patient determined to have an intraepithelial lesion of high grade, or exceeding a high grade, the laboratory must review all normal or negative gynecological specimens available within the previous five years for potential misdiagnosis. If significant discrepancies are found that would affect patient care, the laboratory must notify the patient's physician and issue an amended report.

Reports and records are required by many of the CLIA regulations. The laboratory must, for example, document an annual statistical evaluation of the number of cytology cases examined, reporting the volume of patients by diagnosis, number of discrepancies found, and so on. The laboratory must also document an assessment that contrasts the results of case reviews of each individual who examines slides against the laboratory's overall statistical values. Any discrepancies, including reasons for deviation and corrective action taken, must be documented. The laboratory report must clearly distinguish specimens or smears that are unsatisfactory for diagnostic interpretation. The report must contain narrative descriptive nomenclature for all results, and must indicate the basis for correction on any corrected laboratory report issued. The laboratory must retain all slides for five years from the date of examination. Slides may be loaned to proficiency testing programs, if the laboratory obtains written documentation of the receipt of the slides by the recipient program and if the slides are retrievable upon request.

Because of the unique issues associated with cervicovaginal cytology, this area is discussed separately.

Cervicovaginal Cytology

Cervicovaginal cytology is, to a certain extent, a victim of its own success, as the public perceives it to be 100 percent foolproof. However, this screening procedure is useful in the reduction of cervical cancer only to the degree that it is properly collected, handled, and interpreted. This section addresses the overlap of quality improvement concepts and risk management principles as they apply to cervicovaginal cytology and discusses the responsibilities of women, healthcare providers, and laboratory personnel.

The pap smear is a safe, noninvasive, cost-effective screening procedure. A healthcare provider (obstetrician or gynecologist, family practitioner, internist, nurse clinician, and so on) collects (scrapes) the specimen, composed of cellular material, from the cervix and places it on a glass slide. The specimen is then specially preserved and processed for microscopic evaluation.

Cervicovaginal Cytology Screens

The individuals usually responsible for the initial evaluation and interpretation of the cervicovaginal cytology specimen are cytotechnologists. In some laboratories, a pathologist may perform the initial screening and interpretation and the ultimate diagnosis of the cellular sample. Cytotechnologists are highly skilled individuals. Since 1988, a baccalaureate degree has been required as a prerequisite to the certification examination in cytotechnology. The certification examination is a rigorous national examination administered by the American Society for Clinical Pathology (ASCP). The cytotechnologist evaluates whether the sample is adequate and satisfactory and determines if the cellular sample is within normal limits or negative. A report is then issued to the healthcare provider. If the cytotechnologist detects an abnormality or determines the cellular sample to be positive, the slide is reviewed by a pathologist who renders a final diagnosis. High-risk patients may have all of their samples routinely examined by the pathologist.

Despite the successes of cervicovaginal cytology, it is important to understand its limitations. False negatives may occur as do false positives. A false negative may occur when a patient has a cervical lesion, but the abnormal cells are not present on the slide. This could be because the lesion is small and was not sampled when the pap smear was taken. False negatives also occur when abnormal cells are present on the slide, but the cells are either missed or misinterpreted or misdiagnosed. Even in a high-quality laboratory that follows all the CLIA 1988 requirements and other published standards, abnormal cells will occasionally be missed. Two-thirds of false negatives are attributed to sampling and specimen collection errors. This emphasizes the role of the primary caregiver who performs the pelvic examination and obtains the specimen.

All laboratories that perform cervicovaginal cytology should use a widely accepted reporting nomenclature called the Bethesda System. Using the Bethesda System reduces the chance a clinician will not fully understand the patient's condition, resulting in delayed, inadequate, or omitted treatment.[23]

The healthcare provider is generally responsible for recommending that pap smears be performed. It is imperative that the healthcare provider instruct female patients as to the optimal time for performing a pap smear, for example, not during menses. Patients should not use vaginal creams, contraceptive foams or jellies, douche, or tampons twenty-four to twenty-eight hours prior to a pap smear. Having intercourse within that time frame or while affected by a vaginal infection can hinder accuracy due to associated creams, blood, douches, etc. All of these variants can remove or contaminate the cells necessary for proper evaluation. The task of collecting an adequate sample and ensuring that it is properly labeled and preserved belongs to the provider who collects the specimen. This professional is also responsible for providing the laboratory with a pertinent clinical

BOX 10.1   **Breakdown of Responsibilities Regarding Pap Smear**

Physician Responsibilities

1. Educate female patients over the age of 18, particularly those at risk, to have annual pap smears.
2. Keep up-to-date on current testing guidelines promulgated by professional organizations such as the American College of Obstetricians & Gynecologists.
3. Advise patients as to the best time to obtain a pap smear, for example, just before ovulation.
4. Learn to properly collect the cervicovaginal cytology specimen.
5. Send specimens to an accredited laboratory.
6. Provide the laboratory with a pertinent clinical history and information including symptomatology and risk factors.
7. Correlate laboratory findings with clinical observations.
8. Recommend appropriate follow-up promptly; send reminders.

Patient Responsibilities

1. Schedule an appointment for an annual Pap smear with someone who is skilled in taking Pap smears, such as a gynecologist.
2. Properly prepare for the Pap smear.
3. Call the practitioner if results aren't received within a reasonable period of time.
4. Follow the healthcare practitioner's recommendations for follow-up, such as biopsies.
5. Notify new physician of gynecological history if there is a change of healthcare providers.

Laboratory Responsibilities

1. Provide qualified personnel to direct and staff the cytology laboratory.
2. Ensure that all appropriate personnel (cytotechnologists) participate in proficiency testing.
3. Monitor cytotechnologist workload.
4. Ensure that slide interpretations are not reported on unsatisfactory smears.
5. Use a uniform grading system and terminology for reporting.
6. Establish and use a complete quality management program from cervical cytology.
7. Maintain all cervical cytology slides and records in accordance with state and federal law.
8. State results in a standardized manner, clearly indicating when repeat or follow-up testing is needed.

history that includes symptoms and other risk factors. Omitting the clinical history on the requisition for a patient with a history of abnormal pap smears could lead to delayed or missed diagnoses. The laboratory should provide a sample requisition that encourages providers to routinely include the clinical history. The healthcare providers should complete the requisition themselves and not leave it to administrative office staff. Collection sites should maintain a log of all pap smears sent to the laboratory, including the date sent and the date the report is received. If a report is not received in a reasonable time, then the provider should follow up with the laboratory to determine why the delay has occurred.

Current standards recommend a two-pronged approach for certain patients in the detection of cervical cancer, the pap smear and a human papillomavirus (HPV) DNA test. Prudent healthcare providers will keep up-to-date on these recommendations and adjust their practice accordingly.

Ensuring open, high-quality communication between the laboratory and the referring clinician is essential. The laboratory's findings should be correlated with the observations of the clinician who submits patient specimens. The laboratory should report all cytological findings using concise, descriptive, unambiguous terminology. Finally, the clinician should review all cytology reports and communicate the information to the patient. The circle of open, direct communication is then complete, facilitating prompt patient treatment if issues are identified. If the laboratory recommends repeat testing, it is the physician's responsibility to notify the patient verbally and in writing. The physician's office should maintain a log of patients notified of abnormal pap results that require repeat testing or other follow-up. Dates of notification and follow-up appointment or referrals should be logged. The log should be used as a tickler file so that patients may be contacted to remind them of needed follow-up. Any other specific details should also be documented in each patient's medical record. Box 10.1 details the responsibilities of each of the parties involved.

The CLIA 1988 section on cervical cytology outlines the many responsibilities of the laboratory. The following risk indicators are suggested inclusions in a cytopathology laboratory performance improvement program.

- Specimen procurement, including proper identification, clinical information and fixation

- Specimens lost and not received

- Specimen adequacy

- Proper preparation and staining of slides

- Comparison of cytotechnologist interpretation to cytopathologist diagnosis

- Upon review, new or additional cellular findings that are significantly different from the initial report

- Significant discrepancy between cytopathology diagnosis and histopathology diagnosis

Additionally, it might be helpful to set up a system to identify situations when clinicians submit multiple patient specimens in a short period of time. Rescreens of some of these slides may be called for.

New technologies include computerized screening of cervicovaginal pathology specimens. Whereas the FDA has approved only certain specific computerized devices to rescreen negative smears and identify any issues missed by the initial screener, it will be only a matter of time before manufacturers apply and receive approval from the FDA for all initial screening. One concern is that new technology might drive up the cost of pap smears, possibly limiting access to them by lower-income women. New methods for collecting and preparing cervicovaginal cytology specimens have also been developed. For example, liquid-based pap tests, commonly known as *thin prep*, are said to produce specimens with less blood and thick clumping of cells, which makes it easier to identify abnormalities.[24] Before implementing new technology such as automated screens, a laboratory should conduct a thorough performance/benefit analysis of all available testing enhancements, including thin-prep.

Surgical and Hematopathology Responsibilities

There is a tendency in some laboratories to regard these areas as removed from the usual laboratory requirements concerning written procedures, proper reagent use and storage, and so on. In fact, the same principles apply, and the preanalytic and postanalytic aspects of these areas are of particular concern from a risk management standpoint.

In the preanalytic stage, it is important to note that the specimen is much more likely to be unique than is the case with clinical pathology. When a clinical pathology specimen is lost or mislabeled, it is frequently possible to obtain a new sample of blood or urine from the patient. Repeating a surgical biopsy because of mislabeling obviously poses many more concerns. (Refer to the discussion of specimen collection earlier in this chapter.)

The analytic phase of surgical and bone marrow pathology involves microscopic examination of tissue after processing and staining. The processing and staining procedures should be detailed in writing and are subject to CLIA inspection. The examination and diagnostic interpretation is performed by a CLIA-qualified physician, generally a pathologist. Diagnostic interpretation is performed in a manner that is similar to a radiologist's interpretation of an X-ray, and two pathologists may differ in their interpretation of a specimen, just as two radiologists may arrive at different diagnoses based on the same set of X-rays. In some instances, the differences are matters of nomenclature and classification, without clinical import for the patient involved. Others involve diagnostic differences that are of clinical significance.

In pathology, the need for immediate readings by means of frozen sections further complicates issues of diagnostic variance. In this technique, part of a tissue specimen is rapidly frozen with liquid nitrogen, which allows immediate sectioning and limited staining. Thus it is possible to have a microscopically readable slice in minutes, while a patient is still in the operating room and the surgeon is deciding what to do next. The technical drawbacks of the technique include less microscopic detail and the lack of perspective provided by ancillary stains, which are not available. Also, the size and quality of the preanalytic sample is critical because less tissue is available for examination than can later be evaluated in the permanent sections. Thus a diagnostic mistake might occur because the lesion was not present in the limited frozen-section sample or the collection technique itself prevented an accurate reading. Estimates of the variance between frozen and final diagnoses are around 2 to 3 percent. The frozen-section diagnosis should always be compared with the final report, and the bases for differences evaluated. The ordering clinician should always be promptly notified when such discrepancies occur. Indeed, a discrepancy should be treated as a critical value and accorded an equivalent response. Similar to the need to evaluate effectiveness of frozen-section sampling is the need to monitor another rapid technique, touch prep, which is used during breast cancer surgery to estimate tumor margins. Discrepancies between touch prep results and the final diagnosis should always be reviewed through the organization's quality improvement processes.

Even with conventionally processed and stained permanent microscopic sections, there can be interpretive differences between pathologists. In a review of the literature, pathology appears to be operating at about a 2 percent error rate. Significant variances were found in roughly 1 to 5 percent of cases when specimens were reread by at least one pathologist in several formats and it was determined that 1 percent of the subject specimens had a second reading that was different from the first. Thus in a small hospital, with perhaps two pathologists and five thousand surgical pathology specimens a year, one to five specimens per week might be read differently. The level of significant differences may vary between types of specimens, as well. Gross evaluation of breast specimens revealed major discrepancies in 5 percent of the cases and minor discrepancies in 6 percent.[25]

Given the above data, it is recommended that pathologists engage in ongoing education. For example, CAP and other organizations have diagnostic challenge programs, which can help clinicians sharpen skills.

It is also logical to consider some type of rereading (also known as *overreading*) system as part of the laboratory's quality improvement program. This can be done by randomly allocating a certain percentage of specimens for this purpose, similar to the previously described approach to review of cytopathology results, or by concentrating on known areas of interpretive difficulty, such as breast, prostate, and skin. Regardless of the approach used, the lab should track the results by individual pathologist and consider including such data when recredentialing the practitioner, just as postoperative infection rates are evaluated for surgeons. Other submitted data should include the previously noted correlation rate between frozen and final diagnoses.

Whatever the system used, it is important that the selected rereads cover all types of specimens that reach a given pathologist. For a general pathologist, this would mean all types of specimens. In larger departments, a given pathologist might only examine cytology specimens, or bone marrows, and so on. The pathology department should have objective benchmarks based on the literature or on standards set by national professional organizations. As is the case with other laboratory physician positions, the anatomic pathologist(s) must meet CLIA requirements and be properly licensed and credentialed.

Sending specimens for outside consultation enhances the reread program and can result in additional input for quality assessment. This input is, of course, particularly valuable when the outside expert states that a diagnosis is materially different from the one determined locally. In considering variances in pathologists' interpretations, it is important to distinguish two major categories of disagreement. In the first, the original pathologist has doubts about the diagnosis and has requested another opinion from a local colleague or outside expert. Here, a discrepancy is due to professional prudence by the original pathologist rather than error. The second category involves cases for which the first pathologist had no doubts about the diagnosis, but a second evaluation occurred randomly or because the patient or the patient's primary physician requested outside review. In these latter instances, disagreement may indicate error, and third opinions should be sought, if necessary. Such discrepancies should be a regular part of the quality improvement data reported by the laboratory to the facility's quality improvement department, and, as previously noted, they should be used in the medical staff credentialing process.

Tissue and Organ Donor Services

The hospital is obligated to ensure that tissue or organs are donated under the auspices of a licensed tissue bank and organ procurement organization (OPO). There should be formal agreements, and all hospitals are obligated to refer possible organ donors. A TJC standard requires hospitals to monitor the conversion (success) rate of their eligible patients.[26] Hospitals that perform organ transplants should have standard protocols that address a wide range of topics, including consent, delineation of roles within the OPO, safety checks on organ suitability, cadaver and live donor procedures, institutional review boards (IRBs), and so on. Based on the authors' experiences, such programs should include input from the ethics committee and risk management area. A more detailed discussion is beyond the scope of this chapter. For more information on IRBs, see Chapter 5.

Organ and Tissue Transplantation Services

Organ transplantation includes several laboratory areas that must have the previously discussed accreditation(s). These areas of the lab include histocompatibility (tissue typing) and transfusion services. The functions of these areas with regard to organ transplantation are highly specialized, but CLIA requirements still apply.

Tissue Transplantation

The FDA has jurisdiction over tissue storage and transplant.[27] Tissue should be obtained only from a licensed, accredited facility. Storage of tissue should be per supplier's instructions, with continuous temperature monitoring in alarmed refrigerators or freezers for cold storage items. If such storage is in areas not staffed twenty-four hours a day, seven days a week, the alarms need to be remotely connected to a hospital area that is continuously staffed, and personnel in that area must be trained on how to respond if the alarm is activated. Many institutions find that storage in a freezer in the blood bank, which already has an alarm system, is a practical approach. Key administrative processes associated with storage include placing the tissue receipt in a log and documenting the expiration date. For each tissue fragment, a permanent record must be kept, including the receipt, source, type, lot number, and date of transplant or other disposition. This information should also be documented in the patient's chart. The hospital must be able to trace the tissue back to the supplier, in case of a patient reaction. It is equally important for the hospital to be able to locate the recipient in order to follow up if the supplying tissue bank later finds a defect in the particular lot. (The action to be taken under such circumstances is analogous to the previously described lookback process for blood products.)

It is unwise for a hospital to maintain a tissue retrieval or storage bank, even for autologous tissues, unless the facility can fulfill all related regulatory and licensure requirements. Success and complication rates for tissue and organ transplants should be the subject of routine quality improvement reporting for the departments involved.

Bone marrow progenitor cell transplants (bone marrow or peripheral blood stem cell) programs require systems similar to those that support tissue transplantation, as well as extensive processing and storage protocols that are similar to those required of tissue and blood banks, including alarm-monitored storage areas. Properly supported programs may address autologous and donor marrow or stem cell donation, as well as the storage, processing, and transplantation of related materials.

Critical Values

Critical values are as important in anatomic pathology as they are in clinical pathology. With the high volume of outpatient biopsies and surgeries in many settings, mailed reports may go astray or be missed in a busy practitioner's office. Whether by mail, computer interface, or manual messenger, all steps associated with transfer of information have risks of failure. A summary of concepts (and associated tips) regarding laboratory testing appears in Box 10.2. The following list of circumstances that require direct communication with the ordering physician is not intended to be all-inclusive, but rather is intended to stimulate institutions to reexamine their systems:

- Cases with significant variance between frozen section and final diagnoses
- Amended reports based on special stains or testing
- New or substantively changed diagnoses by an outside consultant
- Reports of malignant or possibly malignant tissue
- Recommendations for follow-up or repeat examinations or repeated screening at more frequent intervals
- Placentas submitted for examination that are suspected of being incomplete
- Unsatisfactory specimens

The pathologist should document the direct follow-up in some manner. Some pathologists do this as an addendum to the diagnostic report itself.

The attending or treating physician is usually the person who discloses a changed pathology result or error to the patient. The pathologist is not involved in the discussion. In this era of transparency, consideration should be given to expanding the pathologist's role in this aspect of medical disclosure. Pathologists may feel an ethical obligation to be involved in the interdisciplinary disclosure process, particularly when it involves an error they made, and the disclosure process may benefit from the inclusion of this expertise.

BOX 10.2   **Summary of Concepts and Tips for the Risk Management Professional**

1. Laboratories are highly regulated by multiple entities.

   TIP—Overall JCAHO Hospital accreditation is NOT sufficient for laboratory accreditation.

2. Even in a low-volume setting, if laboratory testing is performed for clinical purposes, then CLIA certification is required.

   TIP—Pay attention to medical center newsletter articles on exciting new testing in a clinical area separate from the main laboratory. Check to see if there are clinical purposes and/or research implications. (See Chapter 5 on clinical research.) Also, find out if the patient is billed. (See Chapter 4 in Volume 3 on corporate compliance). In a large tertiary institution, risk managers may not always be told about small laboratories in departments other than pathology.

   TIP—Contact CMS for a list of laboratories identified with your institution's name and/or address.

3. Regulations and standards frequently change, and can be difficult to follow.

   TIP—Always have and follow a current copy of the CAP inspection checklists or the JCAHO *Accreditation Manual for Laboratories*. If you have a transfusion service, then a current copy of the AABB standards should be in the laboratory. Regulatory changes can also be followed in monthly newsletters, such as *JCAHO Perspectives* and *CAP Today*.

4. Blood transfusion services and banks receive more regulatory oversight when they do more processing, and if they draw blood from donors. If blood is drawn from donors, the provider must perform complex tests for HIV and hepatitis.

   TIP—If donors are drawn, consider "contracting out" these complicated expensive tests for viruses. Contracting services can also shift liability to another organization.

5. Progenitor cells may be kept frozen for many years for potential needs of the intended recipients.

   TIP—Have protocols from the outset defining who owns the cells if years later, they are not needed by the intended recipient.

6. Laboratory activities involve ongoing interfaces with nursing staff.

   TIP—Ongoing committee, task force, coffee chats, and so forth, are essential to establishing effective relationships among nursing and laboratory staff.

7. Transport of specimens has many associated risks.

   TIP—The most common causes of prolonged turnaround in obtaining test results are not intralaboratory (analytic) issues. This issue usually results from delay in receipt of samples (preanalytic), delay in receipt of the result by the physician, or delay in the physician taking action on the result (postanalytic). In each of these areas, a root cause analysis aids in defining underlying systems issues and areas (e.g., lab, nursing, physician, transport), as well as in identifying simple effective solutions.

· · · · · · · · ·
BILLING COMPLIANCE

Billing compliance is discussed in more detail elsewhere in this chapter and series. Of note, laboratories largely perform testing based on orders from primary physicians and may lack access to diagnostic codes justifying the particular order. Various governmental, private insurance, and pathology practice publications should be reviewed regularly to ensure adherence to various compliance-related requirements. Additional review of final reports should be done to reconcile the results of all billed components. For example, a surgical pathology specimen has six special stains billed, but the report contains results for only five. The laboratory should either issue an amended report with the result of the sixth test or credit the patient's account.

· · · · · · · · ·
CONCLUSION

Laboratory testing poses a wide variety of risks to the patient, laboratory, and hospital staff. This is one reason for the rapid evolution of related government regulations and standards of private accrediting organizations, as well as professional organization statements on pertinent matters such as new technology. To be certain that their organizations address the latest standards, laboratory and risk management professionals should monitor publications and other informational resources on an ongoing basis. They should also leverage the valuable multidisciplinary team staffing and interfacing with the laboratory to mine data for quality issues and develop best safety and liability reduction practices in this complex clinical area.

Endnotes

1. "Types of CLIA Certificate." Available at: www.cms.hhs.gov/clia/certypes.asp. (Accessed on December 11, 2005.)

2. *Ibid.*

3. Note: Medicare, Medicaid, and CLIA Programs; Continuance of the Approval of the College of American Pathologists as a CLIA Accreditation Organization, *Federal Register*, 2001; 66(177):47493–47497. See *Federal Register* online via GPO access. Available at: www.phppo.cdc.gov/clia/docs/fr12se01n.htm. (Accessed on December 11, 2005.)

4. "List of CLIA Exempt States." Available at: www.cms.hhs.gov/clia/exemstat.asp. (Assessed on December 11, 2005.)

5. "CLIA General Program Description." Available at: www.cms.hhs.gov/clia/progdesc.asp. (Accessed on December 11, 2005.)

6. *Ibid.*

7. "List of CLIA Approved PT Proficiency Testing Programs 2005." Available at: www.cms.hhs.gov/clia/ptlist.pdf. (Assessed on December 11, 2005.)

8. *op. cit.,* "CLIA Program General Description."

9. U.S. Food and Drug Administration Center for Biologics Evaluation and Research, "Blood." Available at: www.fda.gov/cber/blood.htm. (Accessed on December 11, 2005.)

10. U.S. Food and Drug Administration Center for Biologics Evaluation and Research, "Blood Establishment Registration and Product Listing (BER)." Available at: www.fda.gov/cber/blood/bldreg.htm. (Accessed on December 11, 2005.)

11. U.S. Food and Drug Administration Center for Biologics Evaluation and Research, "Devices Regulated by CBER," Available at: www.fda.gov/cber/dap/devlst.htm. (Accessed on December 11, 2005.)

12. Clinical and Laboratory Standards Institute (CLSI) (formerly known as National Committee for Clinical Laboratory Standards—NCCLS) 940 West Valley Rd., Ste. 1400, Wayne, Pa. 19087–1898, (610) 688–0100. Available at: www.clsi.org/.

13. www.hipaa.org/.

14. Casalino, L. P., D. Dunham, N. H. Chin. "Frequency of failure to notify patients of significant outpatient test results." *Archives of Internal Medicine* 2009; 169:1123–1129.

15. Cram, P., G. E. Rosenthal, R. Ohsfeldt et al. "Failure to recognize and act on abnormal test results: The case of screening bone densitometry." *Journal on Quality and Patient Safety* 2005; 31:90–97.

16. Patient Safety Goals. Available at: www.jcaho.org/accredited+organizations/ patient+safety/05+npsg/05_npsg_hap.htm]. (Accessed on August 18, 2009.)

17. *Ibid.*

18. Patient Safety Goals. Available at: www.jcaho.org/accredited+organizations/ patient+safety/05+npsg/05_npsg_hap.htm. (Accessed on August 18, 2009.)

19. U.S. Department of Health and Human Services, Food and Drug Administration, and Center for Biologics Evaluation and Research. Guidance for the Industry: Notifying FDA of Fatalities Related to Blood Collection or Transfusions. Final Guidance, September 2003. Available at: www.fda.gov/downloads/BiologicsBloodVaccines/ GuidanceComplianceRegulatoryInformation/Guidances/Blood/ucm062897.pdf. (Accessed on March 30, 2010.)

20. Wise, R. P. FDA and CBER. "FDA's Safety Surveillance for Blood and Blood Products" for presentation to the Advisory Committee on Blood Safety and Availability, May 16, 2005. Available at: www.hhs.gov/bloodsafety/presentations/Wise.pdf. (Accessed on March 30, 2010.)

21. Moriarty, A. T., L. Fartheree, R. Laucerico. "Cytology PT: Where We Are, Where To Now." *CAP Today*. January 2009.

22. CLIA Final Rule published February 28, 1992, at 42 CFR 493.1257(b)(1) and (b)(3)(i).

23. The NCI addresses the use of Bethesda System terminology to facilitate pap smear assessment on its Web site at: www.cancer.gov/cancertopics/factsheet/Detection/ Pap-test.

24. "Screening For Cervical Cancer," Guideline Synthesis on the National Guideline Clearinghouse Web page of the AHRQ site. Available at: www.guideline.gov/Compare/ comparison.aspx?file=CvCSCREEN6.inc. (Accessed on March 30, 2010.)

25. Frable, W. J. "Surgical Pathology—Second Reviews, Institutional Reviews, Audits, and Correlations: What's Out There? Error or Diagnostic Variation?" *Archives of Pathology and Laboratory Medicine* 2006; 130:620–625.

26. JCAHO Online. Available at: www.jcaho.org/about+us/news+letters/jcahonline/ jo_01_05.htm. (Accessed on December 10, 2005.)

27. Wells, M. "Implementation of 21 CFR 1251." Available at: www.fda.gov/cber/ summaries/aatb092005mw.pdf. (Accessed on December 10, 2005.)

11

Managing Clinical Risk and Enhancing Patient Safety in Radiology

Sylvia M. Brown

Since Wilhelm Conrad Roentgen discovered X-rays in 1895, professionals associated with the field of radiology have continued to refine a provider's ability to envision the body's inner workings, without breaking the skin.[1] For example, the interventional radiology setting combines characteristics of the operating room and the radiology suite, housing sophisticated technology that helps physicians diagnose complex patients in the least invasive manner possible. At the same time, advanced telemetric communication systems enhance the capability and efficiency of healthcare organizations by allowing radiologists to interpret and read films and studies from the other side of the world. Another important advance is the digitalization of radiology films, which saves storage space and has the potential to interface the film or study directly with the medical record.

Each advance made by radiology is associated with patient safety concerns and potential for liability. Of particular note, alleged failure to properly interpret films and diagnostic studies or to communicate findings have caused dramatic increases in the severity of malpractice awards against radiologists.[2] This chapter will suggest approaches to help the risk management professional work with clinicians to mitigate key risks associated with increased technology, as well as interface with other clinical environments.

TECHNOLOGY

The technology associated with radiology has never been without risk. Following are examples of technology-associated safety issues that have resulted in liability over the years and key strategies with which to alleviate them. Because technology is evolving at a feverish pace, it is hoped that the general approaches suggested here may also be helpful when the risk management professional must address equipment or procedures not yet in existence.

Radiation Exposure

The wonder of X-rays was quickly tempered by fear when many suffered burns as a result of radiant energy. Thomas Edison's own experiments with X-rays came to an abrupt halt when his friend and assistant, Clarence Dally, suffered serious burns which ultimately led to his death in 1904. Dally is widely reported to have been the first X-ray–related fatality in the United States.[3]

Although modifications have reduced the risk, radiation is still a source of safety and liability issues. Two areas of particular concern for risk management professionals and radiologists involve the amount of radiation received by computed tomography (CT) scan patients, especially pediatric CT patients, and the need for proper use of CT equipment. According to the American College of Radiology's Technical Standard for Medical Nuclear Physics Performance Monitoring on PET/CT Imaging Equipment in 2008, "Radiologist medical physicists, radiologic technologists, and all supervising physicians have a responsibility to minimize the radiation dosage to individual patients, to staff, and to society as a whole, while maintaining the necessary diagnostic image quality. This concept is known as 'as low as reasonably achievable' (ALARA)."[4]

CT Concerns

Two studies appearing in the December 14, 2009, issue of the *Archives of Internal Medicine* reveal higher than expected radiation dosage in clinical CT studies and increased lifetime potential cancer risks as a result. Both studies were funded by the National Institutes of Health (NIH) and the National Cancer Institute (NCI).

Using the 2006 Biological Effects of Ionizing Radiation (BEIR) VII risk model, which is based on health data collected from Japanese atomic bomb survivors, the first study projected that CT scans conducted in 2007 alone could result in some 29,000 cancer cases.[5] The second study evaluated the amount of radiation administered in eleven of the most common CT scans, based on actual data from a population of 1,119 patients who were scanned at many centers in the San Francisco Bay Area.[6]

One point of particular concern to the second group of researchers was that within each type of CT study, effective dosage varied significantly both within and across institutions, with a mean thirteenfold variation between the highest and lowest dose for each study type. Another significant finding was that studies that included an assessment of arteries and multiphase studies requiring repeated scans had higher exposures.

This study was criticized for using a model based on atomic bomb survivor data and the fact that there is no proven link between clinical radiation and disease, but the importance of dose reduction efforts are clear. Specific recommendations made to lower risk included the following:

- Standardizing protocols across sites
- Reducing multiple imaging series within each exam (multiphase studies)
- Implementing dose-reduction strategies
- Participating in accreditation programs such as those offered by the American College of Radiology (ACR)

Reducing the number of CT exams is also important because reports suggest that many of the scans administered may be unnecessary.[7] Also, patient dose information should be tracked and monitored.

"A searchable electronic health record will help educate patients and healthcare providers about radiation exposure, and could facilitate activities to minimize dose when possible," wrote the researchers in the second study. "Understanding exposures to medical radiation delivered through actual clinical studies is a crucial first step toward developing reasonable strategies to minimize unnecessary exposures."[8]

Pediatric Concerns

In 2008, the National Cancer Institute published a guide for healthcare providers, citing three unique considerations for performing CT scans on children: first, children may be more sensitive to medical imaging scan radiation than adults; second, children have a longer life expectancy, resulting in a larger window of opportunity for realizing radiation damage; and third, and perhaps most significant, children receive a higher dose than necessary when adult CT settings are used.[9]

Despite this professional guidance, recent research suggests divergent approaches to the dosage of CT radiation in children. Another area of concern for pediatric patients is nuclear medicine. Administered by Boston Children's Hospital, a 2008 survey of practice at thirteen pediatric hospitals, found a twofold variation in radiopharmaceutical doses administered during pediatric nuclear medicine exams. For some radiopharmaceuticals, the reported maximum activity varied by as much as a factor of 10, and minimum activity differed by as much as a factor of 20, suggesting the need for a consensus among nuclear physicians on appropriate doses for young patients.[10] "Clearly, risk management professionals should be aware of their radiology department's approach to pediatric CT and nuclear medicine dosage for pediatric patients, and they should encourage the pursuit of ALARA for this vulnerable population."

Concerns Related to Use of CT Equipment

Equally important is the need for CT equipment to be properly calibrated and used. The same principle applies to other types of radiological equipment, but two glaring misuses have recently illustrated its importance with regard to CT. One situation involved a rural hospital in which a twenty-three-month-old child received 151 consecutive CT scans in the space of sixty-five minutes, clearly an excessively high dosage delivered, the results of which may not be known for years. The hospital was fined $25,000 by the California

Department of Public Health for failing to follow its own procedures.[11] The second recent example of CT radiation overdosage involves delivery of eight times the standard radiation dose in each of 260 CT brain perfusion scans at a large community hospital, from February 2008 to August 2009. A class action suit has recently been filed on behalf of the patients who received the excess radiation.[12] The advanced age and clinical diagnosis of many of these patients make damage determinations from the overdosage difficult.

The following are essential approaches promoting radiation safety:

1. An effective radiation safety committee, which has the input of a physicist, is a critical mechanism for the healthcare facility. As previously noted, the guiding principle of radiation safety is ALARA, or as low as reasonably achievable. With this central goal in mind, routine review of quality objectives by this group is an excellent way to promote radiation safety.

2. Pertinent safety protocols protecting patients and staff will address topics such as appropriate shielding, use of lead aprons, and so on. Key sources of such protocols include the many federal and state agencies that address radiation safety. For example, OSHA standards address worker safety, the U.S. Center for Devices and Radiological Health under the Food and Drug Administration sets standards for new equipment that produces radiation, and the Nuclear Regulatory Commission (NRC) governs the safety of individuals who are exposed to all material produced by nuclear reactors. Of particular note are the NRC standards intended to prevent misadministration of nuclear isotopes. These standards parallel traditional medication safety approaches by requiring patient identification and a physician's written order specifying type, dosage, and duration of each pharmaceutical to be administered, accompanied by a written dosage and directive explaining how to calculate dosage. (Please see the previous discussion regarding need for standardization of pediatric dosage.)[13]

   The ACR, an important source of information on the standard of care in radiology, also has published statements on radiation safety. For example, the *ACR Standard for Diagnostic Procedures Using Radiopharmaceuticals* states that imaging facilities should reasonably attempt to identify pregnant patients before performing any diagnostic examination involving ionizing radiation. The standard also states "There shall be posting of radiation precaution signs in areas where radioactive agents are used or stored [and posting of] warnings to patients to inform the staff if they are or could be pregnant." Regardless of whether ionizing radiation is to be used, it is reasonably prudent to post signs instructing patients to inform the receptionist or technologist if there is any possibility that they may be pregnant prior to a diagnostic radiology study.

3. A biomedical program that provides for preventive maintenance and repair by technicians, who document current equipment-specific training to manage this highly specialized equipment, is another important risk management strategy to bolster radiation safety. In cases in which the biomedical program is contracted, it is particularly important that the contract specify the mechanism for timely repairs and/or replacement of equipment, should that be necessary.

Computed Tomography

Developed in 1972, CT scans enable the provider to view multiple slices of an organ, enhancing the traditional single dimension view produced by X-rays. Risk of cancer is thought to increase with full-body CT scans performed on a regular basis,[14] and this approach is not recommended by the ACR. As previously noted, standardization of evidence-based radiation dosage approaches for pediatric patients and proper use of CTs are of particular important radiation safety strategies. Other liability and safety issues pertaining to CT scans concern failure to perform them at all or misinterpretation of the results. General principles to assist in preventing misinterpretation, which apply to all diagnostic studies, include the following:[15]

1. Other pertinent reports should be available to the clinician.

2. Any limitations in the study should be noted by the clinician, addressed as necessary, and documented in the record.[16]

3. The clinician should be alert to lesions outside the area of interest (e.g., lung mass seen on a kidney–ureter–bladder film).

4. Current training in interpreting the study is critical.

5. It is important for the clinician to recommend any other studies that may be helpful.

Magnetic Resonance Imaging

Of technological advances in the last twenty years, magnetic resonance imaging (MRI) has been associated with the most dramatic risk. Although the use of magnetic imaging reduces risk associated with traditional radiology exposure and provides a valuable diagnostic perspective for the clinician, the force of the magnet has resulted in numerous patient injuries and liability suits. ACR has published detailed white papers[17] on magnetic resonance safety, which includes helpful checklists and practical tips. Risk management professionals, as well as clinicians, should access the ACR Web site for updates as necessary. Basic safety principles include the following:

1. Orientation to MRI safety should be provided for *everyone* who may practice in the environment, from the chief of surgery to the housekeeping personnel.

2. Screening of patients for metallic objects must be routine and thorough. Items that the patient might not think of as problematic should be asked about specifically, for example, the foil associated with drug patches used to administer some medications. Specific checklists to facilitate screening are available on the ACR site.[18]

3. Care devices such as intravenous poles, which appear metallic but have been specially treated to be safe in the MRI, should be color-coded. Staff must be instructed that these are the only such devices to be allowed in the environment.

4. Emergency protocols must include a provision that requires security staff and staff in the MR suite to inform firefighters and other emergency providers of the risk associated with bringing metal equipment into the environment, if the magnet is operational.

5. Mock codes should be run routinely. The relative infrequency of cardiac arrest in the MRI suite makes this a particularly important strategy. Staff should also maintain current competency regarding the complex process of extricating a patient who requires resuscitation. Another important factor is the considerable distance from code teams and other resources that the MRI is often located due to the immense size of many units. The white papers from the ACR referenced above address MRI code practice specifically.[19]

6. In some older units, a malfunction of the MRI may release toxic gas, necessitating the shut down of the unit and immediate removal of all staff and patients from the area. Depending on the equipment involved, mock drills for this eventuality (quench procedure) are also a prudent risk management measure.

Radiological Devices for Breast Cancer Screening and Diagnosis

Failure to diagnose breast cancer has, for many years, been a source of significant professional liability exposure for radiologists. Specific patient safety and risk management concerns are, to a large degree, driven by new technology and professional organization guidance concerning the use of that technology, including recently issued guidelines revising the age at which routine mammography screening should begin.

Technology

Digital mammography was first approved for use in the United States in 2000 and, since then, has come into use in an increasing number of practices. According to statistics from the ACR, approximately 7 percent of U.S. mammography practices had at least one digital system as of April 2005. That percentage gradually rose to 33.6 percent by April 2008.[20]

The increased use of this relatively new technology may be partially attributed to the 2005 published results of The Digital Mammographic Imaging Screening Trial (DMIST) sponsored by the National Cancer Institute. This study contrasted the effectiveness of cancer identification by traditional film mammography with the capability of new digital mammography. The study population included 49,528 women at thirty-three sites through the United States. The research confirmed the general value of traditional film mammograms, and it also determined that digital mammography is more effective at identifying cancer in three populations: (1) patients under age fifty, regardless of level of breast tissue density; (2) patients of any age, with heterogeneously (very dense) or extremely dense breast tissue; and 3) premenopausal or perimenopausal women of any age (defined as women who had a last menstrual period within twelve months of their mammograms).[21] In a second, more recent study, community hospital–based researchers shared the results of four audits, each based on four thousand or more screening exams, conducted immediately before and then annually throughout the conversion to digital mammography. Their work similarly identified an increased ability to identify cancers in patients with dense breasts.[22]

The implications of these findings clearly include the need for primary care physicians and others who refer patients for mammography to consider whether the patient needs a digital rather than a traditional screening mammogram.

Another sort of technology that enhances the radiological ability to interpret mammograms is CAD, or computer-assisted diagnosis. This resource, in effect, gives the radiologist another pair of eyes, because CAD helps identify suspicious areas that may merit a closer look. The ACR is very concerned that some payers classify CAD as experimental. On their Web site, ACR offers an excellent overview of the tool and points that can help make the case for reimbursement to such health insurance organizations.[23]

One example of another diagnostic resource found in the nuclear medicine area is breast-specific gamma imaging (BSGI), which uses contrast media to identify hot spots in the breast. Studies show that BSGI may even be more helpful than MRI in refining questionable mammography results.[24][25] Finally, it is important for patients and providers to be aware that other diagnostic resources, such as breast MRIs, may complement, but usually not replace, mammographic evaluation.

Professional Resources

The standard of reasonable care in mammography is shaped by several important professional standards. These flow from various organizations and are sometimes controversial. For example, the U.S. Preventive Services Task Force (USPSTF), a panel of private-sector experts in prevention and primary care, sponsored by the Agency for Healthcare Research and Quality (AHRQ) for the last eleven years,[26] recently updated the 2002 recommendations concerning screening mammography. Among new recommendations issued November 17, 2009, are the following:

- The USPSTF recommends that the decision to start regular, biennial screening mammography before the age of fifty years should be an individual one and takes patient context into account, including the patient's values regarding specific benefits and harms;

- The USPSTF recommends against teaching breast self-examination (BSE).

- The USPSTF concludes that the current evidence is insufficient to assess the additional benefits and harms of clinical breast examination (CBE) beyond screening mammography in women forty years or older.[27]

Immediately after these recommendations were published, experts around the country took issue with increasing the age at which mammograms are routinely recommended to fifty. For example, Carol H. Lee, M.D, chair of the American College of Radiology Breast Imaging Commission, noted that "These unfounded USPSTF recommendations ignore the valid scientific data and place a great many women at risk of dying unnecessarily from a disease that we have made significant headway against over the past twenty years. Mammography is not a perfect test, but it has unquestionably been shown to save lives — including in women aged forty to forty-nine. These new recommendations seem to reflect a conscious decision to ration care. If Medicare and private insurers adopt these incredibly flawed USPSTF recommendations as a rationale for refusing women coverage of these life-saving exams, it could have deadly effects for American women."[28]

On December 4, 2009, the USPSTF "unanimously voted to update the language of their recommendation regarding women less than fifty years of age to clarify their original and continued intent."[29] Meanwhile, primary care providers and risk management professionals must remain informed as the issue of how to counsel women between the ages of forty and fifty about whether they should have a screening mammogram crystallizes. There will certainly be significant challenges for providers and patients if payers no longer reimburse for such screening.

Another, more accepted professional organization guiding mammographic interpretation is the ACR Breast Imaging Reporting and Data System Atlas (BI-RADS® Atlas). This product of collaboration among representatives of the ACR, the National Cancer Institute, the Centers for Disease Control and Prevention, the Food and Drug Administration, the American Medical Association, the American College of Surgeons, and the College of American Pathologists[30] comprises standardized breast imaging terminology, a report organization, assessment structure, and a classification system for mammography, ultrasound, and MRI of the breast. Safety and risk management considerations are simultaneously addressed through the use of the BI-RADS approach, and radiologists not using it are potentially noncompliant with the standard of care.

Contrast Media

There are several risk management issues associated with the use of contrast media in radiological studies. The radiology staff and risk management professional should be familiar with ACR's recently updated "Practice Guideline for the Use of Intravascular Contrast Media," as it addresses key infrastructure supporting the administration of contrast media.[31] The following are important principles to consider.

1. Technologists who inject contrast media must be certified to do so by a physician, who observes their technique for a specific number of times. They should also be educated on principles of injection, and competencies in both the basic principles and their injection technique should be evaluated annually. When the technologist is injecting, a physician should be proximate and available to assist.

2. A second major issue associated with contrast media is the importance of screening the patient and taking other prudent measures to avoid reactions. Key points to consider include the following:

   a. Any patient who is allergic to shellfish or iodine may also be allergic to contrast media. All patients should be asked about allergies, their responses documented, and any issues followed up with the physician prior to injection.

   b. In general, the higher the degree of osmolarity and the higher the dose of contrast media, the greater the chance of a reaction. Ionic media are high in osmolarity, and radiologists should be consulted about the clinical risk associated with purchasing an ionic contrast medium product.

3. A third concern is contrast-induced nephropathy (CIN), which sometimes affects patients with renal insufficiency but may also affect patients without obvious risk factors. Of particular interest and concern is a recent study indicating that patients who had CIN showed a significantly higher propensity for long-term adverse events, such as stroke, during the following year.[32] Once again higher osmolarity of media may be a precipitating factor for CIN, so low osmolarity media is indicated for patients at risk. Another CIN preventive strategy is hydration with intravenous fluids for patients at risk prior to the procedure.[33]

4. Gadolinium-based contrast agents are commonly used to increase the visibility of internal structures when performing MRIs. The FDA first notified health professionals in 2006 about reports received warning of an increased risk of nephrogenic systemic fibrosis (NSF), a debilitating and potentially fatal disease for patients with severe kidney insufficiency, patients with chronic liver disease, or those patients in receipt or awaiting a liver transplant. In May of 2007, the FDA requested that manufacturers include a new boxed warning on the product labeling. More information on gadolinium-based contrast agents can be found on the FDA's Web site at www.fda. gov/Drugs/DrugSafety/PostmarketDrugSafetyInformationforPatientsandProviders/ ucm142882.htm.

5. Finally, it is essential that staff managing contrast media be thoroughly qualified to manage the emergencies they may encounter. A resource to consider is radiology department–specific life support training, such as the certification offered by the Mayo Clinic.[34]

Anesthesia

Because surgery is now performed in the MRI suite in very sophisticated operations, and radiologists are routinely performing moderate sedation, management of anesthesia is an important factor in addressing risk in the radiology area. Of note, the American Society of Anesthesiologists (ASA) issued new credentialing guidelines in October of 2005, and amended in October of 2006, that specify training and performance improvement activities important for any non-anesthetic provider administering moderate sedation.[35] Another important document offering guidance with regard to anesthetic administration in radiology is a recently released ASA advisory on anesthetics in the MRI suite. This document discusses the importance of collaboration among all providers regarding an anesthetic care plan for the patient. Of particular importance is the management of the airway.[36]

Of great significance in any discussion of moderate sedation is Versed (midazolam), which was first heralded as the "stingless Valium" many years ago and is still frequently used to sedate radiology patients for CT or MRI. Versed first became a source of concern when patients became unresponsive and could not be revived. Since that time, pressure from liability carriers and The Joint Commission (TJC) has resulted in several important principles that must be adhered to in the radiology area, as well as other clinical settings.

1. All providers who administer moderate sedation must meet credentialing requirements established with input of the anesthesiologists.

2. To address the risk of having moderate sedation become deep sedation, the physician must be immediately available, and appropriate reversal agents must be on hand. Subsequent evaluation through performance improvement of any cases in which moderate sedation became deep sedation may be a useful way to evaluate effectiveness of the management of these cases. All such quality improvement information should be evaluated by an appropriate peer review committee to maximize available protection under any applicable law.

The death of Michael Jackson in 2009 brought another commonly used short-acting hypnotic agent into the media spotlight. It is important for providers in the radiology area and risk management professionals to be aware of the benefits and associated risk with the use of propofol (Diprivan). This drug produces few aftereffects, but a lack of effective reversal agents makes it critical that staff who are capable of rescuing the patient be immediately available in case the level of sedation becomes too deep. Nurse practice acts vary regarding whether nurses may administer the drug at all, and the American Society of Anesthesiology has issued a statement[37] that underscores the physician's responsibility to remain immediately available during administration and recovery.[38] The administration of propofol is particularly important for the risk management professional to be aware of because it is often used in pediatric sedation.

Telemedicine

Telemedicine is a broad topic that is comprehensively covered in Chapter 15 in Volume 3, but there is one new practice approach that is particularly important for radiology. This is the practice called *nighthawking*, which entails the electronic transmission of films to be read in other locations. The latest trend in this area involves physicians outside the United States. Issues to be addressed in such arrangements include compliance with HIPAA, the ability to bill the Medicare program for interpretative services delivered outside the country, and the legal amenability of a foreign physician to being joined in a lawsuit if one were brought. The largest concern, which has recently caught the strong interest of Congress, is difficulty in ascertaining the quality of the training that such providers have had and ensuring quality of interpretation.[39]

The Centers for Medicare & Medicaid Services (CMS) has implemented strategies to address this concern, such as requiring each setting that receives telemetric interpretation to credential physicians who provide the interpretation. ACR has taken a similar approach: "Physicians who provide the official interpretation of images transmitted by teleradiology should maintain the licensure required for providing radiologic or telemedicine service at both the transmitting and receiving sites. Physicians practicing teleradiology should conduct their practices in a manner consistent with the bylaws, rules, and regulations for patient care at the transmitting site and receiving jurisdiction."[40] TJC, on the other hand, has taken a different tack, allowing the distant setting to credential by proxy, as long as the home setting has credentialed the provider. Although it is more convenient and less costly for the distant setting to credential by proxy, risk management professionals must consider the potential exposure that this approach may create for negligent credentialing claims against the distant setting, as well as potential issues related to a lack of state licensure on the part of the remote physicians.

· · · · · · · · ·
INTERFACE WITH OTHER CLINICAL AREAS

High patient volume and the acuity of the patients in radiology make effective interaction with other clinical areas an essential risk management strategy. Here are several important issues and approaches.

1. The patient who comes to the radiology area from an intensive care unit (ICU) and is clinically fragile should be accompanied by a registered nurse. Any logistical issues associated with maintaining the level of care required by such patients should be proactively evaluated by the radiology area with key nursing managers.

2. Nursing managers, radiology professionals, medical records personnel, and others, as appropriate, should evaluate the way in which clinical information such as patient allergies, fall risk, and do not resuscitate status, as well as the procedure for which the patient is scheduled, are communicated.

    There are at least three issues underlying this premise. First, although the medical record should always accompany the patient to radiology, this does not always happen. Second, when the record is present, these key points must be easy for the staff to locate in the record. This, too, is sometimes an issue, either because the radiology staffs are not trained where to look or the information is in many different places. Third, some situations require a telephone discussion to facilitate proper planning for the radiology department's management of the patient.

3. Where there are multiple physicians caring for a patient and anesthesia or other medication may be required while the patient is in the radiology area, it must be clear which physician is to write that medication order. This can be a particularly problematic issue in the pediatric area, when the pediatrician assumes that he or she will control the decision about which medication is best to sedate a young child and a radiologist or anesthetist makes the same assumption.

4. There should be a predetermined approach for managing an intravenous line while the patient is in the radiology area. Many patients suffer needlessly, and clinical risk is increased, when intravenous lines must be restarted because the solution ran out or the battery died on an infusion pump.

5. Radiologists should read all emergency department films within twenty-four hours. There should also be formalized way to track the interpretation and follow up. Please see Chapter 12 on emergency department risk management for a suggested approach.

6. As interventional cardiologists and radiologists begin to perform the same types of procedures, it is important that a consistent credentialing process be maintained for both.

7. As the acuity of patients grows, it is essential that the referring physicians work with radiologists to make sure that patients are not too fragile to undergo procedures. Depending on the population of patients, development and monitoring of appropriate criteria may be appropriate.

TRADITIONAL RISK MANAGEMENT PRINCIPLES

Credentialing

It is important for the credentials committee of the organization to review radiology-related medical staff privileges on a frequent basis because they may need to be updated to encompass new technology and procedures. For example, percutaneous coronary intervention (PCI), including percutaneous transluminal coronary angioplasty (also known as PTCA), may now be performed in an interventional radiology lab, followed by a minimum twelve-hour observational stay. A credentialing statement published on the Web site of the Society for Interventional Radiology details the recommendations of a team of interventional radiologists and cardiovascular surgeons concerning training requirements for practitioners.[41]

Another important question for the credentials committee of the organization is whether obstetric practitioners who read ultrasounds on the labor and delivery unit should document competency training and whether test results should be read by radiology professionals trained in ultrasound.

Informed Consent

As radiology and the surgical suite come closer together, the complexity and risk of the procedures performed increases. All patients should be given adequate information to provide informed consent for invasive procedures, according to ACR standards.[42] (Please see Chapter 4 in this volume for more information on the general principles of informed consent.)

Medical Record Documentation

Concerning medical records, there are two major areas of which the risk management professional must be aware. The first is the rapid pace with which picture archiving and communication systems (PACSs) are digitalizing films and eliminating original images. When considering a PACS, points to consider from a risk management perspective include the following:

1. What is the view of the courts in your locale regarding the credibility of electronic imaging?

2. How will the PACS manage documentation associated with the film? Will clinicians be able to access other providers' interpretations? Will they be able to view the order and rationale for a procedure?

3. In general, how will the PACS interface with your existing documentation system?

Risk management professionals with traditional film libraries should be sure, as much as possible, that original films are not released. Once they are gone, they may not be seen again until discovery in a lawsuit. Exceptions to this general rule sometimes include release of films to physicians' offices. There should be a tracking system if such release is allowed, and the risk management professional must recognize that getting a film back from a codefendant physician may be difficult. The other exception is supported by the federal government and requires the release of original mammograms, rather than copies, because copies are too difficult to interpret.

The second major area for risk management of which professionals must be aware is the important role of radiation technologists in documentation. Many radiation technologists do not document in the medical record beyond the fact that they administered contrast medium, and yet they often observe critical changes in patients during the time that they are with them. For example, when asked if they document about a fall in the radiology department, many technologists will respond that they make out an adverse occurrence form. Although this is an important and appropriate approach, it does not take the place of concurrent documentation in the medical record when a case must be defended. Calling the floor nurse and describing what happened is an alternative approach, but the nurse's documentation does not have the same level of credibility as documentation by the person who was there. Also, if a patient experienced dizziness before he or she fell, the physician is unlikely to know this if the information is only on the incident report. Even if the floor nurse is likely to relay it in her documentation, there is still increased likelihood that the information will fall through the cracks.

Performance Improvement

Because radiology interfaces with so many other areas of the organization, it is important that radiology staff participate in housewide performance improvement initiatives. For example, the representative of the radiation safety committee might be part of the organization's performance improvement committee and/or the patient safety committee.

At a minimum, quality indicators reviewed should include those shared with other clinical areas (e.g., nursing units) regarding information received about methicillin-resistant *Staphylococcus aureus* patient status prior to their transport to the radiology area. Quality indicators may be drawn from standards and statements of key regulatory groups based on information gleaned from incident reporting trends and the facts underlying malpractice cases. The active participation of clinicians in developing and implementing quality indicators is critical to success.

· · · · · · · · ·
CONCLUSION

The technological advances in radiology will continue at an incredibly fast pace. The risk management professional can do much to increase the benefit and reduce the risk associated with this important clinical area.

Endnotes

1. "The History of Radiology." Available at: www.northhertsradiologygroup.co.uk/history. html. (Accessed December 16, 2009.)

2. "Medicine's Malediction." *Imaging Economics* 2004; (4):2.

3. "Rediscovering Radiology." *RT Image* 2004; 17(46).

4. "ACR Technical Standard for Medical Nuclear Physics Performance Monitoring of PET/ CT Imaging Equipment." The American College of Radiology. Revised 2008. Available at: www.acr.org/SecondaryMainMenuCategories/quality_safety/guidelines/med_phys/ pet_ct_equipment.aspx. (Accessed March 31, 2010.)

5. Berrington de Gonzalez, A. et al. "Projected Cancer Risks From Computed Tomographic Scans Performed in the United States in 2007." *The Annals of Internal Medicine* 2009; 169(22):2071–2077.

6. Smith-Bindman, R. et al. "Radiation Dose Associated with Common Computed Tomographic Examinations and the Associated Lifetime Attributable Risk of Cancer." *Annals of Internal Medicine* 2009; 169:2078–2086.

7. Redberg, RF. "Cancer Risks and Radiation Exposure From Computed Tomographic Scans: How Can We Be Sure That the Benefits Outweigh the Risks?" Editorial. *The Annals of Internal Medicine* 2009; 169(22):2049–2050.

8. Smith-Bindman, R., et al., *op. cit.*

9. NCI. "Radiation Risks and Pediatric Computed Tomography (CT): A Guide for Health Care Providers." Available at: www.cancer.gov/cancertopics/causes/radiation-risks-pediatric-CT. (Accessed December 12, 2009.)

10. Fromme, A. "Study Finds Huge Variations in Pediatric Nuclear Medicine Dosing." DiagnosticImaging.com. Available at: www.diagnosticimaging.com/news/display/article/ 113619/1179247?verify=0#. (Accessed March 31, 2010.)

11. Domino, D. "California RT gives deposition in CT overdose case." December 10, 2009. AuntMinnie.com. Available at: www.auntminnie.com/index.asp?sec=ser&sub=def&pag= dis&ItemID=88757. (Accessed March 31, 2010.)

12. Barnes, E. "Cedars-Sinai Raises Tally of Radiation Overdose Cases." November 13, 2009. AuntMinnie.com. Available at: www.auntminnie.com/index.asp?sec=ser&sub=def &pag=dis&ItemID=88220. (Accessed March 31, 2010.)

13. *Ibid.*

14. Hampton, T. "Full-body CT Scans Scale Up Cancer Risk." Medical News and Perspectives, *The Journal of the American Medical Association* 2004; 292:1669.

15. Shively, C. "Quality in Management Radiology." *Decisions in Imaging Economics* 2003; 11(6):6.

16. The American College of Radiology. "ACR Practice Guideline for Communication: Diagnostic Radiology." (2005) Available at: www.acr.org/SecondaryMainMenuCategorie s%2fquality_safety%2fguidelines%2fdx%2fcomm_diag_rad.aspx. (Accessed December 16, 2009.)

17. Kanal, et al. "ACR Guidance Document for Safe MR Practices: 2007." Available at: www.acr.org/SecondaryMainMenuCategories/quality_safety/MRSafety/safe_mr07.aspx. (Accessed December 16, 2009.)

18. *Ibid.*

19. *Ibid.*

20. Haygood, T.M. et al. "Timed Efficiency of Interpretation of Digital and Film-Screen Screening Mammograms." *American Journal of Roentgenology* 2009; 192(1): 216–220. Reprint available at: www.ajronline.org/cgi/reprint/192/1/216. (Accessed March 31, 2010.)

21. Pisano, E.D. et al. "Diagnostic Performance of Digital versus Film Mammography for Breast-Cancer Screening." *The New England Journal of Medicine* 2005; 353(17):1773–1783. Available at: http://content.nejm.org/cgi/content/ full/353/17/1773. (Accessed March 31, 2010.)

22. Vernacchia, F.S. et al. "Digital Mammography: Its Impact on Recall Rates and Cancer Detection Rates in a Small Community-Based Radiology Practice." *American Journal of Roentgenology* 2009; 193:582–585.

23. ACR. "Computer-Aided Detection for Mammography (CAD)" Available at: www.acr.org/ Hidden/Economics/FeaturedCategories/ManagedCare/resources_common_coverage/ ComputerAidedDetectionforMammographyCAD.aspx. (Accessed December 12, 2009.)

24. Brem, R.F. et al. "Breast-specific Gamma Imaging as an Adjunct Imaging Modality for the Diagnosis of Breast Cancer." *Radiology* 2008; 247:651–657.

25. "Breast-Specific Gamma Imaging (BSGI) Can Reduce The Number Of Unnecessary Breast Biopsies When Compared To MRI." Dilon Technologies Inc. March 19, 2009. Available at: http://www.medicalnewstoday.com/articles/142818.php. (Accessed March 31, 2010.)

26. Information about USPSTF available at: www.ahrq.gov/clinic/uspstfab.htm. (Accessed December 12, 2009.)

27. U.S. Preventive Services Task Force (USPSTF). "Screening for Breast Cancer: Recommendations and Rationale." Available at: www.ahrq.gov/clinic/3rduspstf/ breastCancer/brcanrr.htm. (Accessed December 12, 2009.)

28. USPSTF. "Mammography Recommendations Will Result in Countless Unnecessary Breast Cancer Deaths Each Year." Available at: www.acr.org/HomePageCategories/ News/ACRNewsCenter/USPSTFMammoRecs.aspx. (Accessed December 12, 2009.)

29. Statement posted on AHRQ Web site available at: www.ahrq.gov/clinic/USpstf/uspsbrca. htm. (Accessed December 12, 2009.)

30. See www.acr.org/SecondaryMainMenuCategories/quality_safety/BIRADSAtlas.aspx. (Accessed April 13, 2010.)

31. "ACR Practice Guideline for the Use of Intravascular Contrast Media." (Revised 2007.) Available at: www.acr.org/SecondaryMainMenuCategories/quality_safety/RadSafety/ OtherSafetyTopics/intravascular-contrast.aspx. (Accessed March 31, 2010.)

32. "Contrast-induced Neuropathy Doubles Risk of Adverse Events." June 25, 2009. Reuters Health New York. Available at: www.acr.org/SecondaryMainMenuCategories/ NewsPublications/FeaturedCategories/CurrentHealthCareNews/More/ NephropathyDoublesRisk.aspx. (Accessed March 31, 2010.)

33. Di Francesco, L. et al. "Prevention of Contrast-Induced Nephropathy." Chapter 32. *Making Health Care Safer: A Critical Analysis of Patient Safety Practices* Evidence Report/Technology Assessment, No. 43 AHRQ. Available at: www.ahrq.gov/clinic/ ptsafety/chap32.htm. (Accessed March 31, 2010.)

34. Mayo Clinic. "Advanced Radiology Life Support-Enduring Material. August 1, 2009-August 1, 2012" Available at: www.mayo.edu/cme/radiology.html. (Accessed March 31, 2010.)

35. "Credentialing Guidelines for Practitioners Who Are Not Anesthesia Professionals to Administer Anesthetic Drugs to Establish a Level of Moderate Sedation." Approved by the House of Delegates on October 25, 2005, and amended October 18, 2006. Available at: www.asahq.org/publicationsAndServices/standards/40.pdf. (Accessed December 16, 2009.)

36. "Practice Advisory for Magnetic Resonance Imaging: A Report by the American Society of Anesthesiologists Task Force on Anesthetic Care for Magnetic Resonance Imaging." *Anesthesiology* 2009; 110(3):3. Available at: http://journals.lww.com/anesthesiology/ Fulltext/2009/03000/Practice_Advisory_on_Anesthetic_Care_for_Magnetic.9.aspx. (Accessed December 16, 2009.)

37. "AANA-ASA Joint Statement Regarding Propofol Administration." Available at: www. asahq.org/news/propofolstatement.htm. (Accessed December 16, 2009.)

38. "Sedation With Propofol: A New ASA Statement." *American Society of Anesthesia Newsletter*. Available at: www.asahq.org/Newsletters/2005/02–05/whatsNew02_05. html. (Accessed December 16, 2009.)

39. "Report of the ACR Task Force on International Teleradiology." Available at: www.acr. org/SecondaryMainMenuCategories/BusinessPracticeIssues/Teleradiology/ ReportoftheACRTaskForceonInternationalTeleradiologyDoc3.aspx. (Accessed December 16, 2009.)

40. "ACR Standard for Electronic Practice of Medical Imaging 2007." p. 8. Available at: www.acr.org/SecondaryMainMenuCategories/quality_safety/guidelines/med_phys/ electronic_practice.aspx. (Accessed December 16, 2009.)

41. "Angioplasty Standard of Practice." Society of Interventional Radiology Standards of Practice Committee, James B. Spies, M.D., Chairman. *Journal of Vascular and Interventional Radiology* 2003; 14:s219–s221. Available at: www.sirweb.org/clinical/ cpg/S219.pdf. (Accessed March 31, 2010.)

42. ACR Practice Guideline on Informed Consent–Radiation Oncology. Rev. 2007. The American College of Radiology. Available at: www.acr.org/ SecondaryMainMenuCategories/quality_safety/guidelines/ro/informed_consent.aspx. (Accessed March 31, 2010.); ACR Practice Guideline on Informed Consent For Image-Guide Procedures. Revised 2006. The American College of Radiology. Available at: www.acr.org/SecondaryMainMenuCategories/quality_safety/guidelines/iv/informed_ consent_image_guided.aspx. (Accessed March 31, 2010.)

12

Emergency Department Risk Management: Promoting Quality and Safety in a Chaotic Environment

David Lickerman
Stephanie Lickerman

The emergency department (ED) is a rapidly changing and intense environment, one of the busiest and most chaotic in healthcare, yet it is also a place where the public has expectations of quality care. This dichotomy creates care issues and exacerbates malpractice risk.

A particularly concerning characteristic of the setting is the volatility of clinical circumstances and the large number of patients. Patients with widely differing severities of illness arrive in an uncontrolled manner, and the ED personnel must apply quick, yet thoughtful decision making and continual reassessment to ensure optimal healthcare for all who arrive at its doors. This activity has great significance to the entire healthcare organization because 60 to 75 percent of hospital admissions arrive through the ED. For the most part, patients who come to the ED do so because they believe they have an emergency and require prompt attention, but other patients come because the ED allows them immediate access to medical care. Ambulance traffic adds to the influx, and unless patients are processed and discharged (or admitted) rapidly, in the inpatient units as in the ED, high numbers of emergency patients will create an ED logjam.

Typically, medical care in the ED is performed in a linear fashion, so if the patient's needs become too complex, if multiple seriously ill or injured patients arrive at once, or if processing by another hospital department is delayed, the process of ED care will be slowed, leading to overcrowded, potentially unsafe conditions and dissatisfied customers.

ED overcrowding is a daily reality for many of the nation's hospitals. The Centers for Disease Control and Prevention (CDC) has reported that although the number of EDs has fallen by 12.3 percent, the number of visits has increased by 26 percent. EDs are seeing increased usage rates for all age groups, especially among people over sixty-five years old residing in an institutionalized setting and for Medicaid patients who receive ED treatment at four times the rate of those privately insured.[1]

In addition to these issues, there are team and schedule discrepancies. Shift changes for all staff positions (physician, nurse, resident, technician) are unsynchronized, and ED staff works all hours of the day, often several days in a row. Staffing of care teams is constantly changing, so ED workers must establish rapport, delineate leadership, and function as a team with a new mix of personnel daily. Further exacerbating this flux in personnel, rising malpractice rates and falling reimbursements have led some hospitals to contract with outside management groups to run EDs, and this can lead to revolving door ED physician staffing. Yet another major liability exposure is created because there are no established relationships between ED physicians and their patients. Because good relationships normally mitigate malpractice risk in private practice settings, caring and active communication are essential risk prevention behaviors for every member of the ED staff.

The multitude of patient safety–related and exposure-related issues require strong risk management approaches and ongoing monitoring of the effectiveness with which EDs function. By optimizing the safe handling of each patient through carefully constructed approaches that recognize the role of the ED as a department and an integral part of the healthcare organization, it is possible to enhance quality and reduce liability.

This chapter will expand on key issues and present practical solutions. The major focus here is on ED care: prehospital care is covered in the next chapter of this book.

· · · · · · · · ·

IN-HOSPITAL EMERGENCY MEDICINE CARE

The ED is the third most common site for significant medical errors, following only the operating room and the patient's hospital room. Considering the time spent by patients in each of these areas, the contribution of the ED is disproportionately large.[2] Because of high volumes, tight time constraints, and a need for ED physicians to act decisively even when hampered by incomplete data, errors are likely. However, some situations and conditions are more prone to error and generation of malpractice claims. As such, they fall into the hospital risk management professional's arena.

The Most Common Causes of ED Claims

The ED is an environment of controlled chaos and rapid decision making that is susceptible to error. An awareness of the changes in patient condition and good staff teamwork can salvage many potentially poor outcomes, but not all ED patient visits end well. Adverse outcomes that lead to malpractice claims occur sporadically, often without pattern in individual institutions, but aggregate national data are available and instructive. Examination of these data yields both general and specific advice for risk management professionals and the clinicians who work in their institutions.

True emergency conditions are limited in number, but to prevent poor outcomes and later litigation, it is imperative that emergency physicians approach all patients as though they possess an emergent condition. Thus each adult patient with chest pain must be regarded as a possible myocardial infarction; each headache must be suspected to be a cerebrovascular accident or meningitis; each abdominal pain must be seen as a potential intestinal obstruction, appendicitis, aortic aneurysm, ectopic pregnancy, testicular torsion, and so on. The problem, from a clinical standpoint, is that many of these conditions can present in an early stage or with unusual symptoms that make them difficult to recognize. This is particularly true of meningitis and appendicitis. However, the cases that are most costly to settle are those that present in a typical manner yet are misdiagnosed or mismanaged. The physician must consider the risks and benefits of diagnostic testing to the patient and balance the necessity of a definitive diagnosis against its cost, the diversion of ED and hospital resources from other patients, and the perils of a missed diagnosis. Even with careful attention to detail, the variable course of human illness and the fallibility of rapid decision making based on partial data have a strong tendency to deliver adverse outcomes that result in malpractice claims.

It is important for the risk management professional to understand both the nature of ED claims and the severity (cost) of the most common cases. National data for malpractice claims are fragmented because of the confidential nature of many settlements and because many institutions are self-insured with little policing of mandatory reporting as required by the National Practitioner Data Bank (NPDB). However, the Physician Insurers Association of America (PIAA) has conducted a large-scale longitudinal study (4,341 closed ED claims from 1985 to 2008) that can serve as a proxy for national data.[3] These data are physician-specific rather than hospital-specific, but hospitals are frequently named as defendants in the same cases. As a specialty, emergency medicine (EM) ranks sixteenth among the twenty-eight major specialties in monies paid and fifteenth in the number of claims reported. Among all specialties, EM claims constituted 3.99 percent of the claims and 2.51 percent of the indemnity payouts. These have increased from 1.6 percent and 1.18 percent, respectively, over the past ten years. When medical misadventures (the most significant contributor to medical error) are considered, errors in diagnosis were the largest category cited in slightly less than half of the claims. The second largest category was no medical misadventure. This category encompassed cases in which the EM physician was not negligent, but was named in the case. However, even in these cases, the EM physician participated in a payment 4.3 percent of the time.

It is important to note that medication errors accounted for less than 4 percent of the total claims, yet addressing medication issues is one of the goals of The Joint Commission (TJC) and National Quality Forum (NQF) for reducing errors in medical care. Although serious in their own right, they are targeted primarily because they are actionable and measurable items and not because they are the most frequent, lethal, or costly types of error according to ED malpractice data.

TABLE 12.1   Claims Category

Failure to Diagnose	*Individual Payout Severity*	*Overall Payout Severity*
Myocardial infarction	Meningitis	Myocardial infarction
Appendicitis	Head and spinal injuries	Meningitis
Abdominal conditions	Septicemia	Chest pain
Chest pain	Pulmonary embolism	Abdominal conditions
Meningitis		Appendicitis

In order of frequency, these are the clinical issues associated with the most common high-dollar lawsuits for failure to diagnose cases:[4]

1. Myocardial infarction (26.7 percent)
2. Appendicitis (26.5 percent)
3. Abdominal conditions (18 percent)
4. Chest pain, not further defined (14 percent)
5. Meningitis (14 percent)

Other insurers report head injury and cerebral condition, spinal injury and condition, obstetric-related, respiratory distress, and infection as categories with significant incidence and dollar losses.[5]

The diagnoses with the highest individual payout (severity) for the ED, in decreasing order, are meningitis, head and spinal injuries, septicemia, and pulmonary embolism. However, because these are not the most frequent causes of malpractice claims, a different group of conditions has the highest overall payout. Myocardial infarction and meningitis head this list, followed by chest pain, abdominal conditions, and appendicitis. See Table 12.1 for categories of claims. Among pediatric patients, failure to diagnose appendicitis and meningitis are the two most liability-prone conditions for emergency room physicians.[6]

Chest conditions, other than myocardial infarction, that result in malpractice claims include ruptured thoracic aortic aneurysm, pulmonary embolism, pneumonia, and cancer. Serious abdominal conditions other than appendicitis that can result in malpractice claims include ruptured abdominal aortic aneurysms, intestinal obstruction, bowel infarctions, abscesses, ectopic pregnancy, and cancers.

The following paragraphs will delineate clinical and risk management issues associated with or surrounding the highest severity conditions, accompanied by risk reduction strategies for risk management professionals.

Myocardial Infarction   Patients with chest pain, and in particular acute myocardial infarction (AMI), constitute the single most costly diagnostic group in EM, accounting for about one quarter of all EM malpractice dollar losses. In addition, chest pain is the most common symptom of patients who come to the ED. ED physicians and nurses must unerringly sort these patients into either minor (costochondral pain, heartburn) or emergent (myocardial infarction) categories, yet the variety of symptoms presented by this group of patients makes this difficult. Among all specialties, emergency medicine ranks third in claims frequency and severity for misdiagnosis or mistreatment of AMI. However, when considering ED cases only, misdiagnosis of AMI is the largest single category and the major condition most likely to result in a paid claim.

Misdiagnosis   The PIAA Acute Myocardial Infarction Study[7] found that 77 percent of AMI patients whose care resulted in a malpractice claim died because of either diagnostic or treatment errors. Projected earnings losses and family hardships result in large awards, especially when a relatively young patient experiences sudden death because of a missed diagnosis. These younger patients are also more likely to survive an AMI, and thus future medical care costs and noneconomic damages may increase indemnity costs. In fact, the age cohort with the highest average indemnity payout is the thirty- to thirty-nine-year-old age group. However, this age cohort represents only about 12 percent of the total number of cases. Claimants in the forty- to fifty-nine-year-old age group make up 58 percent of the total. The diagnosis of a typical AMI patient (male, older age, crushing chest pain, radiation down the left arm) is not often missed, but his care can still be mismanaged. Patients whose presentations are less typical are more frequently misdiagnosed and, consequently, mismanaged.

Myocardial infarction patients who are misdiagnosed tend to be younger, female, and present with other than typical symptoms. According to this PIAA study, one quarter of these chest pain patients were given a gastrointestinal diagnosis and another 20 percent were diagnosed as having rib cage pain. Other common features of these claims included an incomplete history or physical examination, an inexperienced ED physician, and, because AMI was not suspected in 21 percent of cases, no EKG was performed. Inexperienced physicians are also more likely to depend on enzyme tests; however, enzyme levels do not become abnormal for several hours, and a clinical judgment based on early tests provides only false reassurance. Performance of a risk factor assessment has been promoted as a solution, but fails to identify a significant number of patients with heart conditions. Among patients with AMI who sued for malpractice, the PIAA AMI Study found that nearly 70 percent of claimants had no prior history of coronary artery disease, and about half of males (and two-thirds of females) had no history of smoking or hypertension.[8]

Women are more likely than men to have a missed diagnosis of myocardial infarction and are less likely to have been properly treated. This is, at least in part, because women delay coming to the hospital and their symptoms tend to be atypical. Almost half of heart attacks in women present with shortness of breath, nausea, indigestion, fatigue, and shoulder pain, not chest pain.[9] It is clear from the preceding discussion that atypical symptoms should be considered as a typical presentation in order to most reliably diagnose AMI, especially in women.

Delayed Treatment

Misdiagnosis is not the only issue in ED AMI-related malpractice claims. Delayed treatment is also increasingly important. As thrombolytic therapy (clot-busting drugs) and primary angioplasty (cardiac catheterization laboratory intervention) have become established as standard treatment, there has been an increase in the number of suits filed with claims of delayed diagnosis and delayed treatment of AMI. An evolving trend is the allegation that failure to use or delay in the use of these treatments falls below the standard of care and that earlier use would have preserved cardiac function or saved a life. The PIAA AMI Study found that 14.3 percent of all AMI cases that involved treatment errors originated in the ED, with the average payment being 44 percent higher for cases in which thrombolytic use was a factor. The current TJC performance measurement system, ORYX® criteria for acute myocardial infarction (AMI), evaluates an organization's success in using ED-delivered thrombolytic therapy for AMI in thirty minutes or less, or alternatively, angioplasty within ninety minutes or less. These outcome criteria appear to be deceptively simple, but achieving them requires a high degree of focus in the ED, coupled with coordination between the ED and the department of cardiology. For the ED to meet these tight time constraints, a particular series of events has to happen in rapid succession. First, there must be recognition by the healthcare staff that the patient's symptoms represent a possible AMI. Next, an EKG must be taken and assessed and the physician ascertains the necessary treatment. The patient then has intravenous access established, and, finally, either the clot-dissolving drug is administered or the patient is taken to the cardiac catheterization laboratory.

How Can the Risk Management Professional Help?   Enhancing patient safety and reducing malpractice exposure are better achieved if certain resources are available to the ED, first to aid in diagnosing and treating these conditions and second to help move affected patients to a higher level of care promptly, either in the same hospital or by appropriate transfer to another facility. The risk management professional should advocate that the organization address the following points, which are key in meeting these very time-constrained goals:

- Make certain that there are enough EKG machines available in case of multiple simultaneous arrivals.

- Provide education to facilitate the decision of the ED physician to administer thrombolytics without first consulting a cardiologist.

- Make sure that the thrombolytic medications are stocked in the ED and available for immediate use.

- Make certain that there is a rapid retrieval system for obtaining prior EKGs for comparison.

- Make sure that, if direct intervention in the catheterization laboratory is indicated, strategies are in place to do so. Some effective strategies include use of a call schedule identifying a single responsible cardiologist for the day, activation of the catheterization laboratory by ED physicians (rather than cardiologists), establishment of a single-call activation system using a central paging operator to notify the cardiologist and catheterization lab team, and use of prehospital ECGs to identify candidates before they even arrive in the ED.[10] This last strategy can allow bypass of the ED altogether but will still require the ED to activate the catheterization lab team.

- Make sure STAT cardiac blood tests have both a rapid turnaround time and an established feedback route so that the initial ordering physician receives the results in a timely fashion.[11]

Some key strategies for risk management professionals apply to all high-risk conditions:

- Participate in construction of orientation materials for ED physicians. Make sure that clinical and risk management information concerning AMI diagnosis and treatment are part of the program. These programs should emphasize the high number of atypical presentations, the need to carefully evaluate complaints of chest pain, the need to correlate current and past cardiac diagnostic tests, the need to look for cardiac risk factors (family history, smoking, hypertension), and the need to coordinate diagnostic testing with primary care physicians and cardiology consultants. Above all, emergency physicians should be advised to maintain a high level of suspicion for coronary conditions and to admit patients if it is not possible to exclude a diagnosis of active cardiac disease in the ED.

- Participate in quality improvement committees and departmental staff meetings. Present clinical and risk management information to those present and disseminate information to those who are not able to attend the meetings. Encourage the use of data feedback to clinical staff on their performance in relation to the quality targets.

- Speak at hospital grand rounds or arrange for a speaker to address risk management issues with clinical relevance, such as communication, documentation, medical misadventures, and the need to immediately notify the risk management professional of any adverse events.

Meningitis

Meningitis is an infection of the covering of the brain that is difficult to diagnose, disastrous if not treated promptly, and costly to settle when the issue in a lawsuit. The typical symptoms of meningitis include fever, headache, lethargy, vomiting, and neck stiffness. The difficulty associated with diagnosis is due to the fact that these same symptoms are often seen in more common illnesses such as influenza or respiratory infections. The most severely affected patients are often children under the age of two, and they are even more difficult to diagnose, due in part to communication problems. Meningitis may be caused by viruses, bacteria, or fungi. Patients with bacterial meningitis can die within hours to a few days or be left with life-long disabilities that result in high medical care costs. Patients with fungal meningitis are likely to have a more drawn-out course, but have no better clinical results.

Although not the most frequent of cases, meningitis is among the most costly to settle. The PIAA Data Sharing Project (2005) reported on 48,936 cases over ten years that were settled with indemnity payments.[12] Of these, only seventy-three (0.8 percent) concerned meningitis, but indemnity costs for these cases averaged $308,303, whereas the average for all cases was only $163,711. Family practice and pediatric physicians were defendants in 66 percent of the cases and emergency physicians in less than 10 percent, but in 21 percent of the cases the critical incident occurred in the ED. Where the original point of contact for the patient was in the ED, indemnity averaged nearly $1.4 million and accounted for approximately half of the indemnity paid. The claims involving the worst outcomes and highest payouts were much more likely to involve younger ages. Although the median age was two years and 60.3 percent of the patients died, the majority (82.6 percent) of deaths occurred in patients under one year of age. The highest indemnity costs were paid when patients survived the illness but were brain damaged, quadriplegic, or required lifelong care. For these cases, the average indemnity was $2,633,689, and although they made up only 17.8 percent of meningitis cases, they accounted for more than half of the total indemnity costs.

The most common error (70 percent) in these cases was a delay in or failure to diagnose meningitis. Meningitis is commonly misdiagnosed as a viral upper respiratory infection, ear infection, or migraine headache. Delay or failure to perform a diagnostic lumbar puncture was seen in 23.3 percent of cases. In these cases, there were multiple symptoms that should have prompted consideration of a lumbar puncture, but the procedure was not performed in a timely fashion to aid in diagnosis. Delay in admission to the hospital was also cited in 26 percent of cases. Poor communication, telephone treatment, and inadequate documentation were common remediable causes of large settlements. Clinicians should be advised to maintain a high index of suspicion for meningitis and diligently record negative findings.

How Can the Risk Management Professional Help?   The risk management professional can assist the clinical staff by pointing out to key managers that lumbar puncture supplies should be readily available in the ED. In many institutions, radiologists perform lumbar punctures with the help of imaging equipment when emergency physicians encounter difficulties. This resource should be available on a round-the-clock basis. Quality improvement efforts should be focused on reducing delays in diagnosis and treatment, with coordination among emergency physicians, radiologists, and infectious disease specialists in the institution. The risk management professional can facilitate process improvement by setting up a meeting between these physician specialists. Blood test results should be expedited and antibiotics stocked in the ED for ready access. Through orientation materials or risk management education initiatives, clinicians should be reminded of the following actions that reduce losses and improve patient care:

- Maintain a high index of suspicion for meningitis when presented with a patient with a headache, fever, and altered mental status and do not hesitate to order a lumbar puncture.

- Listen carefully to the history provided by the patient and/or family, especially to caregivers of infants.

- Document carefully, including positive findings, significant negative findings, and the treatment plan.

- Thoroughly evaluate patients with suspected meningitis, treat them immediately, and admit them if the diagnosis is not completed in the ED.

- Patients who are discharged should receive clear instructions (verbal and written) about symptoms that should prompt an immediate return.

Appendicitis

Cases involving a missed diagnosis of appendicitis were the second most frequently cited error in diagnosis in the 2009 PIAA study and made up 26.5 percent of the missed diagnosis claim category.[13] However, only 25 percent of appendicitis claims result in an indemnity payment, and these are responsible for only 3 percent of the total indemnity for emergency medicine. Whereas the average indemnity for all ED cases involving diagnostic errors was $255,447, the average for appendicitis cases was lower, at $59,043. Appendicitis is a condition that develops over time and thus affords a greater opportunity to identify the problem at an earlier stage. When fully developed, a case of appendicitis with rupture is easily diagnosed, but treatment at that late stage can result in lasting complications or death. In the earliest stages, when diagnosis and treatment would prevent complications, it is often indistinguishable from common illnesses such as viral gastroenteritis and food poisoning. The classic triad of right lower-quadrant abdominal pain, fever, and elevated white blood count occurs in only one-third of cases, thus making the majority of cases more difficult to diagnose. The pediatric population poses a special problem for the ED physician, in part due to the inability to obtain a history from a child presenting with abdominal pain.

Unfortunately, there is no definitive appendicitis test. Currently, the best test is a computed tomography (CT) scan of the abdomen, which can be falsely negative and is always costly and time-consuming. For these reasons, patients who will be scanned must be chosen carefully from among a larger group of patients who present to the emergency department with abdominal pain. Furthermore, these scans are too complex to be interpreted by most emergency physicians and must be read by a radiologist. Even radiologists' interpretations are not infallible due to anatomic variability, technical difficulty, and errors in human judgment. The well-known difficulties inherent in making an early diagnosis with any degree of reliability and the nonfatal outcomes in most cases of appendicitis contribute to the low average awards for misdiagnosis of this condition.

How Can the Risk Management Professional Help?   The most important action is to advocate for the round-the-clock availability of in-house abdominal CT scans followed by timely radiological interpretation provided to the ED physician. Other actions include the following:

- Provide clinical education for ED physicians so that they recognize the subtlety of early presentations of appendicitis. A high degree of suspicion is essential.

- Encourage ED physicians to specify a short follow-up interval in the discharge instructions when patients diagnosed with gastroenteritis are sent home, and make certain that these instructions specifically name symptoms that should prompt an immediate return to the ED.

- Ensure availability of an on-call surgeon at all times. Implement procedures to facilitate rapid ED to OR transfer to prevent rupture of the appendix in diagnosed patients.

Head Injuries and Conditions

These conditions do not make up a substantial proportion of ED malpractice claims in large studies, but they are high-severity and high-cost conditions when death or disability is the outcome. This group includes acute subdural and epidural hematomas and, to a lesser degree, slower-developing subdural hematomas. Headache is a common complaint among ED patients, and in some cases there is little to distinguish between patients who are innocuously versus emergently affected. Whereas subdural and epidural hematomas are relatively easy to see on head CT scans, early subarachnoid bleeding is not easily visible. Subarachnoid bleeds require a lumbar puncture (LP) for diagnosis, and the decision to perform this somewhat invasive and time-consuming procedure can be a difficult clinical decision for the ED physician. Knowledge of the serious consequences (death, stroke) of missing a subarachnoid hemorrhage may push the ED physician to perform an LP. Any related malpractice cases may be costly because these conditions, if diagnosed early, can be treated with a high degree of success, whereas even brief delays can result in the death of the patient. These conditions have in common the need for a high index of suspicion on the part of the ED physician, ready accessibility of properly interpreted head CT scans, and rapid neurosurgical support.

How Can the Risk Management Professional Help?   Twenty-four-hour availability of head CT scanning and rapid interpretation by neuroradiologists are key to proper diagnosis and treatment for these patients. The risk management professional should investigate the availability of these services in the institution and facilitate their availability when necessary. Other actions might include the following:

- Rapid access to neurosurgical support means having a neurosurgeon on call or having prearranged transfer agreements with another institution when neurosurgeons are not available at your hospital. If your hospital does not have an on-call neurosurgeon, encourage ED staff to affect rapid transfers as soon as these conditions are identified.

- Performance of a lumbar puncture requires the full attention of a minimum of two staff, one to hold and position the patient and the other to perform the LP. Adequate staffing is necessary.

Spinal Injuries and Conditions

Spinal injuries are the result of accidents. They become risk management problems when there is either a failure to stabilize (support) the injured area during transport to the hospital, transfer from stretcher to bed, movement for imaging studies or during treatment, or a failure to recognize the significance of patient complaints of neck or back pain. In many cases, the crucial error was that a stabilizing cervical collar was removed for X-rays and not replaced, thus allowing too much freedom of movement of an unstable fracture or ligamentous injury. Injury to the spinal cord can result in permanent paralysis for the patient and the need for costly medical care for the rest of his or her life. If such a preventable injury occurs during medical care, it will surely result in a costly malpractice claim. Failure to rapidly treat these injuries with high-dose methylprednisolone, though a controversial treatment, may also be the source of a malpractice claim.

Spinal conditions are caused by objects that take up space in the spinal canal, crowding and injuring the spinal cord. These may include herniated disks, vascular malformations, and malignant tumors. These can grow without notice until a critical size is reached, at which time they compress and may irreversibly damage the spinal cord. When a patient presents with symptoms of this type, they must be diagnosed and treated within the narrow window of a few hours. Failure to do so may well create lasting disability for the patient and liability for the healthcare providers and institution. These injuries are best diagnosed with MRI, so around-the-clock availability of an MRI is critical for institutions that handle trauma. ED personnel should also be familiar with size and weight limitations of the hospital's equipment as oversized patients may require expedited transfer for definitive care.

How Can the Risk Management Professional Help?   The risk management professional should advocate for the following:

- Development and adherence to protocols regarding safeguards for patients with back and neck injuries in the field, ED, and radiology department

- Development of specific protocols that delineate the process for clearing a cervical spine injury, including under what circumstances a cervical collar can be removed and by whom

- Education for ED physicians and staff about the importance of early diagnosis for spinal conditions

- Availability of spinal CT and MRI for patients with potential spinal injuries and conditions

- Maintenance of an on-call list for neurosurgeons to facilitate emergency surgical treatment

Medical Procedure Errors

Among medical procedures, errors in intubation are the most common (49 percent), followed by cardiac arrest management (13 percent), vascular line placement (13 percent), restraints (6 percent), and others (19 percent).[14] Errors in performance of skin procedures (primarily laceration repairs) are also important. Excessive severity and high losses disproportionate to the injury are found in cases that involve intubation errors and vascular line placement. Missed foreign bodies in wounds also continue to make up a frequent, and avoidable, cause of emergency medical malpractice claims.

Wounds are a common reason for patients to visit an ED, and they represent up to 24 percent of malpractice claim allegations in some studies. However, they are typically associated with low severity and therefore account for only about 3 to 4 percent of total indemnity.[15,16] Most malpractice allegations that involve wounds are concerned with failure to find and remove a foreign body, failure to diagnose nerve or tendon injuries, and failure to identify and treat infection-prone wounds.[17,18] These cases are remarkable because they are both numerous and easily avoidable. Discharging a patient with a retained foreign body in a wound is both embarrassing and difficult to defend, not to mention aggravating to the patient.

Most foreign bodies can be detected when the proper modality is used. Metallic foreign bodies (including aluminum) and glass foreign bodies that are 2 mm in size or greater can easily be seen on radiographs.[19] Wooden foreign bodies are often difficult to detect clinically but can be well visualized by ultrasound, CT, or MRI.[20] Plastic is particularly well visualized with MRI scanning.

Patients are often sent home from the ED with a full foreign body or partial piece still present that will later be identified when imaging studies are read by a radiologist. Physician responsibility for radiograph interpretation and patient follow-up is frequently an issue in malpractice claims.[21] There must be coordinated action between the departments of emergency medicine and radiology. Potential misinterpretations of X-rays, which are often subtle and often read quickly, necessitate a reliable system for reading by radiologists. The same principle of cross-checking by specialists is also important to consider for EKGs and laboratory results. Patients with discrepant readings or new findings must be notified, and this notification must be documented. The ED's quality improvement program should review all ED discrepancy reports, offering guidance and support to physicians and staff for system and process redesign. Finally, remember that undiagnosed tendon lacerations are an important problem, accounting for 8 percent of all ED diagnostic errors in one study.[22]

How Can the Risk Management Professional Help?   The risk management professional should educate the ED physicians so that they understand the necessity of X-raying or imaging wounds that potentially contain foreign bodies and the likelihood of success when these tests are performed. Other actions might include the following:

- Provide education about the frequency and cost of these claims.
- Establish protocols for the management of all X-ray, lab, and EKG discrepancies, including patient follow-up notification, documentation, and reporting to risk management when injury is sustained.

Diagnostic Interview and Physical Examination Deficiencies

The most basic elements of emergency medical practice (the diagnostic interview and physical exam) are sometimes either not performed or not documented well enough to serve the defense in a malpractice case. When the different components of an ED visit are broken out as procedures, failure to perform a diagnostic interview (patient history) is the most common root cause of claims, with failure to perform a general physical examination identified as another of the most common omissions.[23] History and physical examinations are the mainstays of proper physician diagnosis. They are essential in the process of elimination (ruling out what the patient does not have) and discovering the proper diagnosis (defining what the patient does have). However, many serious conditions can present in an early stage when symptoms might be minimal and physical signs subtle or nonexistent. The role of the history and physical examination should not be underestimated, for this is where the majority of ED diagnoses are made. It is also where the majority of misdiagnoses occur.

Diagnostic testing is critical in sorting benign conditions from emergencies. Although the emergency physician's training and experience come into play in arriving at judicious test choices, ultimately, information obtained during the history and physical determines whether the right diagnostic tests are obtained. It is neither possible, nor economically feasible, to perform diagnostic tests for every condition in every patient; therefore, it is vital to take a complete and thorough history and physical exam (H&P). One of the most important things a doctor can do during the H&P is to listen to the patient and be aware that patients often list the real reason they came to the ED as an addendum, at the end of the history. Attention paid to an "oh, by the way, doc" can help both the physician and patient prevent many hours of clinical sleuthing. Additionally, a 1984 study found that doctors initiating a medical interview wait an average of only 18 seconds before interrupting a patient.[24] The findings of this study received widespread attention, but have resulted in only incremental improvement. A 1999 follow-up study showed the average length of time given patients to itemize their concerns before the first redirection (interruption) was 23.1 seconds per interview or 28 percent longer.[25] Patients who come to the ED often are injured and in pain. Interrupting their train of thought and verbal flow will not help the doctor decipher the patient's problem. The ED physician must use both technical diagnostic and active listening skills during the physical exam to achieve optimum results.

Importance of Discharge Plans

To reduce risk, discharge plans must be carefully constructed to direct patients to the next step in care or prompt a return to the ED. Inevitably, some patients will be sent home without a definitive diagnosis, some will leave with the wrong diagnosis, and some will need follow-up care at a more specialized medical or surgical practice. Discharge plans must specify a physician or practice for follow-up and a definite time interval within which the patient will have follow-up care. This time should be relatively short to limit the adverse effects of a misdiagnosis. Obviously, it is important to include family members in the discharge planning of pediatric patients, but this also needs to be done with geriatric patients because the prevalence of cognitive impairment among elderly patients in the ED is 16 percent.[26] Discharge instructions should provide information about the diagnosis and should include a delineation of symptoms for which the patient should seek immediate physician consultation or return to the ED. Patients retain this information better when they receive it both verbally and in written form. Written information must be carefully evaluated to make certain that the reading level is calibrated for best comprehension by the widest patient audience: this is at about the sixth-grade level. Attaining this comprehension level is nearly impossible to achieve with handwritten instructions. Many EDs use written templates that allow common conditions to be circled or checked, but computerized systems now on the market are more complete and condition-specific in their explanations and advice. Patients with limited reading skills also benefit from a combination of verbal descriptions and visual depictions of their conditions.

··········
TRENDS IN ED MALPRACTICE

The Emergency Medical Treatment and Labor Act (EMTALA) is a federal law intended to prevent *dumping* of uninsured ED patients from one hospital to another. The dumping referred to in the act was the rapid transfer of unstable patients from private to public hospitals without evaluation or provision of stabilizing treatment in an effort to avoid the financial loss associated with an uninsured (or underinsured) patient. Media attention to this practice and consequent public outcry forced Congress to act, and the law was quickly passed in 1986. The act's basic principles have been sustained; however, its language has been subjected to a series of judicial and administrative interpretations. Because it mandates an initial ED medical screening examination (MSE) and stabilizing treatment, with the threat of fines or removal of a hospital from the Medicare program unless such treatment is provided, EMTALA has become the legislative equivalent of an unfunded national health insurance program.

The Department of Health and Human Services, Centers for Medicare & Medicaid Services (CMS), issued the "Emergency Medical Treatment and Labor Act (EMTALA) Revised Interpretive Guidelines" on May 13, 2004.[27] These guidelines define *hospitals with an emergency department* to mean a hospital with a dedicated ED. These regulations further define dedicated emergency department as any department or facility of the hospital that

1. is licensed by the state as an ED;

2. is held out to the public as providing treatment for emergency medical conditions; or

3. treats one-third of those who visit the department in the preceding calendar year for emergency medical conditions on an urgent basis.

The basic tenets in the law that apply to emergency medicine are (1) that all dedicated EDs (free-standing or within hospitals) must provide a medical screening exam

(MSE; a triage evaluation is not acceptable) calculated to determine the presence or absence of an emergency medical condition and (2) that all emergency medical conditions must be treated and stabilized within the organization's capabilities before discharge or transfer. There are two exceptions: unstable patients may be transferred if they require a higher level of care than is available in the present ED or if they request a transfer in writing. Transferring physicians must send pertinent test results and all documentation (including the name and location of the receiving physician and hospital). The law applies to all patients, not just Medicare recipients, and includes any patients presenting within 250 yards of the main hospital buildings.[28] Please see Chapter 1 in Volume 3 for information on statutes, standards and regulations.

EMTALA has created many challenges for the ED. Appropriate patient stabilization may require the services of on-call medical staff. This has created a situation in which physicians have resigned from hospital medical staffs to avoid their on-call obligation, usually because of concern about increased medical malpractice liability, lack of financial compensation, and the time commitment. In the most recent final rule publication by CMS in 2003, physicians are given latitude to be on call for more than one institution, schedule surgeries during on-call time periods, and limit calls when there are only a few physicians on staff to take a call for a specialty. This most recent interpretation has been helpful to hospitals (who are required to supply on-call physicians with no more leverage than medical staff bylaw provisions) in recruiting some physicians to take calls, but at the same time making it difficult to completely fill the call schedule, especially with specialists. Physician specialists, where they are few in number, are off the hook and free to limit their on-call obligations. This is undesirable from an EM and, arguably, a liability standpoint, because the result in many hospitals has been to create gaps in physician specialist coverage, which makes it necessary to transfer patients to hospitals with available physician specialists.

Additionally, the law does not state who (physician, nurse, physician extender) has to perform the medical screening exam (MSE), but compliance is generally ensured if it is done by a physician. Those EDs using nonphysicians for MSEs must have a hospital board–approved plan, and even with this plan, a ruling may be made that a physician should have completed the exam.[29]

It is important to note that admission to the hospital (whether the patient is stable or unstable) or following treatment in the ED such that the patient is considered medically stable, ends the hospital's obligations under EMTALA. An ED physician's judgment that the patient has reached stability should be documented in the medical record prior to discharge. Risk management professionals can contribute to ED efforts to comply with the law by ensuring that the hospital has standing transfer agreements with neighboring hospitals that represent higher levels of care, whether that means possessing on-call specialists, specialized care units, or the services available in tertiary referral centers.

Psychiatric patients, who frequently require transfer to other institutions, present special problems. If acutely ill, they are often not competent to give consent for or refuse transfer. In addition, their psychiatric problems are not typically resolved within the course of ED treatment. Transfer, in the first case, requires documentation of the patient's condition and decision-making incompetence. With regard to the second case, the stabilization required by law has a different meaning than in medical cases: that the patient is rendered unable to harm himself or herself or others prior to discharge or during transport. As detailed in the next section, the disposition of psychiatric patients is a complex issue that includes EMTALA ramifications.

· · · · · · · · ·
MANAGEMENT OF PSYCHIATRIC PATIENTS

Safe handling of psychiatric patients in the ED represents a special challenge. These patients may present with psychiatric complaints or exhibit dangerous and aggressive behaviors, yet have underlying medical problems that require immediate attention.

The Assessment of the Psychiatric Patient

Although screening by psychiatric social workers is a boon to busy ED physicians, EMTALA and reasonable prudence make it desirable that an ED physician personally evaluate the patient. This is particularly true in two circumstances. The first arises if there is any sign of medical illness. Psychiatric patients admitted to the hospital with no sign of acute medical illness can receive more extensive assessment on an as-needed basis as inpatients. Patients who are being discharged from the ED require more careful scrutiny.

The second circumstance for which it is particularly valuable to have physician assessment concerns patients who are depressed and have expressed suicidal thoughts. Under these circumstances, ED physicians must carefully consider the level of risk before deciding that discharge is safe. This is problematic in that it is not possible to be correct 100 percent of the time. Trained psychiatric specialists occasionally underestimate the suicidal potential of their patients. Psychiatric patients can also be a danger to others, which requires that the physician who is discharging such a person has a "duty to warn." When these patients make threats against named persons, the ED doctor has a duty to either detain the patient (admit) or warn the named parties so that they may take necessary action to protect themselves. The advent of the Health Insurance Portability and Accountability Act (HIPAA) has not altered this requirement. Usually, admission is the safest course, in which case an evaluation by the patient's psychiatrist can be made.

The Psychiatric Patient Awaiting Disposition

It is wise to establish ED procedures for handling psychiatric patients so that their care is well reasoned and consistent. The medical record documentation of observation and interventions concerning psychiatric patients are key to the defense of any subsequent medical malpractice action.

Aggressive, agitated psychiatric patients may require restraint or seclusion, making them a high-risk subset of the ED population. TJC requirements include careful assessment of patients in restraints so that the least restrictive measures are used, the indications are clear, and criteria for release are set. Patients must be reevaluated at prescribed intervals. Initial face-to-face physician evaluation is required and must be repeated every four hours. This is true for the use of both physical and chemical restraints. Patients who are in seclusion should have one-on-one monitoring by an ED staff member. Video surveillance of such patients is not a substitute for direct observation, and videotaping without monitoring the patient merely documents neglect if patients harm themselves. All psychiatric patients should be searched for weapons on arrival, preferably by hospital security personnel. Medications and weapons might be concealed in clothing. To enhance the security of patients and staff, patients should therefore be asked to exchange their clothing for paper scrub suits.

Transfer or Discharge of Psychiatric Patients

When psychiatric patients are transferred, it must be done after reasonable measures have been undertaken to stabilize the patient. This may include physical or chemical restraints and should be undertaken with the assistance of ambulance crews who have been trained to prevent either self-harm or elopement. As previously noted, EMTALA forms must be completed and medical record documentation should include clear, objective documentation of any lack of competency to consent.

If these patients are discharged, medical record documentation should reflect a well-reasoned assessment indicating that the patient is medically cleared and emotionally stable.

PROCESS ISSUES

The flow of patients in and out of emergency departments and the EDs' ability to treat those patients successfully and process them correctly carries significant implications for risk management professionals.

Patient Flow

ED patient flow is a significant patient safety issue and is the product of patient volume, illness severity, ED flow, and hospital throughput. National ED annual patient volume has increased steadily from 89.8 million in 1992 to 120 million in 2006.[30] Although not evenly distributed among EDs, this increase has been nearly universal, and EDs have been forced to deal with a higher volume of patients, many of whom are elderly, ill, or both. At the same time, inpatient bed availability has been adversely affected by financial pressures and a shortage of nursing staff. The end result has been that patients stack up in the ED, particularly during evening hours when incoming volume peaks and patients admitted during the day are still occupying ED beds. When the ED becomes overloaded, patients wait for inordinately long periods of time in the waiting room, ambulances are diverted away from the hospital, patients who need care leave against medical advice (AMA) or leave without being seen (LWBS), and the hospital suffers loss of revenue and reputation and patient care diminishes.

In 2006, 2.4 million potential patients (2 percent) walked out of U.S. EDs without being seen, and another 1.3 percent left without completing their care.[31] This is a failure of the ED's function as a safety net for the community's healthcare. The importance of this function has been recognized in the TJC's 2005 focus on ED patient flow as a patient safety issue. This is also a legitimate concern of the risk management professional. As patient care is delayed, there is an increased potential for adverse events in the waiting room, in the crowded ED, and among those patients whose ambulance transport is prolonged. As an example, a University of Texas School of Public Health study found that severely injured patients are twice as likely to die when area Level I trauma centers are on diversion.[32]

ED Process Inefficiencies Resulting in Errors

The ED is adversely affected by an inability to control patient inflow and outflow, by ED staff, by space limitations, and by the need to depend on other departments for rapid turnaround of diagnostic testing. Although all of these factors contribute to delays, the Government Accountability Office (GAO) found that the factor most commonly associated with crowding was the inability to transfer emergency patients to inpatient beds once a decision had been made to admit them as hospital patients rather than to treat and release them.[33]

As previously mentioned, ED patients are typically processed in a linear fashion. The patient enters at the triage desk, proceeds to registration, is placed in an ED bed, is assessed by an ED nurse, and is examined by the physician who then writes orders for patient diagnosis and treatment. Testing and treatment are completed and a disposition is made. Refer to Figure 12.1 for an annual plot of ED patient registration times for a community hospital and Figure 12.2 for ED flow.

This system is vulnerable to catastrophic failure during high-volume periods, and high-volume periods are encountered on a daily basis in most emergency departments.

Several solutions have emerged in EDs across the country to counter these problems.

- Use of real-time information or tracking systems to monitor patient flow accompanied by proactive steps to reduce crowding. This is most efficiently accomplished by using computer tracking systems coupled with preplanned protocols for overload conditions.

- Use of a fast-track system, which diverts patients with minor illnesses away from the main ED to a smaller area with a dedicated physician or midlevel provider and nursing staff. This can significantly reduce treatment time for these patients and unburden the ED of up to 40 percent of the normal volume.

- Flexible staffing of the ED and triage areas. For example, in overload conditions, on-duty staff may be asked to extend their shifts, on-call staff may be called in, a nurse or technician may float to the triage area to handle a large number of simultaneous arrivals, and physicians and nurses in administrative positions may assume temporary clinical roles at triage or in the main ED.

FIGURE 12.1   Emergency Department Patient Registration Time

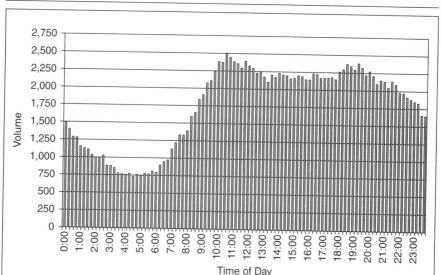

- Use of observation areas. Patients who require extended stays for administration of IV fluids, diagnosis of abdominal pain, evaluation of chest pain, or treatment of resistant asthma episodes can be observed and released from observation units. This not only relieves pressure on the ED, but saves hospital beds for other ED patients who need them. Slightly more than 25 percent of U.S. metropolitan EDs are using observation areas to decrease inpatient admissions, lengths of stay, and costs.[34]

- Creative use of the triage area. Some EDs have used a physician during peak times to perform evaluation and treatment up front in the triage area, thus shortening door-to-doctor times and expediting treatment. Selected patients are not undressed or placed on a stretcher but rather are treated in rolling reclining chairs. A significant number of these patients can be treated and released without ever occupying space in the ED, effectively increasing the area available for treatment of sicker patients in the main department.

- Use of protocols that allow nursing staff in triage and the ED to assess patients, order initial tests, and initiate immediate treatment when necessary. These protocols can be phased to increase nursing responsibility as the ED becomes progressively overloaded and physician arrival at the bedside is predictably delayed. Protocol-driven care is often used for patients with chest pain, respiratory distress (asthma, cardiopulmonary disease, pneumonia), pain, extremity injuries, diabetes, and eye injuries. Protocols are critical for satisfying time-dependent goals such as the ORYX AMI reperfusion and pneumonia standards. They can also be used correctly to initiate testing for patients

FIGURE 12.2   Emergency Department Flow

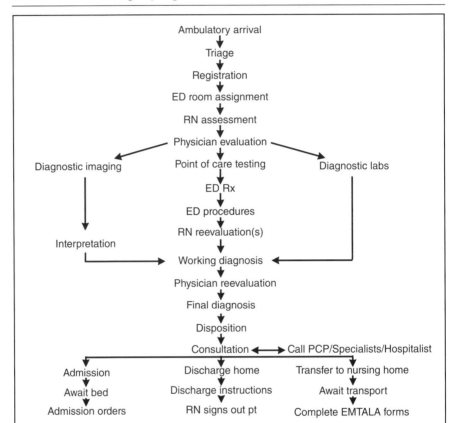

with stroke, abdominal pain, urinary tract infections, and others. If properly chosen tests are completed before the patient is seen by the physician, immediate disposition or discharge is possible at the time of physician evaluation with significant time savings. Protocols must be approved at the departmental level by the ED physicians and should be ordered under the name of the physician(s) on duty in the department at the time the patient is seen.

- Parallel processing of patients. Instead of following a linear sequence, patients can be placed in a room, seen simultaneously by a physician and nurse, and registered at the bedside. This significantly reduces treatment time in EDs where it is a routine practice.

- In-department testing is another important area where time efficiencies can be achieved. A radiology suite in the ED with a dedicated X-ray technologist, the use of a pharmacy technician for processing medication orders and completing a medication reconciliation list, and point-of-care testing (fingerstick blood sugars, hemoccult testing for stool specimens and gastric aspirates, urine pregnancy testing, and rapid urine dip tests) can significantly affect patient flow. Some EDs take these ideas further, performing electrolytes, complete blood count (CBC), cardiac enzymes, and even treadmill stress tests in the department. However, it is important to note that bedside testing carries an economic cost and duplicates laboratory services. Each institution must balance the needs of the ED and the benefits of rapid test turnaround times with redundant costs to the hospital.

A multidepartmental approach to address patient flow is essential.

The inability of patients to move smoothly through the emergency area is sometimes unfairly characterized as an ED problem, when in reality the ED may well be at the mercy of the efficiency (or inefficiency) of the hospital admission or discharge process. Improvements in the ED admission process require a reexamination of nearly every hospital function from admission to discharge, for example, housekeeping, nursing assignments, staffing procedures, and the intricacies of hospital discharge.

Formation of a multidisciplinary committee composed of all participants and stakeholders in the hospitalization process is required to delineate and then streamline the steps of a hospital admission and discharge. On a once- or twice-daily basis, representatives of the hospital's nursing units and ED nursing should meet to discuss patient needs and plan their movements. The ED physician can expedite the admission process by making admission decisions early in the visit, thus alerting the floors to the need to maintain or increase staffing for the next shift.

The Institute for Healthcare Improvement (IHI) has published a set of procedures for sorting through these issues. It also conducts Web-facilitated programs to help hospitals redesign patient flow.[35] TJC has also become involved in this issue and has added managing patient flow to the leadership chapter (LD. 3.3.10.10) of the *2005 Hospital Accreditation Manual*. It states, "The leaders develop and implement plans to identify and mitigate impediments to efficient patient flow throughout the hospital." This standard requires hospital leaders to assess patient movement through the hospital; patient care in temporary bed and overflow locations; shared accountability between the administration and medical staff for patient flow; and use of specific performance indicators to measure components of the patient flow process, to monitor capacity, and to support service processes and the safety of hospital services and areas that receive patients. The standard also specifies that hospitals must improve inefficient or unsafe practices and must develop criteria for ambulance diversion decisions. This is a sweeping mandate with much potential to alleviate the problems of national ED overcrowding and threats to patient safety.

. . . .
POLICY AND PROCEDURE ISSUES

TJC standards require written policies and procedures for high-volume or high-risk conditions. These must be approved by the department and hospital leadership. They should also be reviewed periodically to make certain that they conform to current medical treatment standards. In the case of an adverse outcome, a failure to follow the department policy will predictably become an issue in litigation. Similarly, an outdated policy that does not conform to the current standard of care is hard to defend. It implies that the hospital does not provide quality healthcare to the community. Inclusion of a policy review in staff orientation can prevent medical and risk management misadventures.

Evidence-Based Medicine and the ORYX Initiative

There is a trend in clinical medicine toward implementation of evidence-based care. Some of what has been taught regarding patient care in medical and nursing schools is the result of long experience in the medical profession rather than actual scientific data based on research. When these teachings have been evaluated in a scientific manner, it has often been found that they have no basis in fact. For example, for many years patients who received a LP have been instructed to lie down for a period of hours after the procedure and to drink fluids to avoid a post-LP headache. However, when tested scientifically, these measures do not prevent a post-LP headache. Rather, it is use of a smaller, more narrow needle with a blunt tip that is the primary preventive measure.[36,37] Similar evidence has been used to formulate standards for care of patients with AMI, congestive heart failure (CHF), and community-acquired pneumonia (CAP). These standards have been adopted by the TJC as part of its ORYX initiative and have been implemented in hospitals across the country. As a result, they are becoming national standards of care. Hospital performance on these measures is reported publicly and is being used as a means of comparison. This has both marketing and risk management implications, and risk management professionals are advised to become active in promoting their institution's compliance with these standards.

It is also of note that there have been attempts to make the use of X-ray studies, in particular, evidence-based studies. These include the Ottawa Rules for ankle injuries and the NEXUS studies' rules for X-rays after neck injuries.[38,39] These studies provide recommendations for ordering (or not ordering) X-rays according to set criteria, resulting in a savings of both time and money from a reduction in the number of tests ordered. Reliance on the criteria has been shown to have near-perfect results, suggesting that their use would be quite defensible in the event that a rare adverse outcome became the subject of litigation.

Quality Improvement and Risk Management

Risk management and quality improvement (QI) are closely linked. Each should inform the other. QI is concerned with developing and monitoring processes used to deliver care to ensure that patients receive the maximum benefit and least harm from their visit to the ED. Risk management identifies potential risks and develops means to prevent or reduce their occurrence. QI efforts should enable ED staff to learn from their own errors and those of others to avoid repeating them. Because most errors can be traced back to systemic process failures that ensnare individuals, the ED's processes of care must be tuned to become more predictable for safe outcomes and efficient both in use of time and resources.

Ultimately, improvements in both department-specific and systemwide designs should be expected to improve the safety and effectiveness of patient care. Quality improvement leaders can monitor several parameters (time intervals, census, processes, and outcomes) to assess the efficacy of current processes and the later results of implemented improvements. Overall ED patient care can be judged against earlier measurements or benchmarked against other institutions' performance. The focus of QI activities should change over time: as current goals are reached, new ones should be chosen. The risk management professional can participate in this process by attending ED QI committee and hospital quality council meetings, helping facilitate data collection, and recommending actions to the hospital's administrative team. Use of an ED risk management self-assessment tool is also recommended to highlight areas for improvement.

Risk-oriented topics that might be helpful to include in the ED quality improvement program are depicted in Table 12.2.

The risk management professional should also be concerned with intradepartmental ED issues. Specifically, how are patients in the waiting area supervised? How does the ED change staffing and processes to accommodate increased patient volume during peak times? Are there sufficient resources (ED space, lab, X-ray, and staff) at the appropriate times to meet the basic needs of acutely ill patients? Are patients being admitted and transferred out of the ED in a timely fashion?

Sentinel Events in the ED

Another function of the ED QI program is to analyze adverse events and seek solutions for process errors. As the discipline of quality improvement has matured, focus has shifted from identifying poor individual performance to identifying how poorly designed systems produce errors. Thus adverse events are seen as a source of information that points to areas where redesign is needed. "A sentinel event is an unexpected occurrence involving death or serious physical or psychological injury, or the risk thereof. Serious injury specifically includes loss of limb or function. The phrase 'or the risk thereof' includes any process variation for which a recurrence would carry a significant chance of a serious adverse outcome."[40] Each institution is expected to carefully examine and learn from its own sentinel events. TJC has mandated reporting of sentinel events and maintains a database that is intended to help healthcare organizations learn from each other's mistakes. Even though it is assumed that there is widespread underreporting, a pattern associated with these events has emerged.

The most common root causes of emergency department delay in treatment of sentinel events, listed in order of frequency of occurrence, are issues of communication (84 percent), patient assessment (75 percent), continuum of care (62 percent), orientation and training of staff (46 percent), availability of critical patient information (42 percent), staffing (25 percent), and availability of physician specialists (16 percent).[41] The ED is especially prone to sentinel events and is where over half of all such events occur,

TABLE 12.2   Quality Improvement Assessment

Type of ED QI Assessment	*Example*
Time intervals	Triage to room time
	Triage to physician contact ("door-to-doc" time)
	Triage to analgesic time
	Admission decision to inpatient bed time
	Total ED time (door-to-door time)
Census	By arrival time, day of the week, monthly
	Compared to the previous year
	Ambulatory versus ambulance arrival
	Patients signing AMA or leaving before treatment
Process	Frequency of use of ED protocols
	Frequency of use of inpatient protocols
	Aspirin use for patients with chest pain
	Reperfusion within target for AMI
	Antibiotics within four hours for pneumonia
	Proper evaluation and treatment by physician (disease-specific goals)
	Proper documentation (including repeat vital signs, pain reassessment, etc.)
Outcome	Patient satisfaction
	Cardiopulmonary arrest survival
	Adverse events
	Patient, family, staff complaints

AMA, against medical advice; AMI, acute myocardial infarction, ED, emergency department; QI, quality improvement.

primarily due to delays in treatment that are mostly result of misdiagnosis. Standards for addressing sentinel events are available in the TJC accreditation manual (available online) in the chapter titled, "Improving Organization Performance."

Root cause analysis (RCA) is a special procedure in which all participants (or stakeholders) in a significant adverse event are asked to meet and contribute to a detailed reconstruction of the events that led to the adverse outcome. Each such panel should have a trained facilitator to make certain the process is organized, impartial, and non-punitive. A rigorous examination of all possible contributory factors is conducted with the intent of discovering the single proximate cause of the adverse event. This is termed the *root cause*. It qualifies as such only if, in the opinion of the panel, elimination of this factor would have prevented the adverse outcome. In actuality, there can be several root causes for a single incident. A root cause analysis matrix is available online at www. jointcommission.org. It is expected that the panel's recommendations will be acted upon by the institution to eliminate the root cause(s) so that a similar incident does not occur again. Risk management professionals should participate in RCA sessions so that lessons learned can be applied elsewhere in the organization. The ED QI program's design should also encompass several methods by which the lessons learned are disseminated to the members of the department without compromising patient privacy. Case presentations at department meetings, morbidity and mortality conferences, and department newsletters (e-mail and print) are vehicles to improve the safety of the hospital's future patients.

. . . .

NATIONAL PATIENT SAFETY GOALS AND THE ED

In 2002 TJC presented the first set of National Patient Safety Goals (NPSGs). These goals were developed to promote specific improvements in patient safety. They are based primarily on information derived from TJC's Sentinel Event database. The goals focus on systemwide solutions by delineating problematic areas and formulating specific improvement standards for each safety issue. Those solutions and standards are then used by reviewers to determine compliance and to assign accreditation.[42] Each goal is subdivided into specific requirements and elements of performance. The elements of performance have icons listing scoring category (A or C), if situational decision rules or direct impact requirements apply, if measures of success are needed, and if documentation is required. The goals, which are revised and updated annually, can be found online at www.jointcommission.org. At present, six of these goals (goals 1, 2, 3, 7, 8, and 9) are pertinent to the ED.

Goal 1: Improve the Accuracy of Patient Identification

The purpose and requirement of this goal is to reliably identify the patient and then to match the care and treatment to that same person during the administration of medications, blood products, collection of blood, or other specimens (which should be labeled with two identifiers in the patient's presence), or during the provision of treatments or procedures.

Accuracy of the Patient's Identification Identification is particularly essential for ED patients because they are frequently moved from room to room or to other departments (radiology, cardiac catheterization); patient turnover is rapid so healthcare personnel do not often get to know patients; patient movement may take place during a shift change; and the ED's staff must care for multiple patients simultaneously while being interrupted frequently. All of these factors increase the incidence of mislabeling of laboratory specimens and erroneously administering medications and treatments in the ED. Positive identification avoids errors in test and drug administration, or at worst, notification of death delivered to the wrong family. Reliable methods of identification require active involvement of the patient and/or a designated caregiver if the patient is unable to be involved and at least two different identifiers, but these do not have to be physically separated. A patient ID band with name and date of birth provides two identifiers on one source. Acceptable identifiers include individual's name, an assigned identification number, telephone number, or other person-specific identifier.[43] Room or bed number and patient identification bracelets taped on the bed or placed on the bedside table are not acceptable identifiers. Bar coding that includes two or more person-specific identifiers (not room number) will comply with this requirement, as will biometrics. Scoring of the efficacy of identification processes will be based on the above and how the identifiers are complied with in all phases of patient care, including admitting processes.

Match Identity with Care   When matching the care with the patient, an active verification process that uses facial recognition and verbal affirmation is required before the start of any invasive procedure (percutaneous aspirations, biopsies, cardiac and vascular catheterizations). Challenges to ED patient identification include the unresponsive, confused, traumatized, mentally handicapped, or drug- or alcohol-intoxicated patient. These patients might be unable to state their names or might incorrectly respond affirmatively to the verbalization of another patient's name. Solutions include having a family member, police officer, or EMS personnel identify the patient or assign the patient a temporary name (John Doe) with an associated emergency department or medical record number.[44]

Goal 2: Improve Communication Among Caregivers

Ineffective communication is the most frequently cited category of root causes of sentinel events.[45] Lack of, or ineffective, communication results in more legal claims by patients than does healthcare personnel. There are many reasons for communication errors: different communication techniques, language and cultural barriers, lack of teamwork, informal versus formal communication, and miscommunications. A particularly challenging point is that physicians and nurses are trained to communicate in different ways; doctors learn to diagnose and treat and nurses learn to describe and narrate, not diagnose.[46] Teamwork is not part of the curriculum taught in most medical schools where practitioners are instead instructed to function independently. Most communication occurs informally when clinicians make rounds or read charts. Often it is not structured.[47] Effective communication (timely, accurate, complete, and structured) that is understood by all members of the healthcare team results in fewer lawsuits, increased patient safety, and happier staff. Task-specific communication is now being taught to healthcare providers with positive results for team morale and patient safety. The SBAR technique (situation, background, assessment, and recommendation), developed by Michael Leonard, M.D., is one of these. Another is crew resource management (CRM), first used for critical military aviation applications such as flight crew communication. These techniques teach problem-solving and team communication dynamics so that each member of the team can contribute to the success of the procedure and prevent errors.

SBAR Communication Technique   The elements of the SBAR communication technique are the following:

- Situation: identification of the speaker, patient, and location
- Background: a description of the patient's condition and current problem
- Assessment: the speaker's evaluation of the problem
- Recommendation: the speaker's solution to the problem

SBAR training emphasizes the use of briefings at the beginning of shifts to make sure all clinicians are starting from the same point, teaches the use of assertive language, and emphasizes sharing situational awareness to enhance planning and problem solving.[48]

Crew Resource Management   The key principles of crew resource management are the following:

- Managing fatigue
- Creating and managing a team
- Recognizing adverse situations
- Cross-checking and communication techniques
- Developing and applying shared mental models for decision making
- Giving and receiving performance feedback[49]

Because many aspects of communication are hard to quantify, this goal is currently separated into the measurable tasks of receiving orders and test results; implementing a do not use list of abbreviations, acronyms, and symbols; establishing an acceptable turn-around time for reporting test results; and instituting a standardized approach for handing off communications.

Reporting Test Results   Verbal or telephone orders, or telephonic reporting of critical test results, should be verified by having the person *read back* the complete order or result after writing it down or entering it in a computer. Each organization will determine what test results are critical, but these generally include STAT tests and panic values reports. Electronic reporting (e-mail, text messaging) of orders and results must be verified by the receiver sending an electronic reply to the sender. Verbal orders are discouraged except in emergency situations such as a cardiac arrest, where they should be orally reiterated (*repeated back*). Surveyors will gauge compliance by evaluating performance based on the approach for tracking compliance. This may or may not include documentation, although documentation of verbal orders continues to be critical to the defense of a malpractice case.[50]

Do Not Use List   The do not use list is a short catalogue of medical abbreviations, acronyms, and symbols that are easily miswritten or misread, thus leading to confusion and error. An analysis by MedMarx® of 26,092 error reports from 670 facilities from January 2003 to December 2006 found abbreviations to be a main source of medical errors.[51] Harmful medical errors (along a continuum from temporary harm to permanent harm to death) have consistently been reported at greater than 1 percent for just under a decade.

Pharmacy technicians (38.5 percent), pharmacists (23.7 percent), and pharmacy personnel (5.6 percent) were the staff persons most often involved in 67.8 percent of the cases, with registered nurses involved in 19.2 percent and physicians in 7.2 percent. Distractions were the most frequently reported type of error at 35.4 percent.[52] Each organization is required to establish and document a list of abbreviations, acronyms, and symbols that are not to be used. In addition, this list must also include the official TJC's "Do Not Use" list found online. The Do Not Use list applies to all orders and all medication-related documentation when handwritten, entered as free text into a computer, or on preprinted forms. It also applies to use in any medication-related documentation such as physician notes, nursing admission sheets, and history and physical notes.

Failure to eliminate the Do Not Use abbreviations in medication orders is one of the most frequent (24.6 percent) noncompliance findings during TJC surveys.[53] Institutions are also responsible for ensuring that contractual service providers adhere to this goal and will receive a Requirement for Improvement (RFI) designation if the contracted personnel are noncompliant.[54] The ED is a rapid-paced environment in which physicians and nurses are time constrained, and using abbreviations and acronyms decreases the time required to input patient data. Implementation tips for eliminating dangerous abbreviations are available online at www.jointcommission.org. Use of preprinted order forms or computer-generated templates that use accepted abbreviations, computerized provider order entry (CPOE), posting of the do not use list in physicians' ordering areas, and in-services on this safety issue can reduce the risk of these occurrences. Additionally, the use of bar codes has decreased the number of adverse drug events and dispensing errors by 60 to 96 percent.[55]

Turnaround Times for Results   Turnaround time (TAT) is defined as the amount of time it takes from ordering to receiving a laboratory or test result. Numerous liability suits and patient safety issues relate to turnaround time for laboratory results. Because the ED clinician is usually starting from scratch with often-complex patient health issues and timely action is necessary to avoid adverse outcomes, availability of laboratory results is particularly critical in the ED environment.

TATs for relaying and receiving critical test results should be evaluated and necessary protocols implemented by the organization to enhance timeliness. The organization must define the acceptable length of time between (1) ordering and reporting results and (2) availability and receipt by the responsible licensed caregiver. TJC surveyors will be checking to see that TAT data have been assessed, needed changes to shorten the length of time have been made, and that these changes have been measured and their effectiveness evaluated. Standardization of the chain of communication among caregivers (physician, nurse, ward secretary, and phlebotomists) and departments (lab, messengers, ED, radiology, and so on) and a consistent approach to the use of mechanical forms of relayed information (phone, fax, computer) must be established in protocols. If the ordering caregiver is not available when the test results return, a formal process to make sure that they receive the results should be established. One solution for improved TAT is a *service guarantee* written by diagnostic departments (laboratory, X-ray, others) that promises test results within a specified time interval. Another is CPOE, a process in which physicians input their orders and receive the results digitally. This method decreases the number of steps, people involved, errors, and turnaround times. Although CPOE is expensive to implement for an entire hospital, beginning implementation in the ED offers a less costly way to initiate this key strategy in a critical environment.

Handoffs   *Handoffs* are defined as the transfer of patient care from one healthcare provider to another. In the ED, these take several forms: nursing shift changes; physicians transferring complete responsibility for a patient (sign-outs); physicians transferring on-call responsibility; temporary responsibility for staff leaving the ED for a short time; and nursing and physician handoffs from the emergency department to inpatient units, different hospitals, ambulances, nursing homes, and home healthcare. TJC requires that a standardized approach for handoffs be implemented in all such situations and that they should include the opportunity for personnel to ask and respond to questions. For example, recorded nursing reports may be used as long as there is an opportunity for questions to be answered.

In a study on handoff solutions in high-risk settings done by the Getting at Patient Safety (GAPS) Center in Cincinnati, Ohio, several strategies were observed that improved the effectiveness of handoffs in the healthcare setting. One strategy was the use of an overlap period between the incoming and outgoing caregivers that allowed both sides to ask questions, clarify issues, review patient historical data, update missed patient care that may have occurred during shift change for nurses, enable ED physicians to conclude patient care, and permit a face-to-face final turnover of care. Other strategies include the use of new technologies such as a computerized sign-out form (which caused the error rate to fall by a factor of 3 in one study), digital recorders, and automated records.[56] Many EDs have adopted the above strategies, especially the use of overlap time periods and computerized sign-out forms. Overlap periods in the ED also have an additional benefit in that the original physicians and nurses can complete the care of specific patients rather than handing them off to new staff. This leads to greater patient and staff satisfaction because continuity of care is achieved.

TJC surveyors define an effective handoff as interactive communication that allows questioning between the giver and receiver of patient information that includes up-to-date information regarding the patient's care, treatment and services, condition, and any recent or anticipated changes; has limited interruptions; has a process for verification of the received information (repeat-back or read-back); and allows the receiver to review patient data (previous care, treatment, and services).[57]

Goal 3: Improve the Safety of Using Medications

This goal has three primary requirements, all of them important in the ED. The first is to create a list of look-alike/sound-alike (LA/SA) medicines, accompanied by actions to prevent associated errors. The second is to label all medications, solutions, and containers and discard any that are unlabeled. The third is to reduce possible patient harm from use of anticoagulants.

Look-Alike/Sound-Alike Drugs   The U.S. Pharmacopeia reported wrong dose and prescribing errors more often in the ED than in other areas.[58] Look-alike/sound-alike (LASA) drugs are medications that sound similar (Adderall/Inderal, vinblastine/vincristine), look the same either in the spelling of their name (Celebrex/Cerebyx, Lovenox/Lotronex) or the packaging of the product (Xylocaine-MPF/Shur-Clens, tuberculosis skin tests/influenza vaccines, Brethine/Methergine), or have similar names and similar actions (glipizide/glyburide). LASA medication errors reportedly account for 25 percent of all drug errors, with 12.5 percent of these mistakes being due to medication names.[59] Various medical specialties, such as medicine, orthopedics, oncology, and so on, use certain common medications on a routine basis. The ED is no different in this regard, but ED personnel must also care for patients whose medications might have been prescribed by practitioners from any of the other specialties. The challenge of maintaining this knowledge is further complicated by the introduction of new drugs. With 1,470 LASA medications, it is imperative that a preventive system be in place. The LASA requirement states that individual organizations must create and implement a list containing a minimum of ten LASA drug combinations from the TJC tables available online www.jointcommission.org.

JC surveyors will be looking for the use and implementation of several strategies for each drug combination on every organization's list. (Please refer to Chapter 2 on medication safety for specific strategies that address LASA drugs.)

Additional ways to avoid human error due to attention and memory failures include avoiding fatigue and distractions, having a second person double-check the work, using CPOE and bar coding, enlisting the patient's cooperation, and instilling a culture of safety (institutional commitment and protocols to prevent harm).[60]

Label All Medications and Containers   Labeling of all medications and their containers is critical, but it is especially paramount when the drug is transferred from the original container to another container, such as a syringe, unless it is to be used immediately. If it is not used immediately, the label should contain the drug name, strength, and amount; date prepared and diluents used; date of expiration (if not used within twenty-four hours); and expiration time (if less than twenty-four hours).[61] Measures of success are required for verbal and visual verification by two qualified persons when the person administering the drug is different from the person preparing it, for the retention of the original drug container until the procedure is finished, and when any break or shift change occurs during continued use of the medication.[62] Unlabeled medications and containers are not to be used: they should be thrown out.

Reduce Patient Harm from Anticoagulants   Anticoagulants pose an increased risk for patient harm primarily because the therapeutic range is so narrow, the side effects of being out of range can be disastrous (hemorrhage, stroke), there are multiple interactions with other medications/foods, there are variations in ordering/

dosing, and the requirement of regular monitoring of blood levels is difficult because it is affected by patient compliance. In the ED, 14 percent of all adverse drug events (ADE) and more than 25 percent of all admissions are due to warfarin and insulins.[63] With the combination of digoxin and age, estimates increase to 33 percent of all ADEs in the ED and 42 percent of hospitalizations.[64]

TJC reviewers will be looking for measures of success in the use of approved protocols for anticoagulant therapy and possible drug interactions; notification of dietary services and the use of a food/medication interaction program; and education of patients, staff, and families. Documentation is required that approved protocols for anticoagulant therapy and possible drug interactions are used, as well for a written policy delineating laboratory tests for heparin use.[65]

In reviewing the NPSGs, note that the majority of the safety goals have to do with medication safety. In part this is because medication protocols are readily defined and measurable, but their implementation can also produce meaningful results. With delineation of the main problem areas, patient drug safety can be affected positively. A five-year study of medication errors in the ED showed that

- performance deficit was the number one cause of error;
- wrong administration technique was associated with the greatest percentage of harmful errors;
- wrong dose and prescribing errors were the most common types of error;
- distractions were the leading contributing factor in errors; and
- heparin was the most commonly involved drug, followed by insulin, ceftriaxone, morphine, and acetaminophen.[66]

By using the Institute for Healthcare Improvement's Global Trigger tool (www.ihi. org), institutions have reported approximately forty ADEs for every one hundred admissions (30 to 35 percent of all admission experience ADEs),[67] with the estimated price being $3.5 billion (in 2006 dollars) of added hospital costs.[68] With the cost of ADEs tallied in both lives and dollars, it is important to delineate preventive methods. Automated medication dispensing, unit-based pharmacists, electronic health records, bar coding, trigger tools (software that quickly keys on triggers in patient medical records, such as an international normalized ratio greater than 6 for warfarin patients, to locate ADEs), and computerized medication ordering will help to change the way we handle the medication safety initiatives in the ED. The American Hospital Association (AHA), Health Research & Educational Trust (HRET), and the ISMP have created Pathways for Medication Safety, a modular assessment tool for organizational risk, strategic planning, and medication safety practices that outlines specific tools for use by clinicians and risk management professionals www.medpathways.info/medpathways/tools/tools.html.

Goal 7: Reduce the Risk of Healthcare-Associated Infections

Hospital-acquired infections affect nearly 1.7 million patients with 99,000 deaths annually at a cost of $4.5 to 6.5 billion.[69] ED staff make personal contact with millions of patients each year. Each contact risks transfer of infection to that healthcare worker and then to the next patient. At the same time, healthcare worker (HCW) compliance with hand hygiene practices is only an overall average of 40 to 48 percent.[70]

Hand Hygiene Statistics   Physicians are the least compliant with hand hygiene, having a self-estimated hand washing rate of 73 percent, with an actual rate of 8.6 percent before and 10.8 percent after patient contact.[71] Additionally, when the ranking group member (usually a physician) did not perform hand hygiene, compliance was worse for all healthcare personnel.[72] Good hand washing techniques role-modeled by senior practitioners have been found to increase adherence to hand washing protocols by 34 percent.[73] Not surprisingly, staff compliance increased to 95 percent if the HCW perceived a significant threat to self, such as when caring for an HIV patient.[74]

Lack of time has been identified by several sources as the leading factor for hand washing noncompliance, and it is important to note that the duration of hand washing times by healthcare staff averages only 6.6 to 24 seconds, with an overall average less than 10 seconds.[75] It is also important to note that good hand hygiene has been listed as the single most important preventive measure with which to avoid HCW-to-patient transmission of infection in several studies.[76] Goal 7 has clear risk management implications for the ED's fast-paced, rapid-turnover environment. Requirements for this goal include adherence to the CDC's or World Health Organization's (WHO's) hand hygiene guidelines, implementing evidence-based practices to prevent infections from multiple-drug-resistant organisms (MDRO), documentation of protocols for central venous catheter insertion and cleaning of injection ports/catheter hubs, and treating cases of unanticipated death or major permanent loss of function connected with a healthcare-associated infection as a sentinel event.

Hand Hygiene Guidelines   The CDC's guidelines for hand washing can be found online at www.cdc.gov/handhygiene/. TJC surveyors will be looking for consistent hand washing techniques to be followed by all caregivers as judged by direct observation and staff interviews. Healthcare workers know to wash their hands and why. They just need to do it. This is of particular interest because the TJC compliance trends for adhering to CDC hand hygiene guidelines has steadily decreased from 99 percent in 2004 to 89 percent in 2008.[77] Even though electronic monitoring devices with voice prompts have been shown to affect a modest compliance increase in hand washing, the risk management professional can assist by initiating systemwide strategies aimed at changing culture that sanctions poor compliance behaviors of healthcare workers[78] and ensuring that changes are multifaceted.[79] A monograph with different instruments for measuring hand hygiene adherence authored by the CDC, WHO, TJC, and several other organizations is available at www.jointcommission.org.[80]

Evidence-Based Practices for MDRO Infection Prevention   MDROs are more common in patients who are immunocompromised, have indwelling catheters or ports, and who are elderly. MDROs are on the rise (1 percent in 1999–2000 and 16 percent in 2005–2007 in one study), and patients from long-term care facilities have been found to be reservoirs of resistant strains.[81] Infected patients entering the ED will infect their environment. Staphylococci is easily transferred, and the hands of healthcare workers are the primary transmitting source.[82] Moreover, MRSA has the ability to survive for weeks on nonliving surfaces (plastics, fabrics).[83] Each institution's risk management program should conduct surveillance of MDRO acquisition and transmission through evaluation of compliance rates with best practice guidelines, evidence-based metrics, and outcomes of education programs for staff, patients, and their families in preventive measures. Alert systems should facilitate the identification of new cases.

Documentation of Central Line/Injection Port Protocols   There are approximately one quarter of a million bloodstream infections from central line insertions annually in the United States, causing thirty thousand to sixty-two thousand deaths and total $9 billion in extra costs yearly.[84] Even though the ED is responsible for only short-term care of these lines, many of the elements of performance are pertinent. Education of staff and patients on proper hand washing and the possibility of sepsis; limited use of femoral access; use of a standardized checklist and supply cart, as well as a chlorhexidine-based antiseptic for insertion; and documentation of protocols for central line insertion and insertion port/catheter hub cleansing are required by TJC.

Sentinel Event Infections   When root cause analysis of sentinel event infections is conducted, the ED is not the primary location for discovery of sentinel event infections (cases of unanticipated death or permanent loss of function), but it might be found to be the initial source. For example, when central lines are inserted, or when invasive procedures are done in an emergent manner (under less than optimal conditions), the patient may develop sepsis from the line insertion and die later in the course of hospitalization. The requirement of goal 7 mandates that these be considered sentinel events and that a root cause analysis be completed if the outcome was not the result of the natural course of illness or underlying condition at the time of admission. The analysis questions should include, but not be limited to, Why did the patient become infected, suffer permanent loss of function, or die? TJC surveyors will be looking for improvements that lessen future infection risks due to these sentinel events. Examples of improvements include identification of system and process factors that can be redesigned to decrease negative patient outcomes.

Goal 8: Reconcile Medications Across the Continuum of Care

Most healthcare organizations have experienced great difficult in reconciling medication across the continuum of healthcare. The emergency department is no different. Although goal 8 is not in effect at the present time, TJC will query the facility while on site as to their practices. However, the results will not result in any recommendations for improvement (RFIs), nor will they be addressed in the accreditation report. The requirements of this goal include (1) creating a standardized process for obtaining and documenting a complete list of all medications the patient is taking upon arrival, transfer, and discharge and (2) ensuring that this list is transferred with the patient during transitions of care.

Create a Medication Reconciliation List Reconciliation of medications is defined as the identification of a complete list of medicines each patient is currently taking. This inventory begins with the drugs they are taking at home; continues with the physician's writing of admission, transfer, and discharge orders; and is kept current through all phases of medical care.[85] At a minimum, the final list should be documented and include the patient's name, medication dose, when drug was last taken, and the route and frequency of administration. The function of reconciling medications from the ED to hospital admission, to transfer to nursing home, to outpatient care, to a different service, and to another setting or readmission, is fundamental to preventing medication errors, treatment mistakes, and malpractice claims. Transfers of care are critical points in the reconciliation process because chart reviews show that over half of all hospital medication errors occur at the interfaces of care.[86]

The three-part process of producing a reconciliation medication list first involves collecting the medication history, then ensuring that the medicines and dosages are appropriate, and finally, documenting changes in the medication orders. Because the ED is most often the first contact point for a patient, it is critical for EDs to implement a medication reconciliation form that has been developed in concert with inpatient personnel, the pharmacy, and the medical and nursing staffs. Physicians, nurses, or pharmacists can do the inputting. Implementing medication reconciliation has been shown to decrease the rate of medication errors by 70 percent, reduce adverse drug events by over 15 percent, decrease nursing admission time by over twenty minutes per patient, and reduce pharmacist discharge time by over forty minutes per patient.[87] The ideal vehicle would be a computerized list stored at a central location, accessible to all healthcare providers, and easy to update in outpatient offices, emergency departments, extended care facilities, and inpatient settings.

Reconciliation List with Each Transfer

Whatever form it takes, either written or computerized, the patient's medication list should be reconciled at admission, with each transfer of the patient, and upon discharge. Completion of the form should include the following: patient and family involvement, a comparison of the initial patient list with what providers order, and consideration of the full range of medications as defined in the accreditation manual (prescription medications, sample medications, vitamins, nutriceuticals, over-the-counter drugs, vaccines, diagnostic and contrast agents, radioactive medications, respiratory therapy–related medications, parenteral nutrition, blood derivatives, intravenous solutions, and any product designated by the FDA as a drug).

Reconciliation List and Discharge

Upon discharge a medication list is given to the patient and time is spent educating the patient regarding the medications. This must be documented. These lists can then be transferred to more practical forms such as medication cards. The use of medication cards carried by the patient is especially helpful in emergent situations where the patient is too ill, confused, or psychotic to divulge the necessary information. If the patient cannot supply the medication list, then family members should be queried. Some healthcare organizations have distributed Vial of Life kits, plastic tubes that contain medication lists that patients keep on the shelf of the door of their refrigerators, where paramedics are trained to look for them. This serves a community outreach function and a practical aid to emergency healthcare delivery. Direct access to the patient's electronic medical record supplements (or replaces) these techniques and is efficient and potentially life-saving. With implementation of this goal, electronic versions of the medication reconciliation form will become increasingly available, bringing tangible benefits for patient safety, especially in the ED, one of the first portals of patient entry.

Reconciliation List with Short Duration or Minimal Use Medications

Patients who are seen in the ED for a short duration or in which drugs are used minimally can have a less-detailed reconciliation list (name of current medications but not the dose, route, or frequency).[88] Upon discharge from the ED, these patients are given only the new short-term medication list, unless new long-term medications are prescribed, a change is made in their current medications, or the patient is admitted to the hospital. In these last three circumstances, a full reconciliation list is required.

The TJC requires that the medication reconciliation form is to be used any time orders are rewritten, new orders are prescribed, or the patient changes service, setting, provider, or level of care. TJC surveyors will check for communication from provider to provider, whether inside or outside the organization, and will review the organization's medication reconciliation list for accuracy. Examples of forms in use by other organizations, a how-to guide for getting started in medication reconciliation, and tools for measuring unreconciled medication errors can be found online at the Institute for Healthcare Improvement www.ihi.org.

Goal 9: Reduce the Risk of Patient Harm Resulting from Falls

TJC requirement for this goal has been eliminated for hospitals and critical access hospitals for 2010 and have been moved to the standards section. However, hospitals are still required to assess patients for fall risks, implement individualized strategies to reduce the risk, educate staff on fall prevention, and monitor the effectiveness of interventions and education. The program should include risk reduction strategies/interventions, inservices, and the education of patients and families. The program should also include development and implementation of transfer protocols (for example, ambulance stretcher to bed) when relevant. Falls are the most common cause of hospital admissions for trauma. They affect more than one-third of adults sixty-five years and older, cause the majority of fractures in the elderly, occur more often in women than men, and are the leading cause of injury deaths in the aged population.[89] The average hospitalization fall injury cost is $17,500.[90]

Cause and Incidence of Falls

According to the National Hospital Ambulatory Medical Care Survey (NHAMCS), ED statistics for 1992 to 2002 listed "falls, being struck by or striking against, and motor vehicle traffic incidents" as the injury leaders, resulting in approximately 40 percent of these visits.[91] Although most falls occur in or around the home, a study from the National Center for Patient Safety showed that 20 percent of falls happened in nursing homes and 15 percent in acute care units.[92] Another study showed that the average healthcare cost of a fall for patients aged seventy-two and above averaged $19,440.[93] Patient falls are among the most common occurrences reported, accounting for 10 percent of fatal falls in hospitals.[94]

The ED serves a large volume of patients who are treated on elevated beds, stretchers or gurneys, and rolling recliners. Additionally, patients may be placed in small, confined rooms where they are not easily seen by ED personnel who must care for multiple patients in different locations. ED personnel perform triage for patient severity, which often leaves the older potential fall victim low on the ladder of emergent crises. Patients may be placed in hallways when overcrowding occurs, at which time no staff member is available to sit with someone who needs constant watching. It is clearly essential that ED personnel recognize risk factors and possible solutions to prevent patient falls.

At-risk patients include the following:

- Those with impaired mental status (the most commonly identified factor)
- Those who have already experienced one fall during hospitalization
- Those with impaired mobility and those who need special toilets
- Those with visual or hearing deficits
- Those who are taking certain medications (sedatives, tranquilizers, class 1A antiarrhythmics, digoxin, diuretics, psychotropics, anticoagulants)
- Those who must have assistance transferring from one location to another (usually a bed or chair)
- Those who are sixty-five years of age or older

Environmental risks for falls include the following:

- Poor lighting
- Loose carpeting
- Wet floors
- Bed side rails
- High bed height
- Unlocked wheels on wheelchairs, beds, stretchers
- Cluttered rooms
- Secluded patient spaces
- Use of assistive devices

- Inaccessible or distant nurse call light
- Having the toilet too far from the bed
- Slippery patient footwear and hard flooring[95]

Possible solutions include use of the Morse Fall Scale[96] or the Heinrich II Fall Risk Model,[97] rapid and simple scales to determine a patient's likelihood of falling. The Heinrich model looks at specific risk areas with "confusion, disorientation, and impulsivity"[98] receiving the greatest number of points. In the Morse Fall Scale, points for risk categories are totaled, and those with a high cumulative score receive universal fall precautions and a colored bracelet that identifies them as a high-risk candidate. Putting all bed side rails in the up position is the approach most often used for the cogent patient. Development of a transferable checklist of potential fall information, including history of previous falls, impairment of vision, hearing, cognition, mobility, and other risk factors can also be helpful. Still other risk prevention strategies include bed alarms; having the family sit with the patient; placing the patient in a room close to the nursing station for easier monitoring; padding the patient's hips prophylactically; education of staff, patient, and families on fall prevention; good staff communication; regular walking rounds on patients; and modifying environmental risks.[99]

The best fall prevention programs include the implementation of multiple interventions. The National Center for Patient Safety www.patientsafety.gov has a 139-page publication, *Toolkit to Prevent Senior Falls*, and a fall rate calculator that is downloadable and free.

·········

INTEGRATION OF ED AND HOSPITAL OPERATIONS

Remember that EDs do not function as independent units within the hospital. Because of the time-sensitive nature of their work flow, EDs rely heavily on the services of other departments. These services must be rendered in an efficient and timely manner or the passage of patients through the ED will be impeded. Delays in testing and specialized care constitute a safety risk for both patients in the ED and those who will come to the department in the ensuing hours. ED operations are affected most by health information management systems (HIM), diagnostic services (principally radiology and laboratory services), ancillary departments (respiratory therapy, EKG), operating rooms, cardiac catheterization labs, and inpatient units (general medical–surgical floors, telemetry, ICU, and specialized units). Each of these areas has time-critical functions. (See Figure 12.2.)

Health Information Management Systems

A HIM's main function is to provide past medical history, but for this information to be useful it must be complete and delivered rapidly. Even in the so-called information age, provision of care is often impeded by information gaps, previously collected information that is not available when care is rendered. One study found an information gap in the care of 32 percent of 1,002 ED visits.[100] Past medical history and prior diagnostic test results allow the ED staff to understand the full depth of the patient's condition (often not divulged by the patient), avoid duplication in testing, and identify the patient's primary care providers and consultants. This information is difficult to transport and digest in paper form, and, increasingly, hospitals are using electronic data repositories for this purpose. An effective use of technology, computer-automated HIM serves both clinical and patient safety functions. However, the utility of information is improved if ED physicians can access patients' medical records anywhere within the healthcare system (including physician's offices, pharmacies, and other hospitals). Many multihospital healthcare systems have accomplished this, but broader access to patient data remains more difficult. HIPAA and other privacy law constraints have effectively compartmentalized the patient's medical records, so although providers of direct patient care have the authority to access any patient records necessary to provide care, it is often difficult to obtain them in real time for ED use.

Information retrieval from outside the hospital or system is a cumbersome process that requires providers to do the legwork. Indeed, before any information can be shared, a consent form must be faxed to the information holders with a patient signature so that data can eventually be sent back to those in an active caregiver role. Services that store patient information on the Internet so it can be accessed selectively by healthcare providers with patient (or family) permission are used in other countries, and we are seeing the first use of this approach in the United States. Other solutions, such as smart card–based portable patient records, have been devised but are not yet implemented widely. Ideally, once the patient privacy issues are worked out, national access to electronic patient healthcare records would ensure that the patient's healthcare providers have the necessary information immediately available.

Laboratory

Laboratory services are critical to the function of the ED, because nearly every patient processed in the main ED will require at least one lab test. Results of these tests can radically alter the course of the patient's care. Because of the time sensitivity of these test results, some EDs use point-of-care testing for tests such as hemograms, electrolytes, cardiac enzymes, urinalysis, pregnancy testing, and blood glucose measurements. Strict Clinical Laboratory Improvement Amendments (CLIA) quality-control measures and training requirements increase the difficulty of performing bedside testing and add to the job complexity of ED nurses. Yet, the goal of the process is to deliver the results rapidly to those caring for the patient. Each facility finds its own balance point in this equation, with many relying entirely on services from the laboratory.

Radiology

X-rays or other imaging tests are commonly used for ED patients, with an average of about 0.6 tests per visit.[101] Delays in the process of obtaining radiographs and learning the results of their interpretation significantly affect the duration of ED visits. For billing purposes, a reason for the examination is required for all studies, and for clinical purposes, radiologists should be supplied a history that helps them understand what to look for. Digital imaging is proliferating, allowing ED physicians to view routine X-rays and CT and MRI scans as soon as they are completed. However, a radiologist's interpretation is often required by the ED physician before the next steps can be taken in patient care. In the most efficient systems, radiologists read films and render an opinion to the ED physician immediately, by electronic means. Paper-based systems can be nearly as efficient. Typically, routine film readings are available for the majority of the day, but are not usually available on evening or night shifts. ED physicians are generally adept at reading plain films, but CT and MRI scans require the expertise of a radiologist. It should be obvious, from a risk management point of view, that the services of a radiologist are desirable for as much of the twenty-four-hour day as possible. Because radiologists need to sleep, and prefer to do so at night, hospitals have found many solutions to the problem of how to get films read at night. Some employ radiology residents for night and weekend readings. Others use digital transmission of the images that allows reading at home or at remote sites, and the results are faxed or called back to the requesting ED physician. The physicians who read the films can be medical staff members housed in a location in a different time zone, or the services can be contracted with outside companies who use physicians living in other parts of the world, such as Israel or India. It is important to note that medical staff credentialing processes should address any telemedicine providers. Please refer to Chapter 15 on telemedicine, in Volume 3 in this series.

Respiratory Therapy

Respiratory therapy services are needed by many ED patients and, when required, must be provided immediately. For this reason, ED nurses are often trained to administer initial respiratory updraft treatments, with subsequent treatments administered by respiratory therapists (RTs). For staffing efficiencies, nurses and RTs are sometimes cross-trained for this function, and RTs may also be asked to perform other services such as EKG testing in the ED. In any case, it is essential that respiratory therapy treatments and EKG testing be provided on an immediate basis to those who need them.

Obtaining Rapid EKGs

There is a renewed emphasis on rapid acquisition of EKG data due to the ORYX requirement that rapid reperfusion therapy be provided to patients with AMI. EDs must find strategies to successfully identify these patients rapidly, and EKG data are essential for determining which patients will benefit from such therapies. This is not as simple as it may seem because patients who are ultimately diagnosed with AMI arrive with a wide variety of complaints. However, protocols that mandate EKGs for patients with weakness, dizziness, shortness of breath, and advanced age will capture a larger proportion of the pertinent patients. The ED should also have more than one EKG machine so that multiple simultaneous arrivals can be promptly evaluated.

Emergency Surgery or Cardiac Catheterization

Patients who require emergency surgery, or emergency cardiac catheterization typically have a limited time within which these services must be provided. In some states, a response time is mandated by law for physicians (typically surgeons), and these requirements may place constraints for on-call physicians to live within a travel time–defined radius of the hospital. Trauma centers have the tightest timelines for availability of surgical staff and services, and, in many cases, physicians-in-training who remain on call in the hospital at night are used to satisfy these requirements. ORYX requirements for AMI specify a target time of 90 minutes for opening the affected coronary artery in the cardiac catheterization laboratory, and this requires rapid response from the on-call cardiologist and catheterization laboratory team. Longer response times result in poor patient outcomes and a lower rating for the hospital on publicly available healthcare report cards. It is also important that CMS is currently implementing plans to tie financial incentives to performance.

· · · · · · · · ·
INFORMATION SYSTEMS

Documenting the events of an emergency department visit is important for three primary reasons: clinical utility, billing, and legal purposes. To meet all three needs the medical record must be legible, organized, complete, and retrievable. There are dozens of steps in the process of completing a single ED visit, and documentation of each step is the ideal. However, emergency physicians and nurses must deal with the chaos caused by multiple arrivals, numerous active patients, and disruptive emergency situations. In the midst of chaos, patient care is the highest priority, and documentation sometimes suffers. The plaintiff's attorney's oft-used assertion, "If it wasn't documented, it wasn't done," does not describe the realities of emergency care. However, it is certainly correct to say, "If it wasn't documented, it is difficult to prove it was done." Because of time pressures in the active ED, it is essential that documentation be easy and quick. As with medical record documentation in other parts of the hospital, the staff must be trained to use only approved abbreviations; to cross out errors with a single line; to date, time, and initial error corrections and addendums; and to complete charting at a time that is as reasonably close to the actual occurrence of events as possible.

There are many ED charting solutions in use across the country, and for patient safety, the most complete systems are superior. A handwritten page is the lowest quality solution because it is prone to illegibility and serious omissions. Dictation systems produce a supremely legible document, but they are also vulnerable to omissions and transcription errors and are often not available for editing on the same day as the patient's visit. Speech-to-text systems have improved dramatically and can produce a dictated document in real time but will still have transcription errors that require editing. Many EDs use templates (either paper or electronic) on which positive and negative items in the history and physical can simply be checked off. Finally, there are a growing number of electronic systems for ED documentation. Although more costly than paper-based systems, fully implemented systems are superior for several reasons, which include the following:

- Work is streamlined by eliminating many communication and documentation steps.
- Supports and complements computerized physician (provider, practitioner) order entry (CPOE).
- Clinical information and test results may be retrieved from any linked computer.
- Safety is enhanced by prompts regarding required elements to ensure completion.
- The organization of the medical record is consistent and more easily understandable to clinicians reviewing it.
- Legibility is ensured.
- Multiple users can document in and read the chart simultaneously.
- Communication between members of the ED team in the system is enhanced.
- Automatic timestamps identify all caregivers and time their entries.
- Drug allergies are automatically checked, and duplications are identified, helping to avoid drug interactions and wrong doses and helping to ensure that the right patient receives medication.
- The exchange of information between hospital and office practice systems is facilitated.
- Records of prior visits can be retrieved rapidly.
- Billing and coding are facilitated.
- Medical records cannot be lost in the traditional sense.
- Quality improvement analysis can be automated.
- It is easier to identify addendums and to properly initial, time, and date them.

As one of its three patient safety recommendations, the influential Leapfrog Group for Patient Safety has recommended that CPOE be used to enter medication orders and has set an initial goal of 75 percent compliance.[102] Emergency departments are arguably the place where hospitals could most readily implement this standard. Still, CPOE does not solve all problems associated with the medical record. The medical record is only as complete as it is made to be by healthcare providers, and prompts for required entries cannot reasonably be used for every piece of information. Additionally, data entry might be more cumbersome than paper systems, and significant amounts of customization must be done by the facility. The ED system must interface with hospital billing systems, laboratory and X-ray computers, and HIM systems. Electronic systems require an on-site administrator who can rapidly make changes to fit the department's work flow and the support of the IT department for hardware maintenance and periodic upgrades. Ease of learning the system is important because all full-time and part-time staff must be trained to use the system. Some facilities are struggling with transition systems in which some elements are still on paper that must be scanned in and can be lost. They may also experience confusion about orders that pertain to other departments. Confusion results in delays, which can be costly, and at times, dangerous for the patient. A final consideration is the need for automated backups for the data and a process that allows care to continue on paper during planned or unplanned system downtime. A completely electronic health record that includes CPOE, automated medication reconciliation, cross-referencing error messages, and a full history of the patient's medical health is the ideal.

· · · · · · · · ·

ORIENTATION AND TRAINING OF PERSONNEL

Orientation of new personnel in the ED is very important to ensure the smooth function of the department. A staff member who has not been oriented is of little use in emergency situations and is more likely to commit errors in patient care.

There are many aspects to proper orientation of new ED personnel. New staff needs to be acquainted with the physical layout of the department and hospital; the location of patient rooms, work areas, and supply spaces; and the location of all supplies. Each staff member (technician, secretary, nurse, nurse practitioner (NP), physician assistant (PA), or physician) needs to be well-oriented to the required job functions and up to full speed before stepping into the rushing current of patient flow. In most EDs, this is accomplished by use of a department-specific orientation manual, some classroom work, a demonstration and return demonstration of clinical skills, and preceptorship with an experienced staff member. In preceptorship, new staff works alongside experienced team members at their positions, gradually assuming more responsibility for direct patient care.

Each ED is required by accrediting bodies (state and national) to have policies and procedures that spell out how things are done in the department. New staff should be acquainted with these, not only because many are part of the daily flow of patient care but also because deviation from them can result in adverse consequences for patients. If a lawsuit is filed that alleges substandard care, the fact that the hospital's own policies and procedures have not been followed will only substantiate the claim of negligence. At a minimum, each staff member's orientation should be documented with a checklist that is signed by the staff member and preceptor and kept on file. It is in the interest of the hospital's risk management professional to make certain that proper medical record documentation, policies and procedures, and legal obligations such as EMTALA requirements and HIPAA regulations are part of the formal orientation process. Finally, the most successful hospitals also require new staff to be oriented to the mission of the hospital and the service culture of the institution. It follows from the above discussion that an introduction to patient safety in the ED should be part of new employee orientation (or periodic skills training). This introduction could be taught or written by the hospital's risk management professional.

Training for New Equipment and Refresher Courses

Other types of training should occur in every ED. Periodically, as new equipment is purchased, in-service training should be conducted in the proper use of the equipment. Disaster drills should be held on a regular basis to ensure familiarity with procedures and to maintain the readiness of the department. Formal courses in emergency procedures, such as basic life support (BLS), advanced cardiac life support (ACLS), advanced trauma life support (ATLS), and pediatric advanced life support (PALS), help ensure that every team member knows how to participate in emergency resuscitation events. In some cases, board certification encompasses these training programs, and the requirement may then be waived for ED physicians. However, state regulations may stipulate current certification in the programs for the department's medical director.

Qualifications for ED Physicians

Presently, the nation's emergency medicine physician workforce is a hodgepodge of various medical educational backgrounds and different board certifications. ED physicians may be residency trained and board certified in emergency medicine (60 percent); residency trained in another specialty (usually internal medicine, family practice, pediatrics, or general surgery) and board certified in emergency medicine (8 percent); neither emergency medicine residency trained nor board certified in emergency medicine, but residency trained in another specialty (27 percent); or have no board certification (5 percent). The percentage of ED physicians who are residency trained in emergency medicine has increased from 37 percent in 1997 to 60 percent in 2007. These physicians are not equitably distributed, however, and urban EDs are staffed by emergency medicine–certified physicians at 72 percent, whereas in rural hospital EDs physicians are so trained only 13.5 percent of the time.[103] On average, 32 percent of the doctors working in EDs are doing so without ED-specific training or passage of a national certification exam that tests their ED proficiency and skills. It is no surprise that the current trend is to hire physicians who have either completed a residency in emergency medicine or those that are board certified in emergency medicine. Board certification, which requires that the ED physician demonstrate ongoing competency in a comprehensive and nationally consistent array of topics, is a logical precedent to safer practice. Of particular interest to the risk management professional is a recent analysis of ED malpractice cases showing that non-emergency medicine–trained physicians and residents working in the ED are more likely to generate claims.[104]

Residents in the ED

When emergency medicine residents work in the EDs of teaching hospitals, proper physician supervision is essential. Lack of proper supervision is frequently cited as a factor in malpractice cases in hospitals in which residents are trained. However, in the 2009 PIAA data-sharing study, residents were named in only 4.6 percent of 2,661 malpractice claims.[105] Regardless, residents undoubtedly play a contributing role in a larger proportion of cases.

For example, researchers at Vanderbilt University School of Medicine cited supervision problems as a contributing cause in 31 percent of seventy-four cases.[106] In a recent ED closed-claims study in the Netherlands, residents were involved in 76 percent of the claims, and resident supervision by an attending physician was documented in only 15 percent of the medical records.[107] Supervising physicians must document their own contact with each patient, validate the findings of each resident or medical student, and sign off on each medical record. Serious errors in patient care due to the inexperience of residents can be avoided with proper on-site supervision. This means that attending physicians must work night and weekend shifts alongside their residents.

· · · · · · · · ·
EMS MEDICAL CONTROL IN PREHOSPITAL CARE

Emergency physicians frequently are asked to function as medical control officers for ambulance crews working in the field. This is a serious responsibility to undertake on behalf of patients who are not yet in the ED. However, the movement of these patients falls under both state regulations and federal EMTALA proscription. In both cases, these patients are considered to be under the care of the medical control hospital. However, in most cases, state law allows discretion on the part of the ambulance (emergency medical services, or EMS) personnel to take critically ill patients to the closest appropriate facility, even if it is not the medical control hospital.

An instructive case is *Arrington v. Wong*, an EMTALA case originating in Hawaii in which the physician acting as medical control officer directed the ambulance crew to transport a patient with extreme shortness of breath to a hospital in which he had previously received care, but that was farther away. The patient died shortly after arrival at the receiving hospital, and the Ninth Circuit Court of Appeals ruled that the decision to transport the patient to a more distant facility was a violation of EMTALA. This decision may not be upheld in other jurisdictions, but it reinforces that acting in the best interests of the patient is a highly defensible course of action. It should also be noted that "failure to transport" is the most common reason for EMS lawsuits. It is not permissible to transport an unwilling, yet competent patient, as this is a medical form of kidnapping. It is expected that the crew will attempt to persuade the patient to be transported, and if transport is refused, they should thoroughly document this refusal as part of the prehospital record. In cases where the patient is obviously ill and should be transported, physician intervention (asking to speak directly with the patient) should be undertaken.

Telephone Advice to Call-Ins

Although Poison Control Centers across the United States have an excellent record in fielding calls for cases of accidental or intentional poisoning, the same cannot be said for other medical providers who provide telephone advice. Studies have repeatedly shown that those attempting to treat patients by phone make improper decisions. This is largely the result of collecting incomplete and indirect data about the patient. The inability to physically assess the patient is another important factor in telephone misdiagnosis. Poison Control Centers are effective because they work in a narrowly focused area for which a specific set of information is collected about the patient, and these data serve as the basis for decision making. In addition, the centers are vigilant about follow-up.

Examples of the dangers of telephone advice have been highlighted by the managed-care industry, which uses Ask a Nurse advice lines to perform triage on patients to avoid "expensive" EDs and to channel members to their own network providers. Two medical-legal cases demonstrate the dangers of these systems. In *Adams v. Kaiser Foundation Health Plan of Georgia*, (*Adams v. Kaiser Foundation Health Plan of Georgia*, C.A.F.93VS79895 [1995]), the parents of an ill six-month-old infant were directed to an in-network facility forty-two miles away instead of two closer out-of-network emergency facilities. The infant subsequently died. A similar outcome resulted when a thirty-five-year-old man was instructed to use an antacid for apparent indigestion, then died as a result of myocardial infarction and dysrhythmia before arrival at a hospital (*Cummins v. Kaiser Foundation Health Plan of Georgia*, unpublished decision). These types of errors must be avoided by EDs, all of which receive calls from the public asking for advice.

The problem of managing calls from the public to EDs asking for advice has been addressed by the American College of Emergency Physicians in a policy statement. This statement advises each ED to develop a procedure to identify the nature of incoming calls. Those who have a life- or limb-threatening emergency should be instructed to call 9–1–1 or a similar local emergency medical services system. Calls from patients recently discharged from the ED should be managed using prearranged protocols that include the circumstances in which the patient should return to the ED.[108] The Emergency Nurses Association (ENA) adds one further category, that of providing basic first aid advice. However, this advice should be monitored to ensure that it does not extend beyond the most basic level. The ENA also advises creating a log that includes the caller's name, telephone number, primary care provider, chief complaint, and brief history; advice provided; disposition; and, if possible, the caller's response. To ensure quality advice, the ED should require continuing medical education for those staff involved, and the ED should maintain a continuous quality improvement program for tracking calls.[109]

· · · · · · · · ·
CONCLUSION

The ED is one of the most complex and dynamic environments in healthcare. The high volume of patients, wide variety of problems, and rapid pace of care lend themselves to error. Prevention of harm and reduction of risk in this arena can be accomplished only with a comprehensive approach, which requires the input, oversight, and active participation of the risk management professional.

Suggested Readings

Series

Dunn, R. L. "Uses of Error: diagnosis, detection, and disclosure." *The Lancet* 2005; 365, (9457): 386.

TJC. Healthcare at the crossroads: Strategies for improving the medical liability system and preventing patient injury. 2005. Available at: www.jointcommission.org/NR/rdonlyres/167DD821-A395–48FD-87F9–6AB12BCACB0F/0/Medical_Liability.pdf. (Accessed March 31, 2010.)

Books

Berwick, D. *Escape Fire: Designs for the Future of Health Care*. San Francisco: Jossey-Bass, 2003.

Berwick, D., A. B. Godfrey, and J., Roessner. *Curing Health Care: New Strategies for Quality Improvement*. 1st ed. San Francisco: Jossey-Bass, 2002.

Corrigan, J., L. Kohn, and M. Donaldson, eds. *To Err Is Human: Building a Safer Health System*. 1st ed. Washington, D.C.: National Academy Press, 2000.

Institute of Medicine. *Crossing the Quality Chasm: A New Health System for the 21st Century*. Washington, D.C.: National Academy Press, 2001.

Wachter, R., and K. Shojania. *Internal Bleeding, The Truth Behind America's Terrifying Epidemic of Medical Mistakes*. New York: Rugged Land, 2004.

Resource Web Sites

American Board of Emergency Medicine, www.abem.org/public

American Hospital Association, www.aha.org/aha/index.jsp

Agency for Healthcare Research and Quality, www.ahrq.gov

Association for Professionals in Infection Control and Epidemiology, www.apic.org//AM/Template.cfm?Section=Home

Centers for Disease Control, www.cdc.gov

The Centers for Medicare & Medicaid Services [CMS] is a federal agency within the U.S. Department of Health and Human Services, www.cms.hhs.gov

Food and Drug Administration, www.fda.org

Health, Research and Educational Trust, www.hret.org/hret/about

Institute for Healthcare Improvement, www.ihi.org/ihi

Institute for Safe Medication Practices, www.ismp.org

Joint Commission on Accreditation of Healthcare Organizations, www.jointcommission.org

The Leapfrog Group, www.leapfroggroup.org

Maryland Patient Safety Center, www.marylandpatientsafety.org

Pathways for Medication Safety, www.medpathways.info/medpathways/index.jsp

National Quality Forum, www.qualityforum.org

Society for Healthcare Epidemiology of America, www.shea-online.org

Physician Insurers Association of America, www.thepiaa.org

United States Pharmacopoeia, www.usp.org

Endnotes

1. McCaig, L. F., and C. W. Burt. "National Hospital Ambulatory Medical Care Survey: 2003 Emergency Department Summary." CDC Advance Data from Vital Health and Statistics. 2006; No. 358: 1–37.

2. Leape, L. L., T. A. Brennan, N. Laird et al. "The nature of adverse events in hospitalized patients: results of the Harvard Medical Practice Study II." *New England Journal of Medicine* 1991; 324: 377–384.

3. Physician Insurers Association of America (PIAA). *PIAA Risk Management Review—Emergency Medicine*, PIAA Data Sharing System, 2009. PIAA, Rockville, Md.

4. *Ibid.*

5. Premier Insurance Management Services, Inc., 2005.

6. American Academy of Pediatrics (AAP) Committee on Medical Liability. "Test your knowledge of medical malpractice claims." *AAP News* 2002; (November): 240–241.

7. Physician Insurers Association of America (PIAA). *PIAA Acute Myocardial Infarction Study 1996*. PIAA Data Sharing System, May 1996. PIAA, Rockville, Md.

8. *Ibid.*

9. Patel, H. "Symptoms in acute coronary syndromes: Does sex make a difference?" *American Heart Journal* 2004; 148(1): 27–33.

10. Bradley, E. H., J. Herrin, Y. Want et al. "Strategies for reducing the door-to-balloon time in acute myocardial infarction." *New England Journal Medicine* 2006; 355: 2308–2320.

11. "STAT" in medical terminology is not an acronym; it is short for *statim*, the Latin word for immediately. Available at: Accessed at: ask.yahoo.com. (Accessed January 6, 2006.)

12. Physician Insurers Association of America (PIAA). PIAA Data Sharing Project, 2005. PIAA, Rockville, Md.

13. PIAA, 2009, *op. cit.*

14. Premier Insurance Management Services, Inc.

15. Karcz, A., R. Korn, M. C. Burke et al. "Malpractice claims against emergency physicians in Massachusetts: 1975–1993." *American Journal of Emergency Medicine* 1996;14: 341–345.

16. Western Litigation Specialists. Closed claim data. 2001.

17. American College of Emergency Physicians (ACEP). "Avoidable errors in wound management." *Foresight* 2002; 55: 1–8.

18. Montano, J. B., and M. T. Steele. "Foreign body retention in glass-caused wounds." *Annals of Emergency Medicine* 1992; 21(11): 1360–1363.

19. Ellis, G. L. "Are aluminum foreign bodies detectable radiographically?" *American Journal of Emergency Medicine* 1993; 11: 12–13; Courter, B. J. "Radiographic screening for glass foreign bodies—What does a 'negative' foreign body series really mean?" *Annals of Emergency Medicine* 1990; 19(9): 997–1000.

20. Sutton, D. *A Short Textbook of Clinical Imaging*. London: Springer-Verlag 1990, 400.

21. George, J. E. "Legal issues in emergency radiology. Practical strategies to reduce risk." *Emergency Medicine Clinics of North America* 1992; 10(1): 179–203.

22   Sites, R. L. "Emergency department closed claims: Ohio." *Perspectives–Healthcare Risk Management* Spring: 1990; 1721.

23.   PIAA Risk Management Review-Emergency Medicine, 2009, *op. cit.*

24.   Beckman, H. B., and R. M. Frankel. "The effect of physician behavior on the collection of data." *Annals of Internal Medicine* 1984; 101: 692–696.

25.   Marvel, M. K., R. M. Epstein, K. Flowers, H. B. Beckman. "Soliciting the patient's agenda — Have we improved?" *Journal of the American Medical Association* 1999; 281: 283–287.

26.   Chiovenda, P., G. Vincentelli, and F. Alegiani. "Cognitive impairment in elderly ED patients: Need for multidimensional assessment for better management after discharge." *American Journal of Emergency Medicine* 2002; 20(4): 332–335.

27.   "Clarifying Polices Related to the Responsibilities of Medicare-Participating Hospitals in Treating Individuals with Emergency Medical Conditions." Available at: www.cms. hhs.gov/EMTALA/Downloads/CMS-1063-F.pdf. (Accessed August 18, 2009.)

28.   Centers for Medicare & Medicaid Services (CMS): EMTALA statute — 42 U.S.C. 1395dd. Available at: www.emtala.com/law/index.html. (Accessed August 18, 2009.)

29.   Schecter, J. C. "COBRA Laws and EMTALA." Available at: www.emedicine.com/emerg/topic737.htm. Updated May 26, 2009. (Accessed August 18, 2009.)

30.   Pitts, S. R., R. W. Niska, J. Xu et al. *National Hospital Ambulatory Medical Care Survey: 2006 Emergency Department Summary.* National Health Statistics Report. No. 7, August 6, 2008. Centers for Disease Control and Prevention, Atlanta, Ga.

31.   *Ibid.*

32.   "The Connection, State Report." American College of Emergency Physicians. December 2002.

33.   United States General Accounting Office (USGAO). "Hospital Emergency Departments: Crowded Conditions vary Among Hospitals and Communities." GAO Report No. GAO-03–460. March 2003 Available at: www.gao.gov. (Accessed on March 31, 2010.)

34.   Ross, M., S. Compton, D. Richardson et al. "The use and effectiveness of an emergency department observation unit for elderly patients." *Annals of Emergency Medicine* 2003; 41(5): 668–677.

35.   Institute for Healthcare Improvement. "Optimizing patient flow." 2003. Further information available at: www.ihi.org. (Accessed 8/18/09.)

36.   Walling, A. "Atraumatic vs. standard needles for diagnostic lumbar puncture." *American Family Physician*, May 2001. Available at: www.aafp.org/afp/20010501/tips/6.html. (Accessed August 18, 2009.)

37.   Serpell, M., G. Haldane, D. Jamieson et al. "Prevention of headache after lumbar puncture: Questionnaire survey of neurologists and neurosurgeons in United Kingdom." *British Medical Journal* 1998; 316: 1709–1710.

38.   Stiell, I. G., G. H. Greenberg, R. D. McKnight et al. "A study to develop clinical decision rules for the use of radiography in acute ankle injuries." *Annals of Emergency Medicine* 1992; 21: 384–390.

39. Hoffman, J. R., W. R. Mower, A. B. Wolfson et al. "Validity of a set of clinical criteria to rule out injury to the cervical spine in patients with blunt trauma." National Emergency X-Radiography Utilization Study Group. *New England Journal of Medicine* 2000; 343(2): 94–99.

40. The Joint Commission. Sentinel Event Policy and Procedures. Available at: www. jointcommission.org/NR/rdonlyres/F84F9DC6-A5DA-490F-A91F-A9FCE26347C4/0/SE_chapter_july07.pdf Updated July 2007. (Accessed August 14, 2009.)

41. Manasse, H. R., J. P. Bagian, J. Battles et al. The Joint Commission. Sentinel Alert. Issue 26. June 17, 2002. Available at: www.jointcommission.org/SentinelEvents/SentinelEventAlert/sea_26.htm. (Accessed August 14, 2009.)

42. The Joint Commission. *National Patient Safety Goals Manual*. Chapter JC. Available at: www.jointcommission.org/NR/rdonlyres/31666E86-E7F4-423E-9BE8-F05BD1CB0AA8/0/09_NPSG_HAP.pdf (Accessed August 14, 2009.)

43. The Joint Commission. Two Patient Identifiers, NPSG 01.01.01. Available at: www. jointcommission.org/AccreditationPrograms/LongTermCare/Standards/09_FAQs/NPSG/Patient_ID/NPSG.01.01.0/Two_Patient_Identifiers.htm. December 9, 2008. (Accessed August 14, 2009.)

44. The Joint Commission. *National Patient Safety Goals Manual, op. cit.*

45. Manasse, H. R., J. P. Bagian, J. Battles et al., *op. cit.*

46. Joint Commission Resources. "The SBAR technique: Improves communication, enhances patient safety." *Joint Committee on Patient Safety* 2005; 5(2): 1–2, 8.

47. Arford, P. H. "Nurse-physician communication: An organizational accountability." *Nursing Economics* 2005; 23(2): 72–77.

48. Leonard, M. "The human factor: Teamwork and communication in patient safety." April 14, 2004. Dearborn, Mich. Available at: www.mihealthandsafety.org/2004_conference/Leonardslides.ppt#487,1, The Human Factor: Teamwork and Communication in Patient Safety. (Accessed March 31, 2010.)

49. Grogan, E. L., R. A. Stiles, D. J. France et al. "The impact of aviation-based teamwork training on the attitudes of health-care professionals." *Journal of the American College of Surgeons* 2004; 199(6): 843–848; Moorman, D. W. "On the quest for six sigma." *American Journal of Surgery* 2005; 189: 253–258.

50 The Joint Commission. Accreditation Program: National Patient Safety Goals (see read back orders, p. 4). NPSG 02.01.01. 2008. Available at: www.jointcommission.org/NR/rdonlyres/31666E86-E7F4-423E-9BE8-F05BD1CB0AA8/0/HAP_NPSG.pdf. (Accessed March 31, 2010.)

51. Hicks, R. W., S. C. Becker, D. D. Cousins, eds. "A report on the relationship of drug names and medication errors in response to the Institute of Medicine's call for action." *MEDMARX Data Report* 2008. Rockville, Md.: Center for the Advancement of Patient Safety, U.S. Pharmacopeia.

52. *Ibid.*

53. The Joint Commission. *Improving America's Hospitals: The Joint Commission's Annual Report on Quality and Safety 2008*. Performance Details. November 2008.

Available at: www.jointcommissionreport.org/pdf/JC_2008_Annual_Report-updated.
pdf. (Accessed August 14, 2009.)

54. The Joint Commission. NPSG 02.02.01. "Do Not Use abbreviations." Available at:
www.jointcommission.org/AccreditationPrograms/Hospitals/Standards/09_FAQs/NPSG/
Communication/NPSG.02.02.01/Do+not+use+abbreviations.htm. December 9, 2008.
(Accessed August 14, 2009.) Furthermore, the Institute for Safe Medication Practices
www.ismp.org has joined with the FDA to eliminate error-prone abbreviations by
providing an online toolkit. Available at: www.ismp.org/tools/abbreviations/default.asp
(Accessed August 15, 2009.)

55. The Joint Commission. Accreditation Program: National Patient Safety Goals (see read
back orders), *op. cit.*

56. Patterson, E., E. Roth, D. Woods et al. "Handoff strategies in setting with high
consequences for failure: Lessons for health care operations." *International
Journal for Quality in Health Care* 16(2): 125–132; Wachter, R., and K. Shojania.
"From internal bleeding: Handoffs and fumbles." *MEDscape General Medicine*
2004; 6(2); Excerpted from: *Internal Bleeding: The Truth Behind America's
Terrifying Epidemic of Medical Mistakes.* New York: Rugged Land Publishing,
2004.

57. The Joint Commission. *National Patient Safety Goals Manual, op. cit.*

58. Hicks, R. and Camp, S. "Medication errors in emergency department settings." *US
Pharmacopeia*, 2004. Available at: www.usp.org/pdf/EN/patientSafety/posters052004–
02–20.pdf. (Accessed August 15, 2009.)

59. Lambert, B. L., S. J. Lin, K. Y. Chang et al. "Similarity as a risk factor in drug name
confusion errors: The look-alike (orthographic) and sound-alike (phonetic) model."
Medical Care 1999; (12): 1214–25; Phillips, J. Look-Alike/Sound-Alike (LA/SA)
Health Product Names Consultative Workshop. October 20–21, 2003. Proprietary
Name Evaluation at the FDA, Office of Drug Safety.

60. Keohane, C. A. and Bates, D. W. "Medication safety." *Obstetrics and Gynecology
Clinics of North America* 2008;35: 37–52.

61. The Joint Commission. NPSG 03.04.01 "Labeling in Procedural Areas." Available at:
www.jointcommission.org/AccreditationPrograms/Hospitals/Standards/09_FAQs/NPSG/
Medication_safety/NPSG.03.04.01/Labeling+in+procedural+areas.htm. (Accessed
August 15, 2009.)

62. The Joint Commission. *National Patient Safety Goals Manual, op. cit.*

63. 5 Million Lives Campaign. *Getting Started Kit: Preventing Harm from High-Alert
Medications.* Cambridge, Mass.: Institute for Healthcare Improvement, 2008.
Available at: www.ihi.org. (Accessed August 16, 2009.)

64. Budnitz, D. S., D. A. Pollock, K. N. Weidenbach et al. "National surveillance of
emergency department visits for outpatient adverse drug events." *Journal of the
American Medical Association* 2006; 296: 1858–1866.

65. The Joint Commission. *National Patient Safety Goals Manual, op. cit.*

66. Santell, J., R. Hicks, and D. Cousins. "Medication errors in emergency department
settings — Five year review (1998–2003)." Center for the Advancement of Patient

Safety. Available at: www.usp.org/pdf/EN/patientSafety/posters072004–06–01.pdf. (Accessed August 15, 2009.)

67. Griffin, F. A. and R. K. Resar. "*IHI Global Trigger Tool for Measuring Adverse Events*" 2nd ed. IHI Innovation Series white paper. Cambridge, Mass.: Institute for Healthcare Improvement, 2009.

68. Committee on Identifying and Preventing Medication Errors. Aspden, P., J. Wolcott, J. L. Bootman, and L. R. Cronenwett, eds. *Preventing Medication Errors: Quality Chasm Series*. Washington, D.C.: National Academies Press, July 2006.

69. The Joint Commission Resources. "New Tool in the Fight Against Health Care–Associated Infections: Compendium of Strategies to Prevent Healthcare–Associated Infections in Acute Care Hospitals." *Patient Safety Link e-Zine* 2009; 5(1). Available at: www.jcrinc.com/New-Tool-in-the-Fight-Against-Health-Care-Associated-Infections/. (Accessed August 16, 2009.)

70. Jarvis, W. R. "Handwashing—The Semmelweis lesson forgotten?" *The Lancet* 1994; 344: 1311–1312; Katz, J. "Hand washing and hand disinfection: More than your mother taught you." *Anesthesiology Clinics of North America* 2004; 22: 457–471; Boyce, J. M., and D. Pittet. "Guideline for hand hygiene in health-care settings: Recommendations of the Healthcare Infection Control Practices Advisory Committee and HICPAC/SHEA/ APIC/IDSA Hand Hygiene Task Force." *MMWR Morbidity and Mortality Weekly Report* 2002; 51: 1–44.

71. Arroliga, A., M. Budev, and S. Gordon. "Do as we say, not as we do: Healthcare workers and hand hygiene." *Critical Care Medicine* 2004; 32:(2): 592–593.

72. Lankford, M. G., T. R. Zembower, W. E. Trick et al. "Influence of role models and hospital design on hand hygiene of health care workers." *Emerging Infectious Diseases Journal* 2003; 9: 217–223.

73. Schneider, J., D. D. Moromisato, B. Zemetra et al. "Hand hygiene adherence is influenced by the behavior of role models." *Pediatric Critical Care Medicine* 2009;10(3): 360–363.

74. Katz, J., 2004, *op. cit.*

75. Pittet D. and J. M. Boyce. "Revolutionizing hand hygiene in health-care settings: Guidelines revisited." *The Lancet* 2003; 3: 269–270; Katz, J., *op. cit.*; Boyce, J. M. and D. Pittet, 2002, *op. cit.*

76. Katz, J., 2004, *op. cit.*; Pittet and Boyce, 2003, *op. cit.*

77. The Joint Commission. *National Patient Safety Goal Compliance Trends by Program 2003–2008*.

78. Pittet and Boyce, 2003, *op. cit.*; McGuckin, M. "Hand hygiene accountability." *Nursing Management* 2003; 34(Suppl 4): 2; Swoboda, S. M., K. Earsing, K. Strauss et al. "Electronic monitoring and voice prompts improve hand hygiene and decrease nosocomial infections in intermediate care unit." *Critical Care Medicine* 2004; 32: 358–363.

79. Creedon, S. A. "Healthcare workers' hand decontamination practices: Compliance with recommended guidelines." *Journal of Advanced Nursing* 2005; 51(3): 208–216.

80. The Joint Commission, the Association for Professionals in Infection Control and Epidemiology Inc., the Centers for Disease Control and Prevention, the Institute for Healthcare Improvement, the National Foundation for Infectious Diseases, the Society for Healthcare Epidemiology of America, and the World Health Organization World Alliance for Patient Safety Infection Control. "Measuring hand hygiene adherence: Overcoming the challenges." 2009. Available at: www.jointcommission.org/NR/rdonlyres/68B9CB2F-789F-49DB-9E3F-2FB387666BCC/0/hh_monograph.pdf. (Accessed August 16, 2009.)

81. Pop-Vicas, A., E. Tacconelli, S. Gravenstein et al. "Influx of multidrug-resistant, gram-negative bacteria in the hospital setting and the role of elderly patients with bacterial bloodstream infection." *Infection Control and Hospital Epidemiology* 2009; 30(4): 325–331.

82. Shinefield, H. R. and N. L. Ruff. "Staphlycoccal infections: A historical perspective." *Infectious Disease Clinics of North America* 2009; 23: 1–15.

83. *Ibid.*

84. Clancy, C. M. "Reducing central line-related bloodstream infections." *American Operating Room Nurse* 2009; 89(6): 1123–1125.

85. Institute for Healthcare Improvement. "Reconcile all medications at all transition points." Forms and tools available at: www.ihi.org/IHI/Topics/PatientSafety/MedicationSystems/Changes/IndividualChanges/Reconcile+Medication+Orders+When+Patients+are+Transferred+to+Other+Care+Units.htm. (Accessed August 16, 2009.)

86. Rozich, J. D. and R. K. Resar. "Medication safety: One organization's approach to the challenge." *Journal of Clinical Outcomes Management* 2001; 8(10): 27–34.

87. Whittington J. and H. Cohen. "OSF Healthcare's journey in patient safety." *Quality Management in Health Care* 2004; 13(1): 53–59; Rozich, J. D., R. K. Resar et al. "Standardization as a mechanism to improve safety in health care: Impact of sliding scale insulin protocol and reconciliation of medications initiatives." *Joint Commission Journal on Quality and Safety* 2004; 30(1): 5–14.

88. The Joint Commission. *National Patient Safety Goals Manual, op. cit.*

89. Centers for Disease Control, Injury Center. "Costs of falls among older adults." Available at: www.cdc.gov/ncipc/factsheets/fallcost.htm (Accessed August 17, 2009.)

90. *Ibid.*

91. McCaig L. F. and C. W. Burt. National Hospital Ambulatory Medical Care Survey: 2002 Emergency Department Summary. "Advance data from vital and health statistics" 340: 1–45. Hyattsville, Md.: National Center for Health Statistics. 2004. DHHS Publication No. (PHS) 2004–1250 04–0226.

92. VA National Center for Patient Safety. *Inside the Falls Toolkit Notebook*, 2004, 1–139. Available at: www.patientsafety.gov/SafetyTopics/fallstoolkit/notebook/completebooklet.pdf. (Accessed August 17, 2009.); Rizzo, J. A., R. Friedkin, C. S. Williams et al. "Health care utilization and costs in a Medicare population by fall status." *Medical Care* 1998; 36(8): 1174–1188.

93. Centers for Disease Control, Injury Center, *op. cit.*

94. The Institute for Healthcare Improvement. *Reducing Harm from Falls, Criticality: The Problem of Falls.* Available at: www.ihi.org/IHI/Topics/PatientSafety/ReducingHarmfromFalls/. (Accessed August 17, 2009.)

95. The Joanna Briggs Institute. "Best Practice: Falls in Hospitals." 1998; 2(2): 1–6. Available at: www.joannabriggs.edu.au/pdf/BPISEng_2_2.pdf. (Accessed August 17, 2009.); Bogardus, S. "Another Fall." *Morbidity and Mortality Rounds on the Web, Case and Commentary* 2003. Available at: www.webmm.ahrq.gov/case.aspx?caseID=6. (Accessed August 17, 2009.)

96. Morse Fall Scale. Available at: www.patientsafety.gov/SafetyTopics/fallstoolkit/media/morse_falls_pocket_card.pdf. (Accessed August 17, 2009.)

97. Gray-Miceli, D. Fall risk assessment for older adults: The Henrich II fall risk model. *The Hartford Institute for Geriatric Nursing* 2007; 8: 1–2. Available at: www.ConsultGeriRN.org. (Accessed August 17, 2009.)

98. *Ibid.*

99. Dykes, P. C., D. L. Carroll, A. C. Hurley et al. "Why do patients in acute care hospitals fall? Can falls be prevented?" *The Journal of Nursing Administration* 2009; 39(6): 299–304; Naqvi, F., S. Lee, and S. D. Fields. "An evidence-based review of the NICHE guideline for preventing falls in older adults in an acute care setting." *Geriatrics* 2009; 64(3): 10–13, 26; Institute for Healthcare Improvement. Patient fall prevention and management protocol with toileting program—VAMC Bay Pines. Available at: www.ihi.org/NR/rdonlyres/2D463413–07BF-4B6F-B6F3-A71C70501659/1633/BayPinesVAMCFallProtocol.pdf. (Accessed August 17, 2009.); Agency for Healthcare Research and Quality: Morbidity and Mortality, 2009, *op. cit.*

100. Stiell, A., A. J. Forsters, I. G. Stiel et al. "Prevalence of information gaps in the emergency department and the effect on patient outcomes." *Canadian Medical Association Journal* 2003; 169(10).

101. McCaig, L. F. and C. W. Burt, 2006, *op. cit.*

102. Eikel, C. and S. Delbanco. "The Leapfrog Group for Patient Safety: Rewarding higher standards." *Joint Commission Journal on Quality and Patient Safety* 2003; 29(12): 634–639.

103. Marco, C. A., V. C. Patrick, D. A. McKenzie et al. "A study of the workforce in emergency medicine: 2007." *American Journal of Emergency Medicine* 2009; 27(6).

104. Physician Insurers Association of America (PIAA). *Research Notes. Emergency Departments.* Summer 2001. PIAA, Rockville, Md.

105. PIAA *Risk Management Review—Emergency Medicine*, 2009, *op. cit.*

106. White, A. A., S. W. Wright, R. Blanco et al. "Cause-and-effect analysis of risk management files to assess patient care in the emergency department." *Academic Emergency Medicine* 2004; 11(10): 1035–1041.

107. Elshove-Bolk, J., M. Simons, J. Cremers et al. "Description of emergency department-related malpractice claims in The Netherlands: Closed claims

study 1993–2001." *European Journal of Emergency Medicine* 2004; 11(5): 247–250.

108. ACEP Policy Statement #400100, Approved by the ACEP Board of Directors, July 2000.

109. Emergency Nurses Association. Telephone advice (Position Statement). Approved September 1998. Available at: www.ena.org/SiteCollectionDocuments/Position%20 Statements/Telephone_Advice_-_ENA_PS.pdf. (Accessed March 31, 2010.)

13

Prehospital Emergency Medical Services

Alice L. Epstein
Gary H. Harding

The National Association of State Emergency Medical Services Officials (NASEMSO) and the National Association of Emergency Medical Services Physicians (NAEMSP) define a *medical emergency* as a sudden or unanticipated medical event that requires immediate assistance; *emergency medical services* (EMS) as the provision of services to patients with medical emergencies; and an *emergency medical services system* as a comprehensive, coordinated arrangement of resources and functions that are organized to respond in a timely, staged manner to targeted medical emergencies, regardless of their cause or the patient's ability to pay, to minimize their physical and emotional impact.

An emergency arises, lives are at stake and time is of the essence. Who should respond? How will they know where to go? What can they do to save the life of the injured person? Depending on where you live and work, the answer may be quite different. Lives can be saved and the number of severe injuries reduced if suitable resources are available and when clinical and transport emergency service personnel recognize and act upon their responsibilities in a prompt, efficient, and clinically appropriate manner. This chapter presents the organization of EMS, how they vary from locale to locale, and the inherent risks in the delivery of prehospital emergency services. Discussions of the clinical aspects of EMS (for example, how to assess and treat cardiac pain) are beyond the scope of this chapter, except as they relate to liability and risk management. Also excluded are disaster planning and response, exposure to hazardous materials, and the Emergency Treatment and Labor Act (EMTALA) because they are covered elsewhere in this series.

Although emergency medical services, systems, and the personnel who work in them are discussed in this chapter, content regarding systems operations does not purport to be exhaustive. This discussion is intended to provide background and information to familiarize risk management professionals with risk exposures associated with prehospital emergency medical services and systems and arm them with proactive tactics to minimize associated risk. Risks related to responding to and transporting emergency patients can result in professional liability, general liability, or products liability. Following are examples of exposure-prone areas in EMS:

- Clinical care
- Emergency medical technician (EMT)/paramedic care
- Driver/pilot performance
- Transport craft design, maintenance, and manufacturer
- Dispatch
- Air traffic control
- Operating organization/agency performance
- Helicopter pad operator practices
- Obstruction avoidance
- Weather determination and decision making.

Whether by ground or air, means and operation of transport is just as important as that of the EMS professionals in attendance because any vehicular malfunction or accident aboard the transport vehicle may cause more injuries, or even the death of the patient, operator, and/or clinician(s).

· · · · · · · · ·
LEGAL DUTIES

Duties of prehospital EMS personnel and systems include the obligation to ensure that personnel are trained to a performance standard that is consistent with what another reasonable professional in this arena would do under same or similar circumstances. To achieve a reasonable approach, the system must be sure that it is capable of expeditious, safe response, with suitable equipment and personnel. There is no duty to provide every technology available or the highest level of training for every crew. The duty of "reasonable prudence" is owed to any patient that the system undertakes to treat.

Very few professional liability claims studies have been performed for EMS services. Two published studies during the 1970s and 1980s identified very similar rates of claims filed per number of patient encounters. During the decade between 1972 and 1982, Dade County Fire Rescue handled 265,060 patient encounters, and sixteen claims were filed with the Risk Management Division of Dade County. The claims were produced by 11 patient encounters, which yields a rate of 1 per 24,096 patient encounters. The two greatest causal factors identified were inadequate recordkeeping and management of "gray zone" patients who do not fit any particular protocol.[1] A retrospective review of all claims brought against a large metropolitan EMS system that focused on paramedic–patient encounters during a twelve-year period (1976–1987) revealed a similar incidence of malpractice claims. During this period, EMS units responded to approximately two million calls and transported more than one million patients. During a ten-year period (1976–1985), sixty claims occurred. The overall litigation rate was one lawsuit per 27,371 patient encounters and one lawsuit per 17,995 patient transports.[2]

In a third, more recent study, all claims made against an urban 9–1–1 ambulance service, whether or not a lawsuit resulted, were analyzed for the ten-year period ending in 1993. Eighty-two claims resulting in eleven lawsuits were filed. Motor vehicle accidents involving an ambulance produced the overwhelming majority (72 percent) of claims and 53 percent of the dollars paid out. Medical negligence claims were few, but were the next-largest cause of dollars lost (35 percent).[3]

EMS lawsuits can be complex, because there are often a myriad of individuals, agencies, and organizations named and thereby involved in the claim. Providers of emergency medical services might include volunteer firefighters, police officers, ambulance drivers, paramedics, 9–1–1 dispatchers, and hospital staff, such as physicians and nurses. Personnel providing emergency services may be government employees, private-company employees, or a combination thereof. The 9–1–1 dispatcher may be a federal, state, or local governmental employee who dispatches police and fire assistance, as well as privately owned ambulances. Private providers may be under contract to the city or county, a service provider, or a parent company, or they may act independently. EMS cases can also be complicated by questions about the applicability of sovereign immunity.

Professional liability issues that EMS providers face include failure to obtain consent, failure to diagnose, misdiagnosis, provision of inaccurate information to decision makers, negligent medical care (failure to properly assess, intubate, or stabilize the patient), and unnecessary delay in transport or treatment, among other issues. Additional examples of successful negligence allegations include

- patient transportation to a medical facility without specialty care, including trauma level support, needed by the specific patient;
- failure to properly maintain equipment, supplies, or vehicles;
- inadequate staff hiring, training, and supervision; and
- driving negligently or recklessly.

Liability may also be based on theories other than negligence and filed as a civil rights case, for causes including the following:

- Abandonment: Improper termination of medical care or turning care over to less-qualified personnel, resulting in injury to the patient.
- Assault or battery: Physical contact with a person without the person's consent or against his or her wishes.
- Delayed response: Unacceptable and injurious delay due to such factors as the dispatch process involving more than one dispatcher. For example, the local police department may take the initial call and then be required to turn the call over to a

private ambulance company serving the area under government contract, resulting in delay.

- False imprisonment: Intentional detention of an individual against his or her wishes.
- Breach of confidentiality: Sharing medical information with those who do not have a "need to know." In this regard, it should be noted that EMS providers do have a legal responsibility to report certain medical and other personal information to government agencies. For example, cases that are usually reportable under state law include neglect or abuse of children and the elderly, rape, gunshot wounds, stab wounds, animal bites, and certain communicable diseases.

Government immunity may protect state, county, local, and other governmental entities from litigation for negligent acts of their employees. However, many states have discarded this doctrine or have limited the extent to which it applies. Good Samaritan legislation exists in some form in all fifty states. It is intended to encourage people to help others in an emergency without fear of litigation. However, these laws do not generally protect healthcare professionals from acts of

- gross negligence;
- reckless disregard; and
- willful or wanton misconduct.

There are several theories under which liability actions can be brought against EMS providers, including vicarious liability against the EMS organization. The risk management professional's starting point for addressing risk within the organization should be helping providers deliver care that is timely, adequate, and safe. The following sections provide more insight into EMS operations, related risk management issues, and suggested risk reduction strategies.

BRIEF HISTORY OF EMS SYSTEMS

EMS and EMS systems claim their roots in military medicine. It was recognized that early intervention in wartime injury could reduce deaths and improve "soldier outcome," thereby increasing the number of troops available for war. As one of the first efforts to improve the timeliness of medical intervention, some military operations brought medical specialists to the battlefield. Modern battlefield standards include dedicated vehicular emergency medical transport, rotary-wing and fixed-wing air evacuation, and mobile surgical hospitals.

The evolution of the public EMS system lagged behind the military system because of the financial and political implications and because of the massive size of the undertaking. Before the mid-1960s, due to the lack of any national standards or motivation, emergency medical service could be excellent in one locale and be virtually nonexistent in others. Structure and operations might be reasonable and logical in one area, but poorly thought out and prone to failures in others. Prehospital emergency service providers could have been highly trained professionals with dedicated equipment, or the first responder might have been your neighbor because your neighbor's automobile was the fastest way to get a patient to the local hospital.

A 1966 National Academy of Science National Research Council publication, "Accidental Death and Disability: The Neglected Disease of Modern Society," identified the gross inadequacies in our emergency healthcare systems, citing diversity, lack of standards, and the lack of a systemized approach. Based on these findings and the efforts of many, including those within the emergency medical service profession, the Highway Safety Act of 1966 resulted in formation of the National Highway Traffic Safety Administration (NHTSA). NHTSA was charged with assisting others to develop their own local emergency services programs. The Emergency Medical Services Systems Act of 1973 further exposed the issue of discontinuity in EMS delivery, provided standards for planning and intervention, and allocated resources to state and local governments for the implementation of comprehensive EMS systems. This program was administered through the Health Resources and Services Administration (HRSA). The original goal emphasized improving response to adult emergencies. Pediatric emergencies received less attention. Thus when the first data were examined, adult outcomes had improved substantially, but pediatric outcomes lagged. In 1993, the Institute of Medicine (IOM) published a report entitled "Emergency Medical Services for Children" (EMSC) detailing these concerns. A flurry of Congressional activity resulted, including Public Law 98–555, as amended, which authorized the use of federal funds for EMSC. This legislation was the origin of two consecutive five year plans aimed at improving EMS to children.

Educational requirements for EMS healthcare responders were outlined in 1993 by a multidisciplinary group acting on behalf of the National Highway Traffic Safety Administration (NHTSA). They developed the National EMS Education and Practice Blueprint to better define the levels of training required for emergency services providers. The goals of the document were to delineate required education and experience and scopes of practice for EMS providers across the country. The blueprint also set out a framework for future curriculum development projects and a strategy to address reciprocity concerns.

In response to professional analysis and opinion regarding emergency response to the September 11 attacks, and the serious shortcomings of the emergency response to Hurricane Katrina, improved performance of our emergency response system has become an important focus for both public and civil servants.

In 2003, the NHTSA published the *Guide for Interfacility Patient Transfer*.[4] Key federal authorities convened to

- identify national EMS priorities;
- establish consensus-based guidelines;
- promote consistent high-quality patient care; and
- identify systematic processes for optimal delivery of care.

In 2005, Congress passed Public Law 109–59, Section 10202, which created the Federal Interagency Committee on Emergency Medical Services (FICEMS). The committee was established to ensure coordination among federal agencies involved with state, local, tribal, and regional emergency medical services and 9–1–1 systems. The Institute of Medicine's Committee on the Future of Emergency Care in the United States Health System convened in September 2003 to examine the state of emergency care in the United States. The committee published a series of three reports in 2006 that look at hospital-based emergency and trauma care, at prehospital EMS, and at the special challenge of providing emergency care for children.[5] Within the treatise entitled, "The Future of Emergency Care: Emergency Medical Services At the Crossroads" the Committee noted that EMS agencies do not effectively communicate and coordinate with dispatch services, emergency departments, trauma centers, public safety agencies and public health departments. They also noted that there are no nationwide standards for the training and certification of EMS personnel and that federal responsibility for oversight of the emergency and trauma care system is scattered across multiple agencies. Resultant recommendations of the Committee specific to EMS include the following:

- The need to create a coordinated, regionalized, accountable system. The emergency care system of the future should be one in which all participants along the continuum fully coordinate their activities and integrate communications to ensure seamless emergency and trauma services for the patient.

- The federal government should create a lead agency in the Department of Health and Human Services (HHS) and support the development of national standards for: emergency care performance measurement; categorization of all emergency care facilities; and protocols for the treatment, triage, and transport of prehospital patients.

The Department of Transportation (DOT) formed The National Highway Transportation National EMS Advisory Council (NEMSAC) in April 2007 as a nationally recognized council of EMS representatives and consumers to provide advice and recommendations regarding EMS to NHTSA. Twenty-five emergency medical services stakeholders were appointed to provide the NHTSA with recommendations and advice. The NEMSAC does not manage programs, develop regulations, or make any decisions directly affecting the programs on which it provides advice.

In August 2008, the NHTSA, Office of the EMS, released the EMS Education Agenda for the Future: A Systems Approach.[6] The agenda notes that the 2006 National EMS educational core content is complete. States have been asked to review their statutes and administrative rules relative to the Educational Scope Model. NHTSA originally planned to have the final standards available in early 2009, but the publishers indicated it will likely be at least two years after that before the first textbooks and supporting materials are available. Because many of the educational activities require action by state EMS agencies, the National Association of State EMS Officials (NASEMSO) is leading the effort to develop education agenda implementation strategies and timetables. NASEMSO, a voluntary, nonprofit organization, is focusing on strategies to achieve accreditation for all paramedic education programs (including discussions of how fire service-based, vocational education–based, and other similar programs can achieve accreditation) and transition to the education standards that will move existing EMS personnel to the new standard operating procedure levels. As part of its ongoing collaboration with national EMS partners on education agenda implementation, the National EMT Registry (a voluntary, nonprofit organization funded by user fees) is moving to implement the final two components of the agenda: EMS education program accreditation and national EMS certification.

As recommended in the EMS Education Agenda and in the Institute of Medicine report, the issue of implementing national EMS program accreditation continues to be addressed by the collective EMS community. For the paramedic level only, the NREMT board of directors is presently targeting the date of January 1, 2013, to begin requiring certification as a prerequisite for accreditation. Paramedic training programs in many states are already engaged in related efforts.[7]

At their June 2009 meeting, the Federal Interagency Committee on Emergency Medical Services (FICEMS) adopted a position on the National Health Security Strategy (NHSS). In a letter to HHS secretary, the position was stated as follows: "It is the intent of FICEMS that EMS systems be fully integrated and coordinated with public health systems to address challenges to national public health security. Federal funds may be used to support EMS activities and target capabilities, such as the Emergency Care Enterprise, which implement the priorities of the NHSS."[8]

EMS STRUCTURE AND ORGANIZATION

As evidenced in previous discussion, structural support and coordination-enhancing efforts for the EMS system are in progress. Although this is a step in the right direction, and tangible improvements in the quality of care and response of the EMS system may be on the horizon, many issues that were problematic in the past remain so. It must also be noted many of the recommendations recently made by the government, professional organizations, and the EMS industry are the same as those first made in the mid-1980s.

Because there is still no central EMS coordinating authority that enjoys jurisdiction in all locales, one could rightly assume that there are countless different EMS structures in place throughout the country. There also continue to be differing opinions among healthcare organizations, emergency services providers, and communities on several issues, including the most appropriate sponsor of prehospital services: for example, should emergency services function under the auspices of a medical facility, a fire service, or as a volunteer organization? Similarly, there is no definitive response to the question of which qualifications should be required of personnel who work within and direct EMS, what equipment to use in EMS, and what protocols should guide EMS operations. There are even multiple clinical approaches for the same injury or illness.

Among points that all parties agree on is that effective provision of emergency medical services requires coordination among emergency medicine providers, public health and safety agencies, and medical facilities. Another is that, regardless of the structure of the system, the response must meet the need. One of several organizational approaches currently in place is a statewide entity responsible for many local EMS systems, including dispatchers, prehospital emergency care providers (ground and perhaps air), and base station operations. Other approaches seeking to enhance coordination include systems run by volunteer personnel and privately held EMS companies. A comprehensive organizational chart of the current EMS structure is a valuable tool for emergency services administrators and can also assist the risk management professional to better understand accountability, and thus the potential exposure for various parties.

· · · · · · · · ·
EMS RESPONSE

In general, public health needs, from the occurrence of the emergent injury or illness through treatment and final disposition, can be met if the following stages of a comprehensive response system are in place.

Prevention

When possible, steps are taken to reduce the likelihood of emergent injury or illness from occurring. Examples may include public education emphasizing electrical safety in the home, poison and drug childproofing, the importance of routine physical exams, and so on.

Detection

Most emergent injuries and illnesses that require prehospital emergency medical services are detected by laypersons at or near the scene of occurrence.

Notification

Once detected, many locations, although not all, now have access to a local 9–1–1 service. In some locales, there is still the need to notify the law enforcement department dispatcher who, in turn, notifies the ambulance crew. A majority of calls are from laypeople, perhaps the individual detecting the injury or illness or a bystander who is directed to "Get an ambulance! Get help! Call 9–1–1!"

Dispatch

Although some emergency calls are found later not to be emergencies requiring hospital services, reasonable prudence dictates that EMS dispatch a team to assess, treat, and transport the patient, if necessary. It is important to recognize that the dispatcher may call for ground or air response, or both.

Pre-arrival

It always takes time for the emergency team to arrive on the scene. Hence the dispatcher has a secondary responsibility to provide immediate assistance to the caller and, if applicable, the first responder and any willing bystanders, concerning the actions they can take to respond to the injury or illness. These steps include support for the patient and emotional and crisis control support for the bystander volunteers.

On-Scene

Once the prehospital emergency response team arrives, they assess and provide treatment to stabilize the patient, if possible, in consultation with more experienced and more highly trained medical professionals who might be available on the scene or via communication systems. The initial assessment is an opportunity to validate which facility the patient should be taken to and might result in a decision to take the patient to a more acute setting.

Transport and Facility Notification

Primary responsibilities during transport are to maintain patient stabilization, respond to new emergent problems, and, as rapidly as practicable, get the patient to a higher level of treatment capability. The team might or might not be in contact with the receiving facility during transport, depending upon the locale and situation. The team might have contacted the receiving hospital earlier, while they were en route to the scene. Or, the responsibility for contacting the receiving caregivers might have been assumed by other members of the EMS team, such as the dispatcher or medical control representative.

Emergency Department

Once the transport vehicle arrives at the receiving facility, treatment is most often initiated within the emergency department (ED), although prior communication should have alerted the facility to the need for immediate surgery or other treatment (for example, hyperbaric therapy for a dive injury) not typically available in the ED.

Interfacility Transport and Follow-Up

With admission to the ED documented by EMS representatives who participated in the care of the patient, the role of EMS comes to an end, with two exceptions. If the patient requires interfacility transfer, the providers who brought in the patient might well be the ones to make the transfer. Also, EMS follow-up to determine the effectiveness of care, through quality improvement monitoring, may entail review of the patient's course during hospital care, rehabilitation, discharge, and follow-up.

The remaining sections of this chapter will deal primarily with the risks inherent in EMS processes from notification through transport. Also addressed will be risk-prone aspects of EMS care, such as consent, management of medical equipment, and staffing.

. . . .

FEDERAL GUIDELINES

As previously noted, there is no centralized federal authority that dictates all aspects of EMS systems. However, the following federal agencies do provide important resources or influence EMS in other ways.

- Centers for Disease Control and Prevention (CDC): The CDC is responsible for addressing, among other issues, communicable diseases and their treatment. The CDC often provides information and guidance about emerging infectious diseases, nosocomial infections, and bloodborne pathogens, such as hepatitis A, B, and C.[9]

- Food and Drug Administration (FDA): The FDA has several subsidiaries that may affect the EMS. Through its Center for Devices and Radiological Health (CDRH), the FDA regulates medical devices, their manufacturers, and users. These devices range in complexity from very simple items such as bandages and gloves to defibrillators, transport incubators, and even ambulances. Furthermore, CDRH has the authority to require equipment manufacturers and users alike to report medical device–related adverse events to the FDA under the Safe Medical Device Act (SMDA) through the MedWatch FDA Safety Information and Adverse Event Reporting Program.[10] Healthcare professionals may research the MedWatch database for information about a particular medical device manufacturer, type of device, or even a specific type of event.[11]

- Federal Interagency Committee on Emergency Medical Services (FICEMS): This body was established to ensure coordination among federal agencies involved with state, local, tribal, and regional emergency medical services and 9–1–1 systems.

- National Highway Traffic Safety Administration, Office of the EMS (NHTSA-EMS): According to the NHTSA Office of EMS, their mission is to reduce death and disability by providing leadership and coordination to the EMS community in assessing, planning, developing, and promoting comprehensive, evidence-based emergency medical services and 9–1–1 systems.

- Occupational Safety and Health Administration (OSHA): OSHA often operates under its general duty clause, which requires the employer to provide a safe workplace. This allows OSHA representatives broad leeway to determine what practices are unsafe, making it possible for them to perform unannounced audits of the workplace. Specific areas overseen by OSHA relating to EMS may include bloodborne pathogens,[12] ergonomic practices,[13] and emergency response in the workplace.[14] Note that the regulations of state organizations that are the equivalent of OSHA, such as California OSHA (CalOSHA), may be prescriptive and take precedence over federal guidelines.

- Health Resources and Services Administration (HRSA): HRSA has responsibility for key programs such as HIV/AIDS Services, the Ryan White CARE Act, Primary Health

Care, Health Professions, Special Programs, and Rural Health Policy. Guidance documents provided by this agency, such as "Integrating EMS Into Rural Health Systems,"[15] provide valuable resources for EMS providers.

- National Institutes of Health (NIH)—The NIH is the steward of medical and behavioral research for the nation. NIH publications such as "Research on Emergency Medical Services for Children"[16] and the extensive information available under NIH auspices through the National Library of Medicine, online, are invaluable to all healthcare professionals, including EMS providers.[17]

- Federal Emergency Management Agency (FEMA): FEMA is an independent agency that reports to the president. The charge of FEMA is to plan for, respond to, and assist in recovery from disaster. Most often, FEMA is responsible for mitigating the impact of catastrophes such as the series of hurricanes experienced by the United States in 2005. An example of the proactive role of FEMA is the requirement that state and local off-site response organizations demonstrate their ability to address injured members of the public, who might have been contaminated by exposure to radiation, through annual drills. The authority under which such exercises are carried out is found in FEMA regulations at NUREG-0654/FEMA-REP-1, Rev 1.[18]

- Department of Transportation (DOT): This agency participates in the development of the curricula by which the EMT is certified and recertified.

- Health and Human Services (HHS), Centers for Medicare & Medicaid Services (CMS): One particular matter under CMS purview, which recently received attention, is the responsibility to alert the public to the potential for fraud by ambulance companies. In a fraud flyer intended to help beneficiaries recognize fraudulent practices in the Medicare program, CMS advised beneficiaries to be suspicious of ambulance companies that bill for trips that are not emergent in nature. CMS subsequently recognized that the statement was misleading and published the following revised statement: "Nonemergency ambulance services are covered by the Medicare program when reasonable and necessary."[19]

Other federal government agencies, such as the Environmental Protection Agency (EPA) and the National Institute of Occupational Safety and Health (NIOSH), are responsible for resources relevant to EMS. For example, NIOSH is responsible for the requirement that all healthcare organizations have available material safety data sheets (MSDS) to make employees aware of how to safely handle hazardous materials. NIOSH also provides guidance on the selection of sharps waste disposal units.

State Requirements

The definition of basic emergency medical services, and associated requirements, varies among the states. Also variable are state approaches to clinical issues such as the use of automatic external defibrillators (AEDs).[20] This chapter will not explore the various state regulations.

·········

ACCREDITATION

Although many EMS organizations have not sought voluntary accreditation of services available from private organizations, they should consider the standards of such organizations as the basis for their own audit. Such self-evaluation can be extremely helpful for risk reduction and can enhance quality improvement efforts.

An example of an acceptable accreditation process that can assist EMS systems in assessing practice is found in the standards of the Commission on Accreditation of Ambulance Services (CAAS), an organization originally developed by the American Ambulance Association. The accreditation process includes a comprehensive self-assessment and an independent outside review of the EMS organization. CAAS standards address risk issues such as vehicle maintenance, management of employees, disposition of the patient's personal property, key aspects of clinical care, incident reporting, and loss control. The process emphasizes the importance of coordination among public safety agencies and local EMS providers as a key factor in providing high-quality healthcare. For example, standards evaluate the effectiveness of operation among agencies during a disaster. Important principles addressed in this regard are conflict resolution and inter-agency dialogue.

Human resource practices recognized by CAAS to be critical to success of EMS organizations include credentialing, discipline or corrective action, problem resolution, training, and performance evaluations.

The Commission on Accreditation of Medical Transport Systems (CAMTS) was founded by a group of air medical professionals to promote high-quality medical air transport. The commission offers air ambulance providers the opportunity to have their program assessed by a private outside organization to determine compliance with nationally accepted accreditation standards. Several states, including Michigan, Arizona, and New Mexico, accept CAMTS accreditation in lieu of state licensing of the air ambulance operation.

·········

STAFFING

Staffing volume, training requirements, and infrastructure vary dramatically, in keeping with the many forms of EMS structure discussed earlier. However, there are several key positions found in most EMS operations, including the medical director, emergency medical response professionals, dispatch team, and base station staff.

Medical Director Responsibilities

Organization and provision of EMS requires the participation of physicians, although EMS systems do not routinely use physicians on ambulance staffs to provide prehospital emergency medical care. Every prehospital service provider should designate a physician medical director. The primary responsibility of this position is to ensure quality of patient care by directing the design, operation, evaluation, and any necessary modification of system processes such as notification, dispatch, prehospital care, and transport to the ED.

The medical director should oversee all clinical features of the EMS. To accomplish this, the medical director must have a defined position within the EMS system that encompasses the responsibility to oversee development of medical policies and procedures. The position description should also state the medical director's responsibility and authority to address any deviation from established clinical standards of care or compliance with required training standards of those under his or her supervision.

On a day-to-day basis, medical direction of prehospital emergency care involves developing and overseeing prospective and retrospective approaches that meet accepted standards, in addition to support of prehospital providers at the scene or by voice communication or through online support. Key prospective approaches that should be overseen by the medical director include training, testing, and certification of providers and development of protocols, policies, and procedures. Day-to-day support of these efforts can be provided by the medical director or by others, such as ED physicians or nurses, under the direction of the medical director. Examples of important retrospective approaches include medical audit and review of care, direction of remedial education, and changes in clinical procedures to address any negative clinical outcomes. Various aspects of these approaches can be handled by committees functioning under the medical director, with representation from applicable medical and EMS personnel.

Medical directors should have a license to practice medicine or osteopathy and experience in emergency medicine or prehospital emergency care of the acutely ill or injured patient. Board certification in emergency medicine is optimal. They should be familiar with the design and operation of prehospital EMS systems. Other advantageous experience includes training in medical direction of prehospital emergency units. It is essential to have experience or training in the following: instruction of prehospital personnel and in the EMS quality improvement process, EMS-related laws and regulations, dispatch and communications, and local mass casualty and disaster plans. Also important is experience or training in labor relations, management, and fiscal oversight of healthcare organizations.

The NAEMSP indicates that the medical director should oversee dispatch, including the following aspects:

- The level of medical training of call-takers and dispatchers
- Caller inquiry protocols
- Prearrival patient care instructions
- Ranking of call priority and triage according to potential medical significance of the patient complaint
- Criteria for dispatch of first responders, basic life support (BLS), and advanced life support (ALS) personnel
- Criteria for emergency and nonemergency response
- Criteria for implementation of the disaster or multiple casualty plan

- Procedures for reviewing and updating dispatch protocols
- Qualified direct (online) medical direction and implementation and evaluation of related protocols
- Development and implementation of a system for critical incident stress management

The medical director should also oversee field clinical practice, including medical training and credentialing of out-of-hospital personnel and periodic testing to verify skill proficiency. Protocols should be developed for transport and nontransport personnel. These protocols should include criteria to help determine destination and transport methods. Such protocols should also address patient-initiated refusals and patient safety.

The medical director should oversee the development of medical standards that promote higher levels of patient care quality. It is for this reason that the oversight responsibility must include authority to limit the medical activities of patient care providers who deviate from established clinical standards of practice or who do not meet training standards. In addition, the medical director should oversee staff education, including requirements for initial training and continuing education. Also important are medical competency evaluations for prehospital providers to ensure that an adequate knowledge base and skill proficiencies are maintained.

The medical director should demonstrate leadership by establishing standards for online medical direction, including requirements for field experience for the physicians who provide online support and training of others to whom the authority for medical direction may be delegated, such as RNs and other dependent allied health personnel. Also important is the education of all base station personnel regarding their specific responsibilities for support of online medical direction.

Although all of the above parameters are important and desirable, note that there is no specialty certification by the American Board of Medical Specialties for EMS medical directors. Moreover, not all EMS systems have a medical director.

Prehospital Emergency Medical Care Personnel

The ambulance staff is responsible for delivery of all emergency care from the time they first see the victim through transportation and transfer to the care of a physician. These positions may be staffed by employees or volunteers. In Public Law 105–19, the Volunteer Protection Act of 1997, certain protections from lawsuits were established for volunteers, nonprofit organizations, and governmental entities based on the activities of volunteers. For example, protection is provided from litigation relating to harm caused by an act or omission of volunteers if the volunteers were acting within the scope of their responsibilities and were properly licensed, certified, or authorized to practice in the state in which the harm occurred. To qualify for this protection, it is also essential that harm must not have occurred as the result of willful or criminal misconduct, gross negligence, reckless misconduct, or a conscious, flagrant indifference to the rights or safety of the individual. In addition to becoming knowledgeable about this act, risk management professionals should refer to state-specific Good Samaritan laws.

The skills needed by prehospital emergency personnel vary widely. It is important to recognize that the need that requires emergency response can range from an uncomplicated fall by an elderly person to mass and severe casualties from a large catastrophe. Prehospital personnel must be able to appraise the extent of the injury and carry out whatever additional measures will make it safe to move the victim and minimize morbidity and mortality. They must operate the emergency transport vehicle safely and efficiently and maintain communication among personnel at the scene of the emergency, with dispatch, and with the ED. They must render additional emergency care en route while transmitting additional information to the physician. In some situations, the role of the prehospital provider is filled by a first responder (someone with forty hours of appropriate training) who is capable of handling certain minor needs. However, other prehospital medical emergencies are handled on-scene by highly trained, highly specialized nurses and physicians. Discussion of the clinical training for physicians, except for the medical director and online medical control, is beyond the scope of this chapter. However, the following provides additional information about the role and training of typical prehospital emergency medical providers.

Although there are national guidelines for the education of emergency medical response providers, the job titles, training, and experience of prehospital emergency providers vary from state to state. Typical titles and certifications include First Responder, Emergency Medical Technician-Basic, Emergency Medical Technician-Intermediate, and Emergency Medical Technician-Paramedic. Additional certifications available from the American Heart Association include basic life support (BLS), pediatric advanced life support (PALS), advanced cardiac life support (ACLS), among others. This list of designations represents progressively higher levels of training in CPR and advanced life support. Although there is a National Registry of Emergency Medical Technicians, there is no national requirement that personnel on the prehospital emergency medical provider team have these designations. However, most states do require one or a combination of these designations.[21] The National Fire Protection Agency (NFPA) has developed two voluntary standards:

1. NFPA 1710, Standards for the Organization and Deployment of Fire Suppression Operations, Emergency Medical Operations, and Special Operations to the Public by Career Fire Departments
2. NFPA 1720, Standard for the Organization and Deployment of Fire Suppression Operations, Emergency Medical Operations and Special Operations to the Public by Volunteer Fire Departments.

The NFPA does not have regulatory authority, but many communities use NFPA standards as the basis for building code and other public safety standards. Municipalities may also mandate compliance with NFPA codes related to response times and staffing, which may influence a jury's determination as to whether the standard of care was met in a related negligence case. Key NFPA provisions require two EMT-Basic courses for providers responding to BLS incidents and attendance of two EMT-Paramedics for ALS incidents. NFPA 1710 requires a response time of four minutes (240 seconds) for first responder arrival and eight minutes (480 seconds) for ALS unit arrival. Departments are to achieve this with 90 percent reliability. Departments must evaluate compliance with the standard annually and consider geography within the jurisdiction as they consider how to meet the objective. A quality management program is required, and it must include review of response times and other clinical care issues.

There are state-specific requirements for certification of each level of provider. Certification requires successful completion of a state-approved training program in addition to passing a written and practical examination.[22] Many states require recertification, which may include an examination or evidence of continuing medical education. Often, states do not have reciprocal agreements for paramedic certification. For example, a paramedic certified in Florida does not have reciprocity in Arizona. The paramedic must take an Arizona refresher course before receiving an Arizona certification.

Some basic recommendations for the development of training programs for prehospital emergency response team members are discussed next (state requirements are, of course, a starting point). Didactic training, combined with development of skills, based on actual clinical performance, is a highly effective way to achieve regulatory compliance. Didactic training should be considered for clinical aspects of care such as anatomy and physiology; trauma types, systems, and mechanism of injury; hemorrhage and shock; burns; clinical specialty issues (such as pulmonary, cardiology, obstetrics); airway management and ventilation; environmental conditions; infectious and communicable diseases; and behavioral and psychiatric disorders. Also important to include in a training program is education that addresses such topics as illness and injury prevention, medical and legal issues, therapeutic communication, history taking, techniques of physical examination, patient assessment, clinical decision making, communication, documentation, ambulance operations, medical incident command, rescue awareness and operations, hazardous materials incidents, and crime scene awareness.

Practical skills training should include skills important to the provision of prehospital emergency care, such as ventilatory support, CPR, peripheral venous cannulation, cardiac monitoring, bleeding management, bandaging, defibrillation and cardioversion, spinal immobilization, patient extrication devices, splinting and traction, and medication administration. Clinical training in the hospital and the field is recommended. The aim is to develop entry-level competence in psychomotor skills and enable the trainee to apply skills and knowledge to actual patient situations. Trainees should log adequate patient contact experience to serve as a basis for future clinical decision making and should demonstrate to educators their ability to perform key procedures, including safe medication administration and effective physical assessments, on several types of patients.

A special issue for prehospital emergency providers is the need to be aware of what action they should take if a medical device might have contributed to a patient injury or death. To the extent practicable, equipment should not be touched. It may be removed from the patient if it continues to present a hazard (such as an electrical shock), but it should not be turned off and settings should not be changed unless it is necessary to do so. EMS prehospital providers should be cautioned that they are not experts on device performance and malfunction and that they should avoid any use or handling of the equipment that might destroy evidence. The best approach is to sequester the equipment, that is, set it aside in a secure place, until it can be assessed by biomedical professionals. It is also important to tag the equipment or device so that it is not inadvertently reused. If it is necessary to turn the device off, the operator should document observations such as all settings, measurements on displays, condition, and so on. Mandatory device reporting (MDR) requirements under the Safe Medical Device Act need to be understood by all EMS personnel so that there is compliance with the necessary reporting of a medical device that has caused the death or serious injury of any patient within ten working days to the FDA and manufacturer. See Chapter 3 for more information on biomedical technology.

Emergency Medical Dispatch

Efficient emergency medical dispatching is critical to the proper operation of the prehospital emergency medical system.[23] The first communication of an emergent situation from a layperson at, or close to, the location of the incident typically is routed to an emergency medical dispatch center. The emergency medical dispatcher (EMD) who takes the call has the daunting task of obtaining key information about the emergency from a potentially hysterical layperson untrained in medicine, determining personnel and vehicular resources to dedicate to the emergency, and providing instructions to the caller concerning treatment and life support that can be provided before the arrival of the EMS professionals. The dispatcher must be able to

- Identify the true nature and the urgency of the emergency in a manner that facilitates selection of the best response; and
- Understand the philosophy and psychology of interview techniques and telephone interventions and use lay terminology to acquire a favorable response.

Such abilities help preserve lives and prevent further injury. Without these skills, too few resources might be dispatched for major problems or excessive resources might be mobilized for minor problems, potentially depriving others in need. Training, certification, and recertification of personnel in dispatch life support (DLS) should be required.

Emergency medical dispatch tools include use of predetermined questions, prearrival telephone instructions, and preassigned response levels and modes, all of which should be approved by the medical director. With these tools, the EMD obtains a telephone history and dictates emergency medical care, including instructions to laypersons on the scene. The EMD can also eliminate gaps that might otherwise occur between the time of the call and initiation of treatment upon EMS team arrival. Telephone instructions based on preapproved medical protocols provided by the EMD to the caller can help protect the patient from further harm and initiate life-saving treatment.

Dispatch prioritization must reflect the appropriate level of response including personnel (First Responder, BLS, ALS), transport resources (number, type of vehicles), and mode of response (lights, siren). Poor dispatch decisions place patients at unnecessary risk and can result in significant liability. However, through use of standard protocols, the EMD can reduce exposure.

All medical care policies and procedures used by the medical dispatch center must be developed in conjunction with, and be reviewed and approved by, the medical director of the system. Routine medical review of dispatch center operations should be performed. Dispatch review committees should provide quality assurance oversight and, ideally, include prehospital EMS physicians, medical control, dispatch supervision and management personnel, dispatchers, and EMTs. Liability for dispatch centers commonly results from lack of essential skills, such as ability to operate and troubleshoot complex communication equipment, and to effectively use basic radio and telephone communication techniques.

Base Station Operations

Emergency medical systems base station operations typically are housed within a hospital, often in the ED. The base station role in the emergency medical system is to provide medical control, consultation, and oversight to field personnel. When the emergency field personnel are nonphysician healthcare professionals, direction of their assessment and treatment efforts must be provided by a physician. Ultimate responsibility for medical control rests with the medical director, who may delegate authority to surrogates (physicians, nurses, or others) on duty in the ED. The medical director may be online, which can mean either on the scene or available by voice communication (such as radio, telephone). However, it is so common for the medical director to be offline (because of other duties or because no one can cover twenty-four working hours in the day) that it is usual practice to identify an online medical physician who might not be the medical director.

Protocols should address the potential for other parties (such as the patient's personal physician or a physician bystander) to be present at the scene. Whereas reasonable prudence dictates that control of medical care at the scene be the responsibility of the individual who is most knowledgeable about prehospital emergency stabilization and transport, the patient's personal physician may assume responsibility, as long as that physician's orders do not conflict with established EMS protocols. If there is a conflict, the personal physician should be placed in direct contact with the online medical physician. Prehospital emergency providers do not have authority to displace the personal physician. If the online medical physician and the personal physician cannot agree on treatment, the personal physician has the option of assuming responsibility and accompanying the patient to the hospital. The personal physician may also defer care to the online medical physician.

If there is an intervener (bystander) physician on the scene who is willing to assume responsibility and document acceptable care, and the online medical physician is not available, the prehospital emergency provider should defer to the intervener physician, even if the intervener's care differs from the local protocol. If the online physician is available, he or she has the option of managing the case entirely. Policies must address the respective responsibilities for EMS personnel and bystander physicians concerning transport arrangements, for example, ground or air emergency service transfer, interfacility transfer, and so on. A coordinated effort is clearly essential to patient welfare, and disagreements about appropriate disposition of the patient can result in liability for all parties, including the medical director(s).

Under the guidance of the medical director, the base station provides centralized control of EMS medical resources. The director and base station personnel have an ongoing responsibility to ensure adequate staffing by skilled, competent personnel. For example, all authorities recognize that online medical control must be immediately available twenty-four hours a day. To achieve this goal, organizations may designate physicians, specially trained nurses, or physician's assistants with special training to be responsible for online medical control. It is important to consult state and professional organization requirements when determining which personnel may take on this important role. The online professional is responsible for reviewing and approving all care delivered and for signing the medical record generated for the specific patient.

Other requirements for base station personnel include completion of adequate medical and procedural training (including field experience), which should be routinely refreshed, and knowledge of the scope of practice for different types of prehospital emergency services providers. Base station performance reviews should be documented on an annual basis, and personnel should participate in routine reviews of ambulance runs. Criteria for such reviews should include timeliness of response, effectiveness of transport, and outcome of response.

It does not follow that, because a base station is located in a particular hospital, patients should be transported to that facility. Patient welfare or logistical issues may result in conveyance to another medical facility. It is also important to recognize that the structure, services, and authorities in one base station's operation sometimes differ significantly from another's. For example, one base station might use only physicians in the online role, and another might use other professionals. Or, one base station might offer services such as real-time telemetry monitoring, and others might offer a lower level of technical support. Still other operational differences may include the way in which quality improvement activities are conducted: one base station might house all such review activities, and another might use a systemwide approach.

Base station–related operations that may result in liability range from clinical decision making to staffing to consent issues to inability to maintain communications. If voice or telemetry communication cannot be initiated or maintained due to equipment performance or shortcomings of architectural design, and these failures could have been prevented, the potential for liability is high.

· · · · · · · · ·
AMBULANCE DIVERSION

There might be occasions when an ambulance must be diverted from what is ostensibly the nearest, most suitable medical facility to a facility that is farther away. This diversion might occur when there is a specific patient or physician request or when triage directs a patient with special needs to a facility that provides a specialized or higher level of care. Another important circumstance that results in redirection of patients occurs when a hospital goes on diversion status because the ED cannot handle current patient volume.

ED diversion due to temporary inability to handle the needs of new patients has increased in frequency.[24] Typically, diversion occurs in large urban areas, but it can occur in rural areas due to a lack of available, adequately trained staff. The negative effects of diversion are many. They include an unacceptably prolonged transport time, necessitating out-of-hospital care when hospital resources are clearly needed, and seriously diminished availability of ambulances in the community. Another concern is that EMS personnel, under such circumstances, might feel forced to take on procedures for which they are not properly trained.

A recent study of data collected in all five boroughs of New York City in 1999 and 2000 found a significant association between time on ambulance diversion and increased mortality resulting from acute myocardial infarction (AMI). Each additional hour of ambulance diversion was associated with a 2.9 to 3.8% increase in AMI outpatient deaths. Days that had an incidence of gridlock, which was defined as at least 25% of hospitals in a borough being on diversion simultaneously, were associated with a 14.1% to 15.7% increase in AMI outpatient deaths. An additional day of gridlock was associated with a 39% to 68.4% increase in AMI outpatient deaths. As a result, there were between 201 and 390 additional AMI deaths during the study period associated with ambulance diversions.[25]

Other factors that increase the frequency of diversion include overcrowded EDs due to increased use of the department for other than emergency care, hospital bed shortages, staff shortages, increasing inpatient severity, hospital closures, and the difficulty of placing patients in nursing homes and skilled nursing facilities. Diversion also occurs because of temporary or long-term lack of available medical specialists, space, technology, or critical care beds. Managed care programs have in the past designated specific hospitals for emergency care. However, the Emergency Medical Treatment and Labor Act (EMTALA) dictates that, in an emergent situation, the patient should be taken to the nearest hospital with appropriate services for the emergency.

With the 2003 revisions to the EMTALA Final Rule, it is important to note that "an individual has come to the ED if that individual is in a ground or air ambulance owned and operated by the hospital, even if that ambulance is not on hospital property" or "if they are in an air or ground ambulance on hospital property, even if the ambulance is not owned by the hospital." However, the revised rule further notes that if "an ambulance that is not owned by the hospital is off hospital property and contacts the hospital stating that they want to bring the individual in for emergency treatment, the hospital is allowed to direct the ambulance to another facility if it is in diversionary status."[26]

According to the American College of Emergency Physicians (ACEP), each EMS system, including all of its component agencies, must develop a cooperative diversion policy designed to include the following:

- Identify situations in which a hospital's resources are not available and temporary ambulance diversion is required.
- Notify the EMS system and hospital personnel of such occurrences. This notification must be communicated to the lead EMS agency or a designated communications coordination center.

- Regularly review and update the hospital's diversion status.
- Provide for the safe, appropriate, and timely care of patients who continue to enter the EMS system during periods of diversion.
- Notify EMS system personnel and affected hospitals promptly when the situation that caused diversion has been resolved.
- Explore solutions to address the causes of diversion and implement policies that minimize the need for such diversions.
- Continuously review policies and guidelines governing diversion.

ACEP also requires that diversion policies require all hospitals and EMS agencies in the EMS system to have working agreements among themselves. Diversion criteria must be based on the defined capacities or services of the individual hospital. When the entire healthcare system is overloaded, all hospitals must open. Diversion should occur only after the hospital has exhausted all internal mechanisms to avert a diversion, and this includes calling in overtime staff. Hospital diversions should not be based on financial decisions. Hospitals should not go on diversion status to save beds for either elective admissions or potential deterioration of hospitalized patients.[27]

The decision to go on diversion status should be made by the emergency physician in the ED in consultation with the hospital's administration, including nursing managers. Appropriate EMS representatives should be notified as soon as possible of the diversion status. All personnel with diversion decision power must be identified and titles communicated to the EMS system's lead agency.

When on diversion status, hospitals must make every attempt to maximize bed space, screen elective admissions, and use all available personnel and facility resources to minimize the length of time on diversion. A record of the diversion should be maintained by the hospital concerning disposition of each affected patient. This log should record the type of diversion, and the reason for it, and should include the appropriate approval. Also documented must be the time that the diversion was initiated and terminated. All patient-specific diversions must undergo concurrent physician review for clinical appropriateness.

· · · · · · · · ·
DESTINATION PROTOCOLS

Destination protocols should be developed to assist EMS providers in the triage of all prehospital emergency patients. These protocols should provide direction to EMS personnel on the following issues: proper use of triage checklists; instructions, including usual dosage, frequency, route, and contraindications for medication administration; circumstances mandating online medical direction; and how to resolve any conflict between the patients' hospital preferences, physician relationships, and the proposed destination facility.

All community and regional EMS agencies should be integrally involved in destination protocol development and review. Due to the varied approaches among EMS services nationally, a single protocol is not suitable for all communities and regions. However, every community and regional protocol should reflect current ability of the receiving facilities to deliver routine and specialty care and information on the hours that these services are available. The National Heart Attack Alert Program (NHAAP)[28] recommends that receiving facilities be categorized in a fashion similar to that used for trauma patient destination decisions. For example, receiving facilities should be classified into one of three levels of care, for example, tertiary, secondary, and primary, and by medical specialty, such as cardiac, trauma, or burn.

In those regions where timely transport to secondary or tertiary care facilities is not available, the highest level of care should be sought and specifics formalized in regional protocols. Acceptable EMS diversion practices should also be strictly defined in regional protocols. As previously mentioned, such protocols should also address issues associated with patient preference.

AIR AMBULANCE SERVICES

Transportation of critical patients can be a formidable task. Problems that affect patient outcome negatively include long transport times, distances to facilities, or transport of patients from inaccessible areas. Determining if air transport of a critical patient is essential and clinically indicated is best determined considering the clinical situation (e.g., emergent condition), time-dependent prognosis (e.g., ability to stabilize on-site versus requiring immediate intervention), and current logistics (e.g., weather, local area landing resources). Unfortunately, some incidents that have occurred have been based on errors in judgment related to each of the above. NAEMSP has identified both clinical and operational situations in which air medical services may provide the fastest, most direct transport to an appropriate regional trauma center. Examples of clinical situations in which air transport may be desirable include a trauma score[29] less than 12, a Glasgow coma score[30] less than 10, spinal cord injury or paralysis of an extremity, major burns, two or more long bone fractures, near drowning, serious trauma to a patient less than twelve or more than fifty-five years of age, and so on.[31] More recently, these guidelines have been broadened to include nontrauma and certain pediatric conditions. Three operational situations identified include mechanism of injury (for example, a vehicle striking a pedestrian at greater than ten miles per hour), difficult access situations (such as wilderness rescue), and time and distance factors (for example, transport time to local hospital by ground greater than transport time to trauma center by helicopter).

There are inherent risks in air medical rescue, particularly rescue using helicopters. The National Transportation Safety Board (NTSB) issued a special report in 2006 addressing the safety issues involved in emergency medical services flight operations[32] from both a procedural and equipment perspective (e.g., implementation of a flight risk evaluation before each mission, formalized dispatch and flight-related procedures, use of night vision and terrain awareness equipment). In 2008 the NTSB intensified its efforts by adding these operations to its 2009 "most wanted" list of federal safety improvements. They noted in a 2008 press release that during the prior eleven months there were nine

EMS accidents resulting in thirty-five fatalities and implied that accidents such as those could have been prevented had the Federal Aviation Administration (FAA) implemented the suggested changes. The FAA noted that although they had not implemented the changes, the agency agreed with the safety intent of the recommendations. They noted that the federal rule-making process takes time and that they preferred to work with HEMS (helicopter EMS) operators to encourage them to adopt better practices, decision-making processes, and new safety technology voluntarily. Since the start of 2009, the NTSB has begun a series of public hearings on recent helicopter air ambulance crashes. The NTSB investigations of the accidents have showed no common underlying causal denominator in these crashes. However, the NTSB is scheduled to make nineteen recommendations regarding HEMS. The proposed recommendations address various safety issues including pilot training; safety management systems to minimize risk; collection and analysis of flight, weather, and safety data; flight data monitoring; development of a low-altitude airspace infrastructure; and the use of dual pilots, autopilots, and night vision imaging systems (NVIS).

In April of 2009, the Government Accountability Office (GAO) heard testimony before the Subcommittee of Aviation, Committee of Transportation and Infrastructure, House of Representatives on air ambulance safety and subsequently released a report entitled "Aviation Safety: Potential Strategies to Address Air Ambulance Safety Concerns." The potential strategies mentioned included obtaining complete and accurate data, increasing use of safety technologies, sustaining efforts to improve air ambulance safety efforts, fully addressing certain NTSB recommendations, adopting safety management systems, clarifying the role of states in overseeing air ambulance services, and determining appropriate use of such services.[33] One professional association has delineated the following four categories of air rescue accidents:

- Aircraft accidents
- Operator error (including so-called rescue fever)
- Equipment failure
- Mother Nature[34]

However, neither guidelines nor FAA regulations can fully anticipate the intricacies and interrelated clinical and operational circumstances of each and every air rescue and medical transport. The local emergency dispatch team members, in close consultation with one another, are likely to be in the best position to determine need because they are familiar with the specific incident and available regional resources. EMS providers and dispatchers should be specifically trained on the operations and respective value of ground and air transport services in their locale so that a timely decision can be made about which to use in a particular situation. For example, stable patients who are ground accessible are probably best transported by ground emergency medical vehicles, whereas patients with injuries and unstable vital signs require the fastest, most direct route to a regional trauma center.

EMS directors and other physicians and administrators should participate in the development of local criteria to facilitate the use of air medical transport resources.

Prehospital emergency personnel, law enforcement, fire and rescue personnel, and agencies of jurisdiction over public use lands should use these criteria to help them determine quickly whether to contact their local emergency medical dispatch team or an air medical service in a specific situation.

As of January 1, 2005, Medicare formalized guidelines for Centers for Medicare & Medicaid Services (CMS) surveyors to help them determine the appropriateness of rural air ambulance services. The determination of appropriateness includes whether the decision to transport was "reasonably made and whether the transport was made pursuant to an approved protocol, or whether the transport was inconsistent with an approved protocol." The "reasonable and necessary requirement" for rural air transport is met when such services are requested by a physician or other qualified medical personnel, based on a reasonable determination that the patient's condition would be compromised if the time to transport by land poses a threat to the patient's survival or endangers health. Other resources to facilitate determination the reasonableness of transport include any already existing state or regional emergency medical services agency protocols.[35]

Specific equipment that has been identified as essential to air medical transport includes oxygen (liquid, internal, external); a monitor, defibrillator, and pacer; an end-tidal CO_2 monitor; pulse oximeter; automated blood pressure monitors or Doppler; ventilators; intravenous (IV) pumps; neonatal isolettes; and balloon pumps. Special considerations include the effect of altitude on hypoxia, liquid and gas interfaces, temperature and humidity on medical equipment, noise and vibration, and acceleration or deceleration forces.

Governmental regulations that apply to air transport include the following. The Federal Aviation Administration (FAA) 135 Air Carrier Certificate is issued for air ambulance operations. It outlines the specific operation standards that an aircraft owner must meet. It is not a federal requirement, however, and many air ambulance operators do not hold this certificate. Some states, such as Florida, issue a state air ambulance license after the provider has completed an on-site inspection. This demonstrates the provider's ability to meet local air medical standards.

Important resources on effective air transport from pertinent professional organizations include the following. The Association of Air Medical Services (AAMS) has developed standards related to basic, advanced, and instructor-level air medical crew training, and the International Association of Flight Paramedics (IAFP) offers a national certification for flight paramedics. The Air and Surface Transport Nurses Association (ASTNA) also provides more detailed guidance on the role of the ground and flight nurse in prehospital transport, and this organization hosts an incident and accident reporting database for air medical services.

Special Issues Applicable to Air and Ground Transport

Both ground and air transport of pediatric patients has received special attention in professional organization statements. The American Academy of Pediatrics Section on Transport Medicine recently published the third edition of *Guidelines for Air and Ground Transport of Neonatal and Pediatric Patients*.

Other areas receiving special attention include bariatric transport and psychiatric transport. Equipment, staffing, training, and protocols for these special transport situations are usually not crafted with the same level of detail as those addressing the transport of infants or cardiac victims.

It is also important that certain legal and ethical issues be addressed by policy and procedure for both ground and air transport. These include (1) refusal to transport, (2) termination of resuscitation during transport, (3) licensure when crossing state lines, (4) medical direction at the scene, and (5) flight prioritization of air ambulance runs.

·········
RISK OF VEHICULAR EMERGENCY RESPONSE

The vehicle operator has the responsibility to safely and rapidly deliver the prehospital emergency team to the scene and the patient and team to the receiving facility. At the same time, the operator must not jeopardize other drivers or pedestrians. Historically, there has been a high correlation between poor driving records and accident occurrence. Hence, motor vehicle reports (MVRs) should be reviewed prior to employment and, preferably, on all drivers annually. Some organizations may require timely reporting by employees of moving violations, and so on, that are incurred while driving a personal vehicle. Driving-specific reference checks and a hands-on demonstration of skills behind the wheel may also be helpful. Preemployment physicals and drug testing may also offer information regarding possible driver-related exposure to risk.

Lights and sirens have been used to alert other vehicles and pedestrians of an emergency vehicle response for more than fifty years. Unfortunately, medical emergency response vehicles, using lights and sirens, have often been involved in collisions that resulted in serious injury and even death. The financial risk of emergency medical vehicle collisions includes costs associated with damage to property, for example, involved vehicles and structures, in addition to settlements and awards for personal injury. Of course, such expenditures trigger concomitant increases in insurance premiums. Collisions are the largest source of negligence-related losses.[36] Currently, there is no centralized, systematic collection of EMS collision information. For this reason, the extent of the problem may be underappreciated.

The relationship between patient outcomes and the use of lights and sirens has not been examined. However, it is likely that emergency providers' urgency to reach a patient who may be seriously ill (and about whose condition they know little) plays a major role in the decision to use lights and sirens.

NAEMSP and the National Association of EMS Directors have stated that use of lights and sirens should be based on standard protocols that address the acuity of the patient's situation and on other issues such as traffic-related factors. Clinical situations in which lights and sirens are generally considered acceptable include cardiac or respiratory distress, severe airway issues, drowning, breech childbirth, electrocution, or critical trauma. It is important that the use of lights and sirens be monitored. Their improper use, such as during routine return to stations, should be identified and steps should be taken to minimize the likelihood of recurrence. The medical director should direct efforts to collect information about light and siren use, evaluate the frequency of use in the field, and take steps to reduce this practice wherever possible. By evaluating the way that dispatch currently prioritizes the need for lights and sirens against the clinical circumstances being responded to, it might be possible to set up specific criteria for use of lights and sirens. American Society for Testing and Materials' (ASTM's) Standard F1258, Standard Practice for Emergency Medical Dispatch and related guidance documents[37] caution emergency medical dispatch personnel against using previous personal experience to determine the severity of a current situation and note that red lights and sirens are not always necessary. Of course, responses to nonemergent situations or emergent situations that are already stabilized at the scene do not require lights and sirens. Potential operators should be screened to ensure that they have adequate training in this area and no record of improper use of lights and sirens.

Remember that the operator of an EMS vehicle is not generally relieved of the responsibility to operate it with due care for the general public, including others on the highway. Vehicular manslaughter charges and convictions can and do occur, as have related civil cases. In addition to requiring screening of potential employees' driving records, proactive loss prevention strategies include requiring that all vehicle operators attend an emergency vehicle operators course (EVOC). Such a program educates drivers based on standardized, nationally accepted content.[38] These courses include classroom work, experience on a driving course, and on-the-job performance recommendations. ASTM also provides guidance for ambulance operators in its F1517–94 Standard Guide for Scope of Performance of Emergency Medical Services Ambulance Operations.

· · · · · · · · ·
GROUND AMBULANCE OPERATION

Several areas of ground ambulance operation have implications for risk management. These areas include vehicle safety, issues regarding patient equipment and supplies, and user training and problem reporting for ambulance personnel who use medical devices.

Vehicle Safety

The General Services Administration publishes requirements for ambulance operation in its federal specification for KKK-A-1822E ambulances and other similar publications.[39] For EMS services to be effective, vehicles must be prepared and able to respond when the system is notified of an emergency and when the dispatcher decides the level and magnitude of the response. If the notification and dispatch aspects of the system function properly and the vehicle fails to roll, a poor patient outcome may result and the system may be subject to liability.

Periodic critical item inspections may help the organization maintain safe vehicles. Such inspections focus on the issues most often identified as causing or contributing to accidents and may include brakes, the steering and suspension system, tires and wheels, lights, windshield and windows, windshield wipers, mirrors, and horn. Frequency of the inspection should be based on vehicle use. If it is in use twenty-four hours a day, inspections should be more frequent. Other items that affect vehicle operation, such as the batteries, fluid levels, and heat source for the ambulance compartment should also be routinely assessed. Drivers should keep vehicle inspection report copies and current documentation of the need for repairs and the completion of those repairs.

Vehicle maintenance is typically defined to include preventive maintenance, demand maintenance, and crisis (breakdown) maintenance. Although the majority of these tasks are the responsibility of the operator, base operations should also maintain related documentation to make sure that an adequate number of properly functioning vehicles remain available. Preventive maintenance and repair records should be meticulously maintained and reviewed on a periodic basis to make sure that the vehicle remains reliable and to help determine when it needs to be replaced. Mechanical breakdowns and inability to respond due to weather or road conditions should be reported to base control and documented there. Although adherence to the federal motor carrier safety regulations (FMCSR) is not mandatory, it is prudent to log vehicle and performance information for each trip to ensure that the resolution of any problems is documented.

Patient Equipment and Supplies

For the vehicle to be capable of rolling once proper personnel are in place, adequate equipment and supplies must be on board. Requirements for specific equipment and supplies to be carried by emergency vehicles vary by state and response mode, for example, ground versus air burn-patient transport.[40]

It is common practice for home base hospitals or receiving hospitals to restock ambulances with drugs and supplies used during the transport so that the ambulance is ready for the next call. Items typically assessed and provided in this process include appropriate medications and supplies, such as intravenous tubing and catheters. Hospitals should collaborate to ensure compatibility of equipment used in local emergency rooms. Of particular importance for risk management professionals, the HHS/OIG published a final rule at the end of 2001 establishing safe harbor protection for ambulance restocking arrangements. Numerous requirements apply to these safe harbor provisions, and risk management professionals should ask legal counsel to provide guidance on developing adjunct policies and procedures.[41]

Most ambulances carry basic communication devices, such as a two-way radio for medical communication, a disaster communication device, and a cellular telephone. Consumable supplies such as gloves, bandages, and thermal blankets are usually available. When requisitioning supplies, remember the need for latex-free alternatives; safety products, such as safety needles and syringes; and other protective devices, including masks, eye protection, and a sharps container. Basic-level provider equipment, such as ventilation and airway equipment, monitoring and defibrillation equipment, and immobilization devices, is usually on hand. It is also important to be sure that equipment and supplies on ground ambulances are adequate for the range of patients likely to be encountered; for example, adequate equipment and supplies must be available for pediatric patients, even newborns.

Advanced level provider supplies and equipment, such as vascular access devices and solutions, specialized airway and ventilation equipment, cardiac equipment, and monitoring devices such as pulse oximeters, may also be required. Some ambulances may also carry advanced equipment such as antishock garments, extraction devices, and specialized equipment and supplies. Medications that must be available for advanced level support are specified by the American Heart Association's Emergency Cardiac Care Committee, and providers receive information about these drugs in the Advanced Cardiac Life Support Course offered by AHA (The American Heart Association). Current information may also be obtained from the ACEP, the American College of Surgeons, and the National Association of EMS Physicians. All medications should be in unit-dose packages, and injectables should be preloaded to reduce the risk of medication errors.

In July 2009, the American Academy of Pediatrics, in conjunction with others, released the policy statement "Equipment for Ambulances," which covers principles of pediatric prehospital care, including supplies and equipment for children. This guidance arguably defines the standard of care by addressing, for example, optional medications, interfacility transport, and extrication equipment.[42]

One very important recent technological advance is the development of the automatic external defibrillator (AED). This device includes a computer function that automatically detects and interprets the electrical activity of the patient's heart. If AED detects ventricular fibrillation, it will prompt a decision about whether to defibrillate. If the user elects to defibrillate, the device will automatically determine when to provide the shock. As with other defibrillators, there is coincident risk of shock to operators and bystanders who are in physical contact with the patient when defibrillation takes place. Therefore, it is important to train providers about clinical and personnel safety implications of AED use and to develop appropriate supportive protocols.

The AHA makes available AED-related education programs that promote the use of AEDs in public areas such as sports arenas, gated communities, office complexes, doctor's offices, shopping malls, and on airplanes. The Cardiac Arrest Survival Act (CASA) became law in November 2000. The law requires placement of AEDs in federal buildings and provides nationwide Good Samaritan liability protection for anyone who attempts to save someone's life with an AED. The AHA recommends that public and private organizations implementing AEDs notify the local EMS office and have a licensed physician or medical authority oversee training and operations. This role is often fulfilled by the EMS medical director and EMS system personnel. AHA further suggests that laypersons be educated in cardiopulmonary resuscitation principles and the use of AED equipment. Since 2003, AHA has supported the use of AEDs on persons as young as one year of age as long as pediatric attenuated pads, which reduce the energy delivered by an adult AED, are used.

The FDA requires purchasers of AEDs to present a physician's prescription.

Although the AHA notes that the perceived potential for a lawsuit has in some cases been a deterrent for nongovernmental organizations considering a public access defibrillation (PAD) program, they also observe that suits have not been filed to date against users of AEDs. On the other hand, suits have been filed against airlines and the proprietors of public entertainment settings alleging that they were negligent in being unprepared to respond to a cardiac arrest. Users of AEDs that adhere to AHA recommendations may be in a better position to defend care rendered and should also bear in mind that a plaintiff bringing suit would first have to overcome other previously discussed immunity provisions.

Medical Device Training and Problem Reporting

As in the hospital setting, training for equipment users is essential. For example, current competence in the use of equipment such as defibrillators is particularly critical.

Because EMS equipment is just as necessary as hospital equipment, it is essential that EMS medical equipment maintenance checks and repairs be performed by trained biomedical engineers functioning under the auspices of a comprehensive biomedical program. The remote locations in which EMS equipment is used make this a particularly urgent priority because device failure in such settings leaves few care options. Biomedical services may be accessed through a hospital affiliate's biomedical engineering program or by participating in a shared services arrangement with other EMS operations. Another alternative is an individual contract with a biomedical services preventive maintenance firm. Information, program, and detailed device problems and evaluation reports may be found on the Web site of ECRI Institute, an independent nonprofit healthcare research operation, at www.ecri.org.

EMS personnel should also identify and promptly address any malfunction. There should be a formal process for notifying personnel of defective devices that they may encounter in the field, such as defective pacemakers that were implanted in numerous patients.[43] There should also be a formal recall process to respond to issues such as defective patient monitors that EMS may already have in service.[44]

. . . .

COMMUNICATION SYSTEMS

Communication systems are essential to mobilizing and coordinating EMS. These communication systems must address incoming reports of emergencies from members of the public, vehicle dispatch and coordination, medical direction and control, and interservice communications, which enable all public services to collaborate. The scope of EMS communication goes beyond the radios in the vehicle, base station, and receiving facility. Also part of EMS communication are cellular and computer-based communication products (e.g., handheld, laptop, and similar cellular, Internet, and texting products; GIS; GPS positioning and locating products), repeater towers, and biomedical monitoring stations, which are used to transmit twelve-lead ECG results to the ED. Other telemetric devices used to transmit vital signs may also be considered aspects of EMS communications.

From a regulatory perspective, it is important that all telecommunication systems not under the auspices of the federal government are subject to rules established by the Federal Communications Commission (FCC). EMS communications personnel should be familiar with FCC regulations regarding technical aspects of communication devices, such as appropriate wavelengths, and qualifications for operators. This information can be found in FCC documentation and in the appendixes of the American Society for Testing and Materials (ASTM) Standard F-1220 (www.ecri.org).

From a risk management perspective, several key points relate to communication. EMS communication systems should meet recognized performance standards that address systems planning and design,[45] and EMS communications should be compatible with, and not interfere with, other communication systems, including EMS operations, within the originating community or neighboring communities. An interesting and important related issue that may be addressed by the state, federal government, or the international communications community in the near future is telemetry.

Allegations of negligence may arise if an emergency call comes in and communications systems fail or are unavailable due to improper use, for example, personal conversations among staff. Risk reduction strategies to lessen this exposure include documentation of adequate system maintenance, implementation of applicable backup communication resources, such as cell phones, use of correct communications protocols, and staff education.

· · · · · · · · ·
CONFIDENTIALITY

Numerous threats to patient confidentiality exist in prehospital care. EMS providers are routine recipients of sensitive information. Indiscriminate discussion or unauthorized release of such information presents both ethical and legal risks. All information that is encountered by prehospital personnel must be considered confidential. Information should be communicated only to those who are assuming direct care of the patient and on a need-to-know basis. The only information that should be discussed over the radio is that which is necessary to provide for optimal care of the patient.

The Health Insurance Portability and Accountability Act (HIPAA) and its associated procedural changes apply to EMS providers just as they do to any other healthcare provider. All EMS providers should be educated about the implications of this important federal privacy law. This is particularly important, because HIPAA has been modified by the HITECH Act, an aspect of the recovery legislation that was signed into law in 2009. Among many other provisions, HITECH creates accountability for individual employees of healthcare organizations and makes them potentially responsible for fines ranging from $100 to $50,000, with maximum total fines of $1.5 million annually for repeated egregious offenses. (Please see Chapter 16, in Volume 3 in this series for more information.)

Among other aspects of the HIPAA/HITECH program, it may also be desirable to require that EMS personnel sign a confidentiality agreement. This approach raises their awareness of the importance of maintaining confidentiality.

· · · · · · · · ·

DOCUMENTATION

The prehospital care report (run report) documents the objective data gathered at the scene, in addition to the subjective findings of the field personnel.

It is the only full medical record of the care provided in the field and in transport. As such, it may be used by insurance carriers, defendants, or plaintiffs in criminal or civil liability cases or by law enforcement personnel when investigating child or elder abuse, rape, and death by questionable means.

It is essential that the record accurately and objectively reflect the patient's condition and support the treatment provided. Poor medical record documentation can lead to costly damage awards and compliance issues associated with billing practices.

Important risk management documentation practices include the following:

- A prehospital care report form should be completed for every call, whether or not a patient is found, even if services are not needed or the trip is cancelled en route. A report should be generated for every interfacility transfer.
- If services are cancelled at the scene, EMS providers should document the cancelling authority, time of cancellation, and the circumstance.
- Each patient must have a separate form.
- The form should be initiated by the first EMS provider on the scene.
- The report should be completed at the scene whenever possible.
- The report should be reviewed and checked for complete and accurate content.

The documentation should include the following components:

- Relevant observations about the patient
- Treatment appropriate for the observed medical condition of the patient
- All care provided
- All information needed by others who rely on the record for ongoing patient care, for example, the existence of allergies
- Ability of the receiving facility to manage the patient's condition

To see whether or not the report achieves its goals, EMS providers should periodically try to recreate the run at a later date with the information provided.

The prehospital care report may help ED staff gather additional patient information after paramedics have left the hospital, or it may help a paramedic recall a long-forgotten incident in a court of law. If the prehospital care report presents a comprehensive picture of the events surrounding the incident, it dramatically enhances the defensibility of any case with which the EMS personnel may be involved. An inaccurate or incomplete EMS run form will often expose the EMS provider to legal liability. Not only is the clinical documentation paramount, but the dispatch/transport times and documentation are also critical. If a later malpractice case alleges negligent delays in dispatch, arrival, treatment, or transport, the plaintiff may attempt to use any redundant or inconsistent documentation of times to make it appear that such times were manipulated to match the estimated on-scene arrival time, in other words that the paramedics fabricated the record to cover a delayed response. Ultimately, the safest approach is simply to insist on accurate, unambiguous, and complete documentation. Other potentially relevant documentation that may raise credibility issues includes the real-time dispatch computer log, police reports, fire and safety department reports, medical first responders' run sheets, dispatch logs, and any other documentation generated in the normal course of the provider's business.

· · · · · · · · ·
CONSENT AND REFUSAL TO ACCEPT SERVICES

EMS patients have a right to understand their injury or illness, the steps that may be taken to address the injury or illness, the risks of those steps, and the risks of refusing care. A cognizant patient may refuse all care or certain aspects of care.

Unless there is a life-threatening emergency in which the patient is not cognizant or conscious, prehospital emergency care providers must have either explicit or implied consent before they can perform procedures. It is highly desirable to obtain explicit consent from the patient and the patient's signature on a consent form, if possible. The patient may be deemed to have implied consent to routine types of procedures, for example, blood pressure checks, if they allow these to be done without objection.

Care must be used in applying the emergency exception that is intended to facilitate care of a patient who is in jeopardy and unconscious or otherwise incapacitated. It is not intended to pertain to all cases of intoxication, limited mental capacity, and psychiatric illness. In situations in which EMS personnel are unsure about whether to proceed with treatment, the input of the medical director should be sought. The objective observations and interventions, in such situations, should also be carefully documented in the prehospital record. These include patient condition, results of pertinent assessment, and discussion with the medical control director. (Please see Chapter 4 for more information on informed consent.)

A mentally competent adult has the right to refuse care, even if refusal would result in death or permanent disability. Refusal may be based on religious beliefs, fear, or lack of understanding of medical procedures. If the injured party does not agree to treatment, the EMS provider should document the refusal and the condition of the patient in concise, objective language, based on discussion with the medical director. If patients refuse care, the EMS provider should reassure them that they may call again for help, despite their initial refusal.

Closely related to refusal of care, patients refuse hospital transportation in 5 percent to 25 percent of out-of-hospital calls.[46] In a study of seventeen advanced life support (ALS) ambulance agencies servicing northeastern Illinois during July 1993 and February 1994, 30 percent of all runs resulted in refusal of transportation. Patients who most commonly refused transportation were asymptomatic, eleven to forty years old, involved in a motor vehicle crash, with no past medical history, normal vital signs, and normal mental status. Patients generally signed for their own releases after evaluation.

A thoroughly objective and comprehensive record is the best defense in any related litigation. This record is important because prehospital refusals are often precipitators of malpractice cases.

If the call is of a nonemergent nature, the decision not to treat or transport may be a mutual agreement between the patient and provider. Otherwise, the provider should consult the online medical director for guidance. It should be noted that there has been an increase in the numbers of homeless who avail themselves of ambulance services for minor clinical problems, thus diminishing the availability of ambulances for true emergencies.

The circumstances in which care is refused are often challenging because the prehospital EMS provider is the eyes and ears of the emergency medical director who is not on site, helping him or her assess the patient's decision-making ability. Competencies that delineate assessment skills that are specific to this situation should be developed and maintained. EMS staff should also routinely receive training to augment these skills.

. . . .

DO NOT RESUSCITATE OR COMFORT CARE

Terminally ill patients (such as those with end-stage cancer or AIDS) are commonly encountered in prehospital emergency medical response because of the growing number of hospice programs and home healthcare systems that are replacing the hospital's role in caring for these patients. There are also an increasing number of persons without terminal illnesses who are executing do-not-resuscitate (DNR) wishes through living wills or advanced directives. However, as death draws near, family, friends, or even the patient may call emergency medical services (EMS) personnel to provide comfort care or to transport the dying patient.

In states without legislation that delineates DNR options, the EMS provider might need to initiate resuscitation, even when notified of the DNR request. EMS providers must be thoroughly familiar with pertinent state regulations and any DNR-related EMS protocol.

In addition to pertinent state regulations, several resources may be used to develop policies and procedures. For example, ACEP has developed "Guidelines for 'Do Not Resuscitate' Orders in the Prehospital Setting." Another potentially helpful resource is a *Journal of the American Medical Association* article entitled, "Guidelines for Cardiopulmonary Resuscitation and Emergency Cardiac Care, Part VIII: Ethical Considerations for Resuscitation" by the Emergency Cardiac Care Committee of the American Heart Association.[47] The guidelines incorporated in this publication address, among other things, the difficult topic of discontinuing cardiopulmonary resuscitation (CPR) when there is a valid no-CPR order.

According to the "National Guidelines for Statewide Implementation of EMS 'Do Not Resuscitate (DNR) Programs,' " DNR policies should do the following:

- Recognize that life support may not be necessary or beneficial.

- Provide the basis for a prospective educational program for the public and the medical communities about appropriate use of the EMS system in treating terminal medical conditions.

- Emphasize presumption in favor of resuscitation when patient wishes are not known.

- Define conditions under which a DNR order should be implemented, taking into account patient competency and the role of acceptable surrogates in making an informed decision.

- Identify clinical procedures to be withheld, along with other medical therapies, including comfort care, which may be clinically indicated and should not be withheld.

- Define the manner in which the DNR order is to be carried out and the role of the EMS.

- Define response for the circumstance in which a patient decides to revoke a living will or other formal statement of their wishes.

- Identify information to be contained in a do not resuscitate order and the procedure for periodic review.[48]

Some states have implemented prehospital DNR forms. In these settings, it is recommended that EMS provide public information sessions concerning how they may be used. These forms typically require a statement by and the signature of the attending physician, acknowledging that the condition is terminal or advanced and that recovery is not expected; the patient is capable of making or has made an informed decision; a statement by and signature of the patient that, in the event of cardiac or respiratory arrest, no resuscitation efforts should be undertaken; and a date of issue and expiration. Forms in some locations may be filed with the EMS prospectively. Other methods whereby EMS personnel may be alerted to DNR status include wallet cards, bracelets, or necklaces. However, these are not substitutes for DNR orders. For any other situations, or where there is any doubt about how to proceed in such difficult circumstances, providers should contact the online EMS medical director.

Also clearly important for EMS staff to have when caring for dying patients is formal guidance on bereavement so that they can assist grieving family members and friends. It is important, as well, to formalize guidance for termination of resuscitation in the field.

· · · · · · · · ·
DISCONTINUATION OF LIFE SUPPORT EFFORTS

On occasion, transport to an ED is delayed or prolonged for reasons beyond the control of the EMS personnel, and life support efforts must be discontinued. The Rural Affairs Committee, NAEMP, National Association of EMS Physicians, and EMS standards recommend that advanced life support (ALS) and basic life support (BLS) procedures, once initiated in the field, be discontinued only if (1) the patient recovers; (2) the patient is pronounced dead by a physician; (3) the rescuers are exhausted; (4) procedures place providers at risk; or (5) there are significant delays in transport.

Most hospital EDs and some EMS agencies have adopted guidelines for the discontinuation of prolonged use of ALS or BLS procedures. Such guidelines may contribute to developing a reasonable basis for making informed decisions in the field, where circumstances might be complicated by the need to transport a patient to a receiving facility far from the emergency scene.

All EMS providers should be familiar with the following, which are specific clinical principles supporting the discontinuation of life support efforts:

1. Defibrillation: Generally, defibrillation is required to reverse cardiac arrest and restore functional cardiac activity. It can be effective when applied soon after the onset of cardiac arrest. Chest compressions do not produce enough effective circulatory function to sustain adequate tissue perfusion when continued for long periods.

2. Prolonged cardiac life support: Most medical authorities currently agree that if cardiac arrest is sustained for longer than thirty minutes without any return of a spontaneous pulse, there is no reasonable chance for functional recovery in patients with normal core temperatures, and further application of ALS or BLS procedures provides no significant benefit to the patient.

3. Prolonged ventilatory support: Functional recovery can and does occur after prolonged ventilatory support without chest compression when a patient has functional cardiac activity but does not have adequate spontaneous ventilation.

Protocols addressing the transport of a patient who has suffered a cardiac or respiratory arrest and undergone prolonged resuscitative efforts should not be rigid. They should, however, provide guidance to prehospital emergency providers in this difficult circumstance. Field protocols should be developed by EMS physicians, using available professional organization–generated and other related resources. Such protocols should routinely be reviewed to ensure that they incorporate current clinical standards of care.

When possible, the decision to discontinue life support efforts should be the responsibility of the online physician. A means should also be specified for pronouncement of death, disposition of the body (including desired organ donation procurement), and grief counseling.

DOA Policies

Dead on arrival (DOA) policies should guide medical directors and EMS personnel in determining which patients should not undergo resuscitation because the effort would be futile. Like guidance for the decision to stop resuscitative efforts, such policies should not be rigid. For example, they should not state that resuscitative measures are *never* to be undertaken when specific conditions are present. However, objective criteria, such as the time that has elapsed since the patient became unresponsive, and so on, can diffuse bias that prehospital emergency care providers might harbor related to patient age, type of illness, or social standing.

· · · · · · · · ·

BLOODBORNE PATHOGEN CONSIDERATIONS

Because of the potential for blood splashes in many prehospital emergencies, EMS personnel are particularly vulnerable to bloodborne pathogen exposures. It is important that all who might come into contact with bloodborne pathogens be educated about associated risks and the importance of adhering to the OSHA bloodborne pathogens standard (Occupational Exposure to Bloodborne Pathogens; Needlestick and Other Sharps Injuries; Final Rule [2001, January 18]. *Federal Register* 66:5317–5325). When educating providers, it is important to stress that bloodborne pathogen infections can be transmitted from a staff member to a patient just as easily as they can be passed from the patient to the staff member. EMS providers should also be aware of the numerous bloodborne pathogens that are of concern, including HIV and hepatitis A, B, and C. For example, hepatitis B is transmitted annually to more than eight thousand healthcare workers in all settings, and more than two hundred die each year. The cost in human suffering and financial risk is formidable.

Of many important procedures in the OSHA bloodborne pathogens standard, the one requiring use of personal protective equipment is particularly important to EMS workers because they are likely to encounter infected persons. In addition to bodily fluids that they may be exposed to as they treat injured persons at an accident scene or conduct CPR, prehospital providers may also be called to a scene where they might inadvertently handle drug paraphernalia, including intravenous devices. Resources on strategies to enhance the effectiveness of personal protective equipment are available from ECRI Institute, the Service Employees International Union (SEIU), International Healthcare Worker Safety Center (IHCWSC), and the International Sharps Injury Prevention Society (ISIPS).

It is also important for EMS workers to be aware of the key implications of the Needlestick Safety Prevention Act (which became Public Law 106–430 on November 6, 2000). This act, when followed, goes far to enhance the safety of the EMS provider and other healthcare personnel by encouraging approaches such as the use of needleless devices. Although clinicians sometimes perceive that safety syringes are less effective than retractable devices, this perception is unproven. Thus, wherever possible, EMS systems should implement needleless systems. Current ambulance supplies should be reviewed and immediate steps taken to replace any conventional syringes with safety products.

The act also requires identification, reporting, and trending of accidental needlestick injuries, including those that might occur in the provision of EMS. Furthermore, the act mandates participation of frontline workers, such as prehospital emergency care providers, in the selection of safety products.

Other measures that can help reduce bloodborne pathogen exposures include offering prehospital workers hepatitis B vaccinations. Even though the worker may defer the vaccination, making it available will protect some workers and will raise awareness of the issue for all.

A detailed protocol for seeking treatment in the event of accidental needlestick should be developed for prehospital emergency care providers. Emphasized in the policy should be immediate steps that the affected employee should take and the applicable time frames, and a formal counseling program is a valuable adjunct to such a protocol.

All EMS managers and personnel must be educated about the importance of maintaining confidentiality of patient and employee information related to accidental needlesticks and other potential bloodborne pathogen exposures.

· · · · · · · · ·
RISK AND RESPONSIBILITY OF RESPONDING TO VIOLENT SCENES

Prehospital emergency providers are routinely confronted with emotionally distraught, intoxicated, and unruly patients and other parties. They need to understand how to protect the patients and themselves should circumstances warrant such protection.

EMS providers must understand is that there is no duty to place themselves at risk when they encounter danger. If there are no law enforcement officials on the scene, no effort should be made to capture or physically restrain a violent patient until after such officials arrive. EMS providers should also be trained to quickly assess potentially dangerous situations and proactively enlist the support of law enforcement personnel.

Training is essential to enhancing the judgment that EMS providers must apply in such circumstances. If, for example, law enforcement personnel are en route and the patient is not already demonstrating violent behavior, providers should begin verbal de-escalation. Physical or chemical restraint might be necessary, based on established protocols and with the support of the medical director. However, any restraint is, potentially, a violation of patient rights. To maintain patient safety and avoid liability, providers should use the least restrictive approach available, in accordance with applicable TJC and other related standards. It is important that these principles be applied with the awareness that the prehospital environment is prone to a lack of clinical information. For example, if EMS providers do not know what medications the patient takes, whether prescribed or illicit, and have no allergy information, physical restraints might be a safer course than chemical restraints. Once physical restraints are in place or sedative medication has been administered, EMS providers must monitor the patient to ensure the patient's well being.

In any later defense of related litigation, objective and comprehensive documentation of the EMS providers' observations and interventions will be essential. For example, the record should include documentation of specific observations that led the providers to conclude that the patient was potentially a danger to himself or others and efforts to de-escalate the situation verbally. If physical or chemical restraint is used, the provider should document cardiovascular and airway status after initiation of the restraint and periodically thereafter.

Because EMS providers are often called to the scene of domestic violence, it is important they be aware of the unique issues inherent in these situations. For example, if the dispatcher indicates that domestic violence might have precipitated the call, law enforcement should be summoned and EMS personnel should not enter the scene until it has been secured. If the EMS providers do not suspect domestic violence until after they are on the scene, the victim should be removed as quickly as possible.

Domestic violence is a crime. Therefore, the scene must be treated as a crime scene, and standard precautions regarding preservation of evidence should be exercised. Initial and continuing education programs for EMS personnel must incorporate information about domestic violence, including identification of victims, preservation of evidence, ways to maintain safety at the scene, and documentation requirements.

· · · · · · · · ·
LIABILITY INSURANCE

All organizations and professionals that offer medical and healthcare services to the public face the potential of a lawsuit. Recommended insurance coverage includes automobile; equipment; comprehensive general liability, including products and completed operations; and professional liability. Currently, primary policy limits vary. Typical coverage limits are $1 or $2 million for each type of coverage, and the premium is based on the number of patient encounters. Many services carry excess policies in addition to the underlying policy. For more information on insurance, refer to Volume 1, Chapter 9. Insurance: Basic Principles and Coverages.

Many states have specific insurance coverage requirements for ambulance services, as contrasted with regular automobile and public transport coverage. Risk management professionals should also be familiar with certain additional requirements. For example, Missouri requires ambulance service owners to carry coverage for the injury or death of an individual due to the owner's negligence in employing a person who negligently administers emergency care (Section 190.120, RSMo).

In applying for insurance coverage, the liability underwriter is likely to ask for information on the following topics:

1. Vehicle and equipment exposure: Number of owned and leased vehicles by type, year, make, description, insurance value, vehicle identification number, total stated value of all ambulance units and equipment

2. Employee exposures: Full-time equivalents and number of employees by position and responsibility

3. Volunteers: Number of volunteers and hours by position and responsibility

4. Medical director: Qualification and hours worked

5. Financial information: Revenue and expenditures

6. Other exposures: Known or anticipated

7. Additional activities: Sponsor or cosponsor of events (such as health fairs, carnivals, rodeos, demolition derby, haunted houses, and so on)

8. Patient encounters: Number of patients served

9. Regions served: Urban, community, rural

10. Claims history: Number of claims against the service

The organization may also be asked to submit copies of risk management–related programs, including safety; quality improvement; training; operations manual; and clinical policies, procedures, and protocols.

· · · · · · · · ·
CONTINUOUS RISK IMPROVEMENT

Participants in continuous risk improvement (CRI) should include the medical director, dispatch representative, field clinical personnel, drivers, and hospital ED personnel. The CRI process must be integrated into the day-to-day operations, and data should be shared among the participating agencies. Correction of any deficiencies in patient care involves first reviewing any applicable protocol to ensure its appropriateness or need for revision. Second, the particular deficiency must be assessed through a root cause analysis to determine where system improvements can be made. Third, appropriate education should be instituted, and any interventions implemented should be monitored through the CRI program.

The medical director, with the input of all levels of providers, should

- establish measurable standards that reflect the goals and expectations of the EMS system and local community;
- establish a mechanism for data collection that captures information reflecting standards;
- establish and ensure compliance with written patient care protocols and standard operating procedures;
- convey feedback and stimulate necessary changes in the educational process; and
- monitor the effectiveness of EMS interventions, treatments, and system design.

· · · · · · · · ·
ACCIDENT ANALYSIS

Because many liability-related incidents in the EMS arena are related to vehicular and flight accidents, it is important to analyze transport-related accidents. In this regard, an accident review board can be an effective risk improvement tool. To support the activity of the board, it is helpful to develop a central accident database encompassing the factors associated with the accidents, for example, number of hours worked by involved staff. Valuable data to support this effort can be collected through front seat or cockpit monitoring by pilots or drivers. It also might be valuable to profile programs that have not had an accident.

Emergency medical vehicle-related collisions occurring during an emergency response or transport should be evaluated by EMS system managers and medical directors. Specific issues assessed should include whether the dispatch process was clinically appropriate, the patient's condition on arrival at the scene and when the transport began, and the patient's eventual outcome.

· · · · · · · · ·

BENCHMARKS

Risk-related benchmarks should be established for each aspect of EMS to facilitate prioritization of risk issues and monitoring of intervention-related progress. Such measures may include the following parameters.

Staffing

- Qualifications and credentials of management and crew
- EMS crew satisfaction, such as job turnover rate, self-surveys

Equipment

- Quality and maintenance of equipment
- Radio communications ability

Patient or Clinical

- Patient satisfaction and complaints
- Scene triage, for example, the ability of BLS and ALS personnel to prioritize the emergency
- Scene care, for example, proper protocol implementation including minimizing scene time for the critically ill and injured

Public

- Recognition of an emergency: public awareness
- EMS system access: 9–1–1 awareness and availability
- Bystander interventions: bystander CPR, first aid

Dispatch

- Ability to determine severity of call
- Ability to make contact with the right EMS responders

Response

- Timeliness
- Capability to care for emergency
- Lights and sirens use

Transport

- Delivery to suitable medical facility
- Use of aeromedical transport and ALS intercepts
- System recovery, that is, turnaround time to restock and return to service availability

Disposition

- Patients admitted, discharged, transferred, or died at receiving medical facility
- Outcome measures, that is, condition on arrival at hospital and return to premorbid condition

. . . .

PROACTIVE RISK MANAGEMENT

The most effective way to manage risks is to reduce or eliminate them before they occur through the following preloss risk management strategies.

- Protocols: Protocols are uniform responses to specific clinical situations that tend to produce the safest and most reliable outcome. They should be based on objective clinical research rather than anecdotal experience. In any related negligence case, protocols will be considered, along with other information such as expert testimony, as evidence of the system's standard of care.
- Education: Continuing education is critical to reducing risk because it reinforces system protocols and expands providers' knowledge of out-of-hospital medicine. Education should include regular testing to ensure that every person demonstrates proficiency in critical skills. Risk management concepts and customer service skills should be part of all continuing education programs.
- Documentation: The prehospital care report can and will be used in court to support or condemn the EMS provider's, and the agency's, actions.
- Claims analysis: Identification of trends in the types of claims against EMS both on a local and national level will allow a system to proactively evaluate identified issues and modify protocols and training methods.

. . . .

POTENTIAL CLAIM INVESTIGATION AND LOSS MITIGATION

EMS organizations can use several strategies to limit or contain their risk after an incident. The risk management program should provide supportive resources, and the risk management professional may elect to participate in any or all of these processes.

- Investigation: Getting information about an incident as soon as possible dramatically elicits much more reliable data on which to base subsequent actions. The investigation should examine the prehospital care report, incident reports, and tape audits, when available, and should include crew interviews.
- Protocols: When an incident occurs, policies and procedures should be evaluated to see if they were in place and what effect EMS provider compliance or noncompliance had on the event. Determine if the related protocol exists. If it does, determine if it was followed, and if not, find out why.

- Remediation and evaluation: The crew members involved should be educated and tested on their skills competency (for example, intubation skills). Failure to correct clinical deficiencies may exacerbate later allegations of negligence.

· · · · · · · · ·
CONCLUSION

EMS is a critical aspect of healthcare. This arena exhibits constantly evolving clinical techniques and a highly dynamic environment. Although provision of prehospital emergency services is an area with much potential for liability, the public perception that prehospital EMS providers "do good" reduces exposure.

It is essential that the risk management professional address exposures in this out-of-hospital environment in the same way that exposures are managed in the acute-care facility. Risk issues that should receive a high priority include dispatch triage, field assessment, scene safety, biomedical equipment, vehicle safety, and bloodborne pathogen precautions.

Endnotes

1. Soler, J. M. et al. "The ten-year malpractice experience of a large urban EMS system," *Annals of Emergency Medicine* 1985; 14(10):982–985.

2. Goldberg, R. J. et al. "A review of prehospital care litigation in a large metropolitan EMS system." *Annals of Emergency Medicine* 1990; 19(5):557–561.

3. Colwell, C. B., P. Pons, J. H. Blanchet, and C. Mangino. "Claims against a paramedic ambulance service: A ten-year experience," *Journal of Emergency Medicine* 1999; 17(6):999–1002.

4. National Highway Traffic Safety Administration (NHTSA). "Guide for Interfacility Patient Transfer," DOT HS 810 599, April 2006, Available at: www.nhtsa.dot.gov/people/injury/ems/interfacility/images/interfacility.pdf. (Accessed on August 30, 2009.)

5. Institute of Medicine's Committee on the Future of Emergency Care in the United States Health System. "Future of Emergency Care in the United States Health System"; "Hospital-Based Emergency Care: At the Breaking Point;" "Emergency Medical Services at the Crossroads"; and "Emergency Care for Children: Growing Pains." June 14, 2006, Available at: www.nap.edu. (Accessed on August 30, 2009.)

6. Available at: www.nhtsa.dot.gov/people/injury/ems/EdAgenda/final/index.html. (Accessed on December 5, 2009.)

7. An example of paramedic program certification efforts in Texas is available at: www.dshs.state.tx.us/emstraumasystems/jodie2013.pdf. (Accessed December 5, 2009.)

8. Yeskey, K. Federal Interagency Committee on Emergency Medical Services. "Letter to Sebelius," June 26, 2009. Available at: www.nasemsd.org/documents/nationalhealthsecuritystrategy_ficemslettertoSebelius.pdf. (Accessed August 30, 2009.)

9. Available at: www.cdc.gov/ncidod/dhqp/index.html. (Accessed on August 30, 2009.)

10. Available at: www.fda.gov/Safety/medwatch/Howtoreport/ucm085568hcp.html. (Accessed August 30, 2009.)

11. Available at: www.accessdata.fda.gov/scripts/cdrh/cfdocs/cfMAUDE/search.CFM. (Accessed August 30, 2009.)

12. U.S. Department of Labor, Occupational Safety & Health Administration. "Bloodborne Pathogens and Needlestick Prevention." Available at: www.osha.gov/SLTC/bloodbornepathogens/index.html. (Accessed August 30, 2009.)

13. U.S. Department of Labor, Occupational Safety & Health Administration. "Ergonomics." Available at: www.osha.gov/sltc/ergonomics/index.html. (Accessed on August 30, 2009.)

14. U.S. Department of Labor, Occupational Safety & Health Administration. "Emergency Preparedness and Response." Available at: www.osha.gov/SLTC/emergencypreparedness/index.html. (Accessed on August 30, 2009.)

15. Fox, C. E. "Integrating EMS into Rural Health Systems," U.S. Department of Health & Human Services, Health Resources and Services Administration, 1999. Available at: www.mtwytlc.com/ruralEMSBestPractice.doc. (Accessed on August 30. 2009.)

16. "Research on Emergency Medical Services for Children," Department of Health and Human Services. PA Number: PA-05–081. Available at: http://grants.nih.gov/grants/guide/pa-files/PA-05-081.html. (Accessed April 9, 2010.)

17. Available at www.nlm.nih.gov/medlineplus/. (Accessed on August 30, 2009.)

18. REP Program Strategic Review Implementation Products, Final FEMA Policy, Recommended Initiative 1.2—Reduce Frequency of Evaluation, Evaluation of Emergency Medical Services Drills, October 23, 2004.

19. "Medicare Fraud, Detection and Prevention Tips." Center for Medicare & Medicaid Services. Available at: www.medicare.gov/FraudAbuse/Tips.asp. (Accessed on August 30, 2009.)

20. "State Laws on Heart Attacks, Cardiac Arrest and Defibrillators." National Conference of State Legislatures. Available at: www.ncsl.org/programs/health/aed.htm. (Accessed on August 30, 2009.)

21. National Registry of Emergency Medical Technicians, State Office Information. Available at: www.nremt.org/nremt/about/emt_cand_state_offices.asp. (Accessed August 30, 2009.)

22. National Highway Traffic Safety Administration, Department of Transportation, Emergency Medical Technician Paramedic: National Standard Curriculum (EMT-P). Available at: www.nhtsa.dot.gov/people/injury/ems/EMT-P/index.html. (Accessed on August 30, 2009.)

23. "NAEMSP Position Paper for Emergency Medical Dispatch." National Association of EMS Physicians, November 2007. Available at: www.naemsp.org/document/emergencymedicaldispatch-pec.pdf. (Accessed on August 30, 2009.)

24. Hospital Capacity and Emergency Department Diversion: Four Community Case Studies, AHA Survey Results, April 2004. Available at: www.aha.org.aha-content/2004/powerpoint/EDDiversionSurvey040421.ppt. (Accessed on August 30, 2009.)

25. Green, L.V., S. Glied, M. Grams, and N. Yankovic. "No Room at the Emergency Room: Causes and Consequences." Presented at Institute for Operations Research and the Management Sciences 2008 Annual Meeting, Hanover, Md. November 2008. Available at: www.informs.org/article.php?id=1519. (Accessed on August 30, 2009)

26. "Clarifying Policies Related to the Responsibilities of Medicare-Participating Hospitals in Treating Individuals with Emergency Medical Conditions, Action: Final rule." *Federal Register* September 9, 2003; 68 (174). Rules and Regulations Section, Centers for Medicare & Medicaid Services, Medicare Program.

27. "Policy Statement for Ambulance Diversion." Emergency Medical Services, Committee of the American College of Emergency Physicians, October 1999. Reaffirmed October 2006. Available at: www.acep.org/practres.aspx?id=29080. (Accessed on August 30, 2009.)

28. "National Heart Attack Alert Program." National Heart, Lung, and Blood Institute, National Institutes of Health. Available at: www.nhlbi.nih.gov/about/nhaap. (Accessed on August 30, 2009.)

29. The Revised Trauma Score is a physiological scoring system with high interrater reliability and demonstrated accuracy in predicting death. It is scored from the first set of data obtained on the patient and consists of Glasgow Coma Scale, systolic blood pressure, and respiratory rate. Available at: www.trauma.org/index.php/main/article/386/. (Accessed on August 30, 2009.)

30. The Glasgow Coma Scale is the most widely used scoring system in quantifying the level of consciousness following traumatic brain injury. It is used primarily because it is simple, has a relatively high degree of inter-observer reliability, and because it correlates well with outcome following severe brain injury.

31. Available at: www.ssgfx.com/CP2020/medtech/glossary/glasgow.htm. (Accessed August 30, 2009.) Additional information regarding clinical indicators and scoring tools is available at: www.emedicine.medscape.com/clinical_procedures. (Accessed on August 30, 2009.)

32. National Transportation Safety Board. "Special Investigation Report on Emergency Medical Services Operations." Aviation Special Investigation Report, NTSB/SIR-06/01, PB2006–917001, notation 4402E, Adopted January 25, 2006. Available at: www.ntsb.gov/publictn/2006/sir0601.pdf. (Accessed April 13, 2010.)

33. United States Government Accounting Office (USGAO). "Aviation Safety: Potential Strategies to Address Air Ambulance Safety Concerns." GAO-09–627T, April 22, 2009. Available at: www.gao.gov/new.items/d09627t.pdf. (Accessed on August 30, 2009.)

34. Shimanski, C. "Accidents in Mountain Rescue Operations," January 2002. Available at: www.escalade.com.au/rescue/media/ShimanskiJan02.pdf. (Accessed April 9, 2010.) Revised in 2008 and available at: www.mra.org/drupal2/sites/default/files/documents/training/AMRO_rev08.pdf. (Accessed on April 9, 2010.)

35. "Medical Review of Rural Air Ambulance Services." CMS Manual System Department of Health & Human Services (DHHS), Pub. 100–08. Medicare Program Integrity. Transmittal Number R102PI.

36. Colwell, et al. "Claims Against a Paramedic Ambulance Service: A Ten-Year Experience." *op. cit.*

37. American Society for Testing and Materials. "Standard Practice for Emergency Medical Dispatch." Publication No. F1258–90. Philadelphia: American Society for Testing and Materials, 1990; Revised ASTM F1560–00, "Standard Practice for Emergency Medical Dispatch Management" 2006; Also ASTM Standard F1552–94, "Standard Practice for Training Instructor Qualification and Certification Eligibility of Emergency Medical Dispatchers." 2009.

38. "1995 Emergency Vehicle Operators Course (Ambulance)." National Standard Curriculum, National Highway Traffic Safety Administration, Department of Transportation. Available at: www.nhtsa.dot.gov/people/injury/ems/web%20site%20intro.htm. (Accessed August 30, 2009.)

39. "Federal Specification for the Star-of-Life Ambulance KKK-A-1822E." General Services Administration (GSA), Federal Supply Service, June 1, 2002, GSA Automotive. Also Federal Standard Number 307. Ambulance Type I-AD, Conv. Cab-Chassis, Additional Duty. Available at: www.aprs.fss.gsa.gov/vehcilestandards/template.cfm. (Accessed August 30, 2009.)

40. American College of Surgeons. "Essential Equipment for Ambulances," *Bulletin of the American College of Surgeons* 1994; 79(9):19–23; South Carolina: "Ambulance Design and Equipment." Reg No. 61–7 (multiple parts applicable); California: "Comprehensive Emergency Medical Service Equipment and Supplies," Cal Code Regs title 22 § 70457.

41. Department of Health and Human Services, Office of Inspector General 42 C.F.R Pt 1001 RIN 0991-AB05 Medicare and State Health Care Programs: Fraud and Abuse. "Ambulance Replenishing Safe Harbor."

42. "Policy Statement-Equipment for Ambulances, Pediatrics" 2009; 124(1):e166–171. Available at: http://aappolicy.aappublications.org/cgi/content/full/pediatrics;124/1/e166. (Accessed April 9, 2010.)

43. "FDA Announces Guidant's Class I Pacemaker Recall." FDA News Release, P05–46, July 22, 2005. Available at: www.fda.gov/newsevents/newsroom/pressannouncements/2005/ucm108465.htm. (Accessed on August 30, 2009.)

44. "Whistleblower Files Lawsuit Against HP, Agilent." *Device Daily Bulletin* 2005; 2:41. Available at: www.fdanews.com/newsletter/article?articleID=69204. (Accessed August 30, 2009.)

45. National Advisory Commission on Criminal Justice Standards and Goals. *Report on Law Enforcement*, 1973, and *Report on the Criminal Justice System*, 1973. Washington D.C., GPO.

46. Hipskind, J. E., J. M. Gren, and D. J. Barr. "Patients who refuse transportation by ambulance: A case series," *Prehospital and Disaster Medicine* 1994; 12(4):278–283.

47. American College of Emergency Physicians. "Guidelines for do not resuscitate orders in the prehospital setting." *Annals of Emergency Medicine* 1998, 17:1106–1108; Emergency Cardiac Care Committees and Subcommittees, American Heart Association. "Guidelines for cardiopulmonary resuscitation and emergency cardiac care, VIII:

Ethical considerations in resuscitation." *Journal of the American Medical Association* 1992; 268:2282–2288; Adams, J. G. "Prehospital do-not-resuscitate orders: A survey of state policies in the United States," *Prehospital and Disaster Medicine* 1993; 8:317–322.

48. National Association of Emergency Medical Services Directors and the National Association of Emergency Medical Services Physicians "National Guidelines for Statewide Implementation of EMS 'Do Not Resuscitate' (DNR) Programs," April-June, 1994. Reaffirmed May, 2002. Available at: www.naemsp.org/documents/nationalguidelinesforstatewideimplementationofems.pdf. (Accessed on August 30, 2009.)

14

Risk Management and Behavioral Health

Robin Burroughs
Bruce W. Dmytrow

The provision of behavioral healthcare services creates the potential for both traditional and emerging risk exposures. In this chapter, corresponding risk control techniques and activities are discussed. For purposes of this chapter, behavioral health includes diagnoses, behaviors, and symptoms related to disturbances in behavior, mental processes (excluding developmental delays), and those diagnoses, conditions, and behaviors previously referred to as *psychiatric* or *mental illness*. Also included are diagnoses, behaviors, or conditions related to addiction and substance abuse.

Although behavioral healthcare involves risks specific to the services provided, a root cause of patient injury and healthcare-related litigation remains the breakdown in written and verbal communication between providers and patients, as is often the case in other types of healthcare delivery. An effective behavioral healthcare risk control program identifies opportunities to address and implement actions to minimize these risks.

The efficacy of a behavioral health risk control program improves when it is aligned and integrated with the organization's quality improvement and patient safety initiatives. When monitoring activities are needed to follow up on patient-related risk issues, the organization may delegate such monitoring to its quality improvement program. Similarly, when the risk identification process recognizes opportunities for improved patient care and safety, referrals to the appropriate quality improvement-related committees, departments, and individuals are an important aspect of the risk control techniques applied.

This chapter focuses on risk management in the behavioral healthcare setting. It should be noted, however, that patients with behavioral health symptoms and/or diagnoses will be encountered in all areas of healthcare delivery and by all healthcare and ancillary service providers. Therefore, all staff members should be trained in the recognition of behavioral health symptoms and familiarize themselves with the behavioral health resources available to staff and patients throughout their organization.

The specialized needs of behavioral health patients should be considered on an organization-wide basis when considering safety and security needs and during all safety, disaster, and evacuation drills and exercises.

· · · · · · · · ·

HISTORICAL PERSPECTIVE

Over the past several decades, behavioral healthcare has changed dramatically from a long-term, inpatient-based model to one that is primarily outpatient based. Many factors contributed to these changes. During the 1960s and 1970s, healthcare costs for all specialties began to escalate at alarming rates. Long-term, government-funded psychiatric hospitals had become increasingly expensive to run, and there was a growing public perception that the institutionalization of patients was inhumane. Additionally, healthcare reformers were advocating the need for defined patient rights.

Simultaneously, there were significant advances in identifying the physiological causes of some behavioral health disorders. Correlated advances have been seen in the development of new behavioral health chemotherapy. With increasingly effective antipsychotic, antidepressant, and antianxiety medications, patients are more receptive to psychotherapy, and many become appropriate candidates for outpatient treatment.

Inpatient behavioral healthcare or treatment may always be necessary for certain diagnoses, behaviors, and symptoms. However, the ability to safely and effectively manage patients in outpatient settings has increased both the public's access to behavioral healthcare services and society's acceptance of people with behavioral illness.

· · · · · · · · ·

LEGAL ISSUES

Emerging awareness of the potential for abuse of behavioral health patients has resulted in nationwide legislative activity that has codified specific patient rights.

Federal and State Legislation

In 1981, the federal government established the President's Commission on Mental Health and enacted a Bill of Rights for behavioral healthcare patients. Individual states are empowered to implement the patient Bill of Rights, perform ongoing review and revision of the Bill of Rights, and assess provider compliance affecting those rights on behalf of the patient community.

State Legislation   Every state has promulgated behavioral healthcare regulations and mental hygiene laws that govern the provision of behavioral healthcare. Appropriate risk techniques can ensure that

- all behavioral healthcare providers are conversant with the governing mental hygiene laws; and
- facility or organization protocols, policies, and procedures comply with all applicable regulations and laws.

Bill of Rights Title 42, Chapter 102, Section 9501   Behavioral health patients can be a vulnerable population, and healthcare professionals must take all necessary steps to protect their rights. In its patient Bill of Rights (U.S.C.A, Title 42, Chapter 102, Section 9501), Congress directed the states to ensure that mental health patients receive the protection and services they require. In order to preclude the possibility of litigation and control risk, the legal requirements set forth in the Bill of Rights must be fully implemented. Moreover, written protocols, policies, and procedures must ensure the provision of each right.

Appropriate Treatment and Related Services   Once the patient has entered treatment, he or she has the right to receive timely, appropriate, individualized treatment and services according to his or her specific diagnoses, behaviors, symptoms, and individual needs.

Individualized Written Treatment or Service Plans   Each behavioral health patient must have initial medical, psychosocial, and behavioral health assessments that are used in the development of a specific plan of care with measurable goals and achievable treatment objectives. The plan of care is adjusted, as necessary, based on the patient's response to treatment. Initial and periodic health assessments are performed to assist in evaluating complaints and symptoms.

Informed Consent   Informed consent requires a discussion between the patient and the physician that includes the risks, benefits, and alternatives to the proposed treatment, medication, or procedure, as well as the ramifications that may result from refusal to consent to a medical procedure or treatment protocol. The same elements of informed consent are required for behavioral health patients as for any other patient group. This discussion is the responsibility of the physician proposing the treatment, procedure, or medication and may not be delegated to any other person. The physician is responsible for memorializing the discussion and the patient's response in the health information record. Generally, the patient signs an informed consent form to further document understanding of the discussion. The informed consent process is required for any proposed treatment, procedure, or medication that involves a significant risk of patient injury or adverse effect. (Please see Chapter 4 for more information on informed consent.)

Many behavioral healthcare patients are competent to make their own healthcare decisions and to provide informed consent. If a member of the clinical team has questions regarding the patient's capacity to fully understand all the required elements of the informed consent discussion, a competency evaluation should be performed by a licensed physician. The physician's findings related to the patient's ability to provide informed consent for healthcare decisions must be clearly documented. It is important to remember that patients may have the capacity to make decisions regarding their healthcare even if they are not competent in other areas.

If the patient is deemed incompetent to provide informed consent, this should be clearly documented, and the informed consent discussion should be conducted with the patient's legal representative. In the absence of an authorized guardian or representative, the courts may be asked to appoint a legal representative to act on the patient's behalf for healthcare decisions. In some instances, the courts may require directly observed chemotherapy for a behavioral health patient who has been deemed a risk to himself, herself, or others when the patient does not voluntarily take essential medication.

The age of consent varies according to state statute. Many healthcare professionals have begun to recognize the rights of mature or emancipated minors (those nearing the age of maturity or having a clear and in-depth understanding of their illness and diagnosis). This is particularly true of situations in which the parent(s) or guardian gives consent for treatment in the presence of major objections on the part of the mature minor. Of particular concern are treatments or medications that have significant risk or potentially permanent side effects, such as electroconvulsive therapy or antipsychotic medications. When there is conflict between the parent and the mature minor concerning related treatment decisions, appropriate risk control techniques include involvement of the facility's healthcare counsel and/or obtaining a court order to ensure the mature minor's wishes are considered.

Additional information related to the informed consent process can be found in Chapter 4.

Right of Refusal   Competent patients (those who are capable of understanding the risks of refusing proposed treatment) have the right to refuse treatment without fear of reprisal from the involved physician, facility, or other healthcare providers. Risk increases when the refusal of treatment has the potential for serious negative effects on the patient's health, or even the risk of death. When the refusal of treatment has the potential for severe adverse effects on the patient's health, reassess the patient's competence and involve the facility's healthcare legal counsel.

For incompetent adult patients, the legal representative may refuse treatment in accordance with the patient's known wishes at the time they were competent. However, legal counsel, and in some cases the courts, should be involved when refusal of treatment involves the following issues:

- Refusal will or could result in significant adverse effects to the patient.
- Refusal will or could result in danger to the patient or others.
- A parent or guardian wants to refuse clinically indicated treatment for their minor child.

- A parent or guardian wants to refuse clinically indicated treatment for the mature minor, and the mature minor wants to consent to treatment, or the mature minor wishes to refuse treatment to which the parent(s) have consented.

As stated, the patient's right to refuse treatment must be without fear of reprisal by his or her care provider. However, in some cases when a patient refuses clinically indicated treatment, that individual may no longer be an appropriate patient for the present practitioner or facility. In such situations, a revised plan of care must be discussed with the patient and/or his or her representative. Appropriate referrals to practitioners or facilities should be made and documented. Assistance with appropriate referrals should then continue until the patient's transfer is successfully completed or the patient's non-compliance or refusal of referral is documented.

An additional possible consequence of refusal of treatment may be the cessation of health insurance benefits for the involved behavioral health diagnosis. Although patients have the right to refuse treatment, they should be informed that such refusal might have insurance benefit-related consequences that are outside the control of the healthcare provider. Patients refusing treatment should be advised of this possibility, informed that they may be personally responsible for continued charges and fees, and encouraged to contact their insurance carrier. If necessary, the patient should be provided with assistance for this process. Notice of possible loss of benefits and any subsequent assistance provided should be documented in the patient's health information record.

Freedom from Restraint or Seclusion   Patients have a right to receive treatment in an environment free from restraint or seclusion. However, if a patient is deemed to be an imminent threat to himself or others, the practitioner may order physical or chemical restraint or seclusion.

Sound risk control technique requires that the least restrictive, yet effective, restraint be used. Behavioral health organizations maintain specific policies and procedures to govern the ordering, application, release, and documentation of restraints. Such policies should also address how soon the patient is to be seen by a physician following the application or administration of the restraint. Such policies should be in compliance with applicable state and federal standards regarding the use of restraints.

When chemical restraint is clinically indicated and ordered, the pharmacist assesses its appropriateness and makes recommendations if alternative medications or equally effective medications with fewer side effects or adverse reactions are available. The pharmacist may also recommend a new or modified medication regimen to minimize or end the patient's need for periodic chemical restraint.

Humane Treatment   Behavioral healthcare should be delivered by qualified practitioners in a safe, humane environment. Compassionate treatment helps promote a positive therapeutic experience and increases the opportunity for favorable treatment outcomes.

Confidentiality   All patients have the right to confidentiality of their clinical, personal, and financial information. Except in the case of medical or clinical emergencies, healthcare providers and practitioners may not release any patient health information (verbal or written) in the absence of written patient consent or authorization. Even in such emergency situations, providers may release only the information necessary to ensure continuity of care for the acute event.

A general consent for the release of medical information typically used for other types of healthcare services is not sufficient when the patient has received treatment for a behavioral health or mental health diagnosis and/or treatment for drug or alcohol abuse. Behavioral health patients have additional confidentiality protection that requires they specifically consent to the release of any health information that includes treatment related to drug or alcohol use and/or a behavioral health diagnosis.

Access to Behavioral Health Records   Behavioral health patients have the right to review and/or obtain copies of their health information records. On occasion, practitioners may have concerns regarding the potential for adverse effects to a patient upon reading his/her health information record. If this determination is reached, the practitioner should clearly document his/her rationale within the patient's health information record in order to support the decision and communicate this information to other involved providers. However, if the patient continues to request access to their health information record despite being informed that it could be therapeutically harmful, the practitioner may obtain assistance from risk management and/or legal counsel. Each behavioral health organization establishes and implements policies and procedures that govern related processes.

As previously discussed, access to behavioral health records by other individuals and organizations is specifically restricted. In most instances, such information may only be released with written permission of the patient or their legal representative. There are exceptions when the patient is in need of immediate care or treatment, and their behavioral health information records are clinically necessary in order to ensure safe and appropriate continuity of care. These exceptions are to be clearly defined in the organization's policies and procedures.

Should records be released under emergent conditions, appropriate risk technique includes generating detailed documentation regarding the circumstances necessitating their release. Additionally, if the patient is later deemed able to give consent or has been stabilized with treatment, the releasing organization is encouraged to subsequently attempt to obtain the patient's retroactive authorization for the release of his or her information. Retroactive authorization should be clearly documented, with reasons noted for its retroactive nature.

Grievance Process   Patients have the right to object to any or all of their treatment as an infringement upon their rights. This is equally true for patients who have been involuntarily committed and those who voluntarily agreed to treatment. The organization complies with this patient right by providing patients with an impartial and timely fair-hearing process.

· · · · · · · · ·
ACCESS TO BEHAVIORAL HEALTH SERVICES

As a result of improvements in the management and control of behavioral health illnesses and symptoms, the majority of behavioral health patients are successfully integrated into their communities. This development emanated from the creation of readily accessible local services. Even with these improvements, challenges that negatively affect access to care remain.

Commercial Insurance Coverage

Healthcare costs continue to rise, and the increased cost of commercial insurance with coverage for a narrowly defined scope of services creates additional burdens for those suffering from behavioral health conditions. Behavioral healthcare insurance benefits are often separate and/or excluded from standard commercial healthcare insurance, require patients to use insurance-approved providers, or are reimbursed to the patient at a lower rate. Even when some level of coverage or benefit is included, one or more of the factors described here may cause patients to avoid or abandon treatment.

- Annual coverage restrictions: There are often specified benefit limits for inpatient and outpatient behavioral healthcare services within each policy year.
- Lifetime coverage limits: Many insurance policies limit the total benefit for a patient's lifetime behavioral healthcare services. Limits vary widely.
- Restricted medication coverage: Insurance policies may limit coverage benefits for medications to only those included in the insurance provider's approved formulary.
- Deductibles and copayments: Deductibles and copayments may apply for both medications and provider or practitioner payments.
- Complex patient reimbursement procedures: Many patients are required to pay directly for behavioral healthcare services and submit requests for reimbursement. Paperwork required for reimbursement may be complicated.

Risk Control Techniques   Because financial or reimbursement issues can negatively affect access to and patient compliance with care, these matters need to be addressed in the organization's quality improvement, patient safety, and risk control programs. The following risk control techniques are suggested:

- Require comprehensive documentation of the clinical justification for prescribed treatment and medications to meet third-party payer requirements for benefits.
- Establish patient assistance programs to aid patients in applying for and understanding their benefits and submitting documents for reimbursement.
- Assist patients in identifying additional resources and facilitate the patient's transition when primary third-party benefits are exhausted.

Managed Care

Managed care contracts may include the restrictions noted previously and also may include the following additional restrictions, which further limit access to services:

- Restricted to approved locations: Patients may be restricted to specific locations or facilities where the managed care organization is contracted to provide patient services.
- Restricted to approved providers or practitioners: Patients may be restricted to specific providers and practitioners with whom the managed care organization contracts.
- Restricted to approved medication formulary: Managed care organizations may cover only those medications that are included in their approved formulary.

Risk Control Techniques   In addition to risk control techniques addressed in the previous section, an effective organizational risk control program addresses the specific risks involved with managed care–related restrictions. Some of those restrictions and risk control techniques include the following:

- When a patient needs to change providers, avoid allegations of patient abandonment by actively facilitating the referral to an approved provider within the managed care network. Document all assistance efforts in the patient's health information record.
- Even though consideration should be given to delivering the most cost-effective, clinically indicated treatment or medication, the provider is responsible for ensuring that the patient's plan of treatment is based upon their individual needs and not governed by financial or benefit restrictions.
- When it is clinically contraindicated to restrict the patient's medication and/or treatment to those included in the managed care approved benefits, assist the patient in applying for extended or out-of-formulary coverage benefits. Some pharmaceutical manufacturers have programs to assist financially distressed patients using their product.

Greater Reliance on Ambulatory Care

Ambulatory care services are generally more cost-effective, and patients often benefit from obtaining treatment while remaining in the community. However, the countervailing interest of patient or community safety may require a patient to receive care in an inpatient setting.

Ironically, the otherwise successful outpatient treatment model may actually create access issues for these patients. Because outpatient care addresses the clinical needs of the majority of behavioral healthcare patients, inpatient facilities may be less available, and third-party payers may be resistant to providing inpatient benefits for services that they deem can be provided on an outpatient basis.

Risk Control Techniques   The organization's risk control program must address inpatient access issues.

- Require comprehensive documentation of the clinical justification for inpatient treatment that specifies why the patient treatment cannot be safely delivered on an outpatient basis.
- Ensure that the patient's plan of treatment is based on his or her individual needs and not governed by financial or benefit restrictions.
- Assist the patient with the appeals, grievance, and fair-hearing processes required by the insurance company if inpatient benefits are denied. These efforts should be documented in detail in the patient's health information record.

· · · · · · · · ·
SCOPE OF PRACTICE

Behavioral health staff is composed of both employed and independent practitioners and is further delineated by licensed and/or certified and nonlicensed staff.

Licensed Staff

Some aspects of behavioral healthcare can only be provided by licensed and/or certified professionals. Professionals must practice within the scope of their authority. This pertains to both independent practitioners and employed professionals.

Every state licenses professional healthcare practitioners and providers including, but not limited to, physicians, clinical psychologists, social workers, physician assistants, and nurses. Each professional state licensing board also defines the scope of practice for its licensees.

In addition, other levels of behavioral health staff may be certified to practice in a particular state. Examples may include certified nurse assistants, mental health technicians, alcoholism and addiction counselors, and certified medication technicians.

Each state licensing and certification board defines the provider's scope of practice. The scope of practice also includes the level of supervision that is required.

Risk Control Techniques   Risk management professionals should consider these control procedures for purposes of behavioral health staffing:

- As part of the initial application or credentialing process, obtain references and criminal background checks for every professional prior to initial patient contact.
- Every independent practitioner and provider should carry professional liability insurance. In a number of jurisdictions, this is mandated by state law. Some states have imposed caps on losses, so appropriate limits will vary. Generally, practitioners and providers should carry combined limits that respond adequately to the professional liability climate within the state or region.

- Healthcare organizations must develop and implement competency-based performance parameters for each professional category. The scope of competencies required should be in accordance with the state's scope of practice for each professional group.

- The healthcare organization must ensure appropriate supervision of the clinical practice of each of its professionals. This process is frequently included in the organization's credentialing and peer review programs.

Professional Competence

Practitioners must be competent to provide their defined scope of services and are required to demonstrate core competencies in order to attain licensure and/or certification. Behavioral health professionals are responsible for maintaining expertise and obtaining required continuing education credits defined by their professional licensing or certification board. Knowledge of current trends and innovations in the profession represents an added responsibility.

All healthcare practitioners should be trained in identification of patients at risk for behavioral health illness. Additional behavioral healthcare training and educational programs for practitioners in other healthcare delivery sites are especially important where behavioral health patients are more likely to be encountered. These sites include the emergency department, intensive care service, and gerontology units. Nonclinical staff, including security, transport, laboratory, and admissions staff, should be trained to manage situations that may arise when interacting with, or in the presence of, a patient who has a behavioral health illness.

Risk Control Techniques

- Perform competency-based performance assessments for each professional at least annually.

- Address identified lack of competence until the professional's performance reaches a level of acceptable competence.

- Require professional staff to annually submit evidence that they have completed the required number of continuing education credits.

Nonlicensed Staff

Behavioral health staff categories such as nurse's aide or assistant may not require licensure or certification. It is not uncommon for these behavioral health workers to obtain their experience and expertise through on-the-job training. Workers interacting with behavioral health patients such as admissions clerks, security, laboratory, dietary, and housekeeping staff, typically receive on-the-job training as well. When this is the case, the organization employing such workers is responsible for providing appropriate work-related training and ongoing staff education.

Risk Control Techniques   Screen potential staff to identify those candidates who may be appropriate members of the organization's workforce. This is achieved through the following risk control techniques.

Screening every employee, contracted worker, and volunteer in a behavioral healthcare setting, including support staff such as dietary and housekeeping, ensures they are appropriate to work with this potentially vulnerable population. References must be verified and criminal background checks performed with uniform application of applicable barrier crimes. The organization's list of barrier crimes must comply with pertinent state or local laws.

Some states require criminal background checks for certain healthcare personnel by statute. Irrespective of legal requirements, behavioral healthcare facilities should require such checks prior to an employee, contract worker, or volunteer's first day in the facility. Drug testing and checking published lists of registered sex offenders are strongly recommended components of screening behavioral healthcare personnel.

Skills Assessment   Define the skills or competencies required for a person to fulfill each position in the organization. Managers and supervisors should directly observe each staff member's skills and competencies on a regular basis. Skill deficits can be addressed through focused education and staff development programs. Following the implementation of the action plan, the staff member's skills are reassessed until the competency standard is achieved or it is determined that the individual lacks the requisite skills for the position.

Staff Development   Staff will need to continue to develop their skills and areas of competence as advances in behavioral healthcare are developed and become standards of practice. All staff should be required to undergo orientation to the facility's protocols, policies, and procedures at the time of hire and at least annually thereafter. Additional in-service and staff development programs designed to address modifications in the standard of care in behavioral healthcare should be provided regularly. Some areas of increased risk related to behavioral healthcare delivery include patient's rights, reporting of suspected abuse or neglect, physical and chemical restraint use, and confidentiality.

Supervision Requirements   Behavioral healthcare facilities should demonstrate the appropriate supervision for each level of staff. Facility policies and procedures define the type and frequency of supervision, and this may be included in position descriptions and as part of the staff member's performance evaluation. Staff should be routinely supervised through direct observation of their patient care practices and through regularly scheduled competency testing.

Practice Environment and Facility-Based and Affiliated Organizations

Independent practitioners and allied healthcare professionals (psychologists, physician assistants, and psychiatric nurse practitioners) are credentialed as members of the organization's medical staff.

Risk Control Techniques   Risk control techniques for independent practitioners and allied health professional include the following.

Credentialing and Reappointment   Behavioral healthcare organizations are required to employ and contract with qualified clinical staff. Organizations should formally credential and reappoint their professionals at least every two years. The credentialing and reappointment policies and procedures are defined in the medical staff bylaws and rules and regulations. Credentialing criteria should be applied uniformly for each medical staff member.

Delineation of Privileges   Practitioners request, in writing, specific clinical privileges based on their training, experience, and expertise. Steps for approving, reducing, or denying privileges should be outlined in the medical staff bylaws, rules and regulations, and/or credentialing policies and procedures, as appropriate. The bylaws should also include a process for medical staff members to appeal adverse credentialing and privilege decisions or reductions in requested privileges, through a defined fair-hearing process. Any such reductions or denials of privileges should be reported to the National Practitioner Data Bank and to practitioner's state licensing board.

Competency Monitoring   Practitioner competency is most appropriately assessed through the ongoing monitoring and peer review of the quality of services provided to patients. Nonphysicians undergo skills and competency evaluations as defined in their position descriptions or through organizational policies.

Practice Environment—Freestanding Organizations

Freestanding behavioral healthcare organizations, such as community-based clinics and supportive living environments, define the appropriate scope of practice for their employees and independent affiliated clinical practitioners. When assessing the risks associated with the delivery of care in such organizations, it is important to remember that, in the event of litigation, the facility will be held to the same quality and patient safety standards as hospital-based facilities. Freestanding organizations are also subject to essentially the same state department of health and other accrediting agency standards.

Risk Control Techniques   Risk control techniques particular to freestanding organizations include the following.

Contractual Agreements   It is recommended that all independent practitioners provide services to the organization in accordance with a formal written agreement or contract. Such contracts should be carefully developed by the organization's legal counsel to ensure that they include appropriate hold-harmless and indemnity provisions, as well as professional liability insurance requirements.

Professional Liability Insurance   As is the case for hospitals, freestanding organizations must ensure that independent practitioners maintain professional liability insurance in amounts deemed appropriate by the organization and in accordance with any state requirements and the local litigation climate.

Some freestanding organizations require their independent practitioners to include the organization as a named insured on the practitioner's professional liability insurance policy. This provides additional protection for the organization in the event of alleged vicarious liability related to the negligence of one of its affiliated practitioners.

Safety and Security   Ensure adequate security and safety of patients and staff, and provide staff with the ability to summon emergency assistance as needed through the use of alarms, panic buttons, cellular telephones, camera surveillance, and other technical systems.

Independent Practices

Each state defines the scope of practice for each type of practitioner who is licensed to practice independently. Independent practitioners may elect to practice in solo, in a group practice, or with contracted status. Many practitioners maintain private independent practices, while they also practice in freestanding or hospital-based facilities. Most practitioners maintain privileges on a hospital medical staff in the event that their private outpatients should require inpatient services at some point during their courses of treatments.

Risk Control Techniques   Several risk control techniques apply to independent practitioners, regardless of setting.

- Every licensed practitioner is required to obtain and renew his or her license to practice in accordance with state law and regulations.
- Every licensed practitioner is required to maintain his or her professional skills and is responsible for attending continuing professional education programs in accordance with state continuing education requirements.
- The practitioner is required to present proof of such ongoing education when applying for renewal of his or her professional license.
- Practitioners must maintain professional liability insurance in adequate amounts and in accordance with state and/or employer requirements and the local litigation climate.

·········
CLINICAL RISKS

Risk management issues related to behavioral healthcare risks need to be identified, controlled, and monitored just as in any other area of service.

Duration and Continuity of Care

Behavioral healthcare professionals develop and implement a specific plan of care for each patient. The course of treatment must be provided in a clinically appropriate setting, be maintained for the appropriate length of time to meet treatment goals and objectives, and include the coordinated efforts of all involved providers.

Risk Control Techniques   Several risk control techniques apply to continued care and treatment of behavioral and mental health patients.

Development of Treatment Plan   Every patient requires a specific plan of care that includes defined goals and objectives of treatment, the appropriate setting for care, the projected length of treatment, and the support systems and services the patient will need.

The treatment plan is continually evaluated and modified as the patient's condition changes or treatment approaches require revision. The organization's continuous quality improvement process may be the most appropriate mechanism to ensure ongoing assessment of the efficacy of treatment plans.

Each element of the patient's treatment plan and all subsequent modifications to that plan are documented in the patient's health information record.

Management of Missed Appointments   A missed appointment may be an indication of a patient at risk. The behavioral healthcare provider has an obligation to address the issue of a missed appointment.

Patients are initially educated to the requirement that they should contact their provider if they are unable to keep a scheduled appointment. Patients who repeatedly cancel appointments may require a reassessment of their treatment plan.

Organizational protocols, policies, and procedures should define what steps will be taken to contact patients who miss appointments. Providers must consider the patient's diagnosis when determining how aggressive and extensive contact efforts should be. All efforts to contact patients who have missed appointments must be fully documented in the patient's health information record.

Community Support Services   The treatment plan should specify appropriate community services that will support the patient throughout the course of treatment and after discharge. Some examples may include the following:

- Transportation services to and from appointments
- Twelve-step programs for patients abstaining from an addiction
- Directly observed medication administration services
- Family counseling resources
- Medical healthcare resources
- Disability benefits
- Job training or retraining programs

- Employment support programs
- Financial aid

Discharge Planning   Each patient's behavioral healthcare treatment plan should include discharge planning that will support a successful and safe termination from current treatment.

Documentation of each aspect of the discharge planning process is essential to defending the clinical decision-making processes involved and to support the defense of any subsequent allegations of inappropriate discharge from treatment.

Monitoring Interventions for Effectiveness

Every patient's course of treatment requires scheduled monitoring to ensure that it is addressing the patient's specific needs, has been modified in accordance with the patient's progress, and adequately addresses the patient's response to treatment. As each aspect of the patient's treatment is monitored, the risks inherent in that aspect of treatment should also be addressed and managed.

Risk Control Techniques   Several risk control techniques apply to monitoring the course of treatment for behavioral and mental health patients. The following are but a few of those techniques.

Appropriate Use of Medications and Treatment Modalities   Improved psychoactive medications and treatment modalities have revolutionized behavioral healthcare, but they may also carry significant side effects and potential for adverse patient reactions. Consideration of specific patient characteristics and accompanying risks, such as patient age, ability to adhere to the medication regimen, access to the prescribed medication, and likelihood of compliance with monitoring and follow-up, are critical to the determination of appropriate medication and treatment plans. Obtain informed consent for all medications and treatment modalities and frequently assess the patient for their effectiveness, with particular attention to any adverse or negative effects.

De-escalation Techniques   Some behavioral healthcare patients experience episodes of increased activity, agitation, behavioral outbursts, or aggressive behaviors that place them or others at risk for injury. The management of such symptoms should be addressed in the patient's treatment plan in order to ensure the safety of the patient and others. The treatment plan defines what techniques are most appropriate for the particular patient in the event of such symptoms. Some examples of these techniques include

- removal from stimulus or conflict-causing situation or person;
- redirection or refocusing;
- nonstimulating environment, including time-outs or isolation;
- therapeutic activity; and
- physical or chemical restraint, including therapeutic holding.

Appropriate risk control techniques related to de-escalation include verifying the following:

- There is a written practitioner order for de-escalation applications.
- There is a completed and documented informed consent discussion. Such a discussion may be held during the patient's quieter times or retroactively.
- Techniques are applied by trained personnel.
- Techniques are applied in the appropriate manner for proscribed periods of time.

Documentation of de-escalation activities must include a detailed description of the patient behaviors necessitating the use of de-escalation techniques, the techniques applied, and the patient's response.

Participation in Treatment Plans   The effectiveness of treatment plans is often enhanced when the patient, the patient's representative, and significant others are included in the design and implementation of the patient's plan. Even patients thought to have cognitive impairments or who are minors should be included in the treatment planning process to the level of their ability.

As an additional risk control technique, some facilities and practitioners formally contract with patients for their compliance with treatment plans and goals and objectives. Although such treatment contracts are not legally binding documents, they serve as an affirmation of the practitioner's and patient's commitment to the agreed-upon plan of treatment.

Any and all patient, representative, or family participation in treatment plans should be fully documented in the patient's health information record. Whenever appropriate, it is desirable to obtain the patient's signature in agreement with the plan of care.

Documentation of Clinical Outcomes and Changes in Interventions
Documentation is required to reflect the patient's specific response to each treatment modality included in his or her treatment plan. Comprehensive documentation must be provided whenever the patient's response or lack of response results in a change in treatment plan or other type of intervention. The documentation should include a description of the element of care; the analysis and assessment of the patient's response; the proposed change, intervention, or modification; as well as the patient's awareness of and, if appropriate, consent to the change.

Documentation of Referrals for Additional Services   Behavioral healthcare patients may have problems in their daily lives related to their behavioral health diagnosis and symptoms. Such issues may include disruptions within the family or at school, difficulty managing finances, presence of addictive behaviors, or difficulties with the legal system and law enforcement. Social services referrals, initiation of family support services, assistance with obtaining financial support, and referral to legal services may be essential to keeping the patient in treatment.

Referral for a physical assessment is also essential for every behavioral health patient and should be included in the comprehensive treatment plan. All referrals must be documented in the patient's health information record.

Appropriateness and Effectiveness of Discharge Plan   As previously addressed, the patient's discharge needs should be assessed throughout the course of treatment. Failure to plan for discharge services creates significant risk to the patient for relapse or noncompliance with treatment.

As with the treatment plan, it is recommended that the patient's input be considered in the development and implementation of the discharge plan.

Follow-Up on Postdischarge Compliance with Referrals and Continuing Care
Part of the discharge planning process includes follow-up of the patient's compliance with recommended postdischarge activities and services. Documentation should accurately reflect assessment of status, including compliance with postdischarge plans.

Suicide and Homicide Prevention

Behavioral healthcare patients must continually be assessed for the risk of suicidal and/or homicidal ideation or acts. Appropriate clinical interview techniques should be used and the patient should be specifically evaluated for these risks. All such evaluation(s) must be documented in the patient's health information record. Each significant change in a patient's condition or in the response to treatment should be viewed in the context of the patient's risk for suicide or homicide.

Whenever a patient is assessed to be at significant risk for suicidal or homicidal behavior, all steps necessary to ensure the safety of the patient and the community must be implemented. In some cases, this may require a breach of patient confidentiality to warn a potential victim of homicidal ideation or to inform a parent or guardian of the significant risk of suicide and the need for involuntary commitment. Should the behavioral healthcare professional deem it necessary to warn a third party, it may be appropriate to involve legal counsel. The courts have upheld exceptions to the duty of confidentiality in the landmark case of *Tarasoff v. Regents of University of California*, 131 Cal.Rptr.14, 551 P.2d 334 (Cal. 1976). In *Tarasoff*, a psychiatrist was held liable for failing to warn the victim of a mental patient's threat to kill a former girlfriend. The duty to warn of potential danger to others was held to outweigh the public policy favoring protection of confidential communications between a patient and psychotherapist. Most state courts have adopted some variation of *Tarasoff* and many have expanded its meaning to include most behavioral healthcare professionals. Each facility must address this risk with legal counsel and determine the steps to be taken when there is a potential need for a warning.

Risk Control Techniques   Several risk control techniques apply to suicide and homicide prevention for behavioral patients. The following describes those techniques.

Initial and Ongoing Clinical Risk Assessments   Every patient should be assessed for suicidal or homicidal ideation at the time of entry into treatment and regularly thereafter. The risk of suicide and/or homicidal behavior should be a major consideration when selecting the most appropriate treatment facility and the safest, most effective level of care for the patient.

Reassessment of these risks should be performed on a routine basis and whenever there is a significant change in the patient's affect and/or behavior. Sometimes, a sudden peacefulness in a previously agitated and depressed patient may be a sign that he or she has resolved the issue internally and has a specific plan of action regarding suicidal or homicidal behavior.

Suicide Precautions and Treatment Plans   When there is an identified risk of suicide or homicide, the patient must be placed on specific clinical protocols for prevention of such actions and behaviors. Typically, this requires voluntary or involuntary admission to an inpatient facility, at least until the patient can be further assessed, and to implement appropriate suicide or homicide prevention techniques.

The primary consideration must always be to ensure patient and community safety. Any and all necessary precautions and suicide/homicide prevention techniques are to be implemented, even if the patient objects and there is a risk of patient litigation. Some preventive actions include:

- **Close Observation or One-On-One Observation (1:1)**
  The patient is never left alone for any reason and is kept in total visual contact by a staff member at all times, including bathroom and grooming activities, sleep, meals, and at all other times. During a one-on-one assignment, the staff member may have no other assigned duties. Another staff member covers for the one-on-one staff member for breaks.

- **Contraband Controls**
  A suicidal or homicidal patient can be extremely creative and persistent in attempting to carry out the plan of action. Almost any object can be modified into a danger or weapon. Patients should be informed at the time of admission that their rooms and possessions will be initially and periodically searched and, if deemed necessary, they may be required to submit to a body search.

  1. Room searches: When a patient is identified as being at risk for suicide or homicide, there should be routinely scheduled searches and additional focused searches of patient rooms, communal areas, dining rooms, and activities areas. These are essential to ensuring as safe an environment as possible and should be documented.

  2. Personal effects searches: Each patient's personal effects should be searched at the time of admission and periodically thereafter for any object or item that could be used to carry out a suicide or homicide plan. Identified contraband is confiscated and stored in a safe place and, if appropriate, is returned only when the patient is discharged. Weapons or items that could be made into weapons must

be permanently confiscated. Under certain circumstances, such as discovery of a concealed firearm, police involvement is required.

3. Body searches: If a body search is necessary, it should only be carried out by a same-sex professional staff member and should be witnessed and documented by a same-sex staff member. Some organizations stipulate that only medical professionals (physician, nurse) perform body searches.

It may be necessary to carry out an even closer body search, such as a skin search or a body cavity search, for patients at high risk for suicide or homicide. This type of search may be indicated if there is reasonable suspicion that the patient has an object or weapon, medication, and other contraband hidden somewhere on his or her person that could be used to carry out the suicide or homicide plan.

A clinically indicated body search must be conducted by a same-sex professional staff member and witnessed by a same-sex staff member to ensure patient safety and to assist in the defense of the staff and organization if allegations of abuse or injury arise. Both staff members who participate in the search should independently document the details of the search in the patient's health information record.

- **Medication Management**
Behavioral healthcare facilities require stringent controls on medications and biologicals. Inpatients' personal medications should be confiscated and returned only at the time of discharge and only if they continue to be prescribed after discharge. Even though TJC accreditation compliance with National Patient Safety Goal 8 for medication reconciliation is currently not being scored nor addressed in the accreditation report, it behooves accredited behavioral health facilities to review their processes and systems at all stages of care transition and handoff.

Medications prescribed for patients during their inpatient course of treatment are stored in locked areas. Patients are generally required to report to the nursing station or medication room to obtain their medications. Mouth checks should be performed to ensure that patients have swallowed their medication.

Family members and other visitors must be educated to the risks of bringing contraband into the organization and are prohibited from carrying any medications or drugs, even those for their own use, when they are visiting in a behavioral healthcare setting. Even if their family member is not at risk for suicide or homicide, other patients in the setting may be at risk. In some cases, it may be necessary to perform voluntary searches of visitors and/or their personal items such as purses and backpacks and to deny visiting privileges to those who decline to permit search procedures. Individuals known to have provided contraband to a patient may be restricted from visiting.

- **Physical Plant Controls**
Some behavioral health inpatient units are designated as locked units to prevent patients from eloping or injuring themselves or others. Patients at high risk for suicide or homicide, incompetent or confused patients, minors, or other patients unable to

protect themselves in the community require protection from elopement or infliction of injury to themselves or others.

Locking or alarming doors, windows, elevators, and so forth can assist in providing a safe environment. Windows must be locked, nonopening, or adapted to open only one to two inches. Doors leading to lobbies, elevators, and stairways should be alarmed and locked so that staff is alerted to any unauthorized exit attempts. Many behavioral health units use camera surveillance for entrances and exits so that out-of-sight-line areas can be visually monitored. Some facilities include the immediate grounds and parking lots in their camera surveillance capabilities. For more information on behavioral design issues, see Appendix 14.1, Latent Risks in the Built Environment for the Behavioral Health Patients, at the end of this chapter.

- **Visitor Controls**
  Behavioral healthcare facilities must establish specific policies and procedures to govern the management of visitors. Many behavioral healthcare organizations require orientation for all visitors to ensure they do not purposely or inadvertently bring potentially dangerous medications or contraband items into the patient care unit.

  Some behavioral healthcare organizations greatly limit visitors. Others require visitors to pass through metal detectors and undergo voluntary searches.

  When there is significant risk to the patient, the practitioner may order that visitors be completely prohibited for all or part of the patient's course of treatment. The practitioner may require that all or specific visitors be allowed only under the direct one-on-one observation.

- **Clinical Monitoring Protocols**
  There must be ongoing monitoring of the effectiveness of the facility's policies and procedures to identify patients at risk for suicide or homicide. Treatment plans are also monitored to ensure appropriate assessment and treatment for these risks.

  The facility monitors patient injuries, incidents, and accidents related to suicidal or homicidal behaviors to identify gaps in their patient safety program and physical plant controls. When an issue is identified, it must be investigated and a plan of correction immediately developed and implemented. Continued monitoring is then maintained to ensure the effectiveness of the plan of correction.

Reporting Attempted and Completed Suicide or Homicide   Attempted and completed suicide or homicide must be reported to the following:

- Facility risk management department
- Facility administration
- Facility legal department or attorney
- Any person identified by the patient as a potential violence or homicide victim, for example, a third party to whom there is a "duty to warn" (see *Tarasoff v. Regents of the University of California* cited earlier)

- Patient's physician
- Patient's family or representative
- Law enforcement, when appropriate
- State department of mental health
- State department of health
- Professional licensing board, if applicable
- Facility professional liability insurance broker and carrier

Requirements to report suicide or homicide attempts or completed actions are defined in each state's health and/or mental health laws and codes. All reporting activities should be documented in the patient's health information record.

A confidential investigation and analysis of any such event should be carried out immediately. A comprehensive investigation includes assessment of whether the organization's protocols, policies, and procedures regarding the identification of patients at risk for suicide or homicide were properly implemented. If they were not, a detailed plan of correction should be developed and implemented to prevent any recurrence.

Elopement Prevention

For some behavioral healthcare patients, remaining in the protected environment of an inpatient unit is essential to ensuring their safety or the safety of others. It may be necessary to prevent the patient from leaving the inpatient unit even if it requires involuntary or court-ordered commitment and is against the patient's wishes. As noted previously, some behavioral healthcare units are locked or otherwise secured to prevent patients from eloping.

Periodic elopement drills need to be carried out to evaluate the effectiveness of the facility's elopement prevention program. Any gaps or deficiencies identified through the drill process are addressed and the prevention program appropriately modified.

Risk Control Techniques   Several risk control techniques apply to prevent patient elopement. They discussed next.

Initial and Ongoing Clinical Assessments   All behavioral healthcare patients must be evaluated for the risk of elopement at the time of their admission to an inpatient treatment setting. Such assessments should be repeated periodically, as the patient's needs dictate.

Elopement Precautions and Treatment Plans   The patient's treatment plan should include any and all indicated elopement precautions. Some of the methods used to prevent elopement and potential injuries to patients at risk for elopement include the following:

- Close observation (one-on-one): Continuous direct observation of patients at risk for suicidal or homicidal behavior is required.

- Frequent checks: Some patients may not require one-on-one observation, but do require frequent staff checks to ascertain that they remain in the unit and are not in a position to elope. In these instances, patients may be placed on face-to-face checks by staff on a schedule of every five, ten, or fifteen minutes. The staff observes the patient at the appropriate intervals and documents his or her location within the unit (patient's room, activities department, therapy room, and so forth) and that the check was performed.

- Physical environment controls: As described previously, exit doors on some behavioral healthcare units are locked to ensure patient safety. All staff should carry keys to exit doors to ensure that doors can be readily unlocked in the event of a fire or other internal disaster requires rapid evacuation of patients.

- Visitor controls: Because many behavioral healthcare inpatient units require patients to wear regular street clothes, there is a risk of patient elopement where visitors or staff enter or leave the treatment unit. Visitors should be required to show a pass to enter or exit the unit. When visitors are entering and exiting, staff should confirm that elevator doors have fully closed prior to unlocking the unit door.

- Clinical monitoring protocols: Patient treatment plans should be monitored for their effectiveness in preventing patient elopements.

Reporting Elopement   In most states, elopements are reportable events. In addition to notifying the physician, family or responsible party, facility administration, and facility security, the following must be notified:

- Facility risk management department
- Facility legal department or attorney
- Local police department
- State department of mental health
- State department of health

All elopements must be investigated, the method of elopement fully determined and assessed, and a detailed plan of correction developed to ensure that future similar elopements are prevented.

Additionally, an analysis of the patient's treatment plan and the facility's elopement precautions should be completed. Any factors that contributed to the elopement must be addressed to ensure they do not recur. All related efforts should be documented in the patient's health information record.

Chemical and Physical Restraints

Restraints can be effective therapeutic tools, but they may also have an impact on patient rights. Because of the critical nature of patient rights, every effort should be made to provide safe, effective treatment in a restraint-free environment. However, there are times when restraints are clinically required. Based on the particular patient's needs, the specific type of restraint must be ordered by the practitioner and must be implemented, monitored, and removed in accordance with applicable regulations, the written order, and the facility's protocols, policies, and procedures.

The facility must ensure that its protocols, policies, and procedures comply with the Special Conditions of Participation through the Centers for Medicaid & Medicare Services under HFS 124. This regulation requires that a licensed independent practitioner perform a face-to-face evaluation of each patient within one hour of the initiation of an episode of restraint. (Locked seclusion is also included in this regulation. See the portion of this chapter that discusses locked seclusion.) The evaluation includes an assessment of the appropriateness of the intervention, the appropriateness of continuing the intervention, and the identification of any precursors that could prevent further episodes of restraint use.

Physical restraints include individual patient equipment such as wrist restraints and environmental techniques such as locked seclusion. Not all psychoactive medications constitute chemical restraint, including those that are prescribed over an extended period of time for chronic treatment of behavioral symptoms. The same medications, however, may be considered a chemical restraint when used on a periodic or urgent basis (PRN) or in dosages used to significantly alter behavior on an immediate basis.

Risk Control Techniques   Risk control techniques to minimize the risk associated with chemical and physical restraints are addressed in the following points:

Initial and Ongoing Clinical Assessments   At the onset of treatment, the practitioner evaluates both the patient's behavioral and medical needs. The clinical indications and patient safety considerations related to the use of environmental, physical, or chemical restraints must be addressed as part of each patient's initial and ongoing treatment.

Clinical Assessment   Additional patient assessments are required whenever there is a significant change in the patient's behavior or medical condition, whenever the patient responds or fails to respond to prescribed treatment or medication, or whenever there is a change in the patient's plan of care.

Restraint Policy   The protocols, policies, and procedures for the use of chemical and physical restraints must be specifically defined and implemented. At a minimum, they must include the following:

- Specific clinical and patient safety indications for the use of environmental, physical, or chemical restraint
- Informed consent process

- Emergency restraint use
- Practitioner orders for restraint
- Specific restraint to be used
- Specific time limits for the restraint to be used
- Frequency and duration of periodic release of physical restraints
- Indications for discontinuance of the restraint
- Requirements for patient monitoring, periodic removal, and observation during and after the application or use of restraint
- Documentation requirements for all aspects of restraint assessment, application, monitoring, efficacy, and removal

Restraint Reduction Protocols   Restraints may be used only in accordance with facility protocols, policies, and procedures, and practitioner's orders. But when a patient's clinical condition requires that a restraint be used to protect the patient or others, the least restrictive restraint that produces the desired effect should be used. For example, staff may recommend the use of the quiet room before implementing a more restrictive technique. Similarly, practitioners may prescribe less-sedating medications before using major tranquilizers. Efforts to reduce the level or degree of the restraint or to eliminate the need for the restraint altogether should be ongoing, focused, and clearly documented in the patient's health information record.

Documentation of and Compliance with Restraint Protocols and Treatment Plans   The following elements should be addressed in the organization's protocols, policies and procedures for all restraints:

- Informed consent process: Use of restraints requires informed consent, except in cases of emergency when patients are deemed to be a risk to themselves or others.

    Often the symptoms or behaviors that necessitate involuntary restraint are the same symptoms or behaviors that render patients, at least temporarily, unable to control their behaviors adequately to participate in the informed consent process. When a patient is deemed unable to provide consent due to behavioral symptoms, the family or legal representative should be notified and consent obtained through the proxy informed consent process under applicable state law. Patients may be able to additionally provide retroactive consent once they have regained behavioral control.

    Documentation relating to the informed consent process for involuntary restraint must indicate

    1. the specific symptoms or behaviors that rendered the patient unable to provide informed consent;
    2. the steps taken to obtain consent from a parent or legal representative; and
    3. subsequent (retroactive) patient consent, if obtained.

- Practitioner orders: A practitioner's order is required for the use of any restraint.

- Emergency use: Restraints may be used without the patient's consent in instances for which it is determined that a patient is a danger to himself/herself or others. Consent, physician orders, and notification to the family or legal representative is then carried out as soon as practicable.

- Restraint efficacy and patient safety: The efficacy and appropriateness of the restraint in meeting the patient's treatment needs should be documented in the patient's health information record. The patient's safety and well-being, as well as the safety of others, is a paramount consideration, and any adverse patient response must be immediately addressed by the clinical staff or practitioner. Any patient injury resulting from restraint must be reported in accordance with regulatory requirements and facility policy.

- Monitoring and observation protocols: There must be consistent, ongoing monitoring of the patient's behavior and physical condition immediately before, during, and after restraint.

Seclusion

Seclusion, a form of therapeutic isolation, is generally characterized as a restraint. As such, it requires careful monitoring to protect patients' rights while their safety and well-being are ensured. Seclusion can be an effective therapeutic tool for some patients. Conversely, self-isolation may be a problem behavior for others. Therefore, each patient's practitioner is required to provide written orders regarding seclusion. Such orders should authorize staff to impose involuntary seclusion in situations in which the patient is a risk to himself/herself or others. The orders should also indicate whether patients may use voluntary seclusion or quiet rooms. Conversely, in the case of patients for whom self-isolation is a clinical problem, the practitioner may require that they be prohibited from isolating themselves from the general patient community.

Once again, the facility must ensure that its protocols comply with the special conditions of participation through the Centers for Medicaid & Medicare Services under HFS 124, which requires that a licensed independent practitioner perform a face-to-face evaluation of each patient within one hour of the initiation of an episode of locked seclusion. (Physical and chemical restraints are also included in this regulation. See the section of this chapter that discusses physical and chemical restraints.) The evaluation should include an assessment of the appropriateness of the intervention, the appropriateness of continuation of the intervention, and the identification of any precursors that could prevent further episodes of restraint.

Patients may be at greatest risk of injury when they have lost control of their behavior. Seclusion may be an effective technique in assisting the patient in regaining control and providing protection for both the patient and others. Informed consent for seclusion should be obtained whenever possible, even if it is obtained following the seclusion episode. The patient's family or legal representative should be notified when involuntary seclusion is required.

Included in this section is a discussion of desirable characteristics of seclusion rooms that minimize risks. This discussion does not address regulatory or building code requirements. Specific state or federal codes related to behavioral health physical plants are defined by the appropriate regulatory agencies and must be consulted in formulating plans regarding seclusion rooms.

Risk Control Techniques The facility must develop and implement protocols, policies, and procedures to govern the use of therapeutic seclusion. The type of seclusion to be used, seclusion duration, patient observation requirements, and patient monitoring requirements should be clearly defined, adhered to, and documented in the patient's health information record. Levels of seclusion are discussed next.

Locked Seclusion In the most restrictive form of seclusion, the patient is involuntarily placed in a locked seclusion room that is equipped with observation access (shatterproof, safety-glass windows, recessed cameras, and so forth) and patient safety equipment such as a floor mat. The room should be free of all other objects.

There must be no electrical outlets, wires, vents, dropped ceilings, removable screws, etc. The room should be shaped so that staff can visually observe the patient at all times. When less than ideal room characteristics are unavoidable, appropriate alternatives such as multiple cameras or other adaptations will be required.

In cases of severe agitation, it may be necessary to remove the patient's clothing to protect him or her from injury. At the very least, shoes, belts, jewelry, dentures, glasses, and pocket contents are removed before the patient is placed in seclusion.

Other risks requiring observation and prevention include misuse of seemingly safe objects including plastic trash bags, plastic eating utensils, blankets and pillows.

Patients have been known to use virtually any item to injure themselves or to assist in an elopement from seclusion. For example, there have been elopements through air ducts, injuries from screws or nails that were used in the room construction, and injuries from sharpened plastic eating utensils used as weapons. Staff need to consider any object in the seclusion room as a potential danger to the patient or staff.

Staff should enter seclusion rooms only with backup, and all patient encounters involving seclusion should be witnessed by at least one other staff member. Patients should also be periodically removed from seclusion to evaluate whether or not they can be reintegrated into the patient population.

The patient's physical condition must be monitored during periods of seclusion. This may include checking the patient's vital signs and closely monitoring the effects of any psychoactive medications that are given.

Seclusion may never be used as a threat or punishment for a patient's failure to behave in a manner desired by the staff or physician. Seclusion is a major curtailment of a patient's freedom and should be used only when other therapeutic techniques have failed to assist the patient to attain adequate behavioral control.

Regardless of the reason for seclusion, and regardless of the type of seclusion used, all patient encounters, monitoring efforts, and patient assessments during periods of seclusion must be fully documented in the patient's health information record. Staff also must document all steps taken to assist the patient in regaining control of his or her behavior before using seclusion.

Claims related to seclusion are generally based upon allegations of false imprisonment and/or patient abuse. Therefore, all efforts to avoid seclusion and to remove the patient from seclusion must be documented to effectively defend against such future allegations.

Open-Door (Unlocked) Seclusion The moderately restrictive open-door (unlocked) seclusion may be an appropriate environmental restraint for patients who have difficulty maintaining behavioral control but who are not a danger to themselves or others. Patients with these needs may voluntarily enter the seclusion room, but the door, although closed for privacy and decreased environmental stimulation, must remain unlocked.

It is appropriate for patients with behavioral control issues to request open-door seclusion, and it is also appropriate for staff to offer open-door seclusion whenever it becomes evident that the patient is having difficulty maintaining behavioral control.

The same patient safeguards must be employed for open-door seclusion as for locked seclusion. This includes monitoring the patient's response to seclusion, monitoring vital signs as needed, periodically removing the patient from seclusion to assess his or her ability to return to the patient community, and ensuring the absence of any objects that could be a danger to the patient or staff.

The seclusion room should remain locked when not in use. This ensures that staff must permit patient access and decreases the possibility of unsupervised seclusion.

As with locked seclusion, open-door seclusion must be addressed in the patient's treatment plan. Documentation in the patient's health information record should also include the symptoms or behaviors that led to the seclusion, the results of patient monitoring during the episode, the patient's response to the seclusion, and the patient's response to re-entry into the general patient community. The time the patient entered seclusion, the duration of each aspect of the episode, and the time the patient exited should be included in the documentation.

Voluntary Quiet Room Some behavioral healthcare treatment units have a designated area where patients may be alone or away from any significant environmental stimulation. Some facilities allow patients to return to their bedrooms during the day if they need a quiet place. But others, in an effort to encourage patient participation in therapeutic activities, restrict patient access to any isolated area, including their bedrooms. In such cases, there may be a designated quiet room for minimally restrictive seclusion. Patients need to be instructed regarding the use of the quiet room, and all use must be documented in the patient's health information record.

The patient's treatment plan should reflect how often the quiet room may be used, the duration of quiet time, and patient observation and monitoring requirements.

Time-Outs for Minors and Mature Minors Time-outs, another form of minimally restrictive seclusion, are used for minors who have lost control of their behavior while interacting in the patient community. Time-outs generally involve removal from the major activities or source of stimulus in the group, but not from the group's presence. There is often a section of the perimeter of the patient treatment area or a particular chair in the room that is designated as a time-out area.

Often, the patient is encouraged to sit alone for a defined brief period of time. The duration of the time-out should be established at the time the minor is removed from the ongoing activities of the group. When the time-out has expired, the minor patient is asked to rejoin the group. If the time-out was not successful in helping the minor patient regain behavioral control, other de-escalation techniques may be required.

As with all other types of seclusion, time-outs must be documented in the patient's health information record.

Physical Environment Controls   Locking doors is the most common method for controlling the behavioral healthcare environment. Within the behavioral health inpatient unit, doors may be locked to restrict patient access to certain areas, and the unit's exit doors may be locked to prohibit unauthorized entrance or exit. Other environmental controls include alarms or keypad controls on doors and elevators and locked window covers.

Risk control techniques involving the use of environmental controls include ensuring adequate protocols, policies, and procedures for timely evacuation of patients and staff from locked units or areas in the event of fire or other internal disaster. There should also be consideration of the potential need for emergency access to the unit by resources such as fire personnel or a code team.

Environmental controls are used to seclude or restrict patients from accessing high-risk areas. Examples include the following:

- Entrances or exits to the unit or facility
- Elevators and stairways
- Windows
- Nursing stations, staff lounges, or locker room areas
- Seclusion room(s)
- Medication storage, preparation, and dispensing areas
- Examination and treatment areas
- Electroconvulsive therapy treatment and recovery areas
- Patient rooms, except during hours of sleep or rest periods
- Bathing or shower rooms
- Activity or craft areas
- Exercise or gym facilities
- Individual or group therapy rooms
- Housekeeping and laundry supplies and equipment storage areas
- Dietary or kitchen facilities

Seclusion Policy   The following are elements that should be addressed in the organization's protocols, policies, and procedures for all locked and unlocked seclusion areas, as well as quiet rooms and time-out areas.

Informed Consent Process   The use of seclusion requires informed consent, except in cases of emergency when patients are deemed to be a risk to themselves or others.

Often the symptoms or behaviors that necessitate involuntary seclusion are the same symptoms or behaviors that render patients, at least temporarily, unable to control their behaviors adequately to participate in the informed consent process. When a patient is deemed unable to consent because of behavioral symptoms, family should be notified and consent obtained, if possible. Patients may be able to provide retroactive consent after they have regained behavioral control.

Documentation relating to the informed consent process for involuntary seclusion must indicate:

1. The specific reasons or behaviors that rendered the patient unable to provide informed consent

2. The steps taken to obtain consent from a parent or legal representative

3. Subsequent (retroactive) patient consent, if obtained

Practitioner Orders   A practitioner's order is required for the use of any patient-specific environmental restraint, including locked, voluntary, or open-door (unlocked) seclusion or the patient's voluntary use of a quiet room.

As noted previously, involuntary controls may be used without the patient's consent in instances when it is determined that the patient presents a danger to himself/herself, or others. Consent, physician orders, and notification to the family or legal representative must be implemented as soon as it is practicable.

Seclusion Efficacy and Patient Safety   The efficacy and appropriateness of seclusion in meeting the patient's treatment needs must be documented. The patient's safety and well-being (as well as the safety of others) are paramount considerations, and any adverse patient response must be immediately addressed by the clinical staff or practitioner. Moreover, any patient injury resulting from seclusion must be reported in accordance with regulatory requirements and facility policy.

Monitoring and Observations Protocols   There must be consistent, ongoing monitoring of the patient's behavior and physical condition immediately before, during, and after seclusion.

Electroconvulsive Therapy

Electroconvulsive therapy (ECT) has been used for behavioral health patients for decades. Commonly called *shock therapy*, it has been both praised and criticized by behavioral health professionals, patients' rights advocates, and society at large.

ECT and other shock therapies, such as insulin shock, have been, at various times, both popular and controversial. They have sometimes been depicted as cruel and inhumane in the public media. Movies such as *The Snake Pit* from the 1950s, *One Flew Over the Cuckoo's Nest* during the 1970s, and *Girl, Interrupted* in 2000 have given the impression that psychiatric hospitalization and treatments such as ECT were used as a form of punishment or to control a patient's undesirable behavior for the benefit of others. Aside from clinical benefits or detriments associated with ECT, these negative depictions of psychiatric hospitals and/or ECT in the media may have been effective in focusing the general population's attention on the need to ensure behavioral healthcare patients' rights and assuring that all behavioral healthcare patients receive humane, safe, and effective treatment.

Traditionally, ECT treatments are given in a series over a prescribed period of time. The number of treatments in the series will depend upon the practitioner's custom and practice, the patient's response to treatment, the presence and/or degree of adverse or side effects, and the patient's overall therapeutic response to the ECT treatments.

ECT patients receive sedation or anesthesia prior to the controlled application of an electrical stimulus. The resulting convulsive response is controlled to minimize the risk of physical injury or posttreatment discomfort. The treatment is administered by a physician and can be provided in both inpatient and outpatient settings, depending upon the patient's needs. Patients are monitored during the treatment and until they have recovered sufficiently to leave the treatment area.

Risk Control Techniques   The risk control techniques applied to electroconvulsive therapy issues are discussed next.

Informed Consent   As with many medical treatments and procedures, results from ECT and the occurrence of adverse or side effects may vary. The physician must clearly discuss the risks, benefits, and alternatives to ECT with the patient to ensure that the informed consent process is fully implemented.

As noted previously, ECT is typically given through a series of treatments, and the informed consent should specify the number of treatments authorized by the patient. Should additional treatments be needed beyond those included in the initial informed consent, additional consent should be obtained.

Documentation of each informed consent discussion and the patient's resulting decision is critical to the effective defense of any subsequent litigation that may arise. Because some patients receiving ECT complain of memory loss following treatment, it is recommended that, whenever possible, a family member or patient legal representative be included in each informed consent discussion and that his or her witnessing of the patient's consent be documented in the patient's health information record.

Clinical Assessment   ECT patients undergo an assessment that includes

- a detailed description of the patient's clinical condition, including diagnoses, symptoms, behaviors, and past and present treatments, specifically addressing the rationale for the proposed ECT treatment;

- identification of the patient's specific symptoms that align with the organization's clinical indications for ECT; and

- ongoing clinical evaluation of the patient's initial and continuing response to ECT treatment.

Health History and Medical Clearance   Patients must have a complete medical history and physical examination to ensure that they are medically stable and medically appropriate for ECT. Pretreatment anesthesia evaluations are performed to assess anesthesia risk and to determine the appropriateness of the specific type of anesthesia proposed.

Intraprocedure and Postprocedure Monitoring Criteria   The ECT clinical protocol must clearly define the type and extent of clinical monitoring of the patient's medical condition required during and following ECT.

Management of Medical Emergencies   The ECT clinical protocol should address the manner in which medical emergencies during or after an ECT treatment will be managed. During the treatment, a physician and an anesthesia and/or nursing professional should be in attendance, and patients medically monitored. Depending on the ECT unit location, it may be appropriate for the unit to maintain an emergency cart that includes appropriate equipment and medications. Regardless of the type of facility, there should be adequate emergency equipment available for the clinical personnel to establish an airway, provide CPR, administer oxygen, and obtain transportation to an acute medical care setting.

If the ECT is being administered in a behavioral healthcare facility that is contained within a hospital or medical center, it may be clinically appropriate to have an arrangement with the hospital's CPR team to respond to emergencies in the ECT unit. It may also be appropriate for the ECT professional staff to begin emergency treatment, stabilize the patient's medical emergency, and then transport the patient directly to the hospital emergency department.

Documentation of and Compliance with Electroconvulsive Therapy Treatment Plans   Clinical rationale, informed consent discussion, results of monitoring, and the patient's response to treatment must comply with the treatment plan and be documented in the patient's health information record.

Addiction or Substance Abuse Therapies

Persons seeking treatment for addiction, substance abuse, and some related uncontrollable repetitive behaviors are often identified as having behavioral health diagnoses and thus may be appropriately treated in a behavioral healthcare facility. This section of the chapter is not intended to be an in-depth discussion of addiction, substance abuse, or repetitive behaviors, nor does it discuss all their appropriate medical and behavioral health treatments. The focus here is on identified risks and practicable risk control techniques.

The following is a partial list of substances, medications, and repetitive behaviors that may result in the patient's seeking treatment in a behavioral health facility:

- Alcohol
- Narcotics (includes legally prescribed narcotics, illegally obtained narcotics or street drugs, or illicitly produced forms of narcotics)
- Hallucinogens
- Sedatives
- Hypnotics
- Amphetamines
- Antianxiety agents
- Caffeine
- Nicotine
- Gambling
- Sex and sex-related behaviors
- Eating
- Debting
- Cleaning
- Handwashing

Because some substances are illegal, patients may be involved in allegations and/or criminal charges within the legal system. Patients must be notified at the start of their course of treatment that entering treatment is not a substitute for their participation in legal or criminal proceedings that may ensue, nor is it in lieu of criminal charges and/or incarceration, unless so ordered by the courts.

Risk Control Techniques   A discussion of risk control techniques related to addiction or substance abuse therapies follows.

Initial and Ongoing Clinical and Behavioral Assessments   Patients seeking addiction therapies undergo initial and periodic clinical and behavioral assessments. Additional clinical and behavioral assessments should also be performed whenever there are significant changes in the patient's symptoms and/or condition.

Medical Clearance for Detoxification   Patients undergoing detoxification may have coexisting acute or chronic medical conditions that require concomitant assessment and treatment. Withdrawal from a substance, even when managed under clinical protocol, may cause additional stress on the patient's health. It is necessary to establish the patient's underlying medical condition, identify any coexisting medical conditions, and treat them as needed.

Ongoing Medical Management Some patients undergoing addiction therapy will require ongoing treatment of coexisting acute and chronic medical conditions or medical symptoms that result from the detoxification process. Concomitant treatment of coexisting and/or detoxification-related medical conditions or symptoms should be documented in the patient's health information record.

Contraband Controls Addiction therapy patients may suffer severe physical and emotional symptoms during detoxification and throughout the course of their treatment. Such symptoms may occur even with supportive therapy, medication, and stress management. The patient may experience strong cravings for the substance for which detoxification is indicated and may be at increased risk for unauthorized use of that substance.

It is critical to the success of addiction therapy that the patient be completely removed from any access to the substance of choice. The behavioral healthcare addiction therapy unit must employ strict contraband controls in order to ensure a safe, substance-free environment for patients.

Facility protocol stipulates what steps will be taken to discard or otherwise destroy any contraband substances located during a search. Identification of an illegal substance in a patient's possession may require notification of law enforcement. Each facility should consult with its legal counsel to ascertain its legal and regulatory responsibilities related to illegal substances. Such legal advice should then be incorporated in the facility's addiction therapy protocols, policies, and procedures.

Patients should be informed at the time of admission that their rooms and possessions will be initially and periodically searched and, if deemed necessary, they may be required to submit to a body search.

- Room searches: When there is a patient identified as being at risk, routine searches and additional focused searches of patient rooms, communal areas, dining rooms, and activity areas are essential to ensuring a substance-free environment.

- Personal effects searches: Each patient's personal effects must be searched at the time of admission and periodically thereafter for any contraband. Identified contraband must be confiscated and discarded or surrendered to law enforcement as appropriate.

- Body searches: If a body search is necessary, it should only be carried out by a same-sex professional staff member and should be witnessed and documented by an additional same-sex staff member. Some organizations stipulate that only medical professionals (physician, nurse) perform body searches.

It may be necessary to carry out an even closer body search such as a skin search or a body cavity search for patients at high risk for contraband. Such searches may be indicated if there is reasonable suspicion that a substance is hidden somewhere on the body.

It is important to reiterate that whenever any level of body search is clinically indicated, it must be respectfully carried out by a same-sex professional staff member and witnessed by a same-sex staff member. This will assist in defending the staff and organization against any allegations of abuse or injury during a search. Both staff members should independently document the details of the search in the patient's health information record.

Medication Management   Behavioral healthcare facilities need to have stringent controls for the management of all medications and biologicals. Any prescribed or unauthorized medications must be confiscated. Prescribed medication may be returned only at the time of discharge and only if it continues to be prescribed. It is preferable to have the patients sign an acknowledgement of the facility's protocols, policies, and procedures related to the management of both prescribed medications and unauthorized drugs in the patient's possession at the time of admission into the treatment facility. This acknowledgement should also address possession of illegal substances, including the fact that law enforcement representatives may be notified of such possession.

Family members and other visitors must be oriented to the risks of carrying medications or drugs when they are visiting the patient in a behavioral healthcare setting. Even if their family member is not at risk, other patients in the setting may be at risk. If necessary, at-risk patients should be prohibited from having visitors. In some cases, it may be necessary to perform voluntary searches of visitors' personal items such as purses and backpacks and to deny visiting privileges to those who are unwilling to submit to reasonable search procedures.

Physical Environment Controls   Some addiction therapy treatment facilities or units within a facility are designated as locked units to prevent the introduction of contraband and to protect patients from eloping. This concern is particularly applicable for addiction therapy patients who are also at high risk for suicide or homicide, are incompetent or confused, are minors, or have other high-risk factors.

See the elopement section in this chapter for the physical plant controls recommended as risk control techniques.

Visitor Controls   Addiction therapy facilities must establish specific policies and procedures that govern the management of visitors. Such facilities require orientation of all visitors prior to meeting with patients to ensure they have not purposely or inadvertently brought a potentially dangerous medication or contraband item into the facility. Some facilities greatly limit the visitors for addiction therapy patients. Others require visitors to undergo contraband searches.

When there is significant risk to the patient, the practitioner may order that visitors be completely prohibited for all or part of the patient's course of treatment. The practitioner may require that all or specific visitors be allowed only under direct one-to-one observation by staff or when they are participating in a patient care activity.

Clinical Monitoring Protocols   There must be ongoing monitoring of the effectiveness of facility protocols, policies, and procedures designed to ensure that the facility is providing quality care to addiction therapy patients in a safe environment that is free of contraband. There must also be ongoing monitoring of addiction therapy patients' treatment plans to ensure that they are properly assessed and treated.

The facility should also monitor instances in which contraband is identified, used, and/or seized in order to identify gaps in their patient safety and physical plant contraband controls. When an issue is identified, it must be investigated and a plan of correction developed and implemented. Continued monitoring is maintained to ensure the effectiveness of the plan of correction.

Discharge Planning and Referral for Ongoing Supportive Care   Each addiction therapy patient must receive a comprehensive discharge plan that includes appropriate referrals for ongoing supportive care. This is especially important when patients have been admitted for substance detoxification. Such admissions are usually of a limited nature and are confined to the initial withdrawal of the substance. Addiction therapy patients may have a long history of symptoms and also may have lost their housing, employment, and social support systems.

The patient will need referrals for follow-up therapy and medical care as needed. A partial list of potentially appropriate referrals includes the following:

- Emergency or long-term housing assistance
- Financial assistance for living expenses
- Financial assistance or insurance coverage for ongoing behavioral and medical healthcare
- Individual and/or group behavioral health and addiction therapy
- Appropriate twelve-step and other community-based support program(s)
- Medical care provider
- Social agencies for assistance with meals, clothing, and so forth

Documentation of Compliance with Addiction Therapy Treatment Plans   The patient's level of compliance with the addiction therapy treatment plan, including abstinence from his or her substance(s), is documented in the patient's health information record. Documentation of patient compliance with the treatment plan should also indicate which support systems and services have been provided to assist the addiction therapy patient in maintaining abstinence and following the prescribed treatment plan.

Experimental Treatments

The behavioral healthcare research community is continually developing and implementing research protocols, especially in the area of medications. Research directed at developing more effective psychoactive medications and improving behavioral healthcare treatments is regulated by the Federal Food and Drug Administration (FDA). Behavioral healthcare patients may meet criteria for inclusion in one or more ongoing research clinical trials.

There are very specific guidelines and regulations controlling research involving human subjects. This section is not to be considered a comprehensive discussion of clinical research or of the FDA guidelines. Rather, it is a brief discussion of some risks involved in clinical research and suggests a number of risk control techniques that may reduce patient injury or investigator/facility liability. For more information regarding this topic refer to the FDA Web site at www.fda.gov.

Risk Control Techniques   A discussion of risk control techniques associated with experimental treatments follows.

Institutional Review Board Approval of Investigational Protocols   Every clinical trial must meet the FDA's requirements for research involving human subjects. For example, every healthcare organization participating in clinical trials is required to have an institutional review board (IRB) that reviews and approves investigational protocols. IRBs are composed of clinicians, administrators, ethics professionals, clergy, and at least one layperson from the immediate community. Additional information about clinical research and institutional review boards can be found in Chapter 5 of this text.

Investigational Protocols   Every FDA-approved and IRB-approved research protocol must prepare, maintain, and follow written procedures for conducting its initial and continuing review of research by the IRB. The patient's participation in the investigational protocol must be documented in his or her health information record.

Protocol-Specific, FDA-Approved Consent for Participation in Investigational Protocol   Every FDA clinical trial includes a protocol-specific informed consent document. The informed consent process includes a review of the FDA-approved consent information that provides the risks, benefits, and alternatives to the proposed experimental medication or biomedical equipment. Additionally, the consent discussion is required to expressly inform the patient that the treatment is experimental in nature, that there may be no benefit derived from it, and that adverse or side effects may result from the treatment.

Assessment of Clinical Appropriateness for Investigational Protocol   A comprehensive patient assessment is required initially and periodically thereafter, as defined in the protocol, to ensure that the patient meets the clinical criteria for inclusion. An additional assessment is to be performed whenever there is a significant change in the patient's condition.

Medical Clearance and Ongoing Medical Management   Patients participating in investigational behavioral health protocols must have medical clearance to ensure that their medical condition is appropriate for them to participate and to ascertain their baseline health status. In addition to promoting safety, this approach also makes it possible to more accurately evaluate the patient's response to the protocol and/or to identify adverse or side effects related to the experimental treatment.

Concomitant or Subsequently Approved Treatment   Participation in an investigational protocol may include the patient's agreement to forego initiating other known or experimental therapies or treatments pending completion of the protocol.

If this is the case, the informed consent process is particularly essential to ensure that the patient makes an appropriate and informed decision regarding participation in the investigational protocol. As previously noted, the informed consent discussion must include not only the risks and benefits of the proposed protocol, but also information regarding any other alternatives to that treatment.

Reporting of Patient Adverse Effect or Injury   Any adverse effect or patient injury resulting from participation in an investigational protocol must be reported to the FDA and the Department of Health for the state in which the patient is being treated.

Documentation of Patient's Response to Protocol   The patient's response to the investigational protocol must be documented in his or her health information record.

Referral for Ongoing Approved and/or Investigational Treatment   Upon completion of the investigational protocol, the behavioral healthcare patient may require referral for other investigational treatments or for standard, approved therapies. All efforts made to refer the patient for additional treatment or therapy should be documented in the patient's health information record.

Appropriate referrals and documentation of those efforts and of the patient's subsequent compliance may be especially critical for behavioral healthcare patients at high risk for suicidal or homicidal ideation/behaviors, addiction, or with a history of noncompliance with their treatment plan.

ABUSE RISKS

Many behavioral healthcare patients may be at high risk of abuse or exhibit abusive or aggressive behavior themselves. There is also a heightened risk of allegations of abuse when the patient population is composed of vulnerable individuals, such as children, adolescents, developmentally delayed, physically handicapped, and/or geriatric patients. All behavioral health patients must be assessed for the risk of abusive behavior. Additionally, a careful history should be obtained, including queries regarding episodes of abuse in the patient's life.

Each organization should build its foundation on a zero-tolerance philosophy regarding any form of patient abuse. In order to maintain a safe patient environment, prevention efforts must be comprehensive and ongoing. However, once abuse has occurred, risk control techniques must be implemented in a timely fashion.

Because the behavioral healthcare population is composed of known vulnerable groups, there is a potential risk for attracting inappropriate workers. Therefore, all employees, contracted personnel, and volunteers must be fully screened to eliminate potential abusers. Once they are approved to be part of the organizational workforce, they must undergo training in the recognition and prevention of abuse.

Alleged Abuser

Abusers of patients can be other patients, staff, family, or visitors.

Patient–Patient Abuse   Trained staff are responsible for supervising all patient-to-patient contact, including therapeutic and social encounters. In order to minimize the risk of patient-to-patient abuse, staff should consider that any unsupervised encounter may result in actual or alleged abuse.

Staff–Patient Abuse   Staff must be aware that behavioral healthcare patients may have an altered or heightened sense of vulnerability and may experience even appropriate staff contact as abusive or inappropriate. It is important that all staff be made aware of patients with a history of abuse or of having been abused, so that staff may behave accordingly.

When patients act out against staff, there must be emergency procedures and mechanisms to enable staff members to protect themselves from abusive patients.

Visitor–Patient Abuse   Patient visitor encounters should be limited to staff-supervised areas. Family and other visitors who have a history of abusing the patient or being abused by the patient may appropriately be barred from visiting.

Alleged Abuse

The facility must have formal protocols, policies, and procedures relating to abuse. Such policies and procedures should include guidelines for preventing, investigating, correcting, and reporting instances of abuse.

Allegations of abuse or complaints of abuse must be fully reported and investigated, and when substantiated, corrective measures must be taken. In addition to reporting such allegations or instances of abuse internally, many states require that abuse be reported to the state department of health and/or department of mental health.

The facility must also implement clinical and administrative guidelines for managing abusive patients. (See the discussions elsewhere in this chapter on the use of de-escalation techniques, seclusion, and restraint.)

Any staff member found to have been abusive should be immediately removed from the patient treatment area. Facility procedure should require that once allegations of abuse have been verified, the employee must be terminated from employment; reported to any relevant licensing, certifying, or professional monitoring authorities; and, when appropriate, reported to law enforcement.

When abuse is of sufficient degree to be considered a criminal act, notification of law enforcement is generally required. The criminal codes in each state provide legal definitions of the various forms of abuse. Additional legal definitions may also be included in child or senior welfare agency regulations. The organization's legal counsel should be consulted whenever a question of criminal acts may arise.

Physical Abuse   Any unwarranted or unauthorized physical contact that did or could have caused an injury or that was experienced as abuse by the patient should be treated and investigated as abuse.

Sexual Abuse   For purposes of this document, sexual abuse will include any verbal or physical contact of a sexual or inappropriately intimate nature that involves a minor or incompetent adult and any unwarranted or unauthorized contact of a sexual or inappropriately intimate nature between adults when one adult has not consented.

Emotional Abuse   Emotional abuse is perhaps more difficult to define. For purposes of this discussion and establishing a threshold for implementing risk control techniques, it should include any verbal or written event, perceived personal slight, or neglect of a patient's needs or requests that results in patient distress or emotional pain and suffering. Clearly, this definition is articulated from the patient's perspective, but it is the patient's perception of abuse that will lead to allegations and potential litigation.

Reporting Abuse

Any allegation or confirmed instance of abuse must be reported internally as a patient incident. The patient's physician, family, and/or legal representative should be notified of the alleged abuse and informed of the patient's immediate condition. Treat any physical injuries or sexual or emotional abuse and note the treatment in the reports. All allegations of abuse should be additionally reported to the appropriate state agencies pending the results of the facility's and/or law enforcement's investigative findings. The investigation's findings, deeming the allegation either substantiated or unsubstantiated, should also be reported to the involved parties and agencies. Following the investigation, it is essential to develop and implement a plan of correction and report this to the appropriate parties and agencies.

Although reporting requirements may vary from state to state, reports to the following entities are typically required:

- State department of mental health
- State department of health
- Internal or organization-specific requirements, including family, legal representative, and physician
- Law enforcement

Investigation and Documentation of Abuse Allegations

All allegations of abuse must be diligently investigated and the findings reported. Develop and implement a plan to ensure that no further abuse can occur. Any treatment provided to the patient related to alleged or confirmed abuse must be documented in the patient's health information record.

Abuse Prevention Techniques

The organization must have protocols, policies, and procedures that ensure a safe treatment environment without the threat of abuse. Prevention requires learning from past episodes when abuse occurred despite the organization's best prevention efforts. Prevention of future occurrences will require a plan of correction that specifically addresses the contributing factors identified during the investigative process.

Abuse prevention includes ensuring that patients are receiving behavioral healthcare in the appropriate setting. This may require improving an organization's admission or acceptance criteria to more adequately screen patients at risk for abusive behavior and assigning at-risk patients to appropriate units, where such behaviors can be controlled.

Mandatory abuse-related screening for employees, contract personnel, and volunteers should be required. Professional guidelines, organizational manuals, and in-service programs should define and explain appropriate behavior among staff and behavioral healthcare patients. Such programs should also reiterate that termination and/or criminal consequences will result when allegations of abuse are substantiated.

Documentation Practices and Requirements

All actions undertaken to investigate abuse allegations, all investigative findings, and any corrective actions taken must be fully documented in the incident and investigational reports. Patient injuries and resulting treatments should be documented in the patient's health information record.

· · · · · · · · ·

ENVIRONMENTAL RISKS

Every aspect of the patient's environment must be assessed for the risk of patient injury. Patients' rights include the right to privacy, but it is essential that staff is able to view patients in every area. All patient/resident property should be carefully checked for potentially dangerous items and contraband at the time of admission. Unscheduled room checks further protect patients/residents.

- Door locks: Door locks must be designed so patients do not have the ability to lock or unlock any unit door. Conversely, every staff member must have access to keys that lock and unlock every door in the unit.

- Patient rooms: Ideally, patient rooms should be square in shape and not have any blind areas where staff cannot immediately see the location of the patient. Patients' closets should be equipped with break-away hanging rods that support only minimal weight.

- Bathrooms: All unit bathrooms must be equipped with break-away shower rods and showerheads and shatterproof mirrors. Plumbing should be fully enclosed, with no exposed pipes.

- Windows: Windows should be made of shatterproof, break-proof materials. If windows can open, their aperture should be modified to allow one to two inches of space. Some facilities use locked window covers made of wire mesh that allow windows to be safely opened for ventilation purposes.

- Seclusion or quiet rooms: There should be no materials in the room except for a mat or mattress. There should be no patient-accessible electrical outlets, vents, screw-on plates or guards that could be removed. Dropped ceilings should not be used in these areas. The room should be square in shape to allow for a complete view of the patient. If a camera is used, it must be outside of the patient's reach and may not be covered by any material that can be unscrewed, loosened, or dislodged.

- Medication storage areas and administration areas or carts: Medication storage and administration areas should be centrally located and patients should present to that area to receive medications. The behavioral healthcare organization should require a mouth check after every medication is administered. If medication carts are used, they should not be left unattended, even for a moment, and must be kept locked at all times. Ideally, carts should be located in a locked medication preparation or administration room. Medication rooms often have Dutch doors in which the lower portion can remain closed and locked while the upper portion is opened for the staff to provide the patients' ordered medications.

- Housekeeping, maintenance chemicals, and equipment: Housekeeping equipment must be kept under direct observation at all times. Toxic cleaning agents must be locked and protected from unauthorized patient access. Plastic trash can liners or other plastic bags for waste disposal should be prohibited because they represent a risk of suffocation.

- Razor or sharps management: Any object that could be used directly or modified to be used as a cutting tool or weapon for self-injury or to injure someone else must be carefully monitored and should be considered a sharp. All personal effects must be searched at the time of admission and all sharps or potentially dangerous items removed. All sharps must be maintained under locked staff control and should be counted and accounted for. Any situation in which there are missing sharps should constitute an incident, and a total unit search should be conducted until the missing sharp is located.

  Battery-powered razors are recommended, but even they can become a sharp if disassembled. Sharps may not be provided to patients at risk for suicidal or homicidal behavior. If sharps are provided to patients, they must be logged in and out and used by patients under staff's visual supervision to ensure that high-risk patients do not obtain access to a sharp signed out for use by another patient. A time limit should be imposed for each sharp released to a patient. If the sharp is not accounted for within the time limit, it should be considered missing. Once again, a missing sharp constitutes an incident, and a total unit search must be conducted until it is located. Examples of sharps include:

- Razors
- Scissors
- Nail clippers, cuticle clippers, or scissors
- Nail files
- Any form of knife, including butter knives and cooking knives
- Eating utensils

· · · · · · · · ·
CONCLUSION

Behavioral healthcare services have evolved significantly during the past several decades, with the primary shift being the provision of more outpatient behavioral healthcare services. Risk control in the behavioral healthcare arena also has evolved to address changing risks. A successful behavioral healthcare risk control program addresses proper hiring, training, and supervision of staff; well-planned and managed physical facilities; thorough patient evaluations and treatment plans; comprehensive informed consent process; and many other components discussed in this chapter.

Like all risk control programs, the behavioral healthcare risk management program should be constantly evaluated and adapted to meet changing needs and circumstances. Incidents should be investigated, analyzed, and used as learning experiences, with appropriate risk control techniques implemented to prevent future similar events. Risk control is always a process and not just a program. Success can be measured in part by a facility's ability to learn from its own mistakes and from the mistakes of others and to proactively adjust the risk control program in response to those lessons learned.

Suggested Readings

"Bill of Rights" Cornell University Law School Legal Information Institute. Title 42. Chapter 102, Sec. 9501 U.S. Code Collection. Available at: www4.law.cornell.edu/uscode/42/9501.html. (Accessed October 31, 2009.)

"Applicability of National Patient Safety Goals to Behavioral Health." Available at: www. jointcommission.org/NR/rdonlyres/4D0F9019-E4E7–49FD-8191–700688637BB3/0/RevisedChapter _BHC_NPSG_20090925.pdf. (Accessed April 10, 2010.)

Lehmann, C. "AACP Issues Guidelines on Seclusion, Restraint Use." *Psychiatric News, American Psychiatric Association*, 2002; 37(7):12.

Gostin, L.O., 2002."*Tarasoff v. The Regents of the University of California* 551 P.2d 334 (1976)." Chapter 10. "Surveillance and Public Health Research: Privacy and the 'Right to Know.'" In *Public Health Law and Ethics: A Reader*. Available at: www.publichealthlaw.net/Reader/docs/Tarasoff.pdf. (Accessed April 10, 2010.)

Appendix 14.1

Latent Risks in the Built Environment for the Behavioral Health Patients: Concerns for the Healthcare Risk Manager

David M. Sine

If the reader is not a risk manager for a behavioral health treatment facility or a facility that includes a behavioral health treatment unit, it is entirely possible that the latent risks to the behavioral health patient found in the built environment in these facilities have not been closely examined. Because mental disorders are not uncommon in the United States (an estimated 26.2 percent of Americans ages 18 and older, about one in four adults, suffer from a diagnosable mental disorder in a given year), all medical centers and clinics are presumed to receive mentally ill patients.[1] Therefore, this appendix will discuss possible design options to mitigate those risks typically found in the environment of care. We will start with background information intended to inform all risk managers of the potential risks posed by and to behavioral health patients in both psychiatric and non-psychiatric inpatient care settings.

Although mental disorders are widespread in the population, the main burden of illness is concentrated in a much smaller proportion, about 6 percent, or one in seventeen, who suffer from a serious mental illness.[2] Serious mental illnesses include major depression, schizophrenia, bipolar disorder, obsessive compulsive disorder, panic disorder, posttraumatic stress disorder, and borderline personality disorder.[3]

Not all serious mental illness leads to suicide, but suicide is the eleventh leading cause of death in the United States, accounting for 33,300 deaths: an annual rate of 10.9 suicide deaths per 100,000 people. In 2006, suicide was the third leading cause of death for young people ages fifteen to twenty-four, and in that same year, for every 100,000 people ages sixty-five and older, 14.2 died by suicide. An estimated twelve to twenty-five attempted suicides occur for every suicide death.[4,5]

This general information regarding acts of self-harm is enough to cause concern for most any risk manager. The Joint Commission (TJC) and others put an even finer point on it and provide patient data that are specific to the healthcare setting. In 2006,

162,359 individuals were hospitalized for self-inflicted injuries, and in 2005, 372,722 people were treated in emergency departments for self-harm.[6–8] Shapiro and Waltzer reported a wide range of suicide rates: between five and eighty per 100,000 psychiatric admissions in the United States.[9] The American Psychiatric Association has reported that approximately fifteen thousand suicides take place in inpatient hospital units each year, and amazingly, one-third of these took place while the patient was on fifteen-minute checks.[10] A TJC review of inpatient suicides found that 75 percent involved hanging and another 20 percent resulted from patients jumping from a roof or window.[11] Other studies of inpatient suicide include patients who committed suicide while on pass or eloping from the hospital, so it is difficult to discern the methods of those who committed suicide while in the hospital itself;[12–14] however, all report hanging and jumping to be the two most common methods. A recent study of inpatient suicide in Veterans Affairs hospitals found that hanging was the most common method of inpatient suicide (accounting for 43 percent of all inpatient suicides) and that doors and wardrobe cabinets accounted for 41 percent of the anchor points used when hanging was the method of self-harm.[15]

Thus far we have only discussed the risk to the patient. In addition to patient self-harm, patient-to-staff injuries are also a common problem that can lead to significant workers' compensation claims or, absent the protection of sole remedy, lawsuits. The risks to the organization itself are also profound. Patient elopement and acts of self-harm expose the healthcare organization to risks that eclipse premise liability and include professional and general liability, wrongful death, loss of licensure for facility and professional staff, regulatory risk, and reputational risk. Such acts may also trigger state self-reporting requirements and are also a TJC sentinel event (suicide of a person in a treatment setting remains the second most frequently reported sentinel event).

· · · · · · · · ·
RISKS IN THE EMERGENCY DEPARTMENT

The data and the related risks described above may be more apparent (and more anticipated) in a facility or treatment unit intended expressly for the provision of specialty mental health services; in the nonpsychiatric medical setting the risks may be less obvious. Because of the lack of health insurance by as much as 16 percent of the U.S. population, underinsurance for mental disorders even among those who have health insurance, access barriers to members of many racial and ethnic groups, discrimination, and the stigma about mental illness that impede help-seeking behavior, it should not be surprising that many admissions for mental health services initiate in the emergency department (ED).[16] In fact, in 2003 there were 3,718,000 ED visits with a primary diagnosis of mental disorder, and today 8 percent of all ED visits (which include both self-presentation and EMS transports) are related to mental health problems.[17] Clearly, the latent risks for the behavioral health patient in the built environment must be addressed, even in the general medical/primary care settings (clinics and hospitals) that are not intended for the exclusive delivery of mental health services.

Hospital EDs often do not have specialized psychiatric facilities or psychiatric specialists available, and they may find it difficult to place behavioral health patients, many of whom are indigent or uninsured, in outside facilities. ED staff spends more than twice as much time seeking beds for these patients or boarding them than they do those without psychiatric problems.[18] Because of the complexity and abundance of medical equipment in the ED, it is simply not possible to "harden" the built environment or to make clinical equipment tamper resistant to the point that the risks are sufficiently mitigated. For this reason, there is no substitute for observation of those patients with a known or a suspected risk of self-harm. The power cords, lines, points of attachment, ready access to sharps, and a staff that can be distracted by the urgent business of emergency care makes the ED an opportunity-rich environment for a patient intent on self-harm. The model codes adopted by authorities having jurisdiction do, however, require that at least one secure holding room of 120 square feet be provided in the ED "for security, patient and staff safety, patient observation, and soundproofing."[19,20] This room, if code compliant, will have finishes, vent and diffusers, and sprinklers that are all tamper resistant. In addition, the secure holding room is to have "no sharp corners, edges, or protrusions, and the walls are to be free of objects or accessories of any kind" and have no electrical outlets or medical gas outlets.[21] The room door will swing out and have hardware on the exterior side only. In short, it is a room that, although designed for safety, would be difficult in which to provide medical care. If the risk of self-harm is coincidental with a need for emergency medical treatment, then the inability to prevent unwanted access by the patient to potentially injurious medical equipment will mandate continual staff observation of the patient or perhaps protective restraint.

· · · · · · · · ·
RISKS IN THE MEDICAL UNIT

When a patient believed to be at risk of self-harm needs medical services that require admission to a hospital medical unit, a standard hospital room will not do. Although not intended for the exclusive use of behavioral health patients, a hospital sleeping room with extra design considerations in which as many opportunities for self-harm have been removed as is possible is recommended. Many of these recommendations will be similar to those made for a sleeping room in a behavioral health unit or treatment facility. Because of the great amount of electrically powered equipment, sharps, cords, and tubes necessary for patient care, this room should be considered inappropriate for a behavioral health patient unless compliance with a policy to "semiharden" the room by removing unneeded patient care equipment, IV poles, cords, and wires is confirmed immediately prior to and continually during the hospital stay. However, given the impossibility of removing all of the opportunities for self-harm due to the very nature of the care provided, a trained sitter is still required for those patients who are identified as at risk for self-harm. It is recommended that policies on what equipment may be removed, how to safeguard any remaining equipment (such as shortening cords), and policies on the use (and qualifications of) sitters be developed. A list of basic safety precautions is provided at the end of this appendix.

·········
RISKS IN THE BEHAVIORAL HEALTH UNIT

We have discussed the latent risks to the behavioral health patient that may be found in the built environment in the ED and in the medical unit. Obviously, there is at least an equal level of concern for risks in the built environment in a mental health treatment facility or mental health treatment unit. Yet, even in a purpose-built mental health unit, no environment can be perfectly safe or eliminate all risks. The impossibly of eliminating all risks was described by Sine and Hunt[22] with language subsequently adopted by the *Guidelines for the Design and Construction of Healthcare Facilities*:

> A safe environment is critical; however, no environment can be entirely safe and free of risk. The majority of persons who attempt suicide suffer from a treatable mental disorder or a substance abuse disorder, or both. Patients of inpatient psychiatric treatment facilities are considered at high risk for suicide; the environment should avoid physical hazards while maintaining a therapeutic environment. The built environment, no matter how well it is designed and constructed, cannot be relied upon as an absolute preventive measure. Staff awareness of their environment, the latent risks of that environment, and the behavior risks and needs of the patients served in the environment are absolute necessities. Different organizations and different patient populations will require greater or lesser tolerance for risk.[23]

The *Guidelines* has been formally adopted by many jurisdictions and is considered the established standard of care for the design of healthcare facilities. Compliance with the parameters outlined in the *Guidelines* may, therefore, provide a lower level of liability risk exposure for the institution if the design of the built environment is ever needed to be defended in court. If the design varies from these standards, these deviations and the clinical justifications for the deviation should be clearly documented.[24]

·········
A SYSTEMATIZED APPROACH TO MITIGATION OF RISKS IN DESIGN

Behavioral health treatment units (and medical surgical facilities treating behavioral health patients as described above) may rely greatly on patient suicide risk evaluations that use risk factors to develop patient treatment plans. Risk factors for nonfatal suicide attempts by adults include depression and other mental disorders (as well as alcohol and other substance abuse and separation or divorce).[25] Although these risk factors are related to suicidal behavior, they do not necessarily predict individual behavior. Risk managers and architectural designers should be aware that often the intentions of the patient cannot be reliably determined.[26,27] Therefore, a conservative approach is for the facility leadership and design professional to design the space as if all patients admitted to the locked unit are presumed to be at equal risk for self-harm and elopement. Although the law and ethical principles require that providing treatment in the least restrictive setting be an underlying value in psychiatric hospital treatment and design, the architecturally least-restrictive environment should be determined by anticipating the single patient who is most at risk on the unit.[28,29]

There has been a great deal of discussion about the perceived advantages of single-patient bedrooms for psychiatric units. The 2010 edition of the *Guidelines* calls for a maximum of two patients per room (except that four patients are allowed in children's units). A 2007 survey by the National Association of Psychiatric Health Systems communicated three important differences between the psychiatric treatment environment and the medical/surgical environment relative to single-bedroom design.[30] First, patient treatment does not take place in sleeping rooms on psychiatric units. Patients receive group and individual therapy in group rooms or interview rooms. Patients are encouraged to be in the dayroom during their waking hours for therapeutic reasons. Second, infection control is handled differently in psychiatric treatment environments. Isolation is rarely attempted on psychiatric units because of the ambulatory nature of the unit population; thus, the studies that show benefits to single-bed patient rooms in reducing airborne and presumably contact infections are rendered largely moot.[31] Third, families are encouraged to visit psychiatric patients, but hours of visitation are limited and families are encouraged to meet with patients in semipublic areas, not patient rooms. In sum, in the extremely limited research on patient room occupancy, there is no evidence that single-occupancy rooms offer clinical or safety advantages in the nominal psychiatric treatment environment.

Although the *Guidelines* offer a designer good counsel and do establish a de facto "architectural standard of care," psychiatric facilities require an additional framework for proper design. In what may appear at first to be contradiction, it is recommended that although the designer assumes an equal level of risk for all patients in a single treatment unit, not all of the treatment unit should be treated as a homogenous landscape.

Within the unit, some areas present greater risks and design challenges than do others. Four areas, each with increasingly more patient safety concerns and therefore design restrictions, have been identified.[32,33] Staff areas (area 1) are only required to meet applicable building codes and regulations. Areas with easy and direct observation of the nurse station (area 2), such as corridors, require fewer precautions than activity areas (area 3), such as TV lounges where staff may not always be present. The highest levels of concern and design challenge (area 4) are for spaces in which patients will be left alone for long periods of time, including the patient rooms and patient toilets. Seclusion rooms have their own unique requirements, as do admissions screening rooms in which staff interacts with patients who may be initially unknown to them and who may become volatile at any moment. The precautions for each level also require all of the considerations for the lower-numbered levels. Solutions to all of these problem areas will vary depending on the organization's patient population and risk tolerance. A device or feature that is perfectly acceptable for one patient population and healthcare organization may not be acceptable for another.

One example of the variability in design choices within a single treatment unit is provided by cabinet doors and drawers. Patients have been known to hang themselves from objects as close to the floor as 18 inches, and one study found that 50 percent of nonjudicial[34] hangings were from heights below the level of the victim's waist.[35] Therefore, cabinet doors and desk drawers are avoided in all patient private spaces (area 4 above). However, cabinet doors and drawers are acceptable in areas that fall under staff supervision (areas 1 and 2 above). Similarly, furniture for use in a group room (where patients have been known to throw or use furniture to strike staff or other patients) or an exam room may be inappropriate in a patient sleeping room. To reduce the possibility of patients using the furniture to barricade themselves or otherwise stack or pile the furniture, all patient sleeping room furniture should be anchored securely in place, with the possible exception of a desk chair (if provided). This precaution is not necessary in a group room that is attended by staff when occupied.

········

EVIDENCE-BASED DESIGN, RISK, AND THE THERAPEUTIC ENVIRONMENT

A fine line exists between a unit in which physical hazards are eliminated to the point of the environment looking institutional and a built environment that is therapeutic and supportive of treatment. Few studies exist that use well-controlled research designs to determine the effects of environmental factors in inpatient psychiatric settings.[36] The only current agreement seems to be that a more residential and less institutional look for the unit is preferred. Unfortunately, the focus on a residential look and feel for behavioral health units, often based on weak or poorly designed research, has eclipsed the aforementioned lessons learned regarding the risk of acts of self-harm by some behavioral health patients. A postoccupancy survey in a new behavioral health facility that finds increased patient satisfaction, but at the same time finds staff feeling isolated in the new space, cannot be taken as an endorsement of a new design.[37] Unfortunately, some awards for architectural design are based on how things look and not how things work, their functionality, or their context.[38] The real issue here should be a move toward "warm and typical residential" and away from "cold and institutional" through use of appropriate color, texture, and light. The current support in the literature for homelike treatment largely leaves *homelike environment* undefined, and important questions remain unanswered, such as what home (or cultural norm) is to be emulated by the designer.

Some of the conflicts in the evidenced-based design literature between those who call for a homelike environment and those who call for a secure unit can be resolved, however, because some evidenced-based design appears to have validity in the behavioral health setting.[39,40] The risk of patient falls and their causes, always of interest to the risk management professional, have application in behavioral health, and especially so in the geriatric-psychiatric patient population and treatment setting. Studies that link design issues to fall rates have identified doorway placement, hand rails, and access to toilets as potential contributors. Surprisingly, several studies concluded that side rails do not reduce the rate of falls, which may be taken as even more evidence to avoid standard mechanical hospital beds in a behavioral health setting.[41]

The literature also identifies the use of natural light as having a positive effect on treatment.[42] Clearly, building orientation as well as windows play a part in this design goal. Closely tied to the evidence that supports the benefits of increased daylight are the benefits of views of nature. Views of nature have been shown to increase positive feelings of calm and decrease feelings of anxiety and anger.[43] However, both the increase in size and number of windows, as well as the use of interior courtyards to increase light or views of nature, may increase the building's (and occupant's) exposure to risks where there are natural hazards such as seismic activity, windstorms, or flooding.

During such environmental or natural emergencies, it may not be feasible to evacuate patients and residents for days or even weeks. Staff operating under emergency conditions are expected to adapt to a combination of stressors, including high workload, unclear roles, reduced staff-to-patient ratios, lack of sleep, limited resources, and adverse environmental conditions. Staff who are injured, fatigued, hungry, or otherwise physically and mentally stressed are neither effective nor efficient and can make bad choices that exacerbate emergency conditions.[44]

Because most hospitals operate at near capacity, an influx of patients and additional staff during a disaster is difficult to accommodate. These issues cannot be optimally resolved by operational policies and emergency management decisions alone regarding what space to use and for what purpose in an existing building. These are also important design issues that must be addressed during the planning phase of new construction or the major renovation of an existing space. Hazard mitigation measures should be incorporated into building design to reduce risk of injuries and damage, minimize the disruption of hospital operations, and promote the possibility of uninterrupted patient care.

· · · · · · · · ·

CONCLUSION

The healthcare risk manager should be aware of the potential risks that the built environment in any healthcare setting poses to the behavioral health patient. As the behavioral health patient population changes due to changes in demographics, employment, and other factors in the community, so too must the healthcare built environment evolve. Although healthcare facilities are arguably more adaptable than most buildings, the rate of change in healthcare treatment modalities, medical technologies, and inevitable changes in the patient population require a higher rate of change than is found in other structures. A regular, documented assessment by a competent individual of the appropriateness of the built environment and the latent risks therein is necessary if the ongoing changes in the patient population and the ever-evolving risks are to be mitigated by modifications in our thinking about and the design of the built environment.

· · · · · · · · ·

AN ABBREVIATED CHECKLIST FOR A PSYCHIATRIC MEDICAL UNIT

Due to the abundance of pumps, monitors, tubing, sharps, plastic bags, cords, and other medical equipment in the medical-surgical patient room, a trained sitter is required for those patients who are identified as at risk for self-harm. It is recommended that policies on what equipment may be removed, how to safeguard any remaining equipment (such as shortening cords), and the use (and qualifications of) sitters be developed.

- The ceiling should not be of a lay-in type. These ceilings can permit hiding of contraband, provide a convenient place to secure a ligature for self-harm, or may allow the patient access to above-the-ceiling interstitial spaces.

- If the room's outside window is operable, the opening should be limited so a person could not pass through the opening (4–6 inches is considered the architectural standard). Alternatively, a window opening could be protected with a security screen. The limitation of the window's opening should be secured by a device that would require a special tool to remove it from the inside (such as an uncommon screwdriver).

- Window glazing should be shatterproof even if the room is on the first floor.

- The patient's room doorknob should be of a tamper-resistant antiligature design.

- If a hospital bed is used, the electrical power cord on the bed should be secured. It is recommended that the bed cord be replaced with a jumper cord that can be removed by staff, kept in a secure place, and used only when the bed needs to be adjusted (check with bed design to ensure that bed can be mechanically lowered to a CPR position).

- Tamper-resistant screws should be used throughout the room.

- Power cords on the TV should be secured. Note that mounting brackets can be an attachment point for a ligature.

- Cork bulletin boards should be replaced with a dry mark board, thus eliminating use of thumbtacks.

- All glass in nightlights and other lighting fixtures should be of a shatterproof and tamper-resistant design, and light fixtures should be secured to restrict patients' access to bulbs and sockets.

- Grab bars in the bathroom are not appropriate and should be either removable or have the wall gap filled in.

- Coat hook, towel bars, cubicle curtain tracks, and closet poles should be eliminated.

- Electrical outlets should be of a GFIC (ground fault interrupter circuit) tamper-resistant type, and covers that are metal should be replaced with shatterproof non-conductive covers.

- The piping for the toilet and lavatory should be protected.

- Lavatory faucets should be tamper resistant.

- The HVAC (heating, ventilating, and air-conditioning) grills should be tamper resistant.

- The bathroom door and hardware should be appropriate for a behavioral health application.

- If either a shower door or curtain is used, it must be appropriate and not provide a convenient place to secure a ligature for self-harm.
- Shower controls and showerhead must be of a tamper-resistant design.
- Mirror- and picture-glazing material should be shatterproof (e.g., Lexan).

Endnotes

1. Kessler, R., W. Chiu, and O. Demler. "Prevalence, severity, and comorbidity of twelve-month DSM-IV Disorders in the National Comorbidity Survey Replication (NCS-R)." *Archives of General Psychiatry* 2005; 62(6):617–627.

2. *Ibid.*

3. National Alliance on Mental Illness. "What is Mental Illness: Mental Illness Facts." Available at: www.nami.org/template.cfm?section=About_Mental_Illness. (Accessed November 2009.)

4. *op. cit.*, Kessler, 2005.

5. Kessler, R., G. Borges, and E. Walters. "Prevalence of and risk factors for lifetime suicide attempts in the National Comorbidity Survey." *Archives of General Psychiatry_* 1999; 56(7):617–626.

6. *Ibid.*

7. Centers for Disease Control. National Center for Injury Prevention and Control. "Web-based Injury Statistics Query and Reporting System (WISQARS)." www.cdc.gov/ncipc/wisqars. (Accessed November 2009.)

8. Centers for Disease Control. "CDC Fact Sheet on Suicide." www.cdc.gov/ncipc/factsheets/suifacts.htm. (Accessed November 2009.)

9. Shapiro, S. and H. Waltzer. "Successful suicides and serious attempts in a general hospital over a 15-year period." *General Hospital Psychiatry* 1980; 2(2):118–126.

10. American Psychiatric Association. "Practice guideline for the assessment and treatment of patients with suicidal behaviors." *American Journal of Psychiatry* 2003; 160:1–60.

11. The Joint Commission. "Inpatient suicide: Recommendations for prevention." *Sentinel Event Alert*. Available at: www.jointcommission.org/SentinelEvents/SentinelEventAlert/sea7.htm. (Accessed November 2009.)

12. Blain, P. A. and L. J. Donaldson. "The reporting of inpatient suicides: Identifying the problem." *Public Health* 1995; 109:203–301.

13. Proulx, F., A. D. Lesage, and F. Grunberg. "One hundred in-patient suicides." *British Journal of Psychiatry* 1997; 171: 247–250.

14. King, E. A. "The Wessex recent in-patient suicide study, 2: Case-control study of 59 in-patient suicides." *British Journal of Psychiatry* 2001; 178:537–542.

15. Mills, P. et al. "Inpatient suicide and suicide attempts in Veterans Affairs hospitals." *Joint Commission Journal on Quality and Patient Safety* 2008; 34(8):482–488.

16. U.S. Surgeon General. *Surgeon Generals Report on Mental Health: 1999*. Available at: www.surgeongeneral.gov/library/mentalhealth/home.html. (Accessed November 2009.)

17. Institute of Medicine. *Hospital-Based Emergency Care: At the Breaking Point.* Washington, D.C.: National Academy Press, 2006.

18. *Ibid.*

19. Facility Guidelines Institute. *Guidelines for the Design and Construction of Health Care Facilities*, 2006, p. 145.

20. American Institute of Architects. *Guidelines for Design and Construction of Hospital and Health Care Facilities*, 2001, p. 45.

21. *op. cit.*, Facility Guidelines Institute.

22. Sine, D. M. and J. M. Hunt. *Guidelines for the Built Environment of Behavioral Health Facilities.* Washington, D.C.: National Association of Psychiatric Health Systems, 2003.

23. *op. cit.*, Facility Guidelines Institute.

24. Hunt, J. M., and D. M. Sine. "Common Mistakes in Designing Psychiatric Facilities." Available at: http://info.aia.org/journal_aah.cfm?pagename=aah_journal_current. (Accessed November 2008.)

25. Milone, R. D. "Involuntary Hospitalizations." In: D. S. Wahl, ed. *Ethics Primer of the American Psychiatric Association.* Washington, D.C.: APA, 2001.

26. Simon, R. I. "Suicide risk assessment: Is clinical experience enough?" *Journal of the American Academy of Psychiatry and the Law* 2006; 34(3):276–278.

27. Simon, R. I. "Imminent Suicide: The illusion of short term prediction." *Suicide and Life Threatening Behavior* 2006; 36(3):296–301.

28. Peele, R. and R. Chodoff. "The ethics of involuntary treatment and deinstutionalization." In: S. Bloch, ed., *Psychiatric Ethics.* New York: Oxford, 1999.

29. Sine, D. M. "The architecture of madness and the good of paternalism." *Psychiatric Services* 2008; 59(9):1060–1062.

30. McCann, K. *Psychiatric Unit Room Occupancy.* National Association of Psychiatric Health Systems, 2007.

31. Lidwell, O. M. et al. "Nasal acquisition of *Staphylococcus aureus* in a subdivided and mechanically ventilate ward: Endemic prevalence of a single staphylococcal strain." *Journal of Hygiene* 1970; (68):417–433.

32. *op. cit.*, Hunt, J. M.

33. Sine, D. M. and J. M. Hunt. *Design Guide for the Built Environment of Behavioral Health Facilities*, ed. 3.0. www.naphs.org/Teleconference/documents/DesignGuide3.0F INALUPDATED.8.11.2009.pdf. (Accessed November 2009.)

34. ". . . nonjudicial hangings that are extremely common do not entail a drop or a broken neck but cause death by compression of the major blood vessels (with or without airway compromise) of the neck." As found in Dix, J., Graham, M. A., and Hanzlick, R., *Asphyxia and Drowning: An Atlas.* Vol. 3, *Forensic Pathology Series: Causes of Death Atlas Series.* Boca Raton, Fl.: CRC Press, 2000, p. 7.

35. Gunnell, D. et al. "The epidemiology and prevention of suicide: A systematic review." *International Journal of Epidemiology* 2005; 34:433–442.

36. Karlin, B. E. and R. A. Zeiss. "Environmental and therapeutic issues in psychiatric hospital design: Toward best practices." *Psychiatric Services* 2006; 57(10):1376–1378.

37. Tyson, G. A., G. Lambert and L. Beattie. "The impact of ward design on the behaviour, occupational satisfaction and well being of psychiatric nurses." *International Journal of Psychiatric Health Nursing* 2002; 11:94–102.

38. Brand, S. *How Buildings Learn: What Happens After They're Built.* New York: Penguin, 1994.

39. Sine, D. M. and J. M. Hunt. "Following the evidence towards better design: Some patterns of what works in behavioral healthcare environments are emerging." *Behavioral Healthcare* 2009; 29(7):45–47.

40. Ulrich, R. S. et al. "A review of the research literature on evidence-based healthcare design." *Health Environments Research & Design Journal* 2008; 1(3):61–125.

41. *Ibid.*

42. Beauchemin, K. M. and P. Hays. "Sunny hospital rooms expedite recovery from severe and refractory depressions." *Journal of Effective Disorders* 1996; 40(1–2):49–51.

43. Ulrich, R. S. "Effects of interior design on wellness: Theory and recent scientific research." *Journal of Health Care Interior Design* 1991; 3(1):97–109.

44. Sine, D. M. "Staffing in a Crisis: Loyalties in conflict. Lessons learned by behavioral health facilities during major disasters." *HealthBeat* 2007; 7(1).

15

Managing Risk in the Ambulatory Environment

Robert F. Bunting Jr.
Joyce H. Benton

P rimary care focuses on proactive medicine. It is based on the belief that patients can be managed better and more effectively on an outpatient, or ambulatory, basis before diseases reach the point that acute inpatient care is warranted.

As inpatient care increasingly shifts to the ambulatory setting, it is important to be aware that there are several aspects that make up the ambulatory environment. However, their definitions change frequently as the healthcare delivery system evolves to meet the needs of patients, providers, and payers.

Box 15.1 provides a glimpse of the settings that offer ambulatory care.[1,2] They range from the traditional physician's office to newer environments, such as infusion therapy and laser centers. Each setting offers new benefits and risks.

In addition to the variety of settings that characterize the ambulatory environment, innovative treatment modalities are also important vehicles for primary care. Alternative medicine certainly is not a new concept. Some of its affiliate practices have been in existence for centuries. Yet, it is a growing field with several important implications for the risk management professional.

Traditionally, the study of quality, and of the risks associated with healthcare delivery, has focused on the acute-care setting. In 1999, the Institute of Medicine estimated that between forty-eight thousand to ninety-eight thousand hospital patients die annually from avoidable medical error. Regardless of the accuracy of this estimate, it fails to take into account the number of patients treated at ambulatory facilities each year.[3,4]

BOX 15.1   Ambulatory Care Facilities

- Ambulatory surgery centers
- Birthing centers
- Cardiac catheterization centers
- Dental clinics
- Dialysis centers
- Endoscopy centers
- Group medical practices
- Home health agencies
- Imaging centers
- Indian health clinics
- Infusion therapy services
- Laser centers
- Lithotripsy services
- MRI centers
- Mental health centers
- Military clinics
- Mobile healthcare services
- Multispecialty group practices
- Occupational health centers

- Office-based surgery offices
- Ophthalmology practices
- Oral and maxillofacial surgery centers
- Pain management centers
- Physician offices
- Plastic surgery centers
- Podiatric clinics
- Prison health centers
- Public health centers
- Radiation/oncology clinics
- Rehabilitation centers
- Sleep centers
- Sports medicine clinics
- Student health services
- Unconventional medicine centers
- Urgent/emergent care centers
- Women's health centers
- Wound care centers

This chapter will explore the risks associated with delivering care in an ambulatory setting. Whenever possible, appropriate quality improvement activities will be discussed. This chapter is designed to enhance the understanding and appreciation of the more salient points of many topics that, though often considered only in the context of acute care, also apply to the vast array of ambulatory settings.

· · · · · · · · ·
COMMON CONCEPTS

Though each of the ambulatory care facilities listed in Box 15.1 has its own specialized risk areas, they collectively share many aspects of risk. The following topics are presented in a general manner because they apply to various types of healthcare practices in the ambulatory environment.

Professional Liability

Medical services traditionally provided in an acute care setting are now performed in an ambulatory care setting. This transition brings with it an increase in the severity and frequency of professional liability claims in the ambulatory care setting.

The Physicians Insurers Association of America's (PIAA's) Data Sharing Project, which contains medical professional liability claims information on twenty-eight specialties, revealed that obstetric and gynecologic surgeons, internists, and general and family practitioners were the three top specialties in the number of medical professional liability claims reported from 1985 to 2007. The top five medical misadventures most likely to generate medical professional liability claims during this period included improper performance of a procedure, no medical misadventure (situation where there is an absence of an allegation of any improper medical conduct on the part of this insured), errors in diagnosis, failure to supervise or monitor care, and medication errors.

The list has changed little in more than 20 years since PIAA, a trade association of physician owned and operated professional liability carriers, first identified improper performance, diagnostic error, failure to monitor care, performing a procedure not indicated, and medication errors as the most prominent medical mishaps for all specialties combined. The average indemnity award steadily increased from 2002 through 2007. During these five years, the average indemnity paid on behalf of all practitioners increased 9 percent.[5]

According to the National Practitioner Data Bank, physician claim frequencies experienced a decline from 2001 to 2008. During this period, the average size of loss increased at a rate of 3 percent per year.[6]

The incidence of and relationship among adverse events, negligence, and medical professional liability lawsuits have been debated for years, and studies have yielded some interesting findings. Levinson and colleagues were the first to identify specific communication behaviors associated with physicians' risk for medical professional liability claims.[7] Some of the behaviors that were inversely related to the degree of risk included the length of time spent with the patient, orienting the patient about the care delivery process, facilitating conversations with the patient, and conversing in a warm, friendly manner.

Physicians continue to have malpractice-related issues related to key aspects of primary care. Of the thousands of claims against physicians in the PIAA Data Sharing Project, more than fifty-eight thousand claims reported improper performance of a procedure as the primary allegation, and forty-six thousand had their origin in a diagnostic interview, evaluation, or consultation.[8]

Communication

Poor communication is not listed by PIAA as an official cause of medical professional liability claims, but it underlies most medical professional liability actions. Insurance claims administrators and medical professional liability defense attorneys estimate that communication failure is a contributing factor in 80 percent of all professional claims or lawsuits. In 20 percent of the cases, it is the reason for the filing of the lawsuit.[9]

Good communication skills often have been viewed as a personality trait that some people have and others do not. In fact, good communication skills can be learned and improved through systematic practice. The communication approach most commonly used by clinicians is the interview.

A typical clinician conducts more than 160,000 interviews during a professional career. It is possible for physicians to alter their communication behaviors in ways that both increase patient satisfaction and decrease risk. The history of the healing arts has emphasized the role of the physician as an identifier of disease and as an agent of healing. The traditional role of the clinician has been to find the problem and fix it. However, a new model of disease and healing has emerged that also accounts for psychological, sociological, and ever-present behavioral forces. This expanded context has focused attention on the medical interview, and the transactions that occur during the interview, as an area for change.[10]

The following model for physician–patient communication presents specific communication strategies to be used in the interview. Because the four elements of the model begin with the letter *E*, the model is called the E4 component of clinical care. These elements are engaging, empathizing, educating, and enlisting the patient.[11]

Engagement is a connection between the clinician and patient that continues throughout the encounter. These simple techniques can help build rapport with patients in any practice setting.

- Greet the patient by name and shake hands. It is especially important to greet new patients when they are fully clothed.

- Build rapport by being as curious about the person's medical condition as you are about your own.

- Elicit the patient's agenda, which should include their goals for the encounter and all complaints. Patients asked to explain their concerns by a physician were most often interrupted after the first voiced concern and after an average time of only eighteen seconds.[12]

Empathy is an active concern for the emotions, values, and experience of another. The first step in empathy is validating patients' expressed fears, concerns, symptoms, and pain. This step can create a positive atmosphere in the clinician–patient encounter. The second step in empathic communication is to accept the feelings and values of the patient. Third, empathy should convey an impression that the physician is present and with the patient. Physicians should sit down, maintain eye contact, and remove physical barriers between them and patients. The simple act of sitting while speaking with a patient improves the patient's perception of how much time was spent with the physician. Open and relaxed body language should be displayed.

A major component of the physician–patient encounter is to educate patients about the encounter itself, medical diagnosis, etiology of the disease, treatment options, and follow-up requirements. Education occurs when the cognitive, behavioral, and affective needs are addressed. This process should start at the beginning of the encounter and continue through the patient visit. The following guidelines reduce the chance of misunderstanding.

- Assess the patient's current knowledge.

- Assume that there will be questions. Reassure patients that time will be available for them to ask questions.

- Ensure that patients understand the information provided by asking them to restate points that were presented.

Enlistment is an invitation by the clinician to the patient to collaborate in decision making involving the problem and the treatment plan. This final step involves two processes, decision making and encouraging compliance. Most patients make a self-diagnosis. If the clinician's diagnosis differs from the patient's diagnosis, the patient will act based upon his or her own diagnosis. Therefore, it is crucial that the clinician understand and discuss the patient's diagnosis. The following guidelines might improve patient compliance.

- Explain to the patient the specific details for the treatment plan, the expected benefits that will result, and the potential adverse results of patient noncompliance.
- Identify any concerns, fears, resistance, or real-life reasons why the patient might not comply with the proposed treatment.
- Make necessary referrals to assist the patient in obtaining appropriate physical, financial, social, and community support.

Clinicians and patients sometimes bring two very different perspectives to a visit. These different perspectives can result in a breakdown of communication and leave the clinician and patient frustrated. A patient may be seen as difficult to work with by one clinician, but not difficult by another. Therefore, the word *difficult* does not refer to a specific type of patient, but to a clinician's experience

Difficult is defined as "a function of the relationship" and is based on the interactions of two people. Difficulties occur in physician–patient relationships because of three core problems. These are frustrations for the clinician or patient, inflexibility, and misaligned expectations.[13]

Clinicians and staff often have to confront two types of patients in their practices that are hard to manage. These are the angry patients and the noncompliant patients. Even when patients are angry or frustrated with the physician, office staff, their course of treatment, or their response to treatment, there are ways to improve the quality of physician–patient communication.

- Watch for verbal and nonverbal signs of dissatisfaction and frustration. Be aware that anger, dissatisfaction, and frustration can be expressed in many ways.
- Acknowledge patients' anger or dissatisfaction because this is the first step in letting patients know that their concerns are being heard. Establish that the goal is to assist them in expressing and resolving their concerns in the best possible manner.
- Allow patients to express their anger in a private area, away from other patients.
- Demonstrate empathy by listening and maintaining eye contact. Maintain a nonjudgmental facial expression, a neutral tone of voice, and open body language.
- Focus on the content rather than the delivery of the patient's message, and ask for clarification as needed. Remain calm and respond to, rather than react against, the patient's concerns.

- Use self-disclosure, cautiously and only when appropriate, to indicate that one has had similar experiences and understands the patient's response.

- After the patient has vented anger, respond to the content of the message. Identify those issues that can be readily resolved.

- End the discussion with a mutual understanding of what will be done to address and/or resolve the patient's concerns.[14]

A friendly, mutually satisfying relationship with patients is a desirable goal; however, some patients fail to comply with agreed-upon treatment plans. A noncompliant patient can increase the likelihood of a negative outcome. (Refer to Exhibit 15.1 for a sample letter to a noncompliant patient.)

Whenever the physician accepts a patient or renders care to a patient, a physician–patient relationship is created that continues for as long as the patient's condition requires attention. The physician–patient relationship can be dissolved properly only by the mutual consent of the parties or by reasonable notice of the termination. If a physician withdraws services without providing reasonable notice to the patient, or when medical attention is still needed, the patient may sue on grounds of abandonment.

EXHIBIT 15.1   Sample Noncompliant Letter

\<Date\>
\<Patient's Name\>
\<Address\>

\<City\>, \<State\> \<Zip Code\>
Dear \<Patient's Name\>:

The purpose of this letter is to advise you that a recent review of the \<Name of the Organization\>'s records has determined that you are out of compliance with your physician's recommended treatment plan.

As you are aware, your primary care physician, Dr. \<Primary Physician's Name\> referred you to \<Consulting Physician's Name\> for \<Treatment/Procedure\>. Dr. \<Consulting Physician's Name\> has recommended that you undergo \<Treatment/Procedure\>. It is our understanding that at the present time you are opposed to the recommended procedure or treatment.

\<Name of the Organization\>'s primary concern is to accommodate your medical needs and deliver quality healthcare services. Due to your noncompliance with the recommended treatment plan, our ability to assess your healthcare needs in a complete and professional manner is affected significantly.

Should you dispute the content of this letter, you have the right to initiate a grievance. Please address in writing any contrary information you may have to:

\<Appropriate Company\>
\<Address\>
\<City\>, \<State\> \<Zip Code\>
\<Name of the Organization\> looks forward to your cooperation in this matter.

Sincerely,
\<Physician's Name\>
cc: Medical Record

Source: Adapted from Benton, J. and K. Taylor. *Ambulatory Healthcare: Stay a Step Ahead of Diagnostic-Related Claims,* Session Materials from ASHRM Annual Conference, November, 2000.

A physician may decide to terminate the relationship for reasons such as failure to comply with the recommended medical treatment, disruptive behavior, or other indications that the patient will not benefit from the physician's care. The reasons for terminating the relationship should be documented carefully in the medical record, as should conversations with the patient leading to the termination. Terminate the relationship by sending a certified letter requesting return receipt. A copy of the letter should also be sent via regular mail, in the event that the patient does not accept the certified letter. Keep a copy of the letter and mail receipt in the patient's medical record. Document in the record that the letter was sent, and note any subsequent conversations with the patient. (Refer to Exhibit 15.2, Sample Termination Letter.)

When a patient terminates the relationship, the physician should document the patient's decision in the medical record and advise the patient in writing of any incomplete treatment plans. The patient should be advised of any recommendation to continue any unfinished treatment. The physician should offer to forward a copy of the patient's records to the subsequent physician upon receipt of a signed authorization.[15] For a more in-depth discussion of communication, refer to Chapter 15, Volume 1 in this series.

EXHIBIT 15.2   Sample Termination Letter

\<Date\>
\<Patient's Name\>
\<Address\>
\<City\>, \<State\> \<Zip Code\>

Dear \<Patient's Name\>:
I am writing to inform you that I will no longer be available to provide you with medical care for the following reasons.

    \<Insert reasons for withdrawing medical services. Indicate the patient's current health status and include any recommendations you have for medical care.\>

This notice will become effective on \<Specify Date\> or 30 days after you receive this letter, whichever is later.

    I advise you to seek medical care from another physician. You might wish to contact the Member Relations Department of your health plan or physician referral network \<provide telephone numbers if available\> for your referral. My office will forward a copy of your medical records to your new physician after I receive your written authorization on the enclosed release of information form.

    If during this 30-day period you should require urgent care, please do not hesitate to contact my office or proceed to your nearest emergency department.

    Please feel free to contact my office if you have any questions regarding this notice.

Sincerely,
\<Physician's Name\>
Enclosure: Release of Information Form
cc: Medical Record

Source: Adapted from Benton J., and K. Taylor. *Ambulatory Healthcare: Stay a Step Ahead of Diagnostic-Related Claims,* Session Materials from ASHRM Annual Conference, November, 2000.

Medical Records Management

The medical record can be a healthcare provider's best friend or most formidable enemy. Management of the medical record, therefore, is critical. Its primary purpose is to document the course of a patient's illness and the treatment that the patient receives. It is the main communication medium for planning, coordinating, and orchestrating patient care. Although not always practical, it is best to document everything and omit nothing.

Because the medical record can serve as objective evidence that the standard of care was met during the patient's treatment, documenting completely, accurately, and legibly is a crucial risk management skill. It has been found that in medical professional liability suits in which documentation and recordkeeping were judged inadequate, damages were paid in two-thirds of the cases. When documentation and recordkeeping were judged adequate, damages were paid in only one-third of the cases. If a patient's file contains good documentation, the likelihood of a suit even being filed is generally reduced because the plaintiff's attorney knows that a settlement or a favorable verdict in court would be difficult.[16]

All staff should be trained in proper documentation practices, and a policy delineating how to document patient care should be developed and implemented. Refer to chapters elsewhere in this series for more information.

The information included in the medical record is important to both the physician and the patient. The physician owns the original record and is responsible for safeguarding the information in the medical record against loss, defacement, tampering, and unauthorized access.[17] Because of the confidential nature of the information contained in the record, copies of the record usually cannot be released to any other person without appropriate authorization from the patient, the patient's legal guardian, or legal process.

Generally, patients have access to the information contained in their medical records. However, if a patient asks to see his or her medical record, the physician's staff should involve the physician because the physician is the best person to explain the information to the patient. Only rarely should a physician use therapeutic privilege to prevent releasing information to the patient. That privilege is imposed only to protect patients who would be harmed by reviewing their records.

There is both a legal and an ethical basis for the confidentiality of medical information. The legal basis for confidentiality is derived from the physician–patient privilege, which is set forth by state statutes and court decisions. The ethical principle of confidentiality originates from the belief that confidentiality encourages patients to seek needed medical care and to be candid with their physicians about their medical condition. Confidentiality also is necessary to protect the patient's inherent privacy interests.[18]

Ideally, medical records would be kept forever. Because that is not possible, the following issues should be considered when establishing a medical record retention policy:

- Seek counsel regarding state legal requirements, including the statute of limitations and any applicable federal laws relating to record retention.

- Consider the age of the patients, keeping in mind that claims relating to minors might emerge many years after treatment. Identify the patient care, research, and teaching needs of any organizations that might require access to the medical records.

- Weigh the cost of archiving and microfilming records against the potential risk of their destruction.

- Destroy records, if applicable, on a regular schedule governed by written policies and procedures.

- Institute a policy for permanently listing all records that have been destroyed.

Absent other legal authorization or requirements, physicians and their employees should not release privileged information about a patient's treatment or diagnosis without first obtaining a written authorization from the patient or, if a minor, from the parent or legal guardian. Release of information should be carried out in accordance with all applicable state and federal laws and with accrediting and regulatory agency requirements and written practice policy.

A waiver of the confidentiality privilege may be made only by the patient or patient's legal representative. Exceptions to the waiver requirements exist, however, in the context of active litigation where most medical records must be provided in response to a valid subpoena or request for production of medical records in accordance with state law.

Following the September 11, 2001, terrorists' attacks that involved commercial airliner crashes in New York City, Pennsylvania, and Washington, D.C., resulting in the loss of thousands of lives, the United States Congress enacted the Patriot Act in 2001 and the Homeland Security Act in 2002. In a separate action, the Health Insurance Portability and Accountability Act (HIPAA) privacy rule was enacted in 2003. These acts created confusion among healthcare providers and health information management professionals. Therefore, the American Health Information Management Association reviewed these acts and drew the following conclusions.

- The United States government is permitted to access any and all protected health information (PHI) it deems necessary to protect the nation.

- PHI should be released to the requesting authority without delay after proper verification.

- Complete identification of the government official must be obtained and verified, including a copy of identification, office location, and the branch of government requesting the information.

- Although HIPAA was modified significantly by recovery legislation signed into law in February 2009, sometimes called the HITECH Act, HIPAA regulations continue to permit these disclosures. (Please see the Chapter 16 in Volume 3 for more information on HIPAA and HITECH.)

- These disclosures must be recorded in the accounting of disclosures.

- A patient or legal guardian's authorization is not required when a request is responded to under either the Homeland Security or Patriot Acts.[19]

Policies and Procedures

A policy is a predetermined course of action established as a guide toward accepted business strategies and objectives. A procedure is a method by which a policy can be accomplished. It provides the instructions necessary to carry out a policy statement. Policies and procedures provide guidelines, limits or boundaries, alternatives, common understanding, definitions, roles and responsibilities, and internal controls. References for the policy development should be included in the policy.[20]

Policies and procedures are essential to any successful practice, whether it is primary care, an ambulatory surgery center, or other outpatient facility. Policies and procedures must be based on established, authoritative guidelines from nationally recognized entities, such as the Occupational Safety and Health Administration (OSHA), the Centers for Disease Control and Prevention (CDC), or other professional organizations. Sources for policies and procedures include national organizations, regulatory agencies, licensing agencies, experts, texts and journals, and standards in other healthcare entities. Some commercial companies sell policies and procedures to assist organizations that lack the resources to develop them independently. However, any organization that implements a preestablished set of procedures must be sure that the procedures reflect its practice, and they should be individualized as appropriate.

Office practices should have a complete set of operational and clinical policies and procedures in place. All healthcare professionals should be knowledgeable about office protocols and committed to following them. Such protocols set the standard of care for a clinical practice and can be used as a guideline to identify negligence.

General guidelines for policies and procedures include several elements.

- There is a need for consistency in policies within the clinical practice. A consistent format should be used throughout the organization. Policies should not conflict with each other or with national, state, or local standards of care. The policy should identify all affected areas. The format should include a section on authority. The policy should follow a preestablished approval process before it is finalized and implemented.

- Each policy should be dated at its inception. The policy manual itself should have a cover page that displays an annual review and approval date, and a table of contents for easy reference. The manual should be treated as an evolving document that is reviewed, added to, and modified whenever necessary. Policies and procedures should be archived when they are revised. This is important in a medical professional liability suit because the physician practice should be held to the standard of care contained in the policy in effect at the time of the incident, not currently.

- In lieu of a hard copy manual, many practices use an intranet to maintain the policy and procedure manual. Doing so ensures that the latest version is always readily available, and no one need worry about whether the most current document is available.

- Policies must reflect reality or actual practice and should meet the most stringent national, state, or local standard of care.

- Policies and procedures must be analyzed on a regular basis for correctness and compliance.

- Education for all staff must be completed and documented before the policy is implemented.

Patient Rights

Since ancient times, physicians have recognized that they have a responsibility to ensure that the individual rights of patients are honored and that patient rights are restricted only as a last resort to protect the safety of the patient or others. Physicians realize that the health and well-being of patients are a joint effort between the physician and patient.

The American Hospital Association developed a Patients' Bill of Rights, which includes the following:

- The right to considerate and respectful care.

- The right to obtain complete information concerning the diagnosis, treatment, and prognosis in terms that the patient can understand. When it is not medically advisable to give such information to the patient, the information should be made available to an appropriate person on the patient's behalf.

- The right to know by name the physician or other clinician responsible for coordinating the patient's care.

- The right to receive from the physician information necessary to give informed consent before the start of any procedure or treatment except in an emergency. The patient has the right to know the names of the persons responsible for the procedures or treatment.

- The right to refuse treatment to the extent permitted by law and to be informed of the medical consequences of such action.

- The right to every consideration of privacy concerning the patient's own medical care program.[21]

Informed Consent

Informed consent is a legal doctrine that encompasses a communication process, not simply executing a form or document.[22] A patient has the right to receive information about healthcare treatment from physicians and to discuss the benefits, risks, and costs of applicable treatment alternatives. Informed consent frequently is regarded legally as a memorialization of an understanding between the patient and the physician. The law of informed consent varies from state to state, and physicians should become familiar with the law in their state. For a thorough discussion of informed consent, refer to Chapter 4 in this volume.

Patient Complaints

Good technical skills and medical expertise are essential elements of the services an organization provides to the public. Today's healthcare consumers demand more. They want convenience, comfort, courtesy, and respect in addition to competent care. If one or more of these qualities is missing, the customer might complain. A satisfied patient tells four other people about care and service rendered. A dissatisfied patient tells twenty other people about the bad experience. The organization must satisfy five patients for every one patient it disappoints to maintain its positive reputation.[23] Every patient is essential to the well-being of an organization. When complaints are voiced, the organization has a second chance to correct and improve conditions for all customers of the practice.

There are many pitfalls to avoid when handling complaining customers. These include becoming defensive, citing organization policy, listening inattentively, giving the runaround, exhibiting negative nonverbal behaviors, overreacting, and siding against the organization. These actions are nonproductive. They emphasize the notion that the organization is unresponsive, uncaring, and not a place of choice for receiving healthcare services. Patients want to be taken seriously, treated with respect, and listened to attentively. They may seek immediate action, compensation, and someone to be reprimanded. Patients desire to have the problem resolved so that it never happens again.

There are ten fairly simple and easily practiced steps for handling complaints.

1. Listen without interruption.
2. Don't get defensive.
3. Use a "sad but glad" statement. For example, "I'm sad that you are upset, but I'm glad that you have come to me so I can address your concerns."
4. Express empathy.
5. Ask questions to clarify the problem.
6. Find out what the customer wants.
7. Explain what can and cannot be done.
8. Discuss the alternatives fully.
9. Take action.
10. Follow up to ensure customer satisfaction.[24]

Complaints must be documented and tracked so that the organization can identify repeated complaints, patterns that need attention, and preventive actions. A separate complaint form or the facility incident report form may be used.

Professional Staff

Credentialing is the process of assessing and validating the qualifications and competence of a licensed practitioner to offer services in a healthcare setting. Evidence of licensure, education, training, and experience is necessary to determine whether a healthcare professional is competent. This information should be kept in a separate bound file for each professional staff member. Credentialing information is considered confidential. This information should not be disclosed to an outside party without a court order, statutory requirement, or an authorization from the individual.[25]

Office staffs today consist of a variety of professionals, including physicians, physician's assistants, nurse midwives, nurse practitioners, registered nurses, licensed practical nurses, mental health counselors, surgical technicians, radiology technologists, medical laboratory technologists, and phlebotomists. Each of these professions has its own responsibilities and codes of ethics. Some require recertification or license renewal on a regular basis.

Thorough credentialing also requires well-defined job descriptions. Job descriptions should reflect the scope of practice defined by state professional practice acts, state licensing boards, and professional organizations. In some cases, employees may not be covered under the physician's medical professional liability insurance policy. It is important that everyone working under the physician's direction be insured appropriately. For more information on credentialing, refer to Chapter 14 in Volume 1 in this series on physician and allied health professional credentialing.

The United States Congress recognized that the healthcare system depends on the willingness of professionals to participate in reviewing quality of care issues, so it adopted the Healthcare Quality Improvement Act (HCQIA) in 1986.[26] Under the act, immunity for participation in professional review actions by professional review committees is granted from federal and state law claims, except for civil rights violations, if the review actions meet the standards of the act. The act provides that a review activity meets the standards of the act for immunity purposes if it is performed in the reasonable belief that the action is in the furtherance of quality healthcare, a reasonable effort to obtain the facts is made, and notice and a hearing are afforded in the event that an action is warranted by the facts. Though protection afforded by the HCQIA is not absolute, protection can be maximized by performing peer review activities that follow a formal, objective plan.

The act established a national data bank for the collection of data on adverse actions against physicians and other healthcare providers.[27] To protect their immunity for peer review, entities that make malpractice payments or that take adverse professional actions as a result of formal peer review must report adverse professional review actions to the National Practitioner Data Bank (NPDB). Refer to Chapter 1, Volume 3 for more information on the NPDB.

Hospitals and other entities that provide healthcare services and follow a formal peer review process to further quality healthcare are allowed to query the data bank. Hospitals must request certain information from the data bank before granting practice privileges to a new applicant. During the recredentialing process, which normally occurs every two years, a hospital must request information regarding physicians who are already on staff. Individual physicians, dentists, and other healthcare practitioners may query the data bank concerning themselves.

· · · · · · · · ·
CLINICAL AND SAFETY ISSUES

The clinical and safety issues inherent in the delivery of patient care range from safe medication administration and providing a safe physical environment, to ensuring that equipment is in good repair, to being prepared for a wide array of emergencies, both internal and external.

Medication Administration

Medication errors occur in every healthcare setting, including the physician's office and community pharmacies. Though the observed rate ranged from 0 percent to 13 percent, the error rate for prescription medications dispensed by community pharmacists was approximately 1.7 percent, which is equivalent to approximately 50 million community dispensing errors annually.[28] The cost of preventable adverse drug events in the ambulatory Medicare population was estimated to be $1,983 per case in 2000, costing approximately $887 million.[29]

The chance for error is ever present in the prescribing, dispensing, and administering of medications. Common medication-related errors seen in physician office practices include incorrect prescribed dosage, incorrect medication for diagnosis or condition, multiple pharmacy prescriptions, medication incompatibility, inappropriate dispensing of sample medications, and illegible handwriting on prescriptions.

Proactive risk management practices can help prevent medication-related errors and theft of medications or controlled substances. In medication prescriptions and orders, use computer order entry or print in block lettering. The indication for the medication should be put on the order or prescription. The order should be complete, including strength and concentration of the product, and should include route and rate of administration. Abbreviations should be used sparingly if at all. Verbal orders should be used in emergencies only. Prescription pads should be locked or stored away from patient care and reception areas, and they should never be presigned or postdated. Any lost or stolen prescription pads should be reported to local pharmacies, hospitals, and the Drug Enforcement Administration. An internal process to monitor, track, and correct medication errors should be established and reviewed on a regular basis.

There are also proactive risk management strategies for medication storage. The staff should be trained on the applicable state and federal regulatory standards for ordering, storing, and dispensing controlled substances and other medications. Only necessary pharmaceuticals should be stored in the office, and these should be stored away from patient or visitor access. Controlled substances should be double-locked, regularly counted, and have limited access. All administered and discarded doses should be accounted for in writing. Expiration dates should be monitored, and outdated supplies should be properly removed and disposed of. Medication samples should be logged in and out, and manufacturer lot numbers should be tracked. The lot number of any samples given to patients should be recorded in the medical record. Medication containers with potentially lethal doses should be removed from patient care areas, and special controls for potentially dangerous drugs should be instituted.

Employees should be qualified by education or training to administer medications. A medication proficiency exam should be part of the employee skills list. Drug reference materials should be accessible. Patient allergies should be checked before administering any medication. Employees should triple-check the medication against the order, after dispensing, and before administration. The patient's identity should be checked before administering any medication. Staff should be educated to question any medication orders that are incomplete, ambiguous, or illegible. If there are questions about a medication or dose, the prescribing physician or a pharmacist should be consulted. The administered medication, route, and amount of medication should be recorded immediately in the medical record. Patients may remain in the office for a specified time after receiving certain medications such as moderate sedation, other drugs that may impair their abilities, or where the results might need monitoring for allergic reactions or efficacy. It must be noted that moderate sedation should be administered only in settings equipped with appropriate monitoring capability, for example, pulse oximetry; appropriate reversal agent(s) should be on hand; appropriate staff should be currently certified in resuscitation skills; and there should be a procedure supporting the operation's management of a medical emergency.

A comprehensive medication education program for patients should be developed. This information should be documented in the medical record. The principles of informed consent should be considered whenever medications are ordered or changed in the ambulatory care setting. At a minimum, the patient should be educated regarding the purpose of the medication, side effects, adverse effects, and key drug interactions, and this should be documented. Informed consent should be documented formally for medications that carry risk of severe complications or complications that occur frequently.[30]

Adverse Patient Events

Accreditation manuals published by The Joint Commission contain standards that relate specifically to the management of sentinel events. Accredited ambulatory care organizations are responsible for reporting sentinel events to The Joint Commission.

According to The Joint Commission, a sentinel event is defined as "an unexpected occurrence involving death or serious physical or psychological injury, or the risk thereof. Serious injury specifically includes loss of limb or function. The phrase 'or risk thereof' includes any process variation for which a recurrence would carry a significant chance of a serious adverse outcome. Such events are called 'sentinel' because they signal the need for immediate investigation and response."[31] Sentinel events in the ambulatory care setting can include outcomes related to missed diagnosis, delayed treatment, failure to monitor care, and medication errors, among others.

Although it is sometimes difficult for the physician to determine if a patient's signs or symptoms are consistent with an adverse medication reaction, the physician should have a high degree of suspicion and should report any suspected adverse medication reaction via the appropriate mechanism to the pharmacy or drug company. The physician should investigate the patient's drug regimen and history to determine if the signs or symptoms are related to the medication. The reaction should be noted in the patient's medical record, and the patient should be educated about any drug allergies or precautions that are needed.

Disclosure

An important part of the diagnostic or treatment process is to provide the patient or authorized representative with outcome or results information. Sometimes diagnostic tests or treatment results are unplanned or unwelcome outcomes even if the treatment was appropriate. The critical issue is to disclose the results to the patient.

The issues surrounding disclosure of unanticipated outcomes have culminated in new accreditation requirements for hospitals. In 2001, The Joint Commission patient safety standards became effective for hospitals. In addition, the standards for ambulatory care emphasize the importance of disclosure under the proper circumstances.[32] The Joint Commission disclosure standard does not require healthcare professionals to make an admission of liability or error. The disclosure standard is directed at a communication process and is an important patient safety and satisfaction tool.

Safe Environment

An ambulatory care facility should attempt to ensure that the building and parking lot for patients and all staff are adequately lighted and free of potential hazards. Although many physicians do not own or control the building and land used for their office practices, they nonetheless should attempt to reduce the potential for serious physical injury to patients and visitors from accidents such as slips and falls. Often, a physician is named as a codefendant in lawsuits involving these types of general liability accidents even though the facilities are under the direct control and management of another entity, such as the property owner or building management company.

The risk exposures of the physician office facility should be addressed in the office policy manual. The manual should detail safety standards and outline specific inspection parameters and intervals. The policies should address general office safety, hazardous waste and materials, preventive maintenance for clinical and diagnostic equipment, security, personal safety issues, and injury prevention and reporting.

Medical Devices

Under the Safe Medical Devices Act (SMDA) of 1990, healthcare facilities must report serious device-related injuries to the manufacturer, or to the Food and Drug Administration (FDA) if the manufacturer is not known. A MedWatch medical device report by the FDA must be submitted. In addition, the SMDA requires that facilities submit to the FDA an annual summary of all device-related injury reports submitted during the preceding time period. This law currently applies to hospitals, ambulatory surgical facilities, nursing homes, and other facilities where healthcare is provided. The SMDA reporting requirements do not apply to the physician, dentist, chiropractor, optometrist, nurse practitioner, school nurse offices, and the freestanding care unit office. However, it is a prudent risk management strategy to establish and implement a safe medical device policy for the office to ensure patient safety and to reduce any potential liability that might arise from malfunctioning medical devices or equipment.[33]

MedWatch is the FDA's safety information and adverse event reporting program. This program is involved with several products, including

- prescription medications;
- nonprescription (over-the-counter) medications;
- biologics;
- medical devices;
- radiation-emitting devices; and
- special nutritional products.[34]

One of the purposes of the program is to provide a consistent standardized process for monitoring product safety alerts, recalls, and important labeling changes. Reporting can be done online, by telephone, or by submitting the MedWatch 3500 form by mail or fax.[35]

Physicians should carefully monitor the selection, inspection, and maintenance of medical office equipment and devices, because both physicians and manufacturers are often named in liability actions that arise out of patient injuries involving such medical products and devices. To mitigate these types of allegations, a practice should establish, document, and monitor, a procedure for purchasing, inspecting, and maintaining medical equipment and products. Sound medical equipment management involves, at a minimum, the following elements:

- Choosing the appropriate equipment to satisfy clinical needs, while recognizing products' potential hazards and limitations.
- Creating a quality control program for all diagnostic equipment.
- Designing and adhering to preventive maintenance, electrical safety and calibration schedules and policies, as recommended by the manufacturer.
- Establishing emergency procedures in the event of equipment failure.
- Formalizing a reporting process for medical equipment management problems, failures, and user errors.
- Implementing an inspection procedure for receipt of new or repaired equipment.
- Initiating a tracking system and log for product recalls and alerts.
- Maintaining an inventory of all medical devices, regardless of ownership, including manufacturer, model, and serial number.
- Retaining copies of device-specific operator and user manuals and making them readily available to staff.
- Performing regular safety inspections.
- Recognizing product hazards and limitations.
- Training staff on the safe use of devices.
- Using the equipment in a reasonable manner as intended by the manufacturer.[36]

When external vendors are responsible for performing preventive maintenance inspections or repairs, make sure that contracts specify the interval at which the inspections are to be performed and check to make sure that a current certificate of insurance is on file for the company responsible for inspection and maintenance. A policy that directs employees to sequester immediately any equipment involved in a patient injury should be in place. The company responsible for performing inspection and maintenance should not be allowed to examine the equipment until after an independent evaluation has been obtained.

Emergency Response

Healthcare providers need to know their responsibilities in medical and nonmedical emergencies. The scope of medical emergency response activities can range from the provision of basic cardiac life support to more complex medical interventions, depending on the patient populations being served. Regardless of the scope of medical emergency activities undertaken, each ambulatory care practice should establish a formal policy and procedure for the staff to follow in the event of a medical emergency.

Policies and procedures should address the following:

- Certification requirements for basic cardiac life support and annual requirements that certification be updated.
- Inspection and repair record maintenance for all emergency equipment in the office.
- Inspection requirements for an emergency crash cart if one is needed in the office. (It is important to note that a crash cart may be more of a liability than an asset to patient safety if it houses outdated equipment and/or medications, or if it is managed by untrained staff. Most physician's office emergency procedures entail dialing 9–1–1.)
- Training and proficiency requirements for emergency equipment and medications maintained within the office.
- Documentation of such training and proficiency in personnel files.

If an automatic incoming telephone call distribution system is used, it should either allow a patient to speak directly to office personnel in the event of a medical emergency or tell the caller to hang up and dial 9–1–1.

Fire Safety

Fire safety management involves protecting patients, employees, visitors, and buildings from the threat of fire and smoke. Every building is required to be in compliance with the structure and fire protection rules set forth in the National Fire Protection Association's Life Safety Code. Contact the local fire marshal or other knowledgeable authority for information regarding fire safety standards. The practice should establish and maintain an office fire safety program, including emergency evacuation procedures for staff and patients. These should be posted in a conspicuous place in the office. Emergency telephone numbers should be easily accessible to the staff. A fire safety orientation and related annual education program should be held for all employees. Fire drills should be conducted quarterly and results should be evaluated and documented. The building's fire alarm systems should be tested quarterly by a reputable testing service.[37]

Security

The goal of a healthcare organization's security program is to provide a safe environment for employees, physicians, patients, and visitors. A security risk assessment must be conducted as the basis for the development of a security risk exposure plan. Physicians and office staff in clinics and other ambulatory settings are exposed to potentially dangerous confrontation with patients, family members, and intruders. Prevention of violence in the workplace can be aided by the following de-escalation tips:

- Do not argue with or provoke a hostile person. Avoid staring, which could be interpreted as confrontational.
- Be honest about situations; provide honest reasons for delays.
- Keep at least two or three arm lengths away from the hostile person.
- Use a firm tone of voice but not a hostile or angry one.
- Listen and acknowledge concern.
- Separate the hostile person from other patients, if possible.
- Develop an emergency code to alert other office staff that a violent person is on the premises.
- Summon help immediately if a patient or visitor:
  - Uses profanity
  - Makes sexual comments
  - Demands unnecessary services
  - Hints at loss of control
  - Appears tense and angry
  - Appears intoxicated or under the influence of drugs
  - Has a history of violence
- Report serious threats of violence to law enforcement officials.[38]

Infection Control

All healthcare facilities run the risk of healthcare-associated infections (HAIs), which are infections acquired in the facility, and of infections brought into the facility or setting. These infections may be *endemic*, defined as the habitual presence of an infection within a geographical area, which may also refer to the usual prevalence of a given disease within such an area. Infections may be *epidemic*, defined as an outbreak in a community or region of a group of infections of similar nature, clearly in excess of normal expectancy and derived from a common source. Infections may affect patients, healthcare workers, and others who come into contact with patients. The goal of surveillance, prevention, and control of infection is to identify and reduce the risks of acquiring and transmitting both endemic and epidemic infections among patients, employees, physicians, and visitors. Infection control is an organization-wide function.

Basic infection control practices should be implemented in all ambulatory care practices. Each physician's office and practice setting should establish an infection control plan that is written clearly, updated annually and created with staff input. Good personal hygiene and common sense are instrumental to developing an effective infection control program. Most infections are spread by direct contact with unwashed hands. The following are some basic infection control practices that are desirable for all ambulatory care offices:

- Wash hands routinely. Hands should be washed immediately when hands are obviously soiled, after handling soiled equipment, after removing protective gloves, before eating, after using restroom facilities, and before leaving the healthcare facility.

- Employers shall provide hand-washing facilities that are readily accessible to employees.

- Healthcare providers should not eat, drink, smoke, handle contact lenses, or apply cosmetics in work areas.

- Food and drink should not be kept in refrigerators or freezers, or on shelves, cabinets, countertops, or bench tops where blood or other potentially infectious materials are present.

- Mouth pipetting or suctioning of blood or other potentially infectious materials is prohibited.

- Use suitable personal protective devices such as gloves, face shields, masks, goggles, aprons, or impervious clothing when there is a likelihood of contact with potentially infectious materials. These protective devices should be readily accessible in all patient areas.

- Provide mouthpieces, resuscitation bags, or other ventilation devices in areas where the need for resuscitation is predictable.

- Change gloves after contact with each patient.

- Wear gloves when touching contaminated objects, but do not touch items (doorknobs, telephones, test equipment, computer terminals, keyboards) with soiled gloved hands.

- Take precautions to prevent injuries while handling sharp instruments, disposing of used needles, or cleaning used instruments.

- Select safer, better-engineered needles and sharps.

- Sharps should be disposed of in containers that are closable, leakproof, puncture resistant, and properly labeled or color-coded.

- Do not rub eyes or other mucous membranes.

- Treat all body substances from all patients as potentially infectious, and place an adequate barrier between people and the body substance.

- Treat any device that is visibly soiled with patient material, even if dried, as contaminated. Even if a device appears to be clean, do not handle it in an unhygienic manner. Use gloves, a gown, and other personal protective equipment, if indicated.

- Place specimens of blood and other potentially infectious material in a container, seal tightly, and carry in an outer container.

- Disinfect surfaces contaminated with blood or other potentially infectious material with an Environmental Protection Agency–approved (EPA-approved) tuberculocidal disinfectant.

- If a healthcare provider has lesions or weeping dermatitis, the provider should refrain from direct patient care and handling patient care equipment until the condition resolves.

- Personnel having direct patient contact should not use nail polish or artificial nails. Chipped nail polish and artificial nails have been the source of outbreaks of healthcare-associated infections in healthcare facilities.

- The employer should establish and maintain an accurate medical record for each employee that is separate from the personnel file. The employer should also maintain the records as established by state requirements.

The primary regulatory agency in the field of occupational safety and health is the Occupational Safety and Health Administration (OSHA), a federal agency in the U.S. Department of Labor. OSHA regulations are applicable to medical offices, physicians' offices, and other ambulatory care settings. OSHA has conducted numerous inspections of physicians' offices, many in response to complaints. Many infection-control issues are of particular interest to OSHA. To protect workers from occupational exposures to blood and other potentially infectious materials, OSHA enacted the bloodborne pathogen standard in 1992.

Bloodborne pathogens include any microorganism that might be transmitted by contact with the blood or bodily fluids of an infected person. The pathogens of major concern are human immunodeficiency virus (HIV), hepatitis B virus, and hepatitis C virus. The U.S. Congress passed the Needlestick Safety and Prevention Act directing OSHA to revise the bloodborne pathogens standard to establish in greater detail requirements that employers identify and make use of effective and safer medical devices. The act also mandated additional requirements of maintaining a sharps injury log and involving nonmanagerial healthcare workers in evaluating and choosing devices. This standard applies to all employers who have employees with reasonably anticipated occupational exposure to blood or other potentially infectious materials. Staff should be educated about precautions to prevent injuries while handling sharp instruments, disposing of used needles, or cleaning used instruments. An employee exposed to blood or other potentially infectious material is required to report the incident to a designated person within the facility. Evaluations should be available immediately by an accredited laboratory.[39]

Enforcement guidelines that OSHA promulgated for tuberculosis are based on the CDC's "Guidelines for Preventing the Transmission of Mycobacterium Tuberculosis in Healthcare Settings." The agency's latest instructions are that these guidelines would be applied in physicians' offices for personnel present during the performance of high-hazard procedures on suspect or infectious tuberculosis (TB) patients. High-hazard procedures identified in CDC guidelines include sputum induction and administration of aerosolized pentamidine. These procedures should be performed on infectious TB patients only if absolutely necessary.[40]

. . . .
HUMAN RESOURCES ISSUES

The management of human resources entails addressing many complex issues. In large organizations, the duties and responsibilities related to human resources are often assigned to a separate department that takes ownership of that function. In smaller organizations, risk management professionals may have some direct responsibility for human resources.

Employee Handbook

The employee handbook should serve as the official guide for staff in the setting. It should contain work rules and policies pertaining to the personnel employed. At the beginning of the handbook, a bold disclaimer should inform the employee that the handbook is not intended to create an employment contract.[41] The purpose of this statement is to dispel any perception on the part of staff that the organization's obligations to them exceed obligations created by state and federal law. In employment at will states, this statement supports the employer's right to terminate employment for good reason, as long as the organization does not violate antidiscrimination-related and other laws and as long as it complies with its own applicable procedures. It is wise for the organization's risk management professional to review the employee manual and its supporting procedures, with input of counsel as appropriate, because these documents may be critical to defense of a wrongful termination suit. All new employees should receive a copy or at least review the manual and sign a written statement attesting to the fact that they have received a copy or reviewed the information. Current employees should be required to review any additions or changes at least annually with written documentation of the review. The manual should include general information on the practice, wage and salary information, benefits, sick or absence leave, workers' compensation, and disability. Other information on work rules such as hours, dress, confidentiality, smoking, phone calls, and disciplinary procedures, including probation, suspension, and dismissal, should also be included.

Employee Proficiency

Medical personnel need to be qualified to perform their duties so that quality care is provided in a safe manner. A competency and proficiency monitoring process should be an integral part of the practice's quality improvement program.

The employee proficiency process includes the following:

- Implementation of a formalized orientation program for all employees that includes mentoring of new employees.
- Development of criteria-based, written position descriptions for all staff.
- Development and implementation of required skills checklists that reflect the responsibilities and duties of the position.
- Development of employee-prepared performance goals that have been agreed upon with the supervisor.
- Performance of periodic evaluation of employees' competence. This process should include input from the employee and the employee's supervisors and should be based on direct observation of the employee's work. Rewards or promotions should be awarded for high proficiency levels. Evaluation documents should be dated and signed by the employee and reviewer and retained in the employee's file.
- Development and implementation of ongoing education programs for healthcare providers can promote competency, productivity, and efficiency; communicate recommended and consistent behaviors to support quality care; help staff identify actual problems or potential problems; generate ideas and problem-solving methods; and increase staff morale.

Confidentiality   The office practice should adopt a zero-tolerance policy for any staff member who knowingly violates patient confidentiality. This problem is so serious that many practices have made a breach of confidentiality grounds for immediate termination. Exacerbating existing concerns in this area, HITECH, an aspect of the 2009 recovery legislation that modified HIPAA, makes employees personally responsible for fines ranging from $100 to as much as $1.5 million dollars a year for violating HIPAA requirements concerning protection of PHI. A confidentiality statement should be signed upon employment and annually thereafter, and all staff should document that they have received training on HIPAA-related procedures.

Confidentiality extends to more than just inappropriate access and distribution of patient chart data. Breaches of confidentiality can occur over the phone, at the reception area, and interdepartmentally. To avoid serious lapses in confidentiality,

- give patient information only to the patient directly, and do not assume that family members are aware of the patient's condition;
- never leave detailed answering machine messages;
- phone triage should be done in a private area, not in the middle of the office or at a nurses' station; and
- receptionists or other employees who happen to become privy to a patient's health condition should never inquire about the status of it when speaking with the patient.[42]

· · · · · · · · ·
PERFORMANCE IMPROVEMENT

Performance improvement has had many names throughout the years: quality assurance, quality improvement, quality management, and so forth. Regardless of the name, the goal remains the same: improve patient care and outcomes. The concept of quality improvement, which originated in industrial settings, has much applicability to the healthcare arena.

Outcome Measures

The provision of quality services to patients delivered in the outpatient setting can be measured. One important concept in measuring quality is to realize that patients come to healthcare providers with their own expectations for services. Typically, patients do not evaluate the physician and the office staff on their competence in technology and sophisticated medical procedures. Patients evaluate healthcare practices and expertise based on how they are treated and on what they have come to expect in terms of service.[43] The patients' quality measures are often very different from the outcome measurements that the healthcare providers traditionally have used to measure performance improvement.

Outcome is one type of performance improvement measure commonly used by healthcare organizations. Outcomes may be clinical or they may be service focused. Indicators are the specific measures or indices that are collected to quantify the selected quality outcomes. For a performance improvement program to be effective and comprehensive, the indicators must be measurable, clinical, and customer focused.

Healthcare is a service industry similar to many other service segments of the marketplace. In fact, many healthcare organizations use other industries as benchmarks for driving the changes and improvements in their systems. The hotel and hospitality industry may be used as a model to compare the healthcare patient registration process. Environmental engineering companies can be used to compare the decor, lighting, and traffic flows for patient care areas. Every aspect of the healthcare setting should be evaluated for its customer friendliness and its ability to effectively meet customers' needs.

The clinical care delivered by hands-on caregivers should be monitored for quality. The staff that is providing the care accomplishes this monitoring best. The clinical care portion of the quality equation is monitored and evaluated by reviewing the clinical documentation in the medical record, as well as by trending issues identified through sentinel events, clinical area incident reports, and clinical area specific performance improvement indicators.

Specific indicators should be established for the monitoring of care. Many of the national professional organizations have promulgated guidelines, and external regulatory and licensing bodies also may be queried for information. High-risk, high-volume, and problem-prone areas are good places to start the selection process for clinical quality indicators. The areas for monitoring will differ by the kind of clinical practice delivered in that setting. The monitoring and evaluation process must be carefully documented and must evidence follow up on identified issues.

Although diagnosis-specific indicators are helpful, it is also important to evaluate indicators that are common to all diagnoses. Some examples of potentially meaningful generic indicators include the following:

- Adequacy of documentation of medication refills ordered via telephone
- Adequacy of documentation of after-hours telephone calls
- Entries in the clinical record dated and timed by each practitioner who makes an entry
- Legible documentation from all staff and practitioners
- All documents in the record permanently secured in the record binder
- Adequacy of documentation of consultations and referrals, notations regarding review of the consultant's findings, and subsequent modifications, if indicated, in the plan of care
- All diagnostic test results entered in the record and initialed by the ordering physician
- Information of abnormal test results or required changes in plan of care provided to the patient, and the plan of care modified appropriately

A complete, legible, and accessible clinical record is the best tool to demonstrate the adequacy, timeliness, and quality of service that is provided by the organization. To anyone outside the organization who might ever have reason to review the record, if it is not documented, it was not done. Such perceptions hold true regardless of what was actually done or what protocols, policies, and procedures indicate should have been done.

The old quality assurance paradigm identified the "bad apple" and focused intervention with that individual. The new performance improvement model looks at the system rather than the individual. Quality and process improvement focuses on process issues because most inefficiencies and error in organizational settings are the result of process errors. Professional liability claims are often the result of system failures in medical offices. These failures can be identified and corrected more readily in an organization that works to empower its staff.[44]

Participating in data analysis with external sources is one way of benchmarking the organization's progress toward quality improvement and also facilitates meeting certain standards, such as those promulgated by The Joint Commission. Such analysis can identify areas or issues that should be addressed from either a risk management or performance perspective. Many companies provide outcomes-based benchmarking data.

Patient Satisfaction Surveys

Customer satisfaction is a primary goal of any service organization. The practice must survey patients to identify expectations, indicators, variables, or factors that patients feel are important and that they will be using to judge and measure the practice's services. A practice cannot measure whether it is meeting its patients' needs if it is not cognizant of those needs. Patients should be asked about their satisfaction with the services provided at each episode of care. Because patients are more likely to give an honest opinion if that opinion is shared in confidence, it is probably most productive to seek a satisfaction-evaluation process that collects information without asking that patients disclose their identity.

There should be a formal, systematic process for the collection and analysis of such patient satisfaction data and the data should be evaluated through organization-wide performance improvement activities, which result in any appropriate changes. Additional monitoring of perception of interventions should ensure that changes have improved patients' satisfaction with the services being provided. Some measures of patient satisfaction that might be used in this way include waiting time, friendliness and helpfulness of the staff, cleanliness and efficiency of the facility, confidentiality of their medical information, and reasonableness of costs and fees.

Incident Reporting

Reporting of unusual occurrences or incidents is essential to the organization's risk identification program and is important to improving patient care. An incident is any happening that is not consistent with the routine care of a particular patient or a described operation of the facility. Incidents are early warning signs of potentially problematic areas of patient care. The organization should establish a written policy and procedure that sets criteria for the identification of an occurrence and specifies how an incident or occurrence report should be completed and by whom. All incidents or occurrences that fit the established criteria should be documented on a specified form and investigated or followed up by designated individuals. A statement in the policy and on the form should designate the process and form as confidential.

It is difficult to develop an all-inclusive list of occurrences to be reported, but certain events should qualify automatically. Some issues that should always be the subject of incident reporting include the following:

- Patients who fall or sustain an injury on-site
- Patients who experience cardiopulmonary arrest at the office
- All patients who require emergency measures at the office
- Patients who must be transferred by ambulance from the office to an acute-care setting
- Medication errors
- Medication adverse or allergic reactions
- Patients who are injured due to an equipment failure or user error while at the facility
- Patients stating they are pursuing legal action because of their displeasure with an outcome of care rendered by the practice
- Patients who leave the office without being seen
- Patients whose adverse outcome was unexpected
- Patients who experience a near-miss even if there is no injury[45]

Incident report forms are most effective when completed by the person who first becomes aware of or witnesses the event. Once completed, the form should be reviewed and signed by a manager. The form should then be routed to the healthcare risk management professional or otherwise be incorporated in the performance improvement process.

Medical record documentation of the event is also very important. The occurrence should be documented in the medical record, along with any medical steps that were taken to minimize adverse effects. Incident reports should never be filed or alluded to in the medical record. If the event is a potentially compensable event, the healthcare risk management professional should be involved as soon as possible. Depending on insurance policy provisions and previously established internal risk management procedures, the person in that role should notify the insurance company as soon as possible. If a claim is made, the insurance company will then be prepared to take appropriate claims management steps to protect the practice.

Incident reports must interface with the quality improvement program to maximize protection of information and ensure that significant safety issues are addressed in a comprehensive and timely manner. Another approach to providing protection is under the attorney–client privilege, which is also referred to as attorney work product protection. For more information on incident reporting see Chapter 6 in Volume 1, Early Warning Systems for the Identification of Organizational Risk.

·········
ACCREDITATION, LICENSURE, AND REGULATORY ISSUES

Healthcare remains one of the most regulated industries. From governmental entities such as the Centers for Medicaid & Medicare services, to state legislatures, to private organizations such as The Joint Commission, a vast array of regulatory organizations affect healthcare. Here are a few that are particularly important to ambulatory care environments.

The Joint Commission

The Joint Commission established the Ambulatory Healthcare Accreditation Program in 1975 to encourage quality patient care in all types of freestanding ambulatory care facilities (www.jointcommission.org/AccreditationPrograms/AmbulatoryCare). The Joint Commission's standards apply to the full range of ambulatory care providers. A growing number of ambulatory care organizations seek The Joint Commission's accreditation because its standards represent a national consensus on quality patient care. The Joint Commission's Office-Based Surgery Accreditation Program focuses on customer service, improving care and improving health, patient care, patient safety, qualified and competent staff, and responsible leadership.[46]

One surveyor typically conducts on-site surveys for two days. If the volume of the organization is more than ten thousand visits annually, two surveyors will be assigned for two days. The survey includes many activities, some of which are an opening conference, observation of the administrative and clinical activity, assessment of the physical facilities and patient care equipment, and a leadership exit conference.[47]

The Joint Commission updates its goals frequently, and the following indicates the breadth of its 2009 National Patient Safety Goals across the continuum of care:

- Ambulatory care and office-based surgery
- Behavioral healthcare
- Critical access hospital
- Disease-specific care
- Home care
- Hospital
- Laboratory
- Long-term care[48]

Accreditation Association for Ambulatory Healthcare

The Accreditation Association for Ambulatory Healthcare (AAAHC) (www.aaahc.org), incorporated in 1979, is a nonprofit corporation that serves as an advocate for the provision and documentation of quality health services in ambulatory healthcare organizations. AAAHC accreditation is a voluntary process that involves several steps. The first step in accreditation is for the organization to conduct a self-assessment using published AAAHC guidelines. The next step is to participate in an on-site survey conducted by trained AAAHC surveyors. Following the survey, the accreditation team makes recommendations that are reviewed by the AAAHC Accreditation Committee. This committee makes the final accreditation decision. Accreditation may be awarded for six months, one year, or three years, depending on the level of compliance with the published standards.[49]

The AAAHC strives to improve the quality of patient care. According to the association, its members benefit in the following ways:

- Find innovative ways to improve patient care and services.
- Increase efficiency and reduce costs.
- Improve risk management programs.
- Decrease insurance premiums.
- Motivate staff by instilling pride and loyalty.
- Strengthen public perception.
- Recruit and retain qualified professional staff.
- Develop alliances with other provider groups.[50]

Institute for Medical Quality

The Institute for Medical Quality (www.imq.org), much like other accreditation agencies, offers several educational, consultation, accreditation, and certification programs. It also offers a program dedicated to ambulatory care.[51]

American Society of Anesthesiologists

Founded in 1905, the American Society of Anesthesiologists (ASA) (www.asahq.org) serves as an advocate for patients who receive anesthesia. ASA offers many opportunities for improving and monitoring the quality of care provided to patients. The Anesthesia Consultation Program enables experienced consultants to evaluate the care delivered on-site and then issue a written report detailing findings and recommendations.[52]

Association of Perioperative Registered Nurses

The Association of Perioperative Registered Nurses (AORN) (www.aorn.org) is a professional association dedicated to nurses who provide nursing care related to operative patient care. It publishes position statements on topics such as correct site surgery, bloodborne diseases, and numerous personnel issues.[53]

Governmental Accreditation

Voluminous local, state, and federal rules and regulations are enforced by innumerable agencies. Perhaps the best recognized are state inspections of nursing homes. Although the details and impact of these legal issues are beyond the scope of this chapter, they are nonetheless important.

Managed Care Accreditation

Healthcare delivery has undergone significant change since the advent of managed care during the latter part of the twentieth century. What used to be a private matter between patient and physician has become a multifaceted collaboration involving patient, physician, other providers, and purchasers of healthcare. Managed care is a discipline with its own standards and guidelines, but it also has its own risks related to healthcare delivery.

Managed care accreditation is a phenomenon that originated during the early 1990s. The two primary accrediting agencies are the Utilization Review Accreditation Commission (URAC) (www.urac.org) and the National Committee for Quality Assurance (NCQA) (www.ncqa.org).

URAC is a charitable foundation that was founded in 1990. It is a standards-based organization that promotes healthcare performance improvement. The commission has many purposes, but the one that pertains most to the field of risk management is accreditation. Organizations that successfully meet all URAC requirements are awarded a full two-year accreditation. Conditional accreditation may be awarded to organizations that have the necessary documentation but lack some policies and procedures.

The NCQA began accrediting managed care organizations in 1991. It has five different accreditation statuses: excellent, commendable, accredited, provisional, and denied. NCQA uses a triangular approach to evaluating the delivery of healthcare. There is an accreditation process, a member satisfaction survey process, and a measurement process that uses the Healthcare Effectiveness Data and Information Set (HEDIS®). Although the NCQA's processes are voluntary, a majority of health maintenance organizations (HMOs) participate. In addition, approximately 90 percent of America's health plans use HEDIS to measure their performance.[54]

In the latter part of 2002, NCQA reported that there had been "substantial quality improvements, on average, for Americans enrolled in accountable commercial health plans." The improvements were believed to be attributed to "effective and accurate systems for tracking care, quality incentives, and partnerships between health plans and physicians."[55]

HEDIS's effectiveness of care measures are ever growing, but some of them are listed below:[56]

- Adolescent immunization status
- Antidepressant medication management
- Appropriate testing in children with pharyngitis
- Appropriate treatment for children with upper respiratory infection
- Beta blocker treatment after a heart attack
- Breast cancer screening
- Cervical cancer screening
- Childhood immunization status
- Chlamydia screening
- Colorectal cancer screening
- Comprehensive diabetes care
- Controlling high blood pressure
- High-risk medication use in the elderly

Effective risk management programs incorporate or collaborate with, performance improvement programs. By addressing risk management issues through performance improvement processes and using performance improvement monitors to ensure that the issue stays resolved, the organization effectively addresses its own exposure. Benchmarking data generated by such activities against standardized, well-recognized national norms is one of the most effective performance improvement/risk management strategies available.

· · · · · · · · ·

RISK MANAGEMENT ISSUES

One often hears how managed care organizations (MCOs) or health insurance companies refused care for a patient. Such entities are not in the business of providing healthcare but rather paying for services rendered, and such coverage determinations are often the result of negotiations by the employer group that purchased the coverage; therefore, the entity negotiating with the managed care plan should evaluate the terms of coverage very carefully. If the physician or provider disagrees with the MCO's decision regarding coverage, the physician should make every effort to ensure that the MCO has sufficient quality clinical information to make an informed decision. If a denial of benefits is still issued by the MCO, the physician or provider should appeal the decision vigorously, if he or she believes that that decision is flawed and the patient's outcome will be jeopardized. It is ultimately the physician's responsibility to do the best he or she can to ensure the patient receives whatever medical care is necessary.

Contract Management

Healthcare organizations and providers are faced with exposures that arise from contracts they enter into with other parties. Three of the most common contracts that can create risk for the medical practitioner are those (1) with pharmaceutical companies or research organizations to conduct clinical trials on new products, (2) with facilities to assume medical director duties, and (3) with MCOs for the provision of patient care.

To ensure that all contracts are reviewed properly, the ambulatory care administrator or practitioner, who may be the healthcare risk management professional, should develop a contract management system, which should be reflected in the organization's policies. The policies should designate who is authorized to execute different types of contracts, define the review process, establish protocols governing outside contract review, and document compliance with contractual obligations. The policy should also address safety and security of the contracts. Specific issues addressed in this regard include storing all original contracts in a secure, fireproof location in the administrative office and establishing a back-up storage area; forwarding only copies of signed contracts to authorized individuals; and creating security procedures to ensure that only authorized individuals have access to original contracts. There should also be a system in place to identify contracts nearing the expiration date and to ensure that all contracts undergo an annual review at least ninety days before termination.

The best way to ensure the practice or practitioner is not assuming unknown or uncovered liability through a contract is to read all contracts thoroughly before signing them. It is a good practice to have all contracts reviewed by an attorney. In most cases, signing a contract indicates agreement with and acceptance of all the terms and conditions of the contract.[57] For a primer on contract management see Chapter 17 in Volume 1 in this series.

Physicians' Offices and Ambulatory Care Facilities

Operating a physician's office presents several risk management issues. Though some of these concepts apply in to other types of ambulatory care settings, they have more relevance to physicians' offices. Therefore, modification of these examples may be needed before they can be applied to other settings.

· · · · · · · · ·
CLINICAL ISSUES

The following clinical issues include some functions that might, at first glance, appear to be primarily clerical. However, because the physician's office is a healthcare environment, even apparently routine functions can have a profound effect on patient outcome and, therefore, risk exposure.

Patient Scheduling

Patient scheduling practices should be guided by written office protocols. By adhering to protocols, the office staff plays an important role in minimizing the risk of operational system failures and promoting continuity of care and patient safety. Such protocols should include educating new patients about office procedures before initial visits and arranging follow-up appointments. The office schedule should include time to treat unscheduled patients or walk-in visits. Clear guidelines should be developed for triage of emergency and urgent visits. A physician should evaluate all patients who arrive at the medical office for emergency conditions.

Missed appointments should be brought to the attention of the treating physician and documented in the medical record. If hard copy appointment books are used, entries should be made in pen and appointment changes crossed out instead of erased. Included in the medical record should be accurate, objective notation of all attempts made to contact the patient, including telephone calls. Appointment books should be kept as long as clinical records are kept. If computerized logs are used, daily printouts should be saved in chronological order.

Patient Tracking and Diagnostic Follow-Up

Diagnostic-related incidents are associated with the highest frequency and severity of claims. Many of these claims result from a detrimental delay in following a condition.[58] Often the physician is unaware that the patient failed to return as requested, so months elapse and the condition worsens.

Written office policies for follow-up of diagnostic procedures should be developed and adhered to consistently. The importance of a log to track returning laboratory and other pertinent test results cannot be overemphasized.

All follow-up activities should be documented in the medical record. Notify the patients of all test results, not just abnormal results. Office policy should state that it is the office's responsibility to relay test results to patients, not the patient's responsibility to request them. Messages regarding test results should not be left on answering machines, as this might breach confidentiality of the patient's medical information.

Many computer programs have excellent recall and follow-up capabilities. If the office is not computerized, a manual system using a 3×3.5-inch card system with monthly dividers will suffice. Place on the card the patient's name, patient file number, telephone numbers, address, the reason the patient needs to return, and the month and year the follow-up is due. Generally, follow-up attempts should include one phone call, and if that is not successful, a postcard or letter should be mailed. These attempts to reach the patient should be documented in the medical record. If the condition that is the subject of the diagnosis is serious, such as cancer, the physician should consider sending a certified letter with return receipt requested. This receipt should then be filed in the medical record with a copy of the letter.[59]

Primary Care Screening

More care is now delivered in the ambulatory care setting, and more attention is paid to preventive care. The physician's recommendations for screening and preventive care should be based on the patient's medical needs, professional guidelines, and medical judgment. When screening and preventive care are part of the patient care plan, office staff should develop and maintain a tickler system that tracks due dates for recommended preventive care, screening test dates, monitoring results, and physician review and discussion of the results with the patient. Physicians should document the informed refusal of patients who choose not to proceed with recommended preventive care for any reason.

Medication Summary Sheet

A medication summary sheet should be developed for all patients to assist in tracking medications. This sheet should include the date, name of medication ordered, dosage, quantity, number of refills, physician's initials, staff member's initials, and adverse reactions. Allergy information should be included prominently at the top of the sheet.

Referrals and Consultations

When the professional opinion of another party is needed, steps should be taken to prevent miscommunication and lack of coordination among providers and staff. The referring physician should document the formal request for consultation, and a copy of the request should become a part of the patient record. The request should indicate who is primarily responsible for patient care and the duties of each party. Discussions between the physicians, acceptance of the referral by the consulting physician, and time frames for consultation should be documented. The referring office should be instructed to make the appointment for the patient. A copy of pertinent records should be forwarded to the consulting physician; the original records must be retained in the referring physician's office. Consulting reports, including the patient's relevant medical history or physician's summary, should be written, signed, and sent to the referring physician in a timely manner. All patient communication, including the patient's role in the referral process and the patient's understanding and acceptance or refusal of the recommendations, should be documented. A procedure should be developed to monitor the receipt of consultation reports. The physician should review and initial the reports before they are added to the medical record. The plan and actual patient follow-up should be documented in the clinical record.

Patient Education

In the ambulatory care setting, written posttreatment and continuing care instructions are necessary because patients' interaction with healthcare professionals and office staff may be brief and infrequent. The following guidelines for education can assist staff and patients in this process:

- Review all materials for accuracy before adopting them.

- Ensure that teaching tools and other materials are written at the fifth-grade level to ensure comprehension by patients. For example, use the words *give* rather than *administer* and *birth control* instead of *contraception*.

- Maintain a master file of all patient education materials and archive all printed materials, videotapes, or other teaching aids that have been revised or withdrawn from use.

- Have patients confirm their understanding of instructions and perform a return demonstration if the activity is task based.

   Ask patients and provider to sign off on the instructions, indicating the patient's understanding.

- Maintain a signed copy of the patient education and instructions in the medical record.[60]

Advance Directives

All states now recognize various types of advance directives, the most prevalent of which are living wills and healthcare powers of attorney. The latter allows a patient to name an agent to make healthcare decisions when the patient lacks the capacity to do so. Advance directives regarding end-of-life decisions and agents who may make healthcare decisions in the absence of a competent patient generally are matters of state statutory law.[61]

There are various state and federal definitions of competence and various statutory definitions of what is meant by *life support*, that is, whether hydration and nutrition are included or excluded. Also, state laws differ as to the form of execution of such advance directives, with some states requiring only attestation by witnesses in the presence of the declarant of a living will or healthcare power of attorney and other states requiring notarization. Each physician should consult applicable state law concerning the matter.

In the transient society in which we live, it is possible for an individual to come to a medical practitioner with advance directive documents that were executed in another state. Although such documents might have been valid in the state in which they were executed, they may not be valid in the state where the physician is practicing medicine. If possible, new advance directives should be executed in accordance with the laws of the state where treatment occurs. It is recommended that the physician or someone on the physician's staff have a working knowledge of the requirements of the advance directive laws in the state where the physician is practicing and, if possible, maintain generally accepted statutorily prescribed forms for use by their patients.

· · · · · · · · ·
AMBULATORY CARE SYSTEMS AND PROCEDURES

Numerous recent studies have shown that most adverse events can be attributed to issues related to systems rather than to individuals. This underscores the importance of developing effective systems and workflow procedures, and training the staff to ensure that the systems are used correctly on a consistent basis.

Information Flow

Office systems should be established to ensure efficient and appropriate processing and follow-up of clinical information. Office follow-up systems should be able to track and perform required follow-up when patients miss or cancel appointments or fail to schedule or keep recommended appointments for diagnostic testing or specialty consultations. The consulting physician should notify the requesting physician of adverse reports that require immediate attention.

Billing and Collection

The objective of a billing and collection program is to assist the practice with meeting its cash flow needs. Written policies and procedures should be developed regarding the practice's billing and collection process. These should be evaluated on an annual basis and revised as necessary. If handled improperly, billing practices can hinder the relationship between the patient and the practice and can create a negative climate that could lead to litigation.

All fees should be disclosed before services are rendered. Threats of litigation often materialize when a patient receives an unexpected bill. It is best to discuss and agree on the fees before providing the service to avoid creating an environment of distrust. A written fee schedule should be available on request.

Respond immediately to patient calls or letters regarding billing errors. All delinquent accounts and serious complaints regarding billing should be directed immediately to the physician and office manager or risk manager before being turned over to a collection agency. This will allow the physician the opportunity to evaluate the care that was rendered and the validity of the complaint. Other factors such as adverse outcome, which might influence pursuit of payment or collection proceedings, can be taken into consideration. Complaint reviews can also serve as an early warning of legal action and provide the practice with an opportunity to appease the patient. All written and oral communication should be documented in the patient's individual billing file, which should be separate from the patient's medical record.

An attorney should review the collection procedures to ensure that they comply with applicable federal and state laws and regulations. It is also important to send warning letters drafted by an attorney before involving collection agencies and to evaluate the performance of collection agencies on a regular basis.

Practice Coverage

All physicians in practice should have primary and secondary practice coverage arrangements for those times when they are not available. Covering physicians should be of the same medical specialty and have the same hospital privileges as the treating physician, if possible. When the treating physician has contractual agreements with managed care plans that entail specific payment methods or referral guidelines or restrictions, arrangements should be made so that the covering physician's actions comply with that managed care plan's requirements. It is important to ascertain that the covering physician has adequate professional liability insurance, and it is appropriate to ask for documentation of this. The treating physician should also provide information to the covering physician regarding the courses of treatment and anticipated problems in the patient population he or she will be working with. The sharing of this information should be documented in the medical record. Hospitalized patients should be informed of the coverage arrangement and, if possible, introduced to the covering physician. The physician on call should then document all interactions with the patient. The treating physician should notify the hospital and answering service of the names and telephone numbers of the covering physician(s).

Hospitalists

If hospitalists are used in a physician practice, the following guidelines should be followed:

- Explain to patients that the practice uses hospitalists. Describe the credentials of and services provided by a hospitalist, and discuss with the patients whether they will see practice physicians or staff during the hospitalization.

- Evaluate the competence and experience of hospitalists used by the practice, if there is a choice of providers.

- Initiate communication with the assigned hospitalist at the time of a patient's admission and at discharge.

- Communicate specific patient safety issues when transferring care to and from a hospitalist.

- Track patient discharge to ensure follow-up communication and continuity of care.[62]

Locum Tenens Providers and Agency Nurses

Physicians and other providers who deliver healthcare on a locum tenens (temporary replacement) basis create a unique set of risk management issues. Many providers who serve in this capacity are well trained and well respected, but these traits cannot be assumed to exist in all such providers.

Credentialing locum tenens providers is of utmost importance. Although the circumstances that necessitate the need for services of a locum tenens provider often are urgent, the process of using only qualified individuals should not be undertaken with less vigilance than that which is usually applied. Likewise, one must make sure that the care rendered by locum tenens personnel will be covered by an adequate amount of medical professional liability insurance, preferably purchased by the company that provides the locum tenens personnel.

Another issue that arises when using a locum tenens provider or agency nurse is orientation and training. In theory, everyone who delivers care within a specific organizational setting should have similar orientation and training. Unfortunately, this is not the case in many situations. Each organization should develop at least an abbreviated orientation and training program for providers who are new to the organization and will be used only for a short period of time.

Telephone Protocols

Proper telephone protocols should be developed and implemented to promote consistent, accurate, and complete quality care addressing a wide variety of conditions. Such protocols will be scrutinized in medical professional liability lawsuits and so must demonstrate that consistent advice is given for similar patient symptoms. They arguably become the standard of care for that medical facility and, as such, must be developed with great care, using the best evidence available and only implemented by registered nurses who document orientation to principles of telephone triage. Protocols should be developed under physician supervision and signed off before implementation. They are often prepared in checklist format and organized by symptom or patient complaint. Protocols should be reviewed regularly and modified as necessary to reflect changing practice standards.

Policies and procedures addressing the use of telephone triage should be developed and implemented to support written protocols. These policies should also establish telephone hours and the call-back procedure. Protocols, policies, and procedures should always have staff err on the side of caution by making an appointment for the patient or by referring emergent conditions promptly to an urgent care center or emergency room. Patients who request an examination by a physician should be given an appointment. An advisory physician should be available for consultation to the nurses using telephone triage.

The substance of all telephone calls related to patient care, including those that apply telephone triage protocols, should be documented contemporaneously throughout the call. Special preprinted telephone logs may be used, and the policy should require that no blank spaces be allowed. Information that should be documented includes, at minimum, the date and time of the call, the patient's name and date of birth, identity of the caller, identity of the staff member taking the call, the subject of the call, the specific protocol used, and the exact advice given.

Protocol data collection, at a minimum, should identify the patient's symptoms and associated complaints, symptom characteristics and course, history of symptoms, onset, location, aggravating factors, and relieving factors. Information that also needs to be identified during the data collection is the caller's pregnancy status or breast-feeding status (if applicable); allergy history; current and recent medication use; previous medical and psychosocial history; and any history of recent injury, infection, or illness.

A quality improvement program is essential to promoting quality telephone triage. Job descriptions for all employees who perform telephone triage should be compliant with all state practice acts, and the way in which physician supervision will be exercised should be addressed. Employees who perform telephone triage should be formally trained under physician supervision, observed, evaluated, and regularly monitored. As previously noted, receptionists and other clerks can handle administrative calls but registered nurses who have been oriented to telephone triage are the only staff who should address telephone calls that address clinical patient needs. Calls involving symptoms that need to be addressed immediately by a physician should be routed expeditiously to the physician and this should be specified in the written policy. Successful triage is also dependent on the communication skills of the staff member taking the call. Telephone triage education is available through the education departments of medical facilities and colleges or universities.[63]

Closing or Leaving a Practice

When a physician decides to leave a practice permanently, there are a number of steps that need to be followed. To avoid patient claims of abandonment, the physician should notify all patients treated within the past year of the intent to withdraw from practice. Such notification should be in writing and at least sixty days before the date of leaving or closing the practice. A copy of this letter should be placed in the patient's medical record. The termination letter should advise patients of the importance of continued care, the telephone number of the county medical society's referral service, the termination date, and a method and authorization form that enables patients to obtain copies of their medical records. Notices should be placed in the local newspaper.

Requests for release of records can come from many sources. Under most state laws, medical records must be released upon receipt of a valid written authorization, signed and dated by the patient or the patient's authorized representative.

If a physician is withdrawing from practice, patients' records must be retained. The specific length of time that medical records should be retained depends on the statute of limitations in each state and any regulations issued by state regulatory or legislative bodies. If the physician is aware of a possible claim, the record should be kept in its original form as a hard copy until the incident or claim is resolved.

The physician's medical professional liability insurance company should be notified that he or she is closing the practice, and insurance coverage should be evaluated carefully so that the physician has adequate insurance to cover any event that is reported in the future, especially if the coverage is written on a claims-made basis. In all cases, the physician should consult with an attorney to ensure that all regulations have been complied with before leaving practice.[64]

·········

PUBLIC HEALTH DEPARTMENTS AND AGENCIES

The mission of public health departments and agencies is to provide comprehensive public health services that protect, promote, and preserve the health of their citizens and to provide services to all people in their city, county, or district. The structure of the health department can vary from state to state but usually includes a health director who reports to a board of health. Public health departments are usually under a state's department of environment, health, and natural resources or similar entity.

Risks Identified

Health departments traditionally have been considered low-risk operations with few claims. Perhaps for this reason, such departments often lack organized risk management, safety, and performance improvement programs. A claims analysis of a state program was performed during an eleven-year period. Most of the one hundred counties in the state were under the same insurance program. The loss ratio for this program was 1.85 percent.[65] This demonstration of low risk has been attributed to good community relations, low-risk procedures, except for obstetrics, and the practice of delivering care regardless of the patient's ability to pay.

Despite the lack of malpractice claims, there are many opportunities to improve care in this setting, Operational risks identified in public health departments often include polices and procedures that are not reviewed, revised, or kept current on a regular basis. Credentialing of physicians and other allied health professionals is often nonexistent, and peer review is rarely performed. Risk management, performance improvement, safety, and infection control programs and plans are generally not formalized. Usually, there is no designated risk manager. Incident reporting systems may be part of the countywide or citywide incident reporting system and are not specific to health-related risks. Clinical skills checklists and annual evaluations may not be performed on an annual basis. Clinical risks include obstetrical issues such as home deliveries and high-risk obstetrical clinics. Medical emergency policies may not be developed and, if they are, the staff often lacks the expertise to follow established policies.

Risk Management Steps

The risk management steps for public and county health departments and other private sector ambulatory care centers are basically the same. The common concepts and risk management strategies covered earlier in this chapter are applicable to local health departments and should be implemented.

· · · · · · · · ·
AMBULATORY SURGERY CENTERS

As illustrated previously in Box 15.1, there are different types of ambulatory care facilities. Changes to the types of facilities and the services offered occur frequently.

Ambulatory surgery, also known as outpatient surgery and same-day surgery, refers to surgery performed on patients who are discharged home the day of the procedure.[66] It is estimated that in 2003 there were 3,700 ambulatory surgery centers in the United States.[67] Ambulatory surgeries accounted for 15 percent of all surgeries performed in the United States in 1980. By 2000, 70 percent of all surgical procedures were performed in outpatient facilities. The number of surgeries performed in 2000 was 6.7 million, almost a 200 percent increase in just ten years.[68] According to the CDC/National Center for Health Statistics, the number of ambulatory surgical procedures continues to increase because of the continuing need for cost containment; advances in medical technology, including improvements in anesthesia that allow patients to regain consciousness quicker and with fewer side effects; better relief of pain through improved analgesics; and the use in minimally invasive and noninvasive procedures. Most surgeons prefer ambulatory care centers to hospital-based facilities because they can perform two to three times the number of surgeries.[69] According to the American Medical Association, the top five reasons physicians decide to build ambulatory surgery centers are

1. increased efficiency;

2. more control over operations;

3. better access to physical plant, for both physicians and patients;

4. decreased cost to patients; and

5. additional revenue resource.[70]

Anti-Kickback Issues

Most physicians tout the efficiency of ambulatory surgery centers, from both the perspective of the physician and the patient. Almost universally, it is less expensive to have a procedure performed in such a facility than in a hospital-based facility. For this reason, the referral of a patient to a facility must be made with caution because such activity may generate allegations of illegal kickbacks, payments, or other improper financial incentives for referrals.

The safe harbor provisions in federal and state law and regulations pertaining to ambulatory surgery centers are divided into four categories:

1. Surgeon owned

2. Single specialty

3. Multispecialty

4. Hospital or physician owned[71]

Each type of ambulatory surgery center has its own specific requirements that must be met to be afforded the safe harbor protections. It is recommended that legal advice be obtained to ensure compliance, because the financial penalties and damage to public perception associated with related violations can be great.

Anesthesia Care

As in the acute care setting, anesthesia care is a vital component of ambulatory surgery care. Each facility should be equipped to provide all types of anesthesia, including general, regional, spinal, and conscious sedation. All standards of care must be met regardless of the location or setting.

The anesthesia staff should be well-trained and credentialed to perform the services offered. The staffing and workload ratios must meet recognized standards, with appropriate supervision of personnel, such as certified registered nurse anesthetists.

Adequate plans should be in place if a surgical procedure must be aborted emergently. There should be an acute facility nearby in case a patient must be admitted for inpatient services.

Clinical Issues

A preoperative evaluation should be performed on each patient before surgery is performed. Standardized forms should be used and should explore subjects such as previous medical and surgical history, anesthesia history, current medications, and allergies.

Intraoperative monitoring is of paramount importance. Sufficient documentation by the nurse and the anesthesia personnel must be recorded in the patient's medical record. A suitable operative note must either be handwritten or dictated and signed by the surgeon.

Qualified staff must perform postanesthesia care for an adequate period of time. The recovery time might vary based on factors such as the patient's medical history and the type of anesthesia used. Discharge criteria should be used to evaluate the patient before the patient is allowed to leave the facility. Clear and pertinent discharge instructions should also be given to the adult who accompanies the patient home.

In 2002, the U.S. Department of Veterans' Affairs published a study it conducted beginning in 1994.[72] This study revealed that enhanced rapport with patients can be achieved through more personalized service before, during, and after surgery. Providing beepers for family members of surgery patients allows them the freedom to roam, yet remain accessible to the medical team, if necessary. Follow-up telephone calls the day after surgery allow the medical staff to assess the patient's outcome as well as capture valuable feedback and promote a close relationship between the patient and the organization.

These above approaches should allow a facility to minimize its risk exposure while optimizing the quality of care provided to patients. One final key of importance to successfully operating an ambulatory surgery facility is patient selection. Therefore, it is crucial that facilities have appropriate relationships with physicians who understand the importance of performing procedures at an acute care setting if the circumstances warrant doing so.

· · · · · · · · ·
ALTERNATIVE MEDICINE

Traditional medicine refers to the provision of healthcare services before the advent of conventional medicine.[73] Traditional medicine, which was primarily administered by the local physician, was designed to meet the needs of the local community.

Conventional medicine, as practiced in many countries, including the United States, involves care delivered by practitioners schooled at an accredited university and trained in accredited residency programs. Their practice is based on scientific, peer-reviewed studies. These practitioners employ a variety of treatment techniques, including but not limited to medications, physical and occupational therapy, and surgery. During the past two decades, these practitioners have begun to focus more on preventive medicine and wellness programs.

Complementary and alternative medicine (CAM) may either augment or replace conventional medicine. According to the National Center for Complementary and Alternative Medicine (NCCAM), complementary medicine is used together with conventional medicine and alternative medicine is used in lieu of conventional medicine. Integrative medicine combines conventional medicine with CAM therapies that have been proven safe and effective through the same scientific study techniques that conventional practitioners use.[74]

NCCAM classifies CAM therapies into five categories:

1. Alternative medical systems (homeopathic and naturopathic medicine)

2. Mind–body interventions (meditation and mental healing)

3. Biologically based therapies (dietary supplements and herbal products)

4. Manipulative and body-based therapies (chiropractic manipulation and massage)

5. Energy therapies (biofield therapy and bioelectromagnetic-based therapies)[75]

Use of CAM

In 2007, it was estimated that 38 percent of the people living in the United States used at least one CAM therapy.[76] An estimated 38 million adults made more than 350 million CAM visits, and out-of-pocket spending for CAM, including costs for herbal therapies, was estimated to be $34 billion in 2007, representing 1.5 percent of the $2.2 trillion total healthcare spending.[77]

Medical Insurance Coverage

Forty-two states mandate coverage for chiropractic care, and seven states mandate coverage for acupuncture.[78] Many insurance companies now offer coverage for some forms of alternative or complementary medicine.

Organizations and Literature

There are many sources of information on CAM. There are several journals devoted to CAM, with some emphasizing evidence-based medicine. Editorial boards that have an appropriate mix of physicians and nonphysicians publish *Integrative Medicine* and the *Journal of Alternative & Complementary Medicine.* There also is a wealth of information available on the Internet, but as with any online material, caution should be exercised until the validity of the content is verified. Unlike conventional medical literature, there is little data from properly designed and conducted clinical studies.[79]

Legal Cases

Professional liability suits filed against providers of alternative or complementary medicine providers account for only a small percentage of all medical professional liability claims. A comprehensive study published in the *Journal of the American Medical Association* revealed that in the early to mid-1990s, primary care physicians experienced approximately 6.4 claims per one hundred policyholders. During the same period, chiropractors experienced a rate of 2.7. The average indemnity payment per claim averaged $147,853 for primary care physicians and $49,873 for chiropractors. The percentage of claims that resulted in indemnity payments was approximately 31.4 percent for primary care physicians and 49.1 percent for chiropractors.[80]

Generally, medical physicians do not increase their liability exposure simply because they refer patients to other physicians. However, if the referral is made to a practitioner who provides alternative or complementary medicine, liability might be asserted on a basis of negligent referral, negligent supervision, or other similar theories.[81]

Although malpractice claims experience to date does not reflect high exposure for complementary medicine providers, it is clear that providers of alternative medicine must continue to formalize their approaches so that they will meet the standard of reasonably rendered care relative to their peers. Medical physicians must be cautious about referring patients and document their rationale for the referral, as well as appropriate follow up, clearly in the medical record. For a more comprehensive discussion on complementary and alternative medicine refer to Appendix 15.1 at the end of this chapter.

· · · · · · · · ·
CONCLUSION

Risk management in the fields of ambulatory care and complementary or alternative medicine is an important yet often overlooked component of a successful practice. The changes sweeping across the healthcare industry in recent years have affected, and in many cases increased, the exposure of ambulatory settings. This environment is entirely appropriate to the implementation of comprehensive enterprise risk management programs, and healthcare risk management professionals should find implementing such programs both challenging and rewarding.

Suggested Reading

American Society for Healthcare Risk Management. "Physician Office Risk Management Tool Kit." Available from the ASHRM Web site, www.ashrm.org.

Endnotes

1. "Ambulatory Care Accreditation." The Joint Commission. Available at: www.jointcommission.org/AccreditationPrograms/AmbulatoryCare. (Accessed August, 2009.)

2. "Conference Synthesis: Research Agenda for Ambulatory Patient Safety." The Agency for Healthcare Research and Quality (AHRQ). Available at: www.ahcpr.gov/about/cpcr/ptsafety/ambpts2.htm. (Accessed August, 2009.)

3. Kohn, L. T., J. M. Corrigan, and M. S. Donaldson, eds. *To Err is Human: Building a Safer Health System*. Institute of Medicine, Committee on Quality of Health Care in America. Washington, D.C.: National Academy Press, 2000.

4. "Conference Synthesis," *op. cit.*

5. "PIAA Claims Trend Analysis: A Comprehensive Analysis of Medical Malpractice." Data reported to the PIAA Data Sharing Project. Rockville, Md.: Physician Insurers Association of America (PIAA), 2008.

6. *"Hospital Professional Liability and Physician Liability: 2008 Benchmark Analysis."* Columbia, Md.: Aon Global and ASHRM, September 23, 2008.

7. Levinson, W., D. L. Roter, J. P. Mullooly, et al. "Patient-physician communication: The relationship with malpractice claims among primary care physicians and surgeons." *Journal of the American Medical Association*, 277(7), 1997, 553–559.

8. PIAA, *op. cit.*

9. Kelsay, E., et al. *Risk Management: Safeguarding Your Career*. St. Louis, Mo.: TIV, 1997, p. 11.

10. *Clinician-Patient Communication to Enhance Health Outcomes*. West Haven, Conn.: Institute for Healthcare Communication, Inc., 2006. More information on communication workshops is available at: www.healthcarecomm.org.

11. *Ibid.*

12. Marvel, M. K., R. M. Epstein, K. Flowers, and H. B. Beckman. "Soliciting the Patient's Agenda: Have We Improved?" *Journal of the American Medical Association*, 281(3), 1999, 283–287.

13. White, M. K., and V. F. Keller. "Difficult Clinician-Patient Relationships." *Journal of Clinical Outcomes Management*, 5(5), 1998, 32–36.

14. "Risk Management Strategies for the Physician Office." Chicago, Ill.: CNA, 2008, p. 22.

15. *Ibid.* pp. 22–23.

16. Kelsay, *op. cit.*, p. 49.

17. "Risk Management Strategies for the Physician Office," *op. cit.*, p. 16.

18. Davis, K. S., J. C. McConnell, and E. D. Shaw. "Health Information Management." In: Carroll, R., ed., *Risk Management Handbook for Health Care Organizations*, 5th ed. Chicago, Ill.: Jossey-Bass, 2006, Vol. 1, pp. 355–393.

19. "Homeland Security Act of 2002." Public Law 107–296, November 25, 2002. Available at: www.dhs.gov/index.shtm. (Accessed August, 2009.)

20. Page, S. *Establishing a System of Policies and Procedures*. Mansfield, Ohio: BookMasters, 1998, p. 2.

21. *A Patient's Bill of Rights*. Chicago, Ill.: American Hospital Association, 1998. Available at: www.patienttalk.info/AHA-Patient_Bill_of_Rights.htm (Accessed August, 2009.)

22. Rozovsky, F. A. "Informed Consent as a Loss Control Process." In: Carroll, R., ed. *Risk Management Handbook for Health Care Organizations*, 5th ed. Chicago, Ill: Jossey-Bass, 2006, Vol. 2, pp. 53–77.

23. Leebov, W. *Effective Complaint Handling in Health Care*. Chicago, Ill.: American Hospital Publishing Inc., 1990, pp. 1–3.

24. *Ibid*, pp. 14–23.

25. "Staff Credentialing: These Fundamental Principles Can Help Reduce Risk." *In Brief*. Chicago, Ill: CNA, 2007, Issue 2, pp. 1–6.

26. 42 U.S.C. §311101.

27. Title IV of Public Law 99–660, Health Care Quality Improvement Act of 1986, as amended.

28. Flynn, E. A., K. N. Barker, and B. J. Carnahan. "National observational study of prescription dispensing accuracy and safety in 50 pharmacies." *Journal of the American Pharmacy Association*, 43(2), 2003, 191–200.

29. Field, T. S., B. H. Gilman, S. Subramanian, et al. "The costs associated with adverse drug events among older adults in the ambulatory setting." *Medical Care*, 43(12), 2005, 1171–1176.

30. Risk Management Strategies for the Physician Office, *op. cit.*, pp. 36–38.

31. "Sentinel Events Policy and Procedures." Oakbrook Terrace, Ill: The Joint Commission. Available at: www.jointcommission.org/SentinelEvents/PolicyandProcedures. (Accessed August, 2009.)

32. "2009 Standards for Ambulatory Care." Oakbrook Terrace, Ill: The Joint Commission, 2008.

33. Cohen, M. "Statutes, Standards, and Regulations." In: Carroll, R., ed. *Risk Management Handbook for Health Care Organizations*, 5th ed. Chicago, Ill.: Jossey-Bass, 2006, Vol. 3, pp. 413–444.

34. "How to Report a Problem (Medical Devices)." Food and Drug Administration. Available at: www.fda.gov/MedicalDevices/Safety/ReportaProblem/default.htm. (Accessed August, 2009.)

35. *Ibid.*

36. Risk Management Strategies for the Physician Office, *op. cit.*, pp. 39–40.

37. Risk Management Strategies for the Physician Office, *op. cit.*, p. 30.

38. Risk Management Strategies for the Physician Office, *op. cit.*, p. 35.

39. "Frequently Asked Questions." Occupational and Safety Health Administration. Available at: www.osha.gov/needlesticks/needlefaq.html. (Accessed August, 2009.)

40. Centers for Disease Control and Prevention. "Guidelines for Preventing the Transmission of *Mycobacterium tuberculosis* in Health-Care Settings, 2005." *MMWR* 2005; 54(RR-17). Atlanta, Ga.: Centers for Disease Control and Prevention, 2005. Available at: www.cdc.gov/mmwr/PDF/rr/rr5417.pdf. (Accessed August, 2009.)

41. White, P. J. "Employment Practices Liability." In: Carroll, R., ed. *Risk Management Handbook for Healthcare Organizations*, 5th ed. Chicago, Ill.: Jossey-Bass, 2006, Vol. 3, pp. 167–189.

42. *Risk Management Handbook for Medical Personnel: A Collection of Readings*. Chicago, Ill.: Continental Casualty Company, 1995, pp. 38–39.

43. Scott, L. *It's A Dog's World: Leader's Guide*, 2nd ed. Carlsbad, Calif.: CRM Films, 2008, pp. 1–2.

44. "Integrating Risk Management and Quality Improvement." *In Brief*. Chicago, Ill.: CNA, 2006, Issue 1, pp. 1–2.

45. *Ibid.*, p. 2.

46. "Office-Based Surgery." The Joint Commission. Available at: www.jointcommission.org/AccreditationPrograms/Office-BasedSurgery. (Accessed August, 2009.)

47. "Ambulatory Care." The Joint Commission. Available at: www.jointcommission.org/AccreditationPrograms/AmbulatoryCare. (Accessed August, 2009.)

48. "2009 National Patient Safety Goals." The Joint Commission. Available at: www.jointcommission.org/PatientSafety/NationalPatientSafetyGoals. (Accessed August, 2009.)

49. "About AAAHC." Accreditation Association for Ambulatory Health Care. Available at: www.aaahc.org. (Accessed August, 2009.)

50. *Ibid.*

51. "Welcome!" The Institute for Medical Quality. Available at: www.imq.org. (Accessed August, 2009.)

52. "About ASA?" American Society of Anesthesiologists. Available at: www.asahq.org/aboutASA.htm (Accessed August, 2009.)

53. "About AORN." The Association of Perioperative Registered Nurses. Available at: www.aorn.org/AboutAORN. (Accessed August, 2009.)

54. "HEDIS® & Quality Measurement." Available at: www.ncqa.org/tabid/59/Default.aspx. (Accessed August, 2009.)

55. *The State of Health Care Quality 2002: Industry Trends and Analysis.* Washington, D.C.: The National Committee for Quality Assurance, 2002, p. 7.

56. "HEDIS® 2010." Available at: www.ncqa.org/tabid/1044/Default.aspx. (Accessed August, 2009.)

57. "Fundamentals of Contract Review." *In Brief.* Chicago, Ill.: CNA, 2006, Issue 2, pp. 1–2.

58. Weiss, G. G. "Malpractice: Don't wait for a lawsuit to strike." *Medical Economics*, 3, 2002, 83–84.

59. *Ibid.*

60. Risk Management Strategies for the Physician Office, *op. cit.*, pp. 45–46.

61. U.S. Supreme Court, *Cruzan v. Missouri Department of Health.* 497 U.S. 261; 110 S.Ct. 2841; 111 L. Ed.2d 224, 1990.

62. Risk Management Strategies for the Physician Office, *op. cit.*, pp. 52–53.

63. "Telephone and E-mail Communication: Securing Patient Privacy." *In Brief.* Chicago, Ill: CNA, 2008, Issue 2, pp. 1–2.

64. McRae, J. "On 'Signing Off': When a Physician Leaves a Practice." *Risk Management Sourcebook.* Napa, Calif.: The Doctors' Company, 1998, pp. 1–2.

65. CNA Claims Analysis, 1992–2003.

66. Peng, L. "Ambulatory Surgery." Emedicine. Available at: www.emedicine.com/aaem/topic13.htm. (Accessed June, 2005.)

67. "Ambulatory Surgery Centers." *Encyclopedia of Surgery: A Guide for Patients and Caregivers.* 2009. Available at: www.surgeryencyclopedia.com/A-Ce/Ambulatory-Surgery-Centers.html. (Accessed August, 2009.)

68. Derived in part from Jackson, C. "Cutting Into the Market: Rise of Ambulatory Surgery Centers," *Amednews.com*, American Medical Association. Available at: www.ama-assn .org/amednews/2002/04/15/bisa0415.htm. (Accessed August, 2009.)

69. *Ibid.*

70. *Ibid.*

71. Harris, S. "Safe Harbor Rules for Ambulatory Surgery Centers Protect Investment." *Amednews.com*, American Medical Association. Available at: www.ama-assn.org/ amednews/2001/05/07/bica0507.htm. (Accessed August, 2009.)

72. United States Department of Veterans' Affairs. "Addressing the Concerns of Ambulatory Care Patients." Available at: www.va.gov/medical/ambulatorycare.htm. (Accessed August, 2009.)

73. For a detailed review of the issues related to the integration of conventional and alternative medicine, see Washington State Office of the Insurance Commissioner's report. "Issues in Coverage for Complementary and Alternative Medicine Services: Report of the Clinician Workgroup on the Integration of Complementary and Alternative Medicine," January 2000.

74. "What is Complementary and Alternative Medicine (CAM)?" National Center for Complementary and Alternative Medicine. Available at: nccam.nih.gov/health/ whatiscam. (Accessed August, 2009.)

75. *Ibid.*

76. Barnes, P. M., B. Bloom, and R. L. Nahin. "Complementary and Alternative Medicine Use Among Adults and Children: United States, 2007." *National Health Statistics Report*, December 10, 2008. Available at: www.cdc.gov/nchs/data/nhsr/nhsr012.pdf. (Accessed August, 2009.)

77. Boyles, S. "Americans Spend $34 Billion on Alternative Medicine." *WebMD Health News*, July 30, 2009. Available at: www.webmd.com. (Accessed August, 2009.)

78. Dalzell, M. D. "HMOs and Alternative Medicine." *Managed Care*, April 1999. Available at: www.managedcaremag.com/archives/9904/9904.alternativehtml. (Accessed August, 2009.)

79. Fontanarosa, P. B. and G. D. Lundberg. "Alternative medicine meets science." *Journal of the American Medical Association*, 280(18), 1998, 1618–1619.

80. Studdert, D. M., et al. "Medical malpractice implications of alternative medicine." *Journal of the American Medical Association*, 280(18), 1998, 1610–1615.

81. *Ibid.*

Appendix 15.1

Complementary and Alternative Medicine

By Leilani Kicklighter

Complementary and alternative medicine (CAM) is described by the National Center for Complementary and Alternative Medicine (NCCAM) as ". . . a group of diverse medical and healthcare systems, practices and products that are not generally considered to be part of conventional medicine. Although scientific evidence exists regarding some CAM therapies, for most there are key questions that are yet to be answered through well-designed scientific studies, questions such as whether these therapies are safe and whether they work for the purposes for which they are used."[1]

Furthermore, according to NCCAM, many complementary medicine modalities, such as hypnosis to reduce stress or manage pain, are used in conjunction with conventional medicine. Alternative medicine may also be used in place of conventional medicine, such as replacing surgery with focused meditation.

HISTORY OF CAM IN U.S. HEALTHCARE

What is now referred to as complementary and alternative medicine has been a part of the care of the sick by the shaman, the medicine man, and elders for many centuries, predominantly in Asia, East Indian countries, and in American Indian cultures. Many old-time remedies we hear our families speak of, such as the mustard poultice that Grandma used to break up chest congestion, may also be categorized as CAM.

Historically, many poultices, powders, and drinks made from plants were used to treat various maladies. For instance, digitalis was originally made from the foxglove plant. Warfarin is a synthetic derivative of coumarin, a chemical found naturally in many plants, notably woodruff (*Galium odoratum*, Rubiaceae), and at lower levels in licorice, lavender, and various other species. Vitamin K, used to counteract the anticoagulation factor in warfarin, is found in spinach and other vegetables. Many people use lavender and tea tree essential oils as antiseptics and cleaning solutions, as well as deodorants and air fresheners. Essential oils are also used in aromatherapy.

With the invention of anesthetics and antibiotics, conventional medicine shifted its focus to science and turned its back on this traditional type of patient treatment. Only in the last decade or two has organized medicine in the United States begun to move toward accepting CAM as a valuable component of patient care. The opening of complementary and alternative medicine units in hospitals[2] and the development of the division of National Center of Complementary and Alternative Medicine by the National Institute of Health, a part of the U.S. Department of Health and Human Services, are signs that conventional medicine is cracking the door open for CAM. For example, the results of an American Hospital Association survey released in 2008 indicated that 37 percent of U.S. hospitals offer a CAM program of some sort, up from 24.5 percent in 2005.[3]

There are still naysayers, however. For example, in March of 2009, several prominent members of the traditional scientific community demanded that NCCAM be shut down. In a *Washington Post* article, Steven Salzberg, a genome researcher and computational biologist at the University of Maryland, was quoted as saying, "With a new administration and President Obama's stated goal of moving science to the forefront, now is the time for scientists to start speaking up about issues that concern us . . . One of our concerns is that NIH is funding pseudoscience."[4]

This effort was unsuccessful, and there is a great deal of positive momentum behind the formalization of CAM. For example, universities now offer degrees in CAM, and courses in the various components of CAM are available through colleges and universities as continuing education and for-credit courses. Two individuals well known for their involvement in CAM are Deepak Chopra, MD,[5] and Andrew Weil, MD.[6] The visibility of the work accomplished by these two physicians has also helped further the acceptance of CAM by the public at large.

As the debate over CAM continues, the risk management professional must consider how a jury would respond to questions about whether a CAM provider met the standard of care, that is, what a reasonable healthcare provider would have done under the same or similar circumstances. From a safety and liability reduction perspective, the integration of CAM into the conventional medical healthcare setting will be beneficial through use of evidence-based methodology wherever possible to support CAM practice. Also beneficial will be clearly defining the scope of individual provider practice based on review of pertinent regulations, such as those promulgated by the board of medicine, as well as research on the CAM provider's professional organizational standards.

The need for evidence-based analysis of CAM as a priority is illustrated by the large body of research posted on the NCCAM site,[7] and studies are bearing fruit. For example, a survey conducted to determine the effects of therapeutic massage on anxiety and post-procedure pain of patients undergoing insertion of a peripherally inserted central catheter (PICC) and mid-arm catheter insertion found significant improvement in outcomes for patients who underwent therapeutic massage before their procedure.[8] Another example of CAM success is a study that demonstrated that hypnotherapy significantly improved symptoms of patients with irritable bowel syndrome.[9]

One of the most important things that risk management professionals can do to manage associated risks and promote safety is to familiarize themselves with the various aspects of CAM.

· · · · · · · · ·

TYPES OF CAM

NCCAM groups CAM practices into four domains, recognizing there will be some overlap.[10] In addition, NCCAM studies CAM whole medical systems.

Whole medical systems are built upon complete systems of theory and practice and cut across all domains. For example, homeopathy, a system that originated in Europe, seeks to stimulate the body's ability to heal itself by giving very small doses of highly diluted substances that in larger doses would cause illness.

Examples of systems that have developed in non-Western cultures include traditional Chinese medicine. This system is based on the concept that disease results from disruption in the flow of qi and imbalance in the forces of yin and yang. Practices such as use of herbs, meditation, massage, and acupuncture seek to aid healing by restoring the yin-yang balance and the flow of qi. Another such example is Ayurveda, a whole medical system that originated in India. It aims to integrate the body, mind, and spirit to prevent and treat disease. Therapies used include herbs, massage, and yoga.[11]

Mind–Body Medicine

Mind–body medicine uses a variety of techniques designed to enhance the mind's capacity to affect bodily function and symptoms. Some techniques that were considered CAM in the past have become mainstream, such as patient support groups and cognitive-behavioral therapy. Other mind–body techniques are still considered CAM, including meditation, which uses techniques such as focusing attention or maintaining a specific posture to suspend the stream of thoughts and relax the body and mind. Still other CAM modalities include prayer, mental healing, and therapies that use art, music, or dance.

Biologically Based Practices

Biologically based practices in CAM use substances found in nature, such as herbs, foods, and vitamins. Some examples include dietary supplements, herbal products, and the use of other so-called natural, but as yet scientifically unproven, therapies, such as using shark cartilage to treat cancer.

Manipulative and Body-Based Practices

To achieve health and healing, manipulative and body-based practices in CAM are based on movement and manipulation of one or more body parts. Examples include osteopathic and chiropractic manipulation, reflexology, massage, and rolfing, a combination of both manipulation of connective tissue and movement therapy that is geared to improve posture.

Energy Therapies

Energy therapies involve the use of energy fields. They are of two types:

- *Biofield therapies* are intended to affect energy fields that purportedly surround and penetrate the human body. The existence of such fields has not yet been scientifically proven.

- *Bioelectromagnetic-based therapies* involve the unconventional use of electromagnetic fields, such as pulsed fields, magnetic fields, or alternating current or direct current fields.[12]

More resources explaining CAM are listed at the end of this appendix.

·········

SETTINGS OF CAM PRACTICE

The independent office practice setting is the most common setting for practitioners of complementary and alternative medicine; however, many hospitals have begun to create CAM departments as a physical part of the hospital or in a freestanding, but associated setting.

It is also important to note that, with increased public acceptance and use of CAM, more patients are likely to request these modalities while hospitalized. For example, patients may want to continue use of certain supplements and other modalities of CAM, such as medication and self-hypnosis.

·········

CAM PRACTITIONERS

Conventional medicine is practiced or provided by allopathic (medical doctor, MD) practitioners and by osteopathic (doctor of osteopathy, DO) practitioners, as well as allied health professionals such as advanced nurse practitioners (ARNP), physician assistants (PA), registered nurses (RN), physical therapists (PT), and others. Some of these individuals may also be CAM practitioners. Chiropractors are also CAM providers.

Education and Competency Requirements for CAM Practitioners

The education of CAM practitioners varies with the particular modality. Many practitioners are self-taught, others are certified by national organizations after completing educational programs. Still other practitioners may have completed a for-credit or continuing education college-based course or an association-based course. Many CAM disciplines have standardized educational levels, such as a yoga instructor who proceeds to the yoga master level. Still other practitioners, such as chiropractors and homeopathic providers, attend specialized college or university courses.

As previously noted, healthcare organizations that add CAM practitioners to their settings, whether as employees or part of the medical staff, should establish qualifications for such practitioners based on research of professional organization standards and any pertinent state regulatory requirements, such as those of the board of medicine. (Refer to Chapter 14 in Volume 1 for more information on credentialing.)

·········
RISKS RELATED TO CAM

In addition to general awareness of the need for evidence of therapeutic value to support CAM practice and the need to carefully define scope of practice of practitioners, the risk management professional should consider these risks associated with CAM.

Balancing the Benefits and Risks of CAM

It is necessary to define the way in which the CAM practitioner interacts with the organization's care environment and staff. For example, a massage therapist should be accountable to an individual knowledgeable about his or her specialty, and specific criteria should be considered regarding the type of patients treated; for instance, full-term stable infants and children may benefit from pediatric massage, but special consideration applies to neonatal intensive care unit (NICU) patients.[13] As noted by Joy Browne, RN, PhD, with regard to the use of massage therapy in premature infants:

> An expanding body of research has documented the short-term advantages of gentle touch and massage for healthy term infants and some growing and medically stable preterm infants. These findings have provided the impetus for extension of massage techniques to very small, fragile newborns, and have prompted the utilization of new personnel in NICUs specifically to provide massage therapy for newborns. It is important, before engaging in these approaches, for the professional in the NICU to consider the potential impact of massage on the infant and the family. It is also imperative that professionals in the NICU take into account the current growing knowledge base regarding developmental care and the implications for decision making with any provision of stimuli to fragile sick newborns in the NICU.[14]

Among other cautions, Browne notes that it is important for staff to monitor autonomic and behavioral responses during all handling/touch procedures and modify interactions appropriately.

As this example illustrates, CAM-related positive benefits, such as those associated with massage, must continually be balanced against risks, as CAM integrates with conventional care.

CAM-Related Supplements

There is potential for harm due to CAM-related supplements. Some supplements may be contraindicated for certain diseases or conditions or exacerbate the properties of prescribed medications. For instance, echinacea, an herb, is known to have anticoagulant properties and should not be used in conjunction with prescribed anticoagulation medicines such as heparin or Coumadin. St. John's wort is a mood enhancer and should not be used with prescribed mood enhancers or tranquilizers.

It is therefore important that the medical history information is obtained for every patient in all healthcare settings, including the physician's office, hospital, or emergency department, and that any complementary and/or alternative medicines used by the patient, that is, what herbs or supplements the patient is taking, are identified.

Just as important is education for patients on the implications of such supplements and or medicines in regard to the patient's specific clinical condition and how they may interact with prescribed medication. Many patients do not consider herbs, vitamins, over-the-counter (OTC) medicines, and supplements as medications, so when asked what medication they are taking, most patients do not identify these to the practitioner. The practitioner taking the patient's history needs to ask specific questions to gather this important information at each office visit or admission to a hospital, ambulatory surgical center, or emergency department. This information takes on particular significance prior to surgery, when prescribing new medication, or when taking on the care of a new patient not previously seen. Once a thorough history has been obtained, the physician can then emphasize which herbs, vitamins, supplements, and over-the-counter drugs could interact with other medication, surgery, or other diagnostic methods and treatments and instruct the patient to discontinue their use if necessary until further advised. Obviously, the physician should be familiar with herbs, vitamins, OTC medicines, and supplements in order to have a ready knowledge of how they work or interact with prescribed medications, and periodic continuing education on this subject should be considered.

Another aspect of CAM is the risk associated with lack of regulation for herbs and supplements by the FDA. This means that there is no oversight of the substance to ensure standardization, and there have been instances in which certain brands of herbs or supplements contained harmful additives that were detrimental to the patient. Again, querying the patient about all herbs and supplements taken can help to reduce this exposure.

RISK MANAGEMENT PROGRAM IMPLICATIONS

In order for risk management professionals to be able to identify and manage risks to the organization, it is important that they start with a general understanding of the types of services and care provided, including CAM. Knowledge of CAM constitutes another piece of the clinical picture; for example, it may be a cause of an untoward outcome or could be thought to be responsible for an unexplained positive outcome. In all cases, the use of CAM needs to be understood and considered when addressing patient safety. For example, medical record audits in all healthcare settings including the physician's office, ambulatory surgery center, and the hospital should assess whether a patient's use of CAM was identified, documented, evaluated, and acted upon appropriately.

As more healthcare organizations adopt CAM, the risk management professional can assist the organization to minimize risk and enhance patient safety by understanding the modalities used in CAM and identifying the associated risk and benefits. In this manner, the organization supports patient-centered care by allowing those patients wanting to use the practices and techniques associated with CAM to do so, while protecting itself from allegations of negligence. The risk management professional will then be in a position to help the organization assess and address risks proactively in order to maximize clinical benefit.

Suggested Web Sites

Complementary and Alternative Medicine in Cancer Treatment: www.cancer.gov/cancertopics/treatment/cam

Cancer Topics Home Page at the National Cancer Institute: www.cancer.gov/cancertopics/treatment/cam

Aetna InteliHealth on Complementary and Alterative Medicine: www.intelihealth.com/IH/ihtIH/WSC/8513/8513.html

An Introduction to Naturopathy: http://nccam.nih.gov/health/naturopathy

About Research Training and Career Development-Overview: http://nccam.nih.gov/training/overview.htm

CAM Use and Children: http://nccam.nih.gov/health/children

Paying for CAM Treatment: http://nccam.nih.gov/health/financial

Using (CAM) Dietary Supplements Wisely: http://nccam.nih.gov/health/supplements/wiseuse.htm

Tips for Talking with Your Healthcare Providers About CAM: http://nccam.nih.gov/health/decisions/talkingaboutcam.htm

Selecting a CAM Practitioner: http://nccam.nih.gov/health/decisions/practitioner.htm

Are You Considering CAM?: http://nccam.nih.gov/health/decisions/consideringcam.htm

Alternative Medicine, Naturopathic and Alternative Medicines Web Site: www.amna.org

Medline Resources on CAM: http://nlm.nih.gov/medlineplu/complementaryandalternativemedicine.html

Alternative Medicine Alert Available Through American Health Consultants at: www.ahpub.com

American Chiropractic Association: www.acatoday.org

The American Association of Naturopathic Physicians: www.naturopathic.org

National Guild of Hypnotists: www.ngh.com

National Certification Commission for Acupuncture and Oriental Medicine: www.nccaom.org

Association of Ayurvedic Professionals: www.aapna.com

The National Center for Homeopathy: www.homeopathic.org

American Osteopathic Association: www.osteopathic.org

Office of Dietary Supplements: www.ods.od.nih.gov

Suggested Readings

Cox, L., "Why Do We Spend $34B in Alternative Medicine." ABC News Medical Unit. Friday, July 31, 2009, Available at: http://abcnews.go.com/Health/WellnessNews/story?id=8215703&page=1. (Accessed April 18, 2010.)

Liponis, M. "Alternative Therapies that Really Work." *Parade*, December 15, 2008, p. 16. Available at: www.parade.com. (Accessed April 18, 2010.)

Publix Greenwise Market. The Health Center at "Wellness and Pharmacy." Available at www.publix.com/wellness/healthcenter/Home.do. (Accessed April 18, 2010.)

Endnotes

1. The National Center for Complementary and Alternative Medicine. Available at: http://nccam.nih.gov/. (Accessed December 28, 2009.)

2. Abelson, R., and P.L. Brown. "Alternative Medicine Is Finding Its Niche In Nation's Hospitals." *The New York Times*, April 13, 2002. Available at: www.nytimes.com/2002/04/13/business/alternative-medicine-is-finding-its-niche-in-nation-s-hospitals.html. (Accessed December 29, 2009.)

3. AHA. "Latest Survey Shows More Hospitals Offering Complementary and Alternative Medicine Services," September 15, 2008. Press release. Available at: www.aha.org/aha/press-release/2008/080915-pr-cam.html. (Accessed April 18, 2010.)

4. Brown, D., "Critics Object to 'Pseudoscience' Center." *Washington Post*, March 17, 2009. Available at: www.washingtonpost.com/wpdyn/content/article/2009/03/16/AR2009031602139.html?hpid=sec-health. (Accessed December 31, 2009.) Also available from "Maryland Moments," March 2009. at the News Desk of the University of Maryland. Available at: www.newsdesk.umd.edu/facts/mm/08-09/mar.cfm. (Accessed April 18, 2010.)

5. News about Deepak Chopra. Available at: http://topics.nytimes.com/topics/reference/timestopics/people/c/deepak_chopra/index.html. (Accessed December 29, 2009.)

6. News about Andrew Weil, Shaman, MD. Available at: http://topics.nytimes.com/topics/reference/timestopics/people/w/andrew_weil/index.html. (Accessed December 29, 2009.)

7. NCCAM-Funded Research for Fiscal Year 08. Available at: http://nccam.nih.gov/research/extramural/awards/2008/. (Accessed December 29, 2009.)

8. Locke, J., and G. Dennis, G., "PICC and Mid-Arm Line Insertions with Massage in a Community Hospital." AMTA National Convention 2002, Portland, Oreg. Available at: www.massagetherapyfoundation.org/postersession.html#. (Accessed December 30, 2009.)

9. "Effect of Nurse-led Gut-directed Hypnotherapy upon Health-related Quality of Life in Patients with Irritable Bowel Syndrome." *Journal of Clinical Nursing* 2006; June 15(6): 678–684. Abstract available at: www.ncbi.nlm.nih.gov/pubmed/16684163. (Accessed April 18, 2010.)

10. Types of CAM. Available at: http://nccam.nih.gov/health/whatiscam/overview.htm#types. (Accessed December 29, 2009.)

11. *Ibid.*

12. *Ibid.*

13. Browne, J.V., "Developmental Care—Considerations for Touch and Massage in the Neonatal Intensive Care Unit." *Neonatatal Network* 2000; Vol. 19, No. 1. Available at: www.preemie-l.org/massage.html. (Accessed December 30, 2009.)

14. *Ibid.*

16

Risk Management Considerations in Home Healthcare

Kelley Woodfin

Several unique characteristics of delivering healthcare services in the home setting exacerbate liability risk. These include, but are not limited to, the following:

- Lack of direct supervision for home care providers;
- Use of technology traditionally used only in the hospital setting;
- Limited interface with physicians;
- Intermittent nature of scheduled visits;
- Unpredictable level of compliance that can be expected from the patient and family or friends who care for patients on a daily basis.

This chapter discusses the rapid evolution of home care services, identifies specific risk management issues, and recommended strategies to manage those risks. The goal is to enhance the quality of care rendered, reduce exposure to liability, and ensure patient and worker safety.

THE RAPID EVOLUTION OF HOME CARE

At its inception, home care services involved periodic home visits by visiting nurses and private physicians. Nurses generally performed such tasks as obtaining vital signs, wound monitoring, and patient education. Home care providers fall into the following categories:

- Home health agencies
- Hospice agencies
- Home infusion and pharmaceutical services
- Durable medical equipment services
- Independently contracted licensed nurses and nursing assistants

The home care industry has changed significantly since those times. Care provided in the home setting is less expensive than that provided in inpatient facilities. Services now might include a full spectrum inclusive of skilled nursing care, home respiratory care, infusion services that include total parenteral nutrition and chemotherapy, and wound management. Home care also might consist of full rehabilitation services, cardiac care and monitoring, full-scope dialysis services, high-risk newborn care, early maternal and infant discharge programs, and high-risk obstetrical care. The following are some common home health services.

- Nursing assessment
- Bathing and other personal care
- Catheter insertion/care/changes
- Case management
- Enteral/parenteral therapies
- Hospice care
- Infusion therapies
- Medication instruction
- Monitoring of acute/chronic conditions
- Nutrition counseling
- Pain control
- Patient education
- Rehabilitation therapies (physical, occupational, speech)
- Ostomy management
- Wound care
- Monitoring of acute/chronic condition

Steady growth in the nation's senior population has also increased demand for home healthcare services. Although there has been an increase in the number of continuing care retirement communities and stand-alone assisted living and dementia facilities, seniors generally want to remain at home, and family members would rather have their aging relative maintain independence for as long as possible. The term *home and community-based services* is now being used for elder care services that seniors can obtain in locations other than senior care facilities.

There are risks inherent in caring for an elderly person in the home. Cognitive impairment, extensive comorbidities, and physical frailty often result in the inability to follow simple directions and comply with treatment plans and less physical reserve to overcome self-care mistakes. There is also risk related to unrealistic expectations on the part of patient and family, including the assumption that patients are safe in the home as long as they are under the care of a home health services agency.

Another evolving area of home healthcare is telemedicine, which enables the physician to "visit" the home and monitor the patient electronically through the use of equipment including video and integrated peripheral devices such as electronic stethoscopes. Kaiser Permanente Medical Center in Sacramento, California, performed a pilot study of telemedicine in the late 1990s that showed a reduction in care delivery costs, patient satisfaction with videoconferencing, and successful use of integrated peripheral devices that transmit biological data to the physician.[1] Although this study was concluded some time ago, the rapid increase in and sophistication of electronic devices will no doubt contribute to increased provision of remotely located in-home patient supervision and monitoring as a cost-effective, efficient method of providing home care services.

Standards of care for telemedicine in home healthcare and processes for across-state licensing for this type of practice are still evolving, and for this reason, it is not possible to address those issues more completely in this chapter. It is reasonable, however, to forecast an increase in this type of home care in the future and thus a need for both home care providers and risk management professionals to stay abreast of changes in this arena. (Please see Chapter 15, Volume 2 on telemedicine for more information.)

· · · · · · · · ·
STAFFING

In some situations, a home health agency may provide a full spectrum of personnel, such as licensed nurses and home caregivers, in addition to pharmaceutical, durable medical equipment, and durable medical equipment (DME) technicians; respiratory therapists; chemotherapy-certified nurses; ostomy, wound, and pain management interdisciplinary services; perinatal and antenatal clinical services, hospice services; and rehabilitative services professionals, including physical therapists, occupational therapists, and speech therapists. In other cases, the home health agency might subcontract with ancillary services and provide only nurses and home care aides. Hospice services can also be provided for terminally ill patients. These services often include the skills of social workers, psychotherapists, clergy, and licensed nursing personnel.

Although the types of services provided by an agency might differ, several important similarities affect the practice of home care providers:

- All services, from the drawing of venous blood samples to ventilation management, are provided in the home environment, an environment over which the home care worker has limited control.

- Caregivers, licensed nurses, rehabilitation therapists, and other types of home care workers are not directly supervised while providing services in the home and have limited access to collegial support and professional resources, which are readily available in a hospital environment.

- The extent and scope of resuscitative equipment readily available in a hospital setting is not available in the home environment.

- Home care providers must rely on the patient or caregiver to comply with instructions or directions when a home care worker is not in the home. This means that non-healthcare providers are often responsible for suctioning, medication administration, turning and positioning, wound and ostomy care, and other elements of a treatment plan.

- A public that is very concerned about medical error can observe all provider interactions closely in the home care environment.
- The home care provider must consider the potential for community and domestic violence in every setting.

The risk management considerations discussed in this chapter are applicable to any type of healthcare services delivered in the home environment.

· · · · · · · · ·

RISK MANAGEMENT CONSIDERATIONS

The home healthcare environment has grown to be a complex healthcare delivery system that presents significant issues for risk management professionals and includes, but is not limited to, standards of care and duty; outcomes predictability and management; corporate liability; employment and supervision; safety and security; contracts, antitrust, fraud, and abuse; and marketing and advertising activities. Each home health agency should have an enterprise-wide risk management program with a risk manager, policy/procedures, and loss prevention education for all agency staff.

Standards of Care and Duty

The types of legal actions related to this aspect of home healthcare are not dissimilar to those experienced in acute care facilities. Although specific tort law varies from jurisdiction to jurisdiction, home health providers have the same duty to render the degree of care that any healthcare professional with the same training would provide under the same or similar circumstances in the same manner as hospital providers do. Whether the standard of care has been met in an individual case is established by expert testimony based on current professional standards for the same or a similar condition; the agency's internal policies, procedures, and protocols; and standards established by federal and state agencies pursuant to statute. On a national basis, Medicare regulations establish standards for all home health agency interactions with Medicare beneficiaries.

Relevant standards have also been published by professional associations, such as the National Association for Home Care and Hospice (NAHC),[2] a trade association that represents the interests of home care agencies, hospices, and home care aide organizations. This association reviews and approves home care standards for the industry. Standards for physicians, respiratory therapists, registered nurses, vocational nurses, mental health workers, rehabilitation specialists, and other licensed professionals are also established by state regulations governing each profession.

Even though these requirements vary, they may be used in a determination of fact in a negligence claim; thus it is important for each home care worker and provider to be aware of applicable regulations and private organization standards that might pertain to them. Home health nurses should be familiar with their states' nurse practice act, and the organizations that they work for should keep them aware of any pertinent changes both in the organization's own operating policy/procedures and in the relevant practice act and state regulations. Internal guidance documents should be reviewed routinely to ensure that they adequately address local, state and federal practice requirements and that there are no inconsistencies. All new staff should be oriented to these requirements, and the orientation should be documented and regularly monitored by agency management.

A list of home care professional associations and federal regulations are listed at the end of this chapter.

Outcomes Predictability and Management

Individualized goals should be established for each client and monitoring performed to determine patient response and whether changes to the care plan are necessary. For long-term home care clients, an assessment of outcomes should be conducted at least monthly and documented. There should also be routinely documented discussions of communication with the client, his or her family, and the client's physician. Care plan outcomes should be based on realistically achievable goals for each client; establishment of unrealistic goals may make the care plan itself the basis of negligence allegations.

Intermittent contact with clients and the unpredictability of alternative caregiver ability contributes to potential misunderstanding and or failure to implement necessary interventions. These characteristics of home healthcare can make it difficult to achieve the goals specified by individualized care plan. Nonetheless, outcome management as part of a continuous quality improvement program needs to be a part of each client's service, with ongoing assessment of outcomes and changes to the care plan when outcomes are not being met. Education of both client and any alternative caregiver is essential to achieving outcomes. It should be methodically provided, repeated as necessary, and documented by the home health worker.

Corporate Liability

The regulatory and litigious nature of healthcare make home health agencies vulnerable to the same type of corporate liability claims as any healthcare organization, and so it is vital for home health agencies to undertake the same proactive loss prevention activities as a matter of course. The increase in scrutiny of home care's self-monitoring processes[3] and the increase in growth of home health services are factors that drive the importance of developing and implementing an enterprise risk management (ERM) program.

Civil corporate liability claims may involve such allegations as breach of the covenant of good faith, negligent supervision and/or hiring, negligent credentialing, negligent staffing, and so forth. These types of allegations enable plaintiffs to discover information that might not otherwise be available to them in a garden variety negligence action, such as the organization's billing processes, budgeting, executive pay, hiring and disciplinary practices, expenses, and revenues. Another important implication of such actions for the risk management professional is that corporate liability claims require time-consuming review of company policies, procedures, financial statements, financial audit reports, marketing and advertising processes, and other business documents and activities that were applicable during the time frame alleged in the lawsuit. The potential need to produce these items at a much later date illustrates the importance of a well-organized approach to maintaining key organizational documents. In addition, home health agencies are at risk for civil, criminal, and administrative actions in fraud and abuse complaints and IRS or Medicare/Medicaid investigation into accounting and allocation methods.

Employment and Supervision

As previously noted, because home health workers typically work alone, it is incumbent upon a home care agency to use care in interviewing, orientation, training, and supervision processes. The goal of these processes must be clinical proficiency and knowledge, as well as critical thinking skills to facilitate effective problem identification and resolution. Home health workers must be particularly trustworthy, able to communicate with and educate patients and family effectively, and demonstrate reliable clinical skills and judgment.

Basic competencies for each level of worker must be established by the home care agency and used to assess a candidate during an interview. Prior to the interview, for example, the candidate might be asked to complete a checklist indicating the number of times a specific skill or task has been performed in the past year and in the past five years. This document should also contain a provision stating that information provided by the candidate will be used in the determination to hire. Of course, this document does not replace, although it might be the basis for, substantive reference checks.

Regulations that establish hiring requirements in specific areas should be followed. In at least one area, the home agency might even be well served to exceed these requirements. For example, regardless of whether or not a specific state requires a criminal background check on home health workers, criminal and background checks should be performed on each candidate. This process should include verifying that the candidate is not listed on the national sexual offender Web site. Otherwise, the employer risks charges of negligent hiring and retention. The candidate should be advised orally and in writing that employment is contingent on passing this related screening. It is also necessary to check the driving record of candidates when the worker will be using his or her own automobile to drive to and from a patient's home. Common checks performed before hiring a home health provider are as follows:

- Criminal background checks, including fingerprint checks, on applicants for positions involving direct patient care or as required by state statute
- Verification of current residence address and phone number
- Verification of professional licenses and certifications
- Contact of references for personal testimonial
- Contact of previous employers for a period of at least ten years

- Verification of education credentials
- Review of board hot sheets and other professional board notices on problematic professionals

The ability to work without supervision, solve problems effectively, and use good judgment in decision making are critical skills for home care workers. These skills can best be facilitated via a mentoring program. Regardless of their role, no new employees should work alone in the home environment until a qualified mentor has directly observed their work and confirmed that they have the skills necessary to perform their duties without direct supervision. The home care agency may facilitate the hire of qualified individuals by stating a preference in their advertisement for candidates with at least one year of experience in a medical-surgical acute care environment and at least five years of experience in home healthcare. During the interview, it is important to consider the reasons why the person left the most recent job and to ask questions designed to reveal the quality of their decision making, communication skills, and clinical judgment. Vignettes can be very helpful in assessing provider judgment.

Finally, a preemployment physical examination pertinent to the worker's job description and essential functions, such as lifting and moving patients and equipment, should be performed and the candidate advised orally and in writing that their employment is contingent on passing this examination unless reasonable accommodations can be made for any existing disability, according to the Americans With Disabilities Act (ADA).[4] The physical exam should be thorough, and the medical provider who performs it must take into consideration the essential job functions that the worker will be required to conduct safely. The exam should also be specific enough to allow the employer to determine whether the person is physically capable of performing the requirements of the job or to determine reasonable accommodations that might be needed. If the person is deemed unable to perform the essential functions of the job for which he or she applied, and no accommodations are possible, employers would be within their rights to rescind the job offer.

Once a home health worker is hired, the next step should be a thorough orientation to policies and procedures, the company compliance plan, and policies concerning protection of privacy and confidentiality in the home care environment. The range of subjects that should be covered in new hire orientation can be found below.

- Company information and company organization chart
- Supervisory structure and communication with and responsibility of supervisors
- Corporate compliance plan requirements
- Quality improvement plan requirements
- Risk management program requirements
- Privacy and confidentiality in home care
- Company employment practices and policies
- Company operations policy/procedure manual
- Injury and illness prevention program

- Workplace violence prevention policy
- Patient safety
- Standards of care and scope of practice for professional staff
- Standards of care and scope of responsibility for nonprofessional staff
- Documentation standards in home care
- Providing care in the private home and its idiosyncrasies and considerations
- Essential reporting, including incidents, elder and dependent adult abuse, equipment failure

Periodic assessment of medical record documentation and case outcomes should be conducted by supervisors, as should periodic home visits with employees to observe their skills.

Educational in-service programs and attendance at external continuing education programs for professional staff should be supported by management as a means of maintaining and improving skills and knowledge among staff. In addition, a "back to basics" in-service program should be conducted annually for certified and noncertified home health workers to ensure that they keep their skills current. Documentation of courses attended and any related skill checklists should be kept for at least seven years in the personnel file of each employee, although the retention period of such documentation may be longer according to state law or provider agency policy.

The U.S. Department of Labor has established employment standards for the home healthcare industry under the wage and hour standards in the Fair Labor Standards Act (FLSA).[5] These standards apply to persons employed in domestic service in households. In particular, they affect nurses, certified nurse aides, home healthcare aides, and other individuals who provide home healthcare services. Domestic service employees who reside in the patient's house where they are employed are entitled to the minimum wage, but may be exempt from the act's overtime requirements. There are also wage and hour requirements for people who perform companionship services, such as housework, meal preparation, bed making, clothes washing, and other similar personal services. Patients and families should be made aware of these requirements and any exceptions allowable by law. Copies of wage and hour publications may be obtained by contacting the nearest office of the Wage and Hour Division listed in most telephone directories under U.S. Government, Department of Labor. Note, however, that registered nurses are exempt from the FLSA wage requirements where their time is spent in the performance of duties of a nurse, and they are paid on a salary or fee basis as defined by regulations, 29 C.F.R, Part 541.

Safety and Security of the Home Environment

Home health workers are exposed to greater frequency and severity of injuries than other professionals by the inherent difficulty of controlling their work environment. Nearly one in twenty home health workers experience a job-related illness or injury every year according to the Bureau of Labor statistics.[6] The characteristics of home health work, including intensity and speed of work, adverse working conditions, and the necessity of motor vehicle transportation as a condition of work, may be contributors to injury in this setting; for example, the necessity of single-person lifting and moving of patients from their bed, the toilet, their chair, and their bathtub contribute to back, muscle, and ligament injury. The home health professional also risks falling due to household clutter, tight work areas in small rooms with a lot of equipment. Characteristics of the physical environment such as broken concrete on the sidewalk or inclement weather outdoors may also result in injury to the home health worker attempting to access the patient's home while juggling equipment, paperwork, and bags of medical supplies.

Workers alone in remote locations or high-crime areas, including gang territories, may also encounter weapons wielded by patients, family, and/or their friends. Such circumstances clearly increase the chance that a home care provider will be the victim of violence. Workplace violence is defined by the Occupational Safety and Health Administration (OSHA) as violent acts directed toward workers, including physical assault, threat of assault, and verbal abuse.[7] One reference cites the odds for exposure to violence at between 7.2 and 9 times greater for home health workers with moderate to high patient contact, respectively, compared with those healthcare workers with little or no such contact.[8] Guidelines for preventing workplace violence in healthcare and social service workers are available from OSHA (OSHA 3148–01R, 2004).

It is essential that the safety and security of the home care worker and any associated issues that might affect the worker during provision of care in the home be identified in the preadmission assessment. However, even after the patient is admitted for services pursuant to a positive home safety and security assessment, the situation should be reassessed periodically and documented in the patient's home care record. A non-hospital-based home health agency should not rely upon a previous provider's home assessment, even if it is fairly recent. Instead, the new provider agency should perform its own home safety, security, and clinical assessments before admitting a new patient to the service. In addition, and where possible, home safety and security assessments should be performed by a supervisor in the agency so that if unsafe situations are noted, the supervisor will have firsthand knowledge and can work with the patient, family, caregiver, and physician to determine whether these issues can reasonably be overcome. Some of the home safety and security issues to consider are the following.

- General condition of the home environment
- Presence and type of heating, such as wall, space, or central heating
- Presence of air conditioning or installed and/or free-standing fans
- Presence of throw rugs and their condition, and condition of floors in all living areas
- Presence or absence of hot running water and working toilets
- Presence and condition of stairways
- Size and location of patient room within the house
- Adequacy of electrical sockets and source if healthcare equipment is to be used
- Presence or absence of smoke and carbon monoxide detectors and fire extinguishers

- Type and adequacy of lighting in and around the home
- Recent communicable infection of a family member

If deficiencies cannot be corrected, it might be possible for the home care supervisor to construct a workaround plan, which should be developed with the input of the physician and the patient or caregiver. The elements of this plan will depend on the medical condition of the patient and the effect that the identified concern has on the patient's safety and recovery. After consideration, it might be that the only safe environment for the patient is in a skilled nursing or other type of care facility. Medical record documentation of all pertinent discussions is important to support the approach taken.

In addition to the home safety assessment identified above, security of the home and surroundings should be assessed, including but not limited to the following elements:

- Behavioral history of the patient and family members to determine if there have been any past violent behaviors
- Presence and types of locks on doors and windows
- Presence of a working telephone with a listing of emergency numbers for fire, police, physician, hospital, poison control center, and pharmacy
- Presence of firearms in the house, and the ability or nonability to secure them
- Adequacy of outdoor lighting, such as streetlights, porch lights, and alcove lights
- Parking availability adjacent or close to the patient's house or apartment, and lighting in parking areas
- Characteristics of the neighborhood, such as high crime, multiple neighborhood gangs, known drug houses
- Proximity of shrubs and bushes where people might hide.

If the area is determined to be unsafe, a similar approach to that delineated for management of in-home hazards should be taken, including discussion among the home care agency supervisor, the patient's physician, and the patient and caregiver. If an adequate workaround plan is not possible because of the extent of safety and security issues, the patient's physician and patient must be advised that the patient cannot be admitted to home care services. Potential alternative arrangements should then be identified, such as a skilled or assisted living facility or a licensed board and care facility. It may be possible to provide home care services in those settings, until they are no longer needed.

Common sense dictates that, in addition to evaluations and interventions to make sure the environment is safe for a home care worker, it is desirable to share specific guidelines with any new patient or caregiver. These guidelines should particularly address the requirement that firearms and illegal drugs are not allowed in the home while the home care worker is on the job and that there is zero tolerance for any verbal or physical abuse toward the worker by anyone in the home. The home care worker should also make clear that, in addition to the patient, it is desirable to have others present during the visit. Finally, and to the extent possible, it is preferable and less risk-prone to have a home health aide be of the same gender as the patient.

All healthcare providers should ensure that their employees receive comprehensive initial orientation and annual retraining in personal and patient safety and that they demonstrate proficiency after receiving this education and before being sent into the workplace. Part of this ongoing education should include providing employees with a personal safety risk assessment tool and teaching them how to react if they are confronted with a hazardous situation. It is reasonable to develop a threat analysis for some locales, with a response plan for the employee and agency to follow if a personal safety issue arises. Home health workers should be provided by their agency with a means of contacting the agency in an emergency, such as a cell phone, and a code to alert management to the situation so that the proper immediate intervention and assistance can be provided. It is also recommended that any and all events of a personal threat and incidences of actual violence be reported by the worker to the agency promptly so that adequate management and psychotherapeutic support can be provided and a determination made as to how or if the agency can continue to provide services to the patient.

From both an employee and patient loss control standpoint, the cell phone can be an important piece of equipment if properly used in the home care setting. Having a cell phone will allow the worker to call the office or the physician when medically necessary in a timely manner and not necessitate the worker using the patient's phone. A cell phone will allow confidential conversations because the healthcare worker will have the flexibility to call from outside the house, his or her own car, or other location. From an employee perspective, having a cell phone is thought of as not only a time-saver but as a safety outlet. Because home healthcare workers are often not able to choose the location of their patient population, many find themselves in less than desirable neighborhoods.

Workers should be encouraged to call the agency before and after visits when working in neighborhoods that are risky or where the patients and families are difficult. Patient safety is important in home care, but worker safety is equally important. Protocols for the use of cell phones should be developed and implemented. Although their focus is on the larger societal problem of crime, local law enforcement agencies can also be a source of information for home care providers about safety and prevention of or response to a violent situation. Specifically, the community liaison officer may be available to provide related education.

Home care supervisors should also have an open door policy to ensure that workers feel comfortable expressing concern about their personal safety, either in a patient's home or going to and from their work assignments. Even with all these systems in place, the agency should rigorously analyze all incidents and analyze trends for any patterns concerning existing or potential hazards that might result in harm to patients and workers so that appropriate corrective action can be taken to prevent the same or similar situation from recurring.

Defensive driving and driver safety instructions should also be provided to home health workers. In addition, home health workers should notify their automobile insurers if their private cars are to be used for business purposes. Many carriers require that the agency develop and implement a business automobile safety program to reduce the potential for accidents and injuries on the job. As a condition of employment, the agency should require all workers to provide a copy of their driver's licenses and certificates of insurance, with limits that meet predetermined requirements for coverage. As previously noted, each worker's driving history should be reviewed prior to employment and periodically thereafter. Reports to facilitate this process can be obtained from the state or local department of motor vehicles or similar agency. Most state laws permit employers to obtain and use this information to determine whether workers can use their own autos for business or to provide such information to the employers' auto liability carriers for underwriting purposes.

If home health workers must transport patients in their private autos for any reason, their auto policies should cover both driver and any passengers for bodily injury and medical claims. Because most private auto insurance policies do not include significant limits for bodily injury, a preferable approach is for the agency to purchase its own auto liability coverage, including such limits. This strategy can help the agency avoid becoming the "deep pocket" in a lawsuit that might arise from an accident in which a third party was injured. Such coverage should also apply to company-owned vehicles that workers use to transport patients or conduct other business.

All home care workers should be aware that they must contact their supervisors immediately if they are injured on the job, and they must be aware of what initial paperwork to complete and how to submit that paperwork. They should also be required to carry all initial injury reporting paperwork with them in the field so that it is readily available for them to complete. The agency should also be prepared to pick up injured workers and transport them to a designated provider for evaluation and treatment, if the circumstances of the injury indicate this is called for.

Home health managers should also orient staff to the applicability of workers' compensation benefits in their specific state, to report an injury, and how to access related services.

Policies and Procedures

It is important that home health services have both operational and clinical policies and procedures to which all employees are trained. When the services are part of a larger institution, the home health policies and procedures must be individualized to address the unique characteristics of the home healthcare environment. To ensure that all policies and procedures are practical and relevant to the changes in the industry, they must be routinely reviewed and revised, with clinical staff involved in the process of review for clinical procedures.

There continues to be some misperception among providers that it is better not to have procedures, because if there are no procedures, it will be harder for a plaintiff to prove a case. In fact, reasonable care must be rendered, even in the absence of policies, and it is much harder to achieve consistency of approach without them. Also, courts expect that there will be internal policies and procedures relevant to the case under their consideration, and a jury might be instructed to find corporate negligence if there are none. The following are recommended processes to ensure that policies, procedures, and protocols are current:

- Have a system in place for multilevel and multidisciplinary review of newly drafted documents before they are implemented. This review can be as in-depth or cursory as the content requires. It is nonetheless a vital step to ensure that the new policy, procedure, or protocol reflects current standards and is easy to understand and follow. Review should also assure that a monitoring and accountability process is written into the policy.

- Ensure that there is at least a biannual review process for all policies, procedures, and protocols, both administrative and operational.

- If possible, establish an electronic database of retired, new, and existing policies, procedures, and protocols. Even if an electronic database is used, all original policies, procedures, and protocols must be retained according to the agency's record retention policy so that they are retrievable for regulatory review or in the event of a lawsuit.

- Ensure that all policies, procedures, and protocols have the most recent review date noted on the document.

- Ensure that outdated policies are archived separately from those that are current to prevent staff confusion. Archiving is also important because it helps to establish in litigation that the staff members were not using outdated protocols.

- Ensure that new or revised documents are distributed to all applicable workers for review and that there is a mechanism for identifying who has received a copy. A governing policy should require any employee who receives a policy, procedure, or protocol to document that they have read and understand it. They should also confirm in writing that they agree to follow it and to advise management when they are unable to follow it for any reason.

- Implement a mechanism for new hires to become familiar with all existing administrative and operational policies, procedures, and protocols.

- Ensure that monitoring is carried out to determine whether policies, procedures, and protocols are being followed, and involve the staff in this monitoring activity. Such involvement of the staff enhances their understanding of the rationale for policies, and they can be credible advocates to promote enforcement.

- Implement a mechanism for alerting employees to policies, procedures, or protocols that have been revised. Ensure that there is a training session to familiarize them sufficiently with the changes.

- Ensure that there is a process for attaching an applicable policy, procedure, or protocol to an incident report so that the document can be reviewed for relevance and proper action taken where necessary.

Contracts, Antitrust, Fraud, and Abuse Concerns

The home healthcare industry has been scrutinized by federal agencies for fraud and abuse in referral and billing practices for many years. The following are some areas of exposure for home health agencies.

- Exclusive contracts
- Hospital referral arrangements
- Monopolization of home care services in a particular locale
- Certain mergers and acquisitions
- Network price fixing or market allocations
- Predatory practices
- Deep discounts to health systems
- Management contracts

It is an important part of corporate responsibility to develop and implement a compliance plan, and having such a plan is a condition of participating (CoP) in federal reimbursement programs.[9] To minimize exposure of the agency to federal and state fraud investigation, fines, sanctions, and federal lawsuits, the agency must:

- Develop standards of conduct to which all staff are trained and monitor compliance with these standards.
- Implement a conflict of interest statement that all employees of the agency, including executive management, signs, subsequently placing the original in their personnel files.
- Develop and implement a compliance program that sets forth acceptable, legal, and accurate practices for billing and referrals.
- Keep accurate records of billing disputes and corrective actions.
- Implement identity theft surveillance, detection, and resolution processes to protect the identity of clients.
- Keep accurate records of patient referrals from referral sources and to, for example, laboratories, dialysis services, infusion services, pharmaceutical services, and durable medical equipment companies.
- Ensure that no outside services in which an agency director, officer, physician, or staff member has any financial interest are used by the home health agency.
- Have all contracts and affiliation agreements reviewed and approved by legal counsel before they are executed.
- Ensure that all contracts between the agency and other entities include provisions that require that entity to bill separately and to provide evidence of adequate liability coverage, as defined by the agency. Other important contractual provisions include hold-harmless and indemnification provisions, which make clear that the contractor is responsible for the actions of their employees, directors and officers, agents, and subcontractors.
- Ensure that there is a process for obtaining and reviewing the use plan, including preauthorization requirements, of the managed care companies that contract with the home health agency.

- Develop and implement a comprehensive process for identification and reporting of false claims to the applicable governmental agency and to prevent billing errors on the part of the home health agency.

- Develop a process for prompt, thorough investigation of alleged illegal or unethical misconduct by corporate directors, officers, employees, independent contractors, consultants, and licensed professionals.[10]

Marketing and Advertising

To avoid allegations of fraudulent misrepresentation, breach of contract, breach of the covenant of good faith in advertising or other related claims, the home health agency must establish a process requiring legal or risk management review and approval of any advertisements and promotional materials generated by marketing and public relations representatives, whether employed or independently contracted.

Fraudulent advertising and fraudulent misrepresentation are legal claims that, in many states, are associated with the potential for punitive damages that are rarely covered by liability insurance carriers and, where they are not covered losses, must be paid out of the defendant's pocket.

It is not unusual for friction to develop between marketing and legal counsel or risk management when language changes to templates are recommended, but the potential exposure makes it imperative that risk management or legal counsel be the ultimate decision maker regarding propriety of advertising-related language and phrasing. (Refer to Chapter 5 on advertising liability in Volume 3 of this series for other related considerations.)

· · · · · · · · ·

CLINICAL CONSIDERATIONS

The acuity of patients discharged for posthospital care has increased in conjunction with emphasis placed by federal and private payers on decreasing lengths of stay in the acute, subacute, and skilled setting. It is therefore vital that reasonable steps be taken to ensure that each patient is a suitable candidate for home healthcare services and to consider the other clinical issues of home healthcare that have risk management implications.

Admission Process

Intake criteria pertaining to patient selection are essential and should include an assessment of the patient, the home environment, and the ability of a family member or friend to care for the patient in the home worker's absence (Refer to Box 16.1.) A review of physician orders for home healthcare and an assessment of the patient's care needs and level of acuity are also essential.

This approach will help the home health provider determine whether or not the patient is suitable for home care and, if so, what level of worker and expertise is needed. For example, if a family has a brain-damaged infant on a ventilator, a registered nurse

BOX 16.1   Checklist for Patient Referral to Home Health[*]

General Information:

Patient name, date of birth, and medical coverage

Diagnoses for home care

Other diagnoses

Anticipated length of care

In-home relatives or friends

Significant others, including DPOA-HC

Personal Care Needs:

Ambulation

Hearing/sight impairment

Bathing

Housework/meals

Dressing

Medication adherence

Feeding

Toileting

Transport for appointments

Requested Ancillary Care:

Registered nurse

Physical therapist

RN specialist

Occupational therapist

Licensed vocational nurse

Speech therapist

Home health aide

Nutritionist/dietician

Meal delivery

Social worker

Wound care specialist stoma specialist

Dialysis specialist

Enteral/parenteral nutrition therapy specialist

Situations in Which Physician Wants to Be Called:

Parameters for calling re: vital signs, test results, change in condition, noncompliance

Reasons specific to diagnosis

Noncompliance or abusive behavior

Injury the patient may have incurred in an unusual event

Contact Information for Physician:

Physician name, phone number, and specialty

Office hours

Pager number

Office and fax numbers

After-hours phone number

Coverage when physician unavailable

Orders for Care:

Medication dosage, route of administration, frequency, start date, and stop date if applicable

Diet; nutritional counseling

Necessary tests and date due

Infusion therapy, if needed, with specifics on type of IV fluid and rate, any agent to be infused, with dosage and frequency, start date, and, if applicable, stop date

Rehab services, if needed; type and frequency

Care specific to diagnoses, such as wound care, ostomy care, catheter care, etc.

---

[*]*Source:* Adapted from S.L. Montauk, MD, "Home Health Care," *American Family Physician. 1988,* 53(7), Table 5.

with pediatric and ventilator experience will be needed to provide services and periodic visits by a respiratory therapist might be necessary to maintain the equipment or to change settings as ordered by the physician.

Before accepting a patient, the home health provider must obtain information about the pertinent diagnoses, prognoses, and current condition, including clinical and psychological needs. To determine this information, a record of previous hospitalization, the treatment plan, and the physician orders must be reviewed carefully. Physician orders must specify exactly what healthcare services are to be provided, the duration of treatment, and the most suitable professional to provide the treatment, for example, registered nurse, licensed vocational nurse, occupational therapist, physical therapist, and so on. In addition, the home health provider should ensure that the orders for service meet Medicare, Medicaid, managed care plan, or insurer requirements for reimbursement. The prerequisites for Medicare entitlement to home healthcare are the following.

- The patient is under the care of a physician, and a plan of care is rendered under the guidance of this physician.
- The patient requires skilled nursing, occupational therapy, physical therapy, or speech therapy on an *intermittent* basis, and their needs can be met on this basis (defined as no more than twenty-eight hours/week or eight hours in a given day and occurring at least every sixty days). These elements can be extended in some cases, but only with Medicare fiscal intermediary review and acceptance.
- The patient qualifies for Medicare.
- Care is medically necessary and reasonable.
- The patient is homebound.
- The patient resides in a home or facility that does not provide skilled care.

The patient's home health record should reflect whether there is an advance directive or living will, and if so, should contain a copy of it. Every home worker who provides services must be aware of the patient's wishes as expressed in an advance directive or living will. In addition, if there is a durable power of attorney for healthcare (DPOA-HC), a copy should be placed in the patient's home care record with names and contact numbers for all the agent(s) that hold the power of attorney or serve as designees for an advance directive. If there is no healthcare directive such as an advance directive, the agency should arrange a conversation between the home health nurse, the patient, and his or her significant family to discuss the importance of having such a document. The physician should be kept apprised of such discussions, and his or her involvement sought when appropriate.

Once a patient has been accepted into the home health service, the home health provider has a duty to follow the attending physician's orders and communicate any changes in the patient's condition to the attending physician. If the orders are not clear, or if the service provider or the professional staff have any questions or concerns about applicability of an order to the home environment or to the patient after an assessment of needs has been performed, these must be communicated to the physician and resolved before home care service is initiated.

It is essential that the service providers who accept the patient for home care can provide the services ordered. If they cannot, the service providers must not accept the patient into their service.

The worst possible scenario for both patient and agency occurs when the patient is found to be inappropriate for home care after the case is opened and has to be discharged from the service. Often in such situations, the patient must return to a higher level of care. This is clearly disruptive to the patient and the family, and it is no surprise that this result often leads to significant dissatisfaction. In addition, admitting a patient who does not meet the basic admission criteria increases the exposure of the healthcare provider to liability if an adverse outcome results.

Denial of Admission

Denials of admission to home care services should not be undertaken lightly, because they could result in allegations of discrimination or wrongful denial of service. Denial might also anger the family or patient enough to bring a malpractice suit alleging negligence regarding an unrelated clinical matter.

- Location of the patient's home must be within the service provider's geographic service area as approved by their licensing authority.
- Availability of clinical staff and expertise to meet the patient's needs.
- Availability of capable family support if the patient is unable physically, mentally, or emotionally to provide for his or her own care needs.
- Ability of family/caregiver to comprehend and follow instructions for home care and/or to operate any medical devices that might be in use.
- Available working utilities (gas, electric, phone), and evidence that the utility companies have been advised of any equipment the patient needs that must remain operative during a utility interruption.
- Evidence that emergency transport services in the patient's locale have been notified if the patient is using any life-support equipment in the home.
- Safe and reasonably secure home environment that is adaptable to the patient's needs.

By providing clear information about assessment and denial processes, orally and in writing, to new referrals, with a copy to the physician, the organization may limit this exposure. If a preadmission denial becomes necessary, it must be criterion based and not subjective. It must also be communicated to the patients, their families, the referral sources, and the patients' physicians, if those physicians are not the referral source. The notice should be both oral and in writing, identifying the reason(s) for denial and recommending any viable alternatives.

Every reasonable effort should be made to work through issues that might give rise to a preadmission denial before one is issued. To the extent possible, the admission assessment and determination of suitability for service should be performed within one business day of case referral, and denial issued within seventy-two hours of that assessment. Time frames beyond that period might be construed as producing a delay in service, which could expose the home health provider to a lawsuit. A grievance and complaint process should be in place to handle any appeal of a preadmission denial, but those appeals should be few and far between if there has been effective communication with the patient and family, and the reasons for the denial are applicable to the specific case.[11,12]

Withdrawal of Home Health Services for Cause

Before initiating home care services, it is essential to provide the patient or family with information on the agency's policy regarding discontinuing care for cause. Examples of circumstances that might trigger such discontinuation, and that should be communicated prior to the inception of the care relationship, include noncompliance with caregiver instructions, abusive behavior, drug or alcohol use or other behaviors adverse to the patient's health and welfare or the staff's safety, presence of weapons in the home, barriers to home access, safety hazards in the home, nonpayment of invoices, and the potential need for a change in service level if the agency does not have services that the patient requires. In addition, advise the patient and family of the agency's patient rights and responsibilities as well as the agency's procedures regarding withdrawal of home health services, and provide documentation that mirrors these items.

When it appears that it may be necessary to terminate services for cause, unless there are circumstances that would immediately jeopardize the safety of a home care worker, services should continue until the home health provider discusses the issues of concern with the patient, patient's family, and physician. All reasonable actions should be taken to resolve the issues. Should there still be a need to withdraw services, despite remedial actions, other steps should also be taken to avoid allegations of abandonment or other malfeasance. These include working with the patient's physician to ensure continuity of care through referral to another home health provider as evidenced by a letter of acceptance and obtaining a release from the patient or patient representative. Discussions with the physician, patient, responsible party, and pertinent family members regarding the withdrawal of services should be thoroughly and objectively documented in the patient record.

Confidentiality and Privacy

Both state and federal laws protect the confidentiality of medical records and protected health information (PHI). These laws restrict the use and release of certain health information and contain safeguards and restrictions regarding the disclosure of medical records. Home health providers should obtain the advice of a qualified attorney regarding compliance with state and federal laws that cover patient privacy and confidentiality. Home health workers should be aware of the use and disclosure requirement contained within the Health Insurance Portability and Accountability Act (HIPAA/HITECH) Privacy and Security Rules. To mitigate exposure to fines, sanctions, and criminal or civil actions related to improper use and disclosure of protected health information, the agency must do the following:

- Develop confidentiality and privacy policies and procedures.
- Educate staff about HIPAA/HITECH and state laws relative to privacy and confidentiality of patients and patient records.
- Have each home health worker, regardless of level, sign a confidentiality statement.
- Monitor for staff compliance with confidentiality policies and procedures by periodic random concurrent and retrospective auditing.
- Obtain consent to allow for disclosures.
- Establish documentation, record management, and record release procedures that are designed to protect patient records, including the requirement not to transport patient records back and forth in a worker's private auto, and protection of patient records from unauthorized use or disclosure while in the home.

Please see Chapter 16, Volume 3 for more information on HIPAA/HITECH.

Informed Consent and Informed Refusal

Most experienced healthcare professionals understand the importance of consent; however, some might not be able to distinguish between two important types of consent. First, home health providers must have established policies and procedures and forms related to obtaining *general* consent for routine home care services such as medication administration and ostomy, wound, and catheter care. The second type of consent, *informed consent*, must be obtained for nonroutine or specialized risk-prone services such as blood transfusions, renal and other dialysis services, and chemotherapy.

Informed consent is considered by judges and juries to be a process and not simply a piece of paper. A responsibility matrix for obtaining informed consent is particularly critical to help home workers remember who is responsible for ensuring that the informed consent process has taken place and is documented. The matrix should also indicate who is responsible for informing the patient of the risks, benefits, indications, and contraindications of the procedure, as well as who is to obtain the patient or legal representative's signature on the informed consent form, which is used to memorialize the information given and the consent provided.

Before the patient signs the consent, the responsible individual should verify that the patient has received information on which to base consent from the appropriate caregiver and has no further questions. If anyone other than the patient will sign the form, it is essential to verify the identity of any designated legal representative. There should be documentation in the medical record indicating that this individual is responsible for giving consent when the patient cannot give it, for example, when their decision-making ability is incapacitated or the patient is a minor. That person must receive the same information on risks, benefits, indications, and contraindications for the procedure that the patient would receive if they were of age or competent and capable of understanding.

The authorized agency representative may explain information necessary to obtain the general consent for treatment, but the physician must provide information to the patient about the risks and benefits of specific risk-prone services. It is the depth, clarity, and understandability of the information provided that is questioned in a court of law, not just whether a signature was obtained. Informed consent is generally considered to be based on the following:

- The type of and purpose for the treatment
- The general and specific risks and benefits of the treatment
- Alternatives to the treatment and the associated risks and benefits of alternative therapies
- Consequences of refusal

Note that any competent adult has the right to refuse a treatment without refusing all services. For example, home health services should not be withdrawn because the patient refuses a recommended placement of a catheter or some other aspect of treatment. However, this refusal should be informed, meaning that the care provider should disclose to the patient or the patient's legal representative the possible consequences of not allowing the recommended treatment. If the patient's physician is not already aware, the agency should ensure that the physician is notified and that any alternative approach is discussed with the patient or the patient's legal representative.

There may be occasions in which a patient's informed refusal interferes with the agency's duty to provide care. When all reasonable efforts have been made to help the patient understand the possible risks associated with refusing alternatives have been assessed with the patient and physician, it might be clear to the agency that there is no reasonable way to continue care and, hence, the agency would be forced to withdraw services. However, this should be an action of last resort, with clear documentation in the home health record of efforts made by the agency to avoid withdrawal. Associated interventions and follow-up documentation should reflect the principles previously discussed concerning withdrawal of services.

Finally, all activities related to consent or refusal to consent must be objectively documented in the patient's home health record. Please see Chapter 4 on informed consent for more information on informed refusal and consent.

Medical Equipment

Equipment for use in home care, as prescribed by the patient's physician, might be provided by the home health agency or by a durable medical equipment supplier. Any time a supplier is involved, a written contract for services must be completed, including provisions that address what equipment is being supplied, when and how it is supplied, and the respective responsibilities of the agency and the supplier with regard to issues such as equipment maintenance and training. Other contract provisions should, of course, be included as discussed in Chapter 17, Volume 1, on contract review.

An important consideration for both supplier and home care agency is that each must have written procedures on the reporting of medical equipment–related patient serious injury or death pursuant to the provisions of the federal Safe Medical Device Act of 1990 (SMDA) and tracking processes for equipment as required by the SMDA.[13,14] Those workers who use medical devices and home care equipment as part of the patient's treatment plan must be thoroughly trained in the use, handling, cleaning, and adjusting of the equipment. This training is usually provided by the supplier. One element of the written contract between agency and supplier must delineate the supplier's responsibility for training of home health workers and the patient or family in the proper use of the equipment they provide. Training on new techniques or when new equipment becomes available should also be addressed.

To determine the safety and efficacy of having the patient or family be responsible for equipment during the absence of home health workers, patients and their families must receive a periodic evaluation of their knowledge and ability to operate the equipment. It is preferable for the equipment vendor to provide this training because they have the most immediate knowledge of the device involved. The medical record should contain documentation that training was done, as well as assessment of provider and caregiver skills in using the equipment and if any follow-up action is indicated, such as another training session.

The supplier must also provide preventive maintenance and have professionals experienced with the equipment available to answer questions and assist home health workers, as well as the patient and family as required. There should also be support to troubleshoot equipment problems, even after hours and on weekends. The process for these activities must be worked out and identified in the contract before it is signed.

In the preadmission home assessment, the home must be evaluated for safe use of any medical equipment. Refer to Table 16.10 for a list of Common Durable Medical Equipment. It is important to inform the local utilities if life-sustaining equipment is to be used. There should also be a request for protection in the event of rolling blackouts or other utility interruption. Grounded electrical outlets should be available because medical equipment must always be connected to this type of outlet. The amount of electricity being supplied into the household must be adequate, otherwise plugging equipment in and turning it on will result in a blown fuse. No major piece of equipment should ever be plugged into an extension cord with other electrical equipment, such as lamps, fans, televisions, irons, and so on. The home health worker assigned to the case should check to ensure that there is no fraying, splitting, or other damage to medical equipment cords, even though this is primarily the responsibility of the equipment vendor.

Common durable medical equipment includes the following.

- Ambulation aides
- Apnea monitors
- Bedside commodes and other toilet aids
- Bed triangles
- Continuous positive air pressure (CPAP) machines
- Glucose monitor
- Hand-held nebulizers
- Hospital beds, including pressure-reducing mattresses
- Intravenous and total parenteral nutrition infusers
- Lift chairs and stand-left machines
- Liquid oxygen and oxygen concentrators
- Wheelchairs
- Shower aides
- Suction machines
- Oximeters
- Transcutaneous electrical nerve stimulation (TENS) units

In the event of an equipment incident in which the patient is injured or dies, several actions must be taken in the immediate aftermath:

- Contact agency management by phone to report the incident and follow their instructions.

- Ensure no one touches any dials or changes any settings, attempts to continue using the equipment, or tests the equipment to see if it actually failed.

- Do not give the equipment to the family or the manufacturer sales representative or quality manager.

- Ensure that the equipment and all cables, cords, or other pieces are sequestered as evidence for the agency. Arrange for their immediate removal.

- Gather and sequester all preventive maintenance documentation. This information must be maintained with the incident report by the agency's risk management professional or legal counsel.

- If necessary and if a camera is available, take photographs.

- Complete an incident report in which the settings and other characteristics of the equipment at the time of the adverse event are documented, and ensure that the report is routed to the agency's risk management professional or legal counsel no later than the following business day.

- Complete an SMDA report form and route it according to procedure.

- Arrange replacement of the equipment with the equipment vendor or other approved vendor unless death has resulted.

If serious injury or death has resulted, the family will likely demand to know what happened, and they will likely be in significant distress. For the purpose of responding to these requests for information, the agency should use its disclosure policy. The home care worker should not attempt to answer specific questions, but should instead assure the family that the circumstances will be investigated by the agency. The physician should be involved, as required under the policy, and obtaining assistance from an agency social worker or mental health worker might help deal with the family's distress. However, no information about possible cause is to be released until a determination can be made, and then this information should only be released by the agency risk management professional or other designated agency manager, as addressed in the disclosure policy. The agency and equipment vendor should cooperate with each other in the investigation; however, the agency must take action to sequester the equipment so that the vendor representatives may view it but not manipulate or repair it. (Refer to Chapter 3 on biomedical technology.)

The electromagnetic energy that emanates from electronic devices, such as cell phones, has the potential to interfere with equipment operation, resulting in malfunction with potential for patient harm, including inaccurate diagnostic results.[15] All three types of cell phones (analog, digital, and personal communication service) should be treated the same in agency policies and procedures related to cell phones, as should two-way pagers, which function similarly. Walkie-talkies, which generally operate at higher power and lower frequencies when in the talk mode, might pose a greater risk of interference with patient equipment.[16] Because many others over whom the agency has no control could bring cell phones into the home care environment, it is recommended that home health agencies encourage equipment suppliers to provide equipment with a low degree of susceptibility to related interference.

Medications and Infusion Therapy

In most states, certified nursing assistants may apply topical ointments and help a patient open a vial of prescribed or over-the-counter (OTC) medication so that the patient may take it themselves. Injections and the administration of intravenous fluids are, however, within the purview of licensed nurses only. Commonly, intravenous fluids are used in the home environment to facilitate intravenous administration of antibiotics, anticoagulants, and chemotherapeutic agents. Administration of the latter should be performed only by a registered nurse or a certified registered nurse specialist who has received specific training in administration of chemotherapy. In some circumstances, chemotherapeutic agents are administered by a professional from an independently contracted infusion therapy provider.

When anyone other than the home health agency staff is to administer intravenous medications to an agency client, the agency must establish a contract with the specific organization, such as the infusion vendor. Note that the use of peripherally inserted central catheters (PICC) lines is now a common method for infusing medications and chemotherapy in the home. There are many advantages to the use of PICC lines, but there are also numerous associated risks, including catheter-related infection, accidental arterial cannulation on insertion, nerve injury, embolism, cardiac dysrhythmias, and extravasation of fluids and medications. In all states, it is legal for a licensed physician to insert the catheter; in some states, it may be within the expanded role of licensed registered nurses who have been specifically trained and certified in PICC line insertion. Because of the risks inherent to insertion and maintenance of PICC lines, only registered nurses who have been trained and credentialed should insert or maintain a PICC line.[17,18] If these individuals are the employees of an independently contracted vendor, the agency should ask for and maintain documentation of their training.

To the extent that home health workers assist with or administer medications, whether oral, injectable, parenteral, topical, suppository, or inhalation, the agency must establish competency through a medication training program. This approach should require demonstration of technique and written examination before a worker is released to perform a medication task in the home environment. Recognition of medication reactions and proper interventions, communication, and documentation of such events must be addressed in the training program. Obviously, the extent of training will depend upon individuals' certification or licensure and the length of their experience. Registered nurses who specialize in chemotherapy might merely complete a competency list indicating how many times they have administered specific agents in the past five years, and a home health aide would be trained to help a patient self-administer certain medications.

Withholding Care and Other End-Of-Life Issues

End-of-life issues of home healthcare has received significant attention over the recent past as a result of precedent-setting litigation such as in the Terri Schiavo case. The salient issue in the Schiavo case was that the patient did not have a written living will or advance directives to guide caregivers in determining her end-of-life wishes, and this ultimately led to a vehement disagreement between her husband and parents about what Ms. Schiavo would have wanted done for her.

Numerous publications and resources containing information about advance directives, use of durable power of attorney for healthcare DPOA-HC, and do-not-resuscitate orders are now readily available. With continued growth and evolution of high-technology options available for use in home healthcare, home health agencies must be increasingly cautious to ensure that patient wishes and desires related to continuation of care, resuscitative intervention, life-sustaining equipment, referrals to an acute care hospital, organ donation, and maintenance of food and fluids are documented and followed. The federal Patient Self-Determination Act (PSDA) also requires that home care providers ascertain whether advance directives exist "in advance of care provided" and to inform patients in writing of the agency's policies on advance directives and applicable state law.[19,20]

As noted in the section on admission, all home care workers assigned to the patient must be aware of the specific contents of advance directives, of the presence of do-not-resuscitate orders, and of the names and contact numbers for proxy decision makers identified in a DPOA-HC. A copy of all advance directive documents and the DPOA-HC must be inserted in the patient's home care record. However, because the entire record might not be available at the time the information is needed, the originals must be readily accessible to the home care worker in the patient's home. In addition, the presence of such documents and relevant current orders should be incorporated in the patient's care plan so that each assigned worker is aware of and follows the patient's wishes.

The home health nurse should document in clients' medical records if they state on admission that they do not have advance directives and do not wish to have them, and home health workers should reevaluate this position periodically throughout the agency's contact with patients and their families. All discussions should be supported by documentation in the home care record.[21]

To proactively address bioethical dilemmas that arise in the home care environment, it is recommended that each home health agency have contractual arrangements with bioethics consultants and legal counsel available to provide advice and direction.

Initial orientation followed by periodic updates should be provided to each employee to ensure that staff is following the agency's PSDA policies and procedures. Random record reviews should be conducted, as should staff interviews, to validate ongoing staff awareness of and compliance with PSDA requirements.

Cultural Issues in Home Care

Cultural competence is an essential skill set for all home health workers because it enables them to understand the various cultural perspectives and communications of diverse patient populations. Such skills also facilitate individualized care plans, including, where necessary, language interpretation services. Education is critical to attaining and maintaining such skills.[22]

This is particularly the case because home care providers and programs that receive federal funds are bound by the provisions of Title VI of the Civil Rights Act of 1964, which prohibits discrimination based upon a person's national origin. The law also requires reducing or eliminating cultural barriers that restrict a person from receiving effective, individualized social and health services. To avoid fines and sanctions, it is recommended that home health agencies develop and implement related policies and procedures. All staff must be educated on these policies and procedures and subsequently monitored for compliance. One of the processes put in place to ensure compliance should be a contract with a language interpreter service to ensure that interpreters for non-English-proficient patients are available when needed.

The National Center for Cultural Competence has available through its Web site a cultural competency enhancement series that can be downloaded and used to foster cultural awareness and competency of home care workers. The center can also refer home health agency administrators to other cultural competency resources where additional tools and publications can be obtained.[23,24]

Patient and Caregiver Education

Family involvement in a home care patient's life is crucial in helping patients maintain optimal mental functions and feel as though they are still a part of the family. In addition, because home care is by nature intermittent, patients usually cannot remain at home unless there is an available friend or family caregiver who can perform certain tasks for them when a home health worker is not in the home.

Despite the importance of family and caregiver involvement, however, there might be times when these individuals express discomfort with care procedures, or with seeing blood, or with handling equipment. Home health workers can ease this discomfort through teaching and mentoring activities. By demonstrating procedures, obtaining return demonstrations from caregivers, and being sensitive to their concerns, the home care provider can help them reach a point at which they are comfortable with performing the procedure themselves. The same principles, of course, apply to patient teaching.

It is important for assigned home care workers to continue supporting patients and their caregiver families or friends, until they have demonstrated their ability to perform essential care tasks independently. Many of these tasks relate to personal care, suctioning, wound care, hanging new intravenous fluids when a unit has been completed, and administering medications. Written materials on handling specific equipment or performing a specific procedure are very helpful teaching aids and also serve as the basis for documenting teaching activities in the medical record. Such documentation should include what was taught and to whom, an assessment of subsequent ability to perform the task, and whether a return demonstration shows that the patient or caregiver is competent to perform the task in the home care workers' absence.

Transporting Patients

In addition to previously discussed business automobile liability coverage that specifically covers the transport of patients in employee cars, the agency should have written policies and procedures governing how to transport patients safely. If ambulatory assistive devices also are to be transported, the employee must be oriented as to how to embark and disembark patients and their equipment from the car safely. In any case, no home care workers should transport a patient unless they have been cleared to do so by the agency management, based on approval by the agency's business automobile liability carrier and a violation-free driving record.

INFECTIOUS AND HAZARDOUS WASTE MANAGEMENT

Every home health agency should have a comprehensive infection control program that addresses surveillance, prevention, identification, reporting, and control of infections among home care employees and patients. Home health workers must be able to properly and safely handle regulated medical waste and other contaminated items, including soiled patient sheets and clothing and dressings or bandages that are contaminated with blood or other infectious materials, in accordance with applicable local, state, and federal laws. Any receptacle for the safe disposal of medical waste, including red bags and sharps containers accompanied by hazard labels, must be available on the job site for use by the home health worker. The agency should have a policy that prohibits employees from taking a patient's soiled clothing and linen to their own private homes to launder.

In addition, the agency's infection control plan should address preventing spread of infection through universal precautions and use of personal protective equipment and should address managing exposures to blood and other infectious materials. Other points that are important to address in the infection control plan include use of engineering controls to prevent sharps injuries; safe use and disposal of sharps containers; tuberculosis testing, identification, and treatment; HIV testing and prophylactic treatment; and verification of employee immunity to mumps, measles, rubella, tetanus, and diphtheria. All home care workers should know how to identify and report infections and exposures to infection control–related hazards and take proper action in the home care environment to prevent illness and injury. Provision of hepatitis B vaccine should also be provided free of charge to workers who have never had it, and any employees who defer the immunization should be approached periodically about reconsidering their decision.

Training on safety and infection control issues should be provided in terms that are applicable to the language and literacy of the workers and to their job functions. Documentation should be maintained in personnel records, with pertinent program materials, so that these items are readily available for audit by agency management and regulatory entities. Any issues associated with infections and illness or injury, whether patient or worker related, must be addressed under the auspices of the agency's quality improvement and risk management plans, with corrective action directed at prevention of the same or similar incident in the future.

Finally, compliance with all requirements of the agency's infection control program must be monitored for effectiveness. Such monitoring specifically addresses reported illnesses and injuries and incident reports from employees.

Emergency Preparedness

The home care worker will be faced with important challenges in the event of a disaster that affects the household while the assigned worker is present. The hurricanes that affected the U.S. Gulf Coast region recently have illustrated that the three-day food and water standard no longer applies. In fact, it might take much longer for local and national emergency resources to get to the affected area. As it is human nature to relegate disaster planning and emergency preparedness to a lower priority because of the relative infrequency of disasters, it is recommended that all healthcare providers, including home health agencies, ensure that adequate emergency preparedness and disaster response plans are implemented and tested at least annually.

For home care patients who are using life-sustaining equipment (ventilator-dependent or oxygen-dependent patients), it is important that local and county disaster-planning professionals know of the patient's needs so that arrangements can be made ahead of time for transportation and equipment if a natural disaster does occur. Planning is critical to ensure that the necessary services are available.

In the home care environment, the emergency preparedness plan must be designed to ensure that care continuity occurs in a disaster. This means that the assigned worker on duty at the time might well be the person who stays in the patient's home to continue the care if roadways and communications are affected. The plan should address care prioritization, equipment management in a power failure, and communication between home care workers and the home or branch office. Specific attention should be paid to major disasters and to the more common issues of fires, equipment and utility failures, and civil disturbances that might affect the particular home and locale.

Finally, the agency emergency preparedness plan must address business recovery after a major disaster or a situation that adversely affects home and branch office operations. Insurance carriers often have disaster, emergency preparedness, and business recovery staff or consultants available who can assist the agency to develop emergency preparedness and disaster plans.

Discharging Patients

Discharging a patient from care must be undertaken with a rational approach, and the assessment and interventions of the home health staff should be thoroughly documented to mitigate any allegation of abandonment or delay in service. The discharge criteria for hospice facilities are generally straightforward. When the patient dies, the care is terminated. For home health and private duty, the discharge process is more complex. Most home health discharges result from physician certification that the need for home health services no longer exists, such as when antibiotic IV therapy is discontinued or ends, when patients have returned to their preillness conditions and there is no longer a medical need for home healthcare, or when family or independently hired caregivers can take over the personal care needs of the patient.

As discussed earlier in the section on withdrawal of services, it is imperative that the home health provider ensure that patients and their families understand why they are no longer candidates for home care and that they are capable of providing for the patient's needs when home healthcare ends. Clear and realistic written discharge criteria for the agency to follow are important.

Providing the patient with a description of the discharge process on admission to the home health service will minimize misunderstanding when the time for discharge arrives. It is also recommended that aftercare instructions be written for the patient and family to help them understand what, if anything, they need to do once home healthcare ends, including when next to contact their physician. Such instruction should be signed by the patient or legal representative and a copy maintained in the patient's home care record.

A written notice of termination in or reduction of services for Medicare beneficiaries based on Medicare criteria is required for this population.[25]

Incident Identification and Reporting

If an adverse event regarding patient safety or employee injury occurs, staff should know whom to contact for immediate assistance. Subsequent reporting of such circumstances is critical to a proactive loss prevention and control program. More specifically, such a program is dependent upon early incident identification, documentation, confidential reporting, and investigation. All home healthcare workers must be trained regarding the procedures and tools that support these activities. Reportable incidents in home healthcare include, but are not limited to, the following events, in no particular order of importance:

- Incorrect procedure performed or correct procedure performed incorrectly
- Treatment provided without a physician order
- Prescribed treatment not followed
- A treatment or procedure performed is outside the scope of practice of the individual performing it
- Complaint about care or services (including billing) by patient or family
- Medication error or adverse drug reaction
- Development of infection not related to the original home health diagnoses
- Complication of treatment or procedure
- Cardiorespiratory arrest
- Exposure to blood or other potentially infectious materials
- Unscheduled admission to the hospital
- Failure to obtain proper consents
- Injury to patient or family member resulting from malfunctioning equipment

- Development of pressure ulcer or progression to stage III after care initiated
- Loss or damage to personal property
- Unsafe environment for the employee (exposure to criminal activity or weapons, verbal or physical assault by family members during visits, and so on)
- Unsafe environment for the patient (suspected abuse by employees, inadequate care-givers, patient fall, and so on)

The proper protocol for maintaining confidentiality of the documentation must be understood and followed. Incidents not witnessed by the home care worker must still be reported as soon as the worker has knowledge of their occurrence.

Risk management professionals can facilitate incident reporting by making sure that staff members understand that timely reporting is in the best interest of the patients, employees, and the organization and that there will not be punishment or retribution for reporting an incident according to established policy. It is also important that staff understand

- why reporting of incidents is important;
- what to report and required reporting time frames;
- how to report an incident and to protect confidentiality of a report and investigation notes; and
- to whom each type of incident report should be given, for example, risk management or human resources.

Other Reporting

Staff must understand the need for mandatory incident reporting that is required of the risk management professional by such oversight agencies as the department of health and the federal Food and Drug Administration (for medical device reporting where a death has occurred or a significant injury has occurred and the manufacturer is not known). Education of home care providers as to their role, the required time frames in which to report, and their assistance in reporting are vital to help the agency achieve compliance.

Particularly important with regard to external reporting requirements are any instances of suspected or actual child abuse, which must be reported to the applicable state agency. The same is true for suspected or actual elder or dependent adult abuse. Failure to report such circumstances could result in loss of the agency license to operate, or in fines and sanctions. Refer to Chapter 9 in this text on pediatrics for more information on child abuse.

All home care workers must be aware of their abuse-reporting requirements under the law, how to report, and when to report, and they should sign a document for their agency that states that they are aware of and understand their abuse-reporting responsi-bilities. The home health agency should conduct annual retraining to ensure that each worker has had an opportunity to review legal requirements for reporting suspected and actual abuse situations and to review applicable reporting responsibilities.

Medical Record Documentation

Documentation in the home healthcare record is a tool to communicate to others on the care team what care and services patients have received and how they responded. It is also a basis for an audit to ensure that care meets standards in the industry and as established by internal policy and procedure.

Documentation also plays a significant role at trial. It becomes the script in a negligence or malpractice lawsuit, at which time the documentation can either assist significantly in the defense of the case if it adequately reflects what was done for the patient or be detrimental to the case and substantiate a breach in the standard of care. In addition, sloppy and incomplete documentation, although not always specific to a complaint at hand or contributing to allegations in a lawsuit, certainly sets the stage for the plaintiff's attorney to impugn the professionalism of the care provider and makes everyone spend needless time explaining issues that might have been easily corrected.

For these reasons, documentation must be clear, concise, legible, thorough, and descriptive of events that transpire in the patient's care. In addition, each entry must be signed, dated, and the time documented. Errors in documentation may be corrected with one line drawn through the incorrect documentation. That line should be initialed and dated, and the correct information should be documented immediately below. Late entries should be kept to a minimum, and the late entry should be designated as such in the record by adding the words *Late Entry*, followed by the date and time the information is being documented. The agency should keep a log of complete signatures, updated each year, so that initials can be identified later if there is a need to do so.

. . . .

CONCLUSION

Home health services represents one of the fastest growing segments of the healthcare industry and of the United States economy.[26] The job for both licensed and unlicensed personnel can be physically demanding. This chapter has presented many of the risks and associated with delivery of healthcare and services in patient homes, as well as techniques to help the risk management professional and staff minimize the risk and promote safe care.

As the field of home care evolves, it is essential for home care providers to remain abreast of changes in regulations, standards, and guidelines in home healthcare and to network with other agencies to identify best practices that can reduce liability and enhance safety.

Suggested Readings

Schultz, J., *Criminal Background Reports; A Survey of Fifty States*. American Health Lawyers Association Washington D.C.: AHLA; 2002.

"Criminal Background Checks Continuing Care Risk Management Risk Analysis." *ECRI*, 2003, Mar: 1–11.

Equal Employment Opportunity Commission (EEOC) Policy Guidance on the Consideration of Arrest Records in Employment Decisions under Title VII of the Civil Rights Act of 1964, as amended, 42 U.S.C. §2000e et seq. (1982). Available at: www.eeoc.gov/policy/docs/arrest_records.html. (Accessed April 10, 2010.)

"Focus on Home Health Care Worker Safety." *STAT*, 2001, 16:6, 8. Published by Chubb Health Care.

Gorrie, Jan J. "Legal Review and Commentary: Failure to Provide Back-up Power Results in Death and a $450,000 Massachusetts Settlement." *Healthcare Risk Management*, 2005, 27(8): 1–4.

"Home Care Subject to Employee Safety, Workers' Comp Risks." *Hospital Risk Management*, 1993, 15(12):176–81.

Lyncheski, J. E. Esq. and Anne M. Lavelle Esq. "Facing Workplace Violence in the Health Care Industry." *ASHRM Journal*, 2002, Summer: 13–15.

Madeo, James PhD. "A Workplace Violence Prevention Program — An Investment with a Great Yield" Commentary in IRMI Risk Management. Sept, 2003. Available at: www.irmi.com/expert/articles/2003/madero09.aspx. (Accessed March 31, 2010.)

Marrelli, T. M. *Handbook of Home Health Standards and Documentation Guidelines for Reimbursement*. 2nd. ed. St. Louis: Mosby, 1994.

Montauk, S. L., MD. "Home Health Care." *American Family Physician*, 1998; 1:(58): 7.

Office of Inspector General, Department of Health and Human Services. "Compliance Program Guidance for Home Health Agencies." Washington, D.C.: Dept. of Health and Human Services, August 1998.

"Overview of Workers' Compensation." Risk Analysis. *Continuing Care Risk Management ECRI Institute*, 1994, Nov:1–18.

Rozovsky F. and L. Rozovsky. *Home Health Care Law: Liability and Risk Management*. New York: Little, Brown & Company, 1993.

Sherwin, Anne P. "Legal Issues of Concern to Home Care Providers." In: *Handbook of Home Care Administration*, edited by M. Harris. Gaithersburg, Md.: Aspen Publishers, 1994.

Endnotes

1. Sherwin, A. "Legal Considerations in Home Health Care," Chapter 49. In: Harris, M. D. *Handbook of Home Health Administration*, 5th ed. Sudbury, Mass.: Jonas & Bartlett Publishers, 2009.

2. National Association for Home Care and Hospice (NAHC). Available at: www.nahc.org.

3. Sherwin, *op. cit.*

4. Americans with Disabilities home page available at: www.usdoj.gov/crt/ada/adahom1.htm.

5. U.S. Department of Labor Employment Standards Administration.

6. U.S. Department of Labor, Bureau of Labor Statistics, October 2006. Available at: www.bls/gov. Summary 97–4, February 1997.

7. "Guidelines for Preventing Workplace Violence for Health Care and Social Service Workers," Occupational Safety and Health Administration (OSHA), 2004.

8. Canton, A. et al: "Violence, Job Satisfaction, and Employment Intentions Among Home Healthcare Registered Nurses." *Home Healthcare Nurse* 2009; 27(6):364–373.

9. Office of the Inspector General, Department of Health and Human Services. "Compliance Program Guidance for Home Health Agencies," Washington, D.C.: Dept. of Health and Human Services, August 1998.

10. "Overview of Home Healthcare Risks and Liability, Part II: Employee and Business Risk Management." ECRI Institute Hospital Risk Control. Quality and Risk Management 6 May 1996; 10.

11. Montauk, S. L. "Home Health Care." *American Family Physician* 1998; 58(12):7.

12. Health Care Financing Administration HM-11. "Medicare Standards for Home Care," Washington D.C.: Department of Health and Human Services, 1983.

13. Safe Medical Device Act of 1990 (SMDA), 21 U.S.C. §519(3) (i) as amended November 21, 1997.

14. 21 C.F.R. pt. 821 Medical Device Tracking Requirements. Available at: www.washingtonwatchdog.org/documents/cfr/title21/part821.html.

15. "Cell Phones and EMI: Frequently Asked Questions. Equipment and Technology 11.1." Continuing Care Risk Management, ECRI Institute; 2002 Nov:1–3.

16. *Ibid.*

17. "Position Paper: Peripherally Inserted Central Catheters." *Journal of Intravenous Nursing* 1997; 20(4):172–174.

18. Intravenous Nurses Society "Position Paper: Use of Unlicensed Assistive Personnel in the Delivery of Intravenous Therapy." *Journal of Intravenous Nursing* 1997; 20(2):75–76.

19. "Living Wills or Durable Powers of Attorney; Advance Directives." *Federal Register* June 27, 1995; 60(123):33262–33298.

20. *Ibid.*

21. Gates, M. F., I. Schins, and A. S. Smith. "Applying Advance Directives Regulations in Home Care Agencies." *Home Health Nursing* 1996; 14(2):127–133.

22. Nardi, D. A., and S. Siwinski-Hebel. "Cultural Issues in Home Care." *ADVANCE for Nurses* 2005; 7(12): 21–25.

23. Title VI, Civil Rights Act of 1964.

24. U.S. Dept of Health and Human Services, Office of Minority Health. "National Standards for Culturally and Linguistically Appropriate Service in Health Care: Final Report." Washington D.C., Dept. of Health and Human Services, 2001.

25. 42 U.S.C. §1395bbb(a)(1)(E).

26. Meyer, J. D. and C. Muntaner. "Injuries in Home Health Care Workers: An Analysis of Occupational Morbidity from a State Compensation Database," *American Journal of Industrial Medicine* 1999; 35(3):295–301.

17

Risk Management for Retail Clinics

Sara Ratner

THE EMERGENCE OF RETAIL CLINICS

Many healthcare experts believe that the most pervasive, and potentially the most challenging, trend in healthcare delivery today is the "retailization" of healthcare.[1] These experts predict a future in which the consumer is at the center of the healthcare system, actively making informed decisions about the course of care and treatments he or she will receive. In addition, the cost and quality of healthcare services will be known to the consumer, who will use this knowledge to select providers associated with the highest value, as shown by objective criteria.

This future is already alive and well today in many places around the country, as may be seen by the emergence and subsequent national expansion of retail clinics. First started in 2000 in Minneapolis by MinuteClinic, there are now nearly nine hundred retail clinics nationally, managed by sixty-one different operators. Typically, retail clinics are located in retail pharmacies or grocery chains; however, they also are appearing on corporate as well as college campuses, in state capitals, on malls, and within the settings of other healthcare providers.

Central to the original retail clinic model is a limited scope of services. These services vary among operators, but typically provide treatment for illnesses such as strep throat, otitis media, pink eye, and cold sores. In addition, these clinics provide certain vaccinations and screenings for important conditions such as elevated cholesterol, hypertension, diabetes, and obesity. Costs for retail clinic services range from $49 to $89 per visit, which equates to 30 percent to 50 percent less than the costs incurred during a traditional primary care office visit.[2] Most clinic operators accept insurance, including copayments that are equivalent to those paid by patients for primary care office visits.

The quality of the limited scope of services delivered in the retail setting is comparable or, in some cases, superior to the care delivered in the traditional physicians' office setting.[3] Retail clinics are staffed by certified nurse practitioners and physician's assistants who can perform many of the same functions and services as a primary care physician, such as ordering laboratory tests and writing prescriptions. State laws usually require collaborative agreements with physicians, to provide a certain amount of medical oversight.

Recently, retail clinics have begun to expand their model to include more chronic care. For example, Walgreens announced that it is beginning to offer chronic management services for type 2 diabetics.[4] Retail clinics have also begun to offer infusion services.[5] This trend provides a convenient model for efficient management of these high-cost conditions and services. As more people are diagnosed with chronic conditions, retail clinics also provide routine screenings to help increase compliance rates with evidence-based practices addressing the conditions. In addition, these settings can help improve an integrated delivery system's HEDIS® scores. This expanded practice scope, however, also introduces retail clinics to patients with more complex maladies, resulting in increased liability risk.

Retail clinics also leverage another healthcare delivery trend, the electronic medical record (EMR), which is a critical component of any healthcare organization's ability to consistently deliver high-quality care in multiple settings and/or states. Although some retail clinics use an EMR based on a traditional paper medical record, others employ EMR systems that guide the practitioner in diagnosing and treating the patient. Some of these use SOAP (subjective, objective, assessment, and plan) notes or another form of problem-oriented documentation. Often these EMRs accommodate e-prescribing, allowing a prescription to be sent electronically to the pharmacy of the patient's choice. In addition, EMRs can often generate a copy of a visit summary to be sent to the patient's primary care physician, providing valuable updates that reduce fragmentation of care. Such approaches facilitate the role of the retail clinic as an extension of the primary care office, offering the additional hours and weekend coverage needed by patients. Still another trend that EMRs facilitate is the maintenance of medical record copies by patients, who are able to upload their retail clinic visit summaries to medical information portals such as Microsoft Health Vault or Google Health.

The EMR is also an important tool for facilitating physician oversight of treatment. Supervising physicians can electronically review the visit summaries for the patients seen at the clinic to determine if appropriate care was delivered. This approach contributes significantly to quality improvement efforts and promotes practitioner compliance with evidence-based protocols. It also facilitates compliance with certain chart review functions required by state law.

· · · · · · · · ·
EXISTING LAWS GOVERNING RETAIL CLINICS

There are a myriad of existing state and federal laws that govern retail clinics, including those that regulate scope of service,[6] scope of practice,[7] entity structure,[8] self-referrals,[9] and advertising of services.[10] Some of these laws have been written to address traditional ambulatory care environments and hospitals, but they are also being applied to retail clinics because these settings are viewed as akin to physicians' offices. However, other state requirements do not apply to retail clinics. As described below, this legislative tangle makes compliance very challenging for the retail clinic operation.

Scope of Service/Practice

Each state regulates the licensing of healthcare providers operating in their state, as well as the scope of services these professionals are permitted to provide. Many states require the oversight of certain healthcare providers, such as nurse practitioners and physician's assistants. Specific regulations regarding oversight vary from state to state. For example, South Carolina requires a physician-to-nurse practitioner oversight ratio of three to one;[11] in Minnesota there is no oversight regulation;[12] and in Texas physicians are required to be on-site in the retail clinic during 10 percent of the clinic's operating hours.[13] Missouri requires that nurse practitioners "practice with the collaborating physician continuously present" for one month before practicing at a site where the physician is not continuously present.[14]

For an operator in one state, this can be complex, but multijurisdictional entities need to have systems in place to ensure compliance with vastly disparate requirements. For example, Texas's requirement that physicians be on site during 10 percent of operating hours can add significant cost to a model that is primarily staffed by nurse practitioners. Also, Missouri's scope of practice regulations require a practitioner to work in a physician's practice before working at the retail clinic. As a result, the hourly payroll cost to bring on board a new practitioner for the first month is an added cost that cannot be offset by any contribution to revenue.

Corporate Practice of Medicine Considerations

Retail clinics are typically managed by a centralized nonclinical operator. This model is inherently incompatible with the statutory or judicially developed doctrine found in many states, called *the corporate practice of medicine*. The doctrine flows from licensing statutes requiring that only a licensed individual practice medicine or nursing[15] and provides that, because a corporation cannot be licensed to practice medicine, it may not employ individuals in such a capacity. Only those entities that are formed and owned by physicians may employ physicians and/or nurse practitioners. The public policy rationale behind this is to prevent unlicensed individuals from interfering with a professional's judgment.

In states that prohibit the corporate practice of medicine, a for-profit retail clinic operator cannot directly employ healthcare professionals but may engage them only through a separate professional corporation. In these situations, the efficiencies that would otherwise be achieved by spreading administrative resources across multiple entities are likely to be lost. To avoid this result, retail clinics have two options. The first is for a medical provider to enter into a branding arrangement with a retailer and lease space so that care is provided by a professional corporation, yet it has the endorsement and cobranding of the retailer. This arrangement can be seen in several Walmart operations, in which Walmart leases space to a provider based in the Walmart store and that lessee/licensed provider receives the professional fee associated with care provided. The second way in which retail clinics can address the doctrine of the corporate practice of medicine entails a professional corporation (PC) entering into a management agreement that requires the retail clinic operator to provide a wide variety of administrative services to the PC so that it can achieve some of the efficiencies and cost savings generated by a larger management company. Under this arrangement, the management company provides nonclinical resources essential to an operation, such as space, payroll processing, billing/collecting, payer contract negotiating, equipment, and supplies. The professional corporation employs the practitioners and contracts for the collaborating physicians' oversight. However, this arrangement does not completely diffuse limitations on retail clinic operational effectiveness associated with the corporate practice of medicine doctrine because professional fees flow to the PC, not the retail clinic operator.

The corporate practice of medicine doctrine, along with certain fee-splitting statutes, also prohibits a corporation from sharing the professional fee generated by a practice. The rationale is to limit any inducement for the retail clinic to maximize profits through medically unnecessary services. To address fee-splitting concerns, the management fee may be capped at a percentage of revenue and/or, in some states, a PC may only pay the operator a flat management fee.

Fraud and Abuse Laws

Both Stark laws and anti-kickback concerns are potentially raised by certain retail clinic activities, especially those that relate to the clinic's interaction with its host store. The anti-kickback statute "prohibits the offering, paying, soliciting or receiving any remuneration in return for (1) business for which payment may be made under a federal healthcare program; or (2) inducing purchases, leases, orders or arranging for any good of service or item paid for by a federal healthcare program.[16] Remuneration includes direct or indirect kickbacks, bribes and rebates, cash or in-kind payment."[17] In this regard, the proximity of the retail clinic and its host store may be problematic because the convenience associated with proximity may induce providers to steer prescriptions to the host pharmacy. It is therefore important that any existing agreements require that all services be charged at fair market value (FMV) to dispel any implication that below-FMV payments are being made in return for prescription steerage. This strategy can help to minimize potential fraud and abuse concerns. Similarly, a less than FMV lease or administrative fee could create the potential appearance of an impropriety. It is also important for the professional corporation to appropriately disclose to the patient that the prescription may be filled at any pharmacy. This helps to reinforce the patient's freedom of choice. For more information on Stark laws, refer to Volume 3, Chapter 4, on corporate compliance.

The financial nature of the relationship with the collaborating physician also requires close attention. Collaborative agreements must specify that supervising physicians be paid at FMV, and supporting documentation of such payments can help avoid a regulator's conclusion that a payment to a collaborating physician was an attempt to drive his or her referrals. The same principle is equally applicable to physicians owning professional corporations managed by the retail clinics, because any payment they receive above FMV may create the potential for a Stark violation. Clearly, the risk management professional should ensure constant evaluation of all such agreements and the various relationships in the retail clinic setting to avoid potential fraud and abuse violations.

Other Laws and Regulations

Apart from the corporate practice of medicine doctrine, other laws also often impact licensing, advertising, privacy, payer relationships, and the scope of services that can be provided in the retail clinic setting. For example, certain states require retail clinics to obtain a certificate of need (CON) before opening a clinic.[18] The CON process typically demands an extensive filing with the state department of health and requires approval of the clinics for which applications are submitted. Licensing laws specific to retail clinics, such as those Massachusetts is endeavoring to pass, also bear watching, as will shortly be discussed later in this chapter.

As is the case for any healthcare provider today, retail clinics must comply with patient privacy laws. The protection of patient medical information housed by retail clinics is required by federal and state laws, such as the Health Insurance Portability and Accountability Act (HIPAA).[19] HIPAA requires that covered entities, including retail health providers, protect identifiable healthcare information. There are various administrative burdens associated with this mandate, such as security measures for recordkeeping, accounting of disclosures, and safeguards against disclosure. (Please see Chapter 16 in Volume 3, which addresses this topic more specifically.) Recently, the American Recovery and Reinvestment Act (ARRA) enhanced HIPAA's protections by placing greater restrictions on the use of marketing material and the sale of medical information. The applicable sections of ARRA are known as the Health Information Technology for Economic and Clinical Health Act (HITECH). Among many new mandates, HITECH requires notification of patients who may be affected by a breach of protected health information (PHI); adds specificity to HIPAA's requirement that covered entities be able to account for disclosures; and extends statutory accountability for many HIPAA requirements to business associates of covered entities.[20] All retail clinic operators must have policies and procedures in place to address HIPAA/HITECH requirements.

Although HIPAA permits multiple jointly owned covered entities to be designated as a single covered entity through affiliated covered entity (ACE) status, multistate retail clinic providers may have difficulty claiming this status.[21] This is because the designation applies to entities under common ownership or control, and clinics in corporate practice of medicine states may technically not be operating under common ownership. In order to share PHI concerning their patients, such individual entities within a larger retail organization may need to implement business associate agreements with one another.

· · · · · · · · ·

NEW RETAIL CLINIC LAWS

Current and Proposed Laws

In an effort to more closely regulate the retail clinic setting, attempts have been made to amend or otherwise modify the previously described laws and regulations. Many of these efforts potentially hamper the effectiveness of retail clinic operation. For example, some states have attempted to modify the physician/nurse practitioner supervision ratio by requiring a lower ratio of physicians to nurse practitioners.[22] Such changes may significantly impact the operation of retail clinics because they require the operator to hire or contract with a larger number of physicians, which can be quite costly. In one recent instance, Texas amended an existing statute to require that collaborating physicians be on-site 10 percent of the time, rather than 20 percent of the time.[23] Other states have attempted to prohibit the sale of tobacco where healthcare is provided, which directly impacts the retail clinics, their parent company, and/or the host because many retailers sell alcohol and tobacco.[24] In still another example of increased regulatory control, some states have excluded retail clinic settings from legislation expanding the prescribing authority of nurse practitioners or they have modified supervision ratios in settings where nurse practitioners prescribe.[25]

In contrast with what is often said to be unilateral and/or arbitrary regulation of the retail clinic setting, Massachusetts has recently become the first state to comprehensively address retail clinics. In the fall of 2007, the Massachusetts Department of Public Health (DPH) proposed regulations to address retail clinics, and these were finalized in January 2008.[26]

As background, Massachusetts had existing regulations requiring healthcare providers such as retail clinics to be licensed as a small primary care facility. One aspect of the regulations imposes certain physical plant requirements such as the location of bathrooms, certain exhaust ventilation, a janitor's closet, and a patient reception area.[27] To the extent a facility cannot meet any of the requirements, a waiver must be sought as part of the license submission. To address the environment of retail clinics, DPH's proposed regulations codified the waivers necessary to operate such clinics (termed *limited services clinics*, or LSCs, in the regulation) and imposed other operational requirements to ensure quality care.

For example, the physical plant requirements include the following:

- LSCs located on the premises of another entity are not required to provide separate exterior entrances.[28]

- LSCs located on the premises of another entity are not required to provide a separate patient waiting area or reception area that is separate from the public area of the host entity.

- Each LSC shall have a minimum floor area of 56 square feet for each examination room, exclusive of fixed case work.

- LSCs are exempt from the requirement to provide a clean supply storage room and a soiled workroom or holding room.

- LSCs located on the premises of another entity may share toilet facilities with that entity. The LSC's toilet facilities shall be reasonably proximate, based on services provided by the LSC, to the LSC's treatment area.

In addition to modifying physical plant requirements, DPH instituted operational requirements to help ensure that retail clinics operate in a manner that encourages quality and continuity of care, as well as what DPH views as an appropriate scope of services. Examples of specific requirements include the following:

- Each LSC must develop policies and procedures that identify the limited services that the LSC will provide, specify its staffing pattern, address referrals for patients whose needs exceed the clinic's services, identify and limit repeat encounters, and ensure that clinic personnel do not promote the use of services provided by the host retail location.[29]

- The LSC must maintain a roster of primary care practitioners in the area currently accepting new patients.

- Each LSC must provide a copy of the medical record of each visit to the patient at the end of the visit or as soon as available, and, with the patient's consent, provide a facsimile or electronically transmitted copy of the medical record to the patient's primary care practitioner, if any.

- If a LSC is located within a retail location that sells tobacco products, the LSC must prominently post information regarding the danger of tobacco usage, the message of which is to be determined by the department's Tobacco Control Program.

As previously noted, with this legislation, Massachusetts became the first state to enact final regulations governing retail clinics (or LSCs). Interestingly, DPH's regulations are also applicable to all healthcare providers desiring to open a limited service clinic, including integrated delivery systems, community healthcare centers, and hospital systems.

Following Massachusetts's lead, in 2008 Illinois and Oklahoma proposed legislation governing retail clinics. Illinois House Bill 5372 and Oklahoma Senate Bill 1523 were expressly drafted to apply to and govern retail clinics. Some of the provisions are consistent with Massachusetts's regulations, but others are more onerous. For example, the Oklahoma bill requires a physician to own or operate the clinic and that the clinic be accredited by The Joint Commission. The Illinois bill requires a retail clinic to obtain a permit to operate the facility, and as part of that process, the retail clinic must have its services approved by the department of public health. In addition, a physician may not supervise more than two facilities and there must be separate restrooms and a designated receptionist, neither of which most retail clinics have.

Implications of Legislation

In all legislative and regulatory initiatives involving retail clinics, there is tension between regulating the quality of care provided and encouraging or facilitating a new business model that is capable of expanding access and enhancing affordability. Because quality of patient care is of primary concern to legislators, pertinent regulations attempt to ensure continuity of care, access, appropriate triage when the scope is beyond the services provided, and adherence to practice guidelines. All of these strategies are essential to ensuring the quality of care delivered in the setting. However, other regulations, such as those that prohibit the delivery of healthcare anywhere tobacco products are sold, are less relevant to quality of patient care and even appear arbitrary because healthcare is already provided in these settings by the pharmacy.

Additional tension is created by the question of whether retail clinics fit into an existing regulatory framework or require their own niche legislation. Because retail clinics are similar to existing provider arrangements, carving out new regulation in an already overregulated area seems unnecessary. For example, a retail clinic whose host is a healthcare institution may be identical to one whose host is a retail pharmacy. The only variable is the clinic location. To have different regulations solely because of the location of the host is difficult to justify and does not further the universally held goal of patient quality and access.[30]

AREAS OF LIABILITY

Malpractice

Retail clinics face many of the same risks as other healthcare providers. For example, medical malpractice due to allegations such as failure to treat, failure to perform an adequate examination or properly interpret results, and failure to diagnose, remain areas for which prudent policies, procedures, and training, as well as creative strategies such as using risk data in quality analyses can help improve patient safety and mitigate the risk of malpractice liability.

In a medical malpractice action, a plaintiff must prove that the provider had a duty to treat as a result of a patient–provider relationship, that the duty was breached by failing to meet certain standards of care, and that the patient sustained damages as a result of this breach.[31] A critical question for the retail clinic arises regarding when the practitioner/patient relationship begins because no malpractice action is sustainable without such a relationship.[32] It is arguable that once the patient signs into the kiosk, enters the retail clinic, and begins the discussion about symptoms, the relationship exists. However, there are other circumstances that may establish the patient–provider relationship in the retail clinic setting. For example, a patient may peer into the clinic to ask the practitioner if he or she treats a particular condition prior to signing in and deciding to seek treatment at the clinic. That interaction may or may not involve a description of the symptoms and potentially form the practitioner–patient relationship. Additionally, although it is a practice that may potentially increase liability, practitioners often walk in the aisles asking customers if they need help. Questions from customers may arise as to whether a particular medication is appropriate for their condition, what medication is recommended, or whether they should seek care in the clinic. These "aisle consults" should be guided by policies and procedures that define what a practitioner can and cannot communicate to the customer or potential patient, because they clearly create the potential for a practitioner to inadvertently establish the practitioner–patient relationship and a commensurate duty to treat. For example, questions about medications should be referred to the pharmacist. Any detailed discussions should also be documented, if possible, because the practitioner is unlikely to recall a specific interaction if a malpractice action results from a subsequent visit by the prospective patient to an emergency department.

In addition to whether a practitioner–patient relationship and related duty exist, a plaintiff seeking to prove malpractice must show that the standard of care was breached, and much of the litigation may focus on how that standard of care is defined. Generally, the standard of care is derived by examining what a reasonably prudent provider would have done under same or similar circumstances. Examples of evidence that may be involved in answering this question include available evidence-based practice guidelines applicable to the condition or diagnosis involved. State practice acts may also come into play. The clinic's policies, procedures, and bylaws may help to establish whether the staff met the standard of care. In addition, The Joint Commission standards may be presented as evidence. However, one source notes that, although these materials may provide *evidence* toward a standard of care, they are not definitive and are likely of minimal impact in setting a particular standard.[33]

Establishing a standard of care for retail clinics may also be challenging because these clinics provide narrowly defined services in a much more confined environment with fewer resources than a typical primary care office. What a primary care office may treat may not be appropriate for a retail clinic due to the scope of services offered. If a retail clinic is not treating a particular condition, there is a question as to whether it increases its exposure for failing to treat when a primary care practice otherwise would. At this point, it is unclear whether the clinic would be held to the higher standard, that is, what another primary care practice would do in a similar circumstance. To mitigate the potential for being held to a higher standard, it is important that a retail clinic clearly articulate its scope of practice to patients and that there be medical record documentation supporting the communication of limitations on this scope of practice to particular patients. In addition, the practitioner should counsel patients to get the appropriate care when such care is beyond the retail clinic's scope, and this should be documented. This clarifies the role of the clinic to patients and promotes their well-being by conveying that they need to go to a more comprehensive treatment setting. Although this approach does not eliminate all liability, it certainly helps to demonstrate the clinic's reasonably prudent efforts to ensure that a patient reaches a more appropriate care source.

As previously noted, retail clinic operators often operate multiple settings in numerous states. In addition, practitioners in these settings often work solo and are therefore unlikely to have immediate in-person access to other practitioners for the purpose of consultation. This situation may impact quality of care and also obstructs efforts to monitor care to ensure that it is appropriate and within the scope of the clinic's capabilities. Collaborating physicians play a critical role by responding to clinical questions and functioning as a sounding board when needed. However, the existence of these physician relationships does not eliminate malpractice risk. In fact, communication over the telephone about a patient's condition may increase exposure, just as it does in other settings. Remote care, including phone advice and telemedicine, can create liability for treatment in the same manner as if that treatment is provided by a practitioner in the setting.[34] To minimize any confusion about what is being observed on-site and to promote the efficacy of care, which is often based on telephone communication, it is essential that collaborating physicians use the same guidelines as the practitioner to make a treatment decision and that compliance with these guidelines is documented.

The autonomous nature of practice in the retail clinic setting also impacts the ability of a multistate operator to monitor quality and consistency of care. Collaborating physicians must have the ability to perform chart reviews, preferably through a shared EMR, which is often enough to ensure that the care provided is appropriate and within evidence-based guidelines.

An issue that remains unanswered is the potential for practitioners and retail clinics to have per se liability exposure. Per se liability may arise from harm that allegedly arises due to a clinic employee's failure to comply with one of the numerous regulations applicable to retail clinics.[35] If these regulations are construed to establish a particular standard of care, their violation may obviate the need for the plaintiff to prove that the standard was breached.[36] A plaintiff, however, must still establish causation and damages. For example, if a practitioner deviates from the physician supervision requirements, it may be difficult to prove that such an action *caused* any injury experienced by a plaintiff. If, however, a practitioner or corporation failed to have state-required employee health-screening processes in place and a patient contracted a disease such as tuberculosis, this situation could arguably result in a negligence per se claim, in addition to an employee health issue. It is critical that retail clinics have programs in place to monitor compliance with various laws and regulations to mitigate against the potential of a negligence per se claim. It is also important that related audits proactively encourage compliance and not focus solely on remediating violations.

Variations in the relationship between the patient and provider that create a duty to treat on the part of the retail clinic organization include ostensible agency, where a court will imply an employment, or *respondeat superior*, relationship between the parent organization and the practitioner, even if that practitioner is an independent contractor. The key to establishing an ostensible agency case is reliance by the patient on his or her perception that the practitioner is an employee. Even though signs that explain that independent contractors are responsible for their own actions are used in many settings in an attempt to thwart this theory, courts have increasingly used it to impute responsibility to a corporate entity. Similarly, courts have also created a duty on the part of the organization by applying the theory of corporate responsibility, which holds that the entity is responsible for what goes on within its walls. Negligent credentialing and training cases are examples of the use of this theory, which all healthcare organizations, including retail clinics, must be able to rebut through their procedures and processes.

Good Samaritan Liability

Many state laws create immunity for individuals acting in good faith and without compensation when there is an emergency. There are often state-specific guidelines for professionals when acting under this statute; for example, in some states a practitioner must stay with a patient until care is transferred to another competent professional.[37] Perpetrators of wanton, willful, or gross negligent acts are not shielded from a negligence action via the Good Samaritan immunity. Good Samaritan laws often don't apply to a person rendering emergency care, advice, or assistance during the course of regular employment, such as services rendered by a healthcare provider to a patient in a healthcare facility.

With respect to the retail clinic, there is a question as to whether Good Samaritan immunity would protect a practitioner who is called to the pharmacy, an aisle, or parking lot to render care in the event of an emergency. Arguably, the practitioner in this scenario is providing care outside of the course of regular employment; however, arguments can be made that care provided within the walls of a retail host (but outside the clinic) are within the scope of function of clinic employees. Practitioners also need to be mindful when providing care outside the clinic that they may not be immune from liability under the Good Samaritan laws. It is important to work with the malpractice insurance carrier to develop guidelines to help ensure that insurance coverage or Good Samaritan immunity exists for acts outside the clinic, whether in the aisle of the host operation or in an entirely separate setting.

Breach of Contract

For care that is adjudicated to be negligent, a health insurance carrier may seek to recover any fees paid to a retail clinic on the basis of breach of contract. For example, a carrier may argue that there has been a breach of contract if the standard of care has been violated and the contract provides that the clinic's services will meet the appropriate standard of care. It is important to keep this in mind when contracting to provide services under a network agreement, even though the potential for liability is quite limited because, unless there was fraud or an intentional act, any recovery would be limited to fees paid. There is also a small, but tangible chance that a claim for compensatory damages might be made by a payer alleging harm to reputation.

Employer Liability

A retail clinic employer must ensure that it acts to avoid liability from employee claims. These can occur under the theory of negligence for acts or inactions such as failure to protect the employee by not providing certain vaccinations. All healthcare providers, including retail clinics, should have an employee health program in place that requires certain vaccinations to help protect their workforce. They should also have programs to manage injuries and prevent workforce injuries in general. In addition, any employee injury should be assessed with worker's compensation and OSHA parameters in mind.

How to Mitigate Liability

As important as recognizing sources of liability is creating an effective strategy to mitigate against them. Retail clinics provide low-cost, low-margin services; because of this, the high-cost procedures that some traditional providers use to offset their risk does not exist. Costs associated with liability take a great deal of time to recoup, so much emphasis in the risk management program needs to be on prevention.

Credentialing of All Clinical Staff

Risk management in retail clinics begins at hiring. It is important to create an effective employment (recruiting, hiring, credentialing) process that includes appropriate credentialing of practitioners. It is also essential to hire practitioners without adverse clinical practice history. Through a proper credentialing process, the organization can answer such questions as whether the person is properly trained, licensed, able to work in a retail clinic setting without hands-on oversight, and capable of dealing with sensitive patient information. In addition, there may be factors in a practitioner's background that would be of concern in any setting, but are particularly problematic for a retail clinic. For example, a reference check that reveals a practitioner's tendency to disregard advice from physicians or other coworkers is especially alarming for a retail clinic because there is less direct oversight and therefore less ability to identify and address such behavior. Credentialing is just as important for the practitioner staffing the clinic as it is for the collaborating physician. In addition to satisfying the retail clinic operation's responsibility, proper credentialing of a nurse practitioner or other clinical staff may give a supervising physician a higher level of comfort than would otherwise exist. The National Committee for Quality Assurance standards can be used to develop an appropriate credentialing program.[38] In addition, because retail clinics may be staffed with part-time practitioners who may exhibit problem behavior in other settings, it is important to establish a recredentialing policy that includes references from other current clinical positions. As a foundation for credentialing in general, it is critical that there be an ongoing reporting and monitoring system to help ensure that licensure is current for practitioners staffing the clinics and that any clinical practice issues identified for a particular provider are addressed.

One reason that effective credentialing is critical to mitigating risk is that an ineffective credentialing program can be the basis for a negligent credentialing claim.[39] An organization that undertakes the responsibility to credential creates a duty to act reasonably in executing that function,[40] and the risk management professional should review the retail clinic operation's credentialing process to ensure that it is effective and fair.

Monitoring Third-Party Resources

Retail clinics often provide screenings and vaccinations, but the medication necessary to vaccinate and the equipment necessary to perform testing is outsourced to third-party manufacturers. When contracting for these resources, the clinic operator should keep in mind the importance of creating appropriate contractual liability protections. For example, a retail clinic contracting for vaccination materials should be assured that the contract contains concrete indemnification language because the retail clinic is the front line for vaccination administration, and the clinic operator will most likely be a party to any action alleging harm from a vaccination. Indemnification language helps to ensure that the clinic will receive appropriate indemnification if the vaccination material itself, rather than the administration technique, is established to be the source of injury. This important risk management strategy also helps avoid the expense of potentially significant defense against an action, which is a particularly important strategy in light of the low operating margins available to most retail clinics.

The same principle applies to device contracting. For example, a retail clinic that provides cholesterol screenings has the ability to perform thousands of tests. If a device is not functioning properly and yields inaccurate readings that underreport the cholesterol level, the clinic could be advising the patient that their cholesterol is normal when it is actually high and requires further evaluation. In the event a patient is harmed by this, for example, has a heart attack because he/she did not seek care due to the incorrect cholesterol reading, contractual indemnification is critical to ensure that the device manufacturer, not the retail clinic, bears responsibility for failure of the product. Just as in the previously described vaccination scenario, the clinic needs to have a mechanism to shift liability and offset the costs associated with such an exposure.

Another important risk mitigation and care improvement strategy is a quality assurance committee that undertakes aggregate analysis and any appropriate action on chart review results, adverse event reports, and other quality improvement–related trends. A retail clinic organization, which may see thousands of patients a day, must have such a quality review program in place. Such an approach can help the organization determine whether problems are individually focused or more systemic and can facilitate the prioritized development of corrective action. It is also important that an organization with evidence of systemic quality issues, which fails to correct those problems, may be found negligent in the same manner as an individual practitioner who negligently performs a service.

Another resource for quality improvement programs, including credentialing processes, are dashboards that report incidents per thousand, e-prescribing rate, adherence to guidelines, and service excellence, and then extrapolates this information to individual practitioners. An organization that monitors such information and communicates the results, as well as identified issues and corrective action, to practitioners truly engages in quality improvement. Such programs can materially enhance the quality of services provided in response to particular trends, on a local as well as national basis.

Adverse events reported to augment quality improvement monitoring and give the company an opportunity to determine whether the circumstance reported creates a material risk should also be assessed through the quality improvement program, and a priority in such programs is the management of sentinel events. From a risk management standpoint, if a retail clinic is aware of a serious injury or death, it is important to get counsel involved immediately to get advice on how to handle the incident. It is also essential to determine as an organization, with the input of the risk management professional and legal counsel, whether it is necessary to contact the patient, do an investigation that is privileged, set appropriate claim reserves, and execute practitioner remediation or termination. The appropriate handling of such matters is critical, especially in the early stages of any claim.

Whether it is identified during sentinel event evaluation or routine quality improvement review, evidence that a practitioner is not providing care in an appropriate way or is deviating from protocol calls for the retail clinic manager to immediately verify and address the concern. This can be tricky in a retail clinic setting because ability to directly monitor a practitioner is limited. To enhance monitoring ability, a potential practice issue may call for retail clinics to do a higher percentage of chart reviews, track calls to the local medical director, and/or provide a shadow when the practitioner is treating patients. It is also clearly important that such activities be supported by equitable processes that can be applied to all clinicians to avoid any later allegations of wrongful discharge or employment discrimination.

A common mitigating strategy for certain behavioral issues is the determination that additional training or education is required. This points to the general truth that a thorough training process is a critical aspect of risk mitigation. All practitioners should be required to have certain credentials, and it is also essential they be trained on protocols for treating patients in a retail clinic. Because direct oversight does not exist, many retail clinics have strict evidence-based protocols for treating patients, and practitioners must be clear that they are expected to comply with these protocols. Because in-person training capability is more limited in a retail clinic setting, an electronic education program that documents completion of training can be pivotal to ensuring compliance with key protocols. In addition, practitioners must be educated about the philosophy and model of retail clinics. For example, they must understand that retail clinics treat a limited range of services and that patients with needs beyond these services must be triaged to a more appropriate care provider. Even though practitioners may be licensed and trained to provide care beyond what is provided at a retail clinic, it is essential that they understand they must stay within the scope of the setting's practice.

· · · · · · · · ·
CONCLUSION

As retail clinics continue to evolve to treat new and more complex conditions, their risk profile will also change. The risk management professional must address the evolution of liability issues that will certainly continue to parallel those of other primary care providers, that is, expanding and contracting scopes of practice. It is also essential that clinic operators and the risk management professional in the retail clinic environment help build and participate in effective quality improvement programs and that they continuously monitor evolving regulation to ensure compliance.

Endnotes

1. Latkovic, T. and S. Singhal "The Retail Revolution in Health Insurance." *The McKinsey Quarterly*, March 2007. Available at: www.mckinseyquarterly.com/Health_Care/Strategy_Analysis/The_retail_revolution_in_health_insurance_1951. (Accessed April 12, 2010.)

2. "Mercer Study of Retail Clinic Savings on Behalf of Black and Decker" (2005). For a summary see "One-minute drill." *Employee Benefit News* 2007; 21(5). Available at: www.minuteclinic.com/Documents/Press-Releases/MinuteClinic%20Black&Decker%20 Case%20Study.pdf. (Accessed April 12, 2010.)

3. Woodburn, J. D., K. L. Smith, and G. D. Nelson. "Quality of Care in the Retail Health Care Setting Using National Clinic Guidelines for Acute Pharyngitis," *American Journal of Medical Quality* 2007; 22:457–462.

4. Jaspen, B. "Walgreens Clinics to Test Diabetes Treatment Program," *Chicago Tribune*, June 25, 2009.

5. Press Release. "Take Care Health Systems Reiterates Commitment to Year-Round Model in Light of Industry Changes" (noting that Walgreens is piloting a program for infusion therapy). Available at: www.takecarehealth.com/about/press-releases/ press_031009_01.aspx. (Accessed April 10, 2009.)

6. Mo. Reg. 20 C.S.R. § 2150.5–100(4)(c); Ma. Reg. 105 § 140 et seq.; 22 Tx Admin. Code § 193.6(d)(3).

7. *Ibid.*

8. See, for example, NY Educ. Law § 6530(19) and § 6531; NY Educ. Law § 6522; Conn. Gen. Stat. § 33–182a.

9. 42 U.S.C. § 1320a-7b.

10. Various state laws may be enforced through unfair and deceptive trade practices statutes.

11. 40 S.C. Code Sec. 40–33–34.

12. Minn. Session Laws 1999, Chap. 172, §. 2 Subdivision 7.

13. Texas: Stat. § 157.0541. This provision was changed from a 20 percent on-site requirement in Texas SB 532. (Effective September 1, 2009.)

14. Missouri SB 724 (August 28, 2008).

15. See California Business and Professions Code, §. 2400; See *People v. Cole*, 135 P.3d 669, 671 (Cal. 2006); See Ind. Code 25–22.5–1–2(c) (2006); See *Early Detection Ctr. v. Wilson*, 811 P.2d 860, 877 (Kan. 1991); See Mich. Comp. Laws § 450.1251 (2006); See MN Op. Att'y Gen. No. 92-B-11 (Oct. 5, 1955); See N.J. Admin. Code 13, § 35–6.16(f) (2006); See Tenn Code Ann. § 63–6–204(c)(2006).

16. 42 U.S.C. § 1320a-7(b)(1), (2).

17. *Ibid.*

18. Washington D.C. Code Ann. § 44–406.

19. Public Law 104–191, 104th Congress, 1996.

20. Health Information Technology for Economic and Clinical Health ("HITECH") Act 42 U.S.C. §§ 17921 – 17954 Available at: http://frwebgate.access.gpo.gov/cgi-bin/getdoc. cgi?dbname=111_cong_public_laws&docid=f:publ005.111.pdf. (Accessed April 12, 2010.)

21. 45 C.F.R. § 164.105.

22. Ill. HB 5372 (2008).

23. See *supra* note 13.

24. Ill. HB5372.

25. Oh. Rev. Stat. § 4723.48.1

26. 105 C.M.R. § 1400 (Aug. 8, 2007).

27. 105 C.M.R. 140.000

28. 105 C.M.R. § 140.1002.

29. 105 C.M.R. § 140.1001

30. See Federal Trade Commission Letter to the Hon. Elaine Nekritz, State Representative State of Illinois–57th District, May 29, 2008. Available at: www.ftc.gov/os/2008/06/V080013letter.pdf. (Accessed April 12, 2010.)

31. See Furrow. B. R. et al. Health Law § 6–2, at 237–39 (1995).

32. Prosser, W. L., W. P. Keeton et al. *Prosser and Keeton on the Law of Torts*, 5th ed. 1984, § 32, at 174; B. R. Furrow, S. H. Johnson, T. L. Greaney. *Health Law: Cases, Materials and Problems*, 6th ed., 2008. Eagan, Minn.: Thompson/West Publishing.

33. Erline Reilly, Nurses and the Law, 26 New Hampshire B.J. 7, 17–18 (Fall 1984).

34. Compare *McKinney v. Schlatter*, 692 N.E.2d 1045 (Ohio 1997) where advice given over the phone is incorrect, liability exists for telephone advice; with *Oja v. Kin*, 581 N.W.2d 739 (Michigan 1998) the on-call physician did not provide any care, treatment or advice with respect to the patient's condition and therefore no duty existed.

35. See *supra* notes 11 to 15.

36. *Lama v. Borras*, 16 F.3d 473, 480 (1st Cir. 1994).

37. Calif. Health and Safety Code 1799.102; 16 Del.C. §6801 (a); Ariz. Rev. Stat. § 9–500.02; 210 ILCS 50/3.150; Minn. Stat. § 604A.01.

38. See: www.ncqa.org.

39. *Johnson v. Misericordia Community Hosp.*, 1981 99 Wisconsin 2d 708, 301 N.W. 2d 156, 164.

40. *Silver Cross Hospital and Medical Center*, 2007 WL 2141822 (Ill. App.1 Dist.).

18

Managing the Obese Patient: Risks Across the Continuum of Care

Cynthia S. Siders

The World Health Organization (WHO) has identified obesity as an epidemic.[1] Statistics reflect over one billion overweight adults globally with at least 300 million adults that are clinically obese.[2] The Centers for Disease Control and Prevention (CDC) estimates that 67 percent of adults in the United States (33 percent overweight and 34 percent obese) and 20 percent the children (at or above the 95 percentile of the sex-specific body mass index [BMI] for age growth charts) are overweight or obese.[3] According to the CDC, the prevalence of obesity in the United States has dramatically increased in the past twenty years. "In 2008, only one state (Colorado) had a prevalence of obesity less than 20 percent."[4] The American Obesity Association reports an estimated 127 million adults in the United States are overweight, 60 million are obese, and about nine million are severely obese.[5]

An adult BMI of 25.0 to 29.9 is classified as overweight, a BMI greater than 30 is classified as obese, and a BMI greater than 40 is considered extremely obese.[6] BMI is calculated from height and weight and provides a reasonable indicator of weight categories more prone to illness.[7] Numerous sources have reflected the increased health risks of obesity, including chronic diseases such as heart disease, blood lipid abnormalities, cancer (for example, uterus, cervix, ovaries, breast, colon, rectum, and prostate), gallbladder disease, heart disease, type 2 diabetes, stroke, sleep apnea, osteoarthritis, and nonalcoholic fatty lever disease.[8–10]

Sources have estimated that the cost of obesity-related healthcare at $147 billion annually (10 percent of all medical spending).[11,12] According to a joint study by the CDC and the Research Triangle Institute, "Across all payers, obese people had medical spending that was $1,429 greater than spending for normal weight people in 2006."[13] A Purdue University study evaluated 4,574 adults over 20 years and found that obese adults averaged 3.22 hospitals stays with an average length of hospital stay of 10.96 days, as compared to 2.47 hospital stays with an average length of stay of 9.4 days for normal weight patients.[14] Healthcare systems challenged with decreased reimbursement and third-party payer denial of payment for hospital-acquired conditions (for example, infections, falls, deep vein thrombosis, foreign body retained after surgery)[15] have opportunities to minimize clinical, financial, and business risks through proactive patient safety interventions for obese patients.

·········
ENTERPRISE RISK MANAGEMENT APPROACH

Creating a patient-centered and safe environment for the obese patient across the continuum of care requires an enterprise risk management approach. Risks include weight bias and discriminatory care and treatment; failure to provide clinically pertinent patient assessment, monitoring, and treatment; facility design; inadequate, weight-rated medical equipment and supplies; improper patient handling and transfer techniques resulting in patient and staff injury; medication safety; bariatric patient care; provider credentialing and privileging; inadequate staff education and training; lack of multidisciplinary care resources (for example, dietary, physical therapy, respiratory therapy, pharmacy); and legal, licensure and insurance regulations and requirements.

·········
FACILITY DESIGN AND EQUIPMENT

Healthcare organizations must be prepared to care for obese patients across the continuum of care, including diagnosis, treatment, and care management in any department.[16] A March 2009 article in *Bariatric Times* outlined the space requirements for a critical care room and an acute care room for obese patients. "The overall space recommended for a critical care room is 13 feet 7 inches in length and a width of 14 feet. The overall space recommendations for acute care are a length of 13 feet 7 inches and a width of 17 feet."[17] The recommendations are based on "tasks in room, worker space requirements, and equipment space requirements."[18] Although equipment technology and types of equipment change, these three areas are considered critical to creating a safe patient environment for transfers, transport, bedside care, and patient ambulation.[19]

A walk-through and assessment of the facility, starting with the parking lot, is recommended to identify risks for patients and workers. Areas to address include, but are not limited to: the following.

- Parking Lots: Are sufficient handicapped parking spaces available? Do all entrances have ramps and handrails?[20]

- Entrances: Are entrances handicapped accessible? Are oversized/bariatric wheelchairs available at major entrances?

- Weight-Bearing Capacity of Floors: Has the weight-bearing capacity of floors in patient care areas been determined to ensure appropriate capacity to accommodate patient weight, equipment weight, oversized furniture weight, and staff and visitor weight?[21]

- Elevators: Are elevators appropriately weight-rated for morbidly obese patient transport, including equipment, special beds, and additional staff?[22] Are elevators equipped with 46-inch doorways to accommodate a bariatric patient bed?[23]

- Oversized and Bariatric Transport Lifts and Devices: Is a formal process in place for tracking oversized and bariatric equipment throughout the facility? Is the weight capacity of equipment and transport devices identified in a patient-sensitive manner (for example, 25, 50, and 75 for 250, 500, and 750 pounds)?

- Furniture: Are public areas, waiting rooms, conference rooms, dining facilities, and lobbies equipped with oversized chairs, benches, and other furniture?[24]

- Doorways: Will the doorways in diagnostic areas and patient rooms accommodate a 46-inch bariatric bed? Forty-eight inches is recommended for critical care rooms.[25]

- Restrooms: Do restrooms and patient care bathrooms have grab bars and floor-mounted toilets with appropriate weight capacity for the extremely obese patient, staff member, or visitor?[26]

- Patient Care Areas: Do patient care areas have scales of appropriate size and weight capacity,[27] wide blood pressure cuffs,[28] crash carts with emergency airway management equipment for the obese adult and child (as appropriate for clinical area),[29] wide examination tables bolted to the floor,[30] large-sized patient gowns and identification bracelets,[31] patient lifts and lateral transfer devices,[32] and large-sized needles, instruments, and supplies? Providing appropriate equipment to assist the patient in meeting their most basic needs, as well as their mobility, will significantly enhance the patient's care experience. Specialty beds, wide room chairs, floor-mounted toilets, patient lifts, and wide, front-wheeled walkers will help maintain a safer environment for the patient and help prevent patient injury.[33] Creating a patient-friendly environment requires ongoing planning and assessment and committing the financial resources for appropriate equipment purchases and upgrades.[34]

· · · · · · · · ·
PATIENT SENSITIVITY AND WEIGHT BIAS

Weight bias is a frequently mentioned concern of obese patients seeking medical care. Weight bias often reflects negative attitudes and beliefs that can be communicated and displayed as prejudice, discriminatory care and treatment, and negative stereotypes.[35]

Feeling unsupported, disrespected, and berated about their weight, obese patients often cancel or delay necessary appointments, preventive screenings, and early healthcare interventions.[36–38] Studies have reported biases from nurses, physicians, dieticians, psychologists, and medical students.[39–41]

Explicit and implicit measures of bias have even been reported among professionals who specialize in the care of the obese patient.[42] Weight bias often results in the physician spending less time with the patient during appointments, resulting in less discussion, fewer interventions and referrals, and fewer preventive health screenings.[43] Consider using the following strategies to minimize this risk exposure and increase patient satisfaction, participation, and compliance with healthcare delivery:

- Establish a zero tolerance healthcare system policy for insensitivity, discriminatory attitudes and behaviors, and lack of compassion for overweight and obese patients. Include the appropriate action steps that will be taken for noncompliance with the policy.

- Provide competency-based education and training that includes self-awareness of explicit and implicit weight biases, recognition of the difficulty of weight loss, the complex etiology of obesity, communication skills to minimize a negative patient perception, resources to impact lifestyle changes, and facility and community weight loss resources available to the patient.[44,45]

- Consider using larger patients as patient advocates, providing honest feedback about care provider sensitivity, care delivery, and the availability and quality of educational resources.

. . . .

OBESE PATIENT RISK FACTORS

Obesity risk factors and potential comorbid conditions impact every organ of the body; over one hundred thousand deaths in the United States each year are attributed to obesity.[46] The following patient risk factors should be part of a competency-based education and training program for all staff responsible for the care of the obese patient.

Fall Prevention

"Sixty-six percent of obese people suffer from osteoarthritis, a degenerative skeletal condition that becomes more severe in the presence of excess weight."[47] A BMI greater than 40 significantly increases the risk of disability associated with arthritis.[48] Activities of daily living may be difficult or nearly impossible for the obese patient to accomplish. Due to excessive weight, patients may have difficulty ambulating, getting in and out of bed, or even reaching parts of their body during hygiene activities. Providing appropriate equipment that will assist the patient in meeting their most basic needs, as well as their mobility, will significantly enhance the patient's care experience.[49] Obese patients also have an increased risk of developing osteoporosis, which in turn increases their risk for a fracture with a fall.[50] A comprehensive fall prevention program includes a patient assessment for fall risk factors at critical junctures in care (for example, admission, transfer to another unit, change in condition [for some patients this may be every shift], new medications); appropriate interventions to minimize fall risk (for example, appropriate ambulation devices, an individualized transfer and ambulation plan); and patient and family education on fall prevention.

Skin Care

Obese patients are prone to skin breakdown, pressure ulcers, skin irritation, bacterial and fungal infections, and delayed wound healing.[51,52] Malnutrition related to dieting, decreased circulation, and comorbidities (for example, diabetes, immobility, compromised immune system) increase the risk for skin complications.[53] A comprehensive skin safety program includes tools and resources for assessing skin risks, early intervention when skin irritation and breakdown is identified, and evidence-based protocols for the care and treatment of pressure ulcers. Careful assessment of skin folds and pressure points, including the neck, sides of the feet, sacrum, under the breast, abdominal folds, perineal areas, etc., should be a part of each patient's skin safety plan.[54–56] Tubes and catheters can burrow into skin folds and cause skin erosion. Establish protocols to reposition tubes and drains at least every two hours.[57]

Deep Vein Thrombosis

Obese patients and postoperative bariatric patients are at increased risk for pulmonary embolism (PE) and deep vein thrombosis (DVT).[58,59] The American Society for Metabolic and Bariatric Surgery recommends early postoperative ambulation, perioperative use of lower extremity sequential compression devices, and chemoprophylaxis using various anticoagulant regimens, unless contraindicated by patient condition.[60] Prophylactic treatment is recommended as venous thromboembolism can be challenging to diagnose, often presenting without warning signs. "Death due to PE is often immediate or occurs within 1 to 2 hours of onset. In high-risk groups of patients, it is more cost effective to protect against DVT and PE than to treat these conditions when they occur."[61]

A proactive risk management intervention is to establish evidence-based protocols for early recognition, screening, and treatment for deep vein thrombosis. One evidence-based source, entitled *Medical Guidelines for Clinical Practice for the Perioperative Nutritional, Metabolic, and Nonsurgical Support of the Bariatric Surgery Patient*,[62] is available from the National Guideline Clearinghouse, www.guideline.gov.

Medication and Pain Management

Excess body fat can affect the way that medications are absorbed, distributed, metabolized, and excreted.[63,64] Medications can impact respiratory, cardiac, metabolic, hepatic, and renal functioning.[65] Some medications are calculated using actual body weight (a drug that distributes well in fatty tissue),[66] whereas other medications are calculated based on ideal body weight (a drug with a low affinity for fatty tissue).[67,68] "Careful monitoring of clinical end points, signs of toxicity, clinical response, and serum drug levels are strongly advised when giving medications to morbidly obese patients."[69] A clinical pharmacist should be a critical member of the care team providing multidisciplinary assessment and intervention for the obese patient.

Respiratory and Airway Management

Respiratory functioning is often significantly compromised in an obese patient. The chest wall's ability to expand can be impacted by enlarged size, fat deposits in the diaphragm and intercostal muscles, and the enlarged size of the abdomen.[70] A shorter, fleshy neck and difficulty seeing anatomic landmarks (for example, vocal cords) can impact intubation.[71] Sleep apnea, obesity hypoventilation syndrome, and Pickwickian syndrome are common in obese patients.[72] Studies have reported that over 50 percent of obese patients have moderate or severe sleep apnea.[73] A respiratory care plan would include an assessment of risk factors on admission, preoperative and postoperative status, and with new medications and changes in clinical condition; patient education on deep breathing, coughing, and the importance of early ambulation; and interventions and treatments such as continuous positive airway pressure (CPAP) and maintaining the bed in a 30-degree to 45-degree semirecumbent position.[74]

Obese patient risk factors necessitate appropriately equipped and trained emergency response teams. Ensure that correctly sized pediatric and adult endotracheal tubes (standard endotracheal tubes may be too short), blood pressure cuffs, needles, and intravenous catheters are available on emergency carts. Ensure adequate personnel are in attendance for moving and positioning the patient, including placing the backboard. Consider including anesthesia personnel, specifically trained in intubation of obese patients, as critical members of the emergency response team.[75]

· · · · · · · · ·

PREPARING FOR OBESE PATIENTS

Emergency Department

Trauma is the fifth leading cause of death in the United States.[76] According to the American College of Emergency Physicians (ACEP), superobese patients present the most significant challenges to emergency medical care "from prehospital care through hospital admission."[77] A recent study of over fifteen hundred trauma patients "revealed that patients with higher BMIs had significantly increased lengths of stay in both the intensive care unit and the hospital, and also required more days of ventilator support."[78] Obese trauma patients often require additional staffing and specialized equipment for injury stabilization (air splints, braces, and cervical collars are often not available in appropriate sizes for obese patients),[79] trauma evaluation, and transport. Supporting heavy limbs and the patient's excess body weight may make it difficult to perform assessments, obtain intravenous access, and/or perform intubation on the patient. Special consideration should be given to the weight capacity of stretchers, gurneys, and ambulances. Bariatric ambulances are often required for patients who weigh more than four hundred pounds. Due to the high cost, the availability of bariatric ambulances is limited.[80]

As with the emergency response team, obese patient risk factors necessitate appropriately equipped and trained emergency department teams. Ensure that appropriately sized pediatric and adult endotracheal tubes (standard endotracheal tubes may be too short), blood pressure cuffs, needles, and intravenous catheters are available on emergency carts. According to ACEP, the average emergency medical service worker lifts only 100 pounds;[81] ensure that appropriate personnel are in attendance for moving and positioning the patient. Include emergency or anesthesia personnel, specifically trained in intubation of obese patients, as critical members of the emergency care team.[82]

Risk managers can assist ED physicians, administrators, and clinicians in evaluating facility equipment and supplies, ambulance equipment and supplies, transfer agreements and protocols, and clinician knowledge and expertise in caring for the obese patient.[83]

Obstetrics Department

The care of the obese gravid patient poses unique risks for obstetric departments. Facilities must assess their overall capacity to manage high-risk maternal and fetal clinical presentations, including triage and timely transfer when appropriate. Additionally, facilities must assess, plan, and strategize for patients and conditions that may present infrequently, ensuring that the necessary resources (staffing, providers, and equipment) are in place to facilitate optimum care for patients with emergency medical conditions.[84]

Obese patients have an increased risk for gestational hypertension, preeclampsia, gestational diabetes, stillbirth, cesarean delivery, infectious morbidity, and fetal macrosomia.[85,86] Labor and delivery problems seen in the obese patient include difficulty in fetal monitoring, dysfunctional uterine contractions with longer labors, higher cesarean section rates (reported rates of 47 percent with a BMI above 35), and more VBAC (vaginal birth after cesarean) failures.[87,88] Postpartum risks include wound infections and disruptions, deep vein thrombosis, endometritis, and ultimately greater length of stays with more intense nursing care.[89,90] Proactive risk reduction strategies include comprehensive patient assessment, monitoring, appropriate maternal transfer, and preparation for emergencies.

Surgical Department

A Prepared Patient A prepared obese surgical patient will have been informed about the risks and benefits of the proposed surgery and anesthesia plan, including possible complications and possible limitations in correcting comorbid medical conditions. The preoperative assessment provides an opportunity to identify cardiac, respiratory, circulatory, metabolic, and anesthesia risk factors, including a history of deep vein thrombosis, sleep apnea, and diabetic complications. Patient education during the preoperative preparation provides an opportunity for the patient and family to be prepared for the hospital experience, including respiratory care, early ambulation, wound care, pain management, and nutrition support. The preoperative period also provides an opportunity to refer the patient to other members of the multidisciplinary team for presurgical assessment and postoperative treatment planning (for example, respiratory care, physical therapy, nutrition, and dietary management). A well-planned discharge process will begin before the patient is hospitalized.

A Prepared OR Team   Establish a formal training and competency-based educational process for clinical staff responsible for the care of the clinically obese surgical patient and the bariatric patient. Core elements of an orientation, training, and educational program should include, but are not limited to the following:[91]

- Sensitivity Training: Clinical staff should complete sensitivity training to avoid negative attitudes and beliefs that can be communicated and displayed as prejudice, discriminatory care and treatment, and negative stereotypes

- Respiratory Care: Care includes assessing and monitoring respiratory functions as well as airway management.

- Recognition of Common, Potential Comorbid Condition Complications (for example, diabetes, cardiac, respiratory, vascular): According to the Association of Perioperative Registered Nurses (AORN), "Morbidly obese patients are at increased risk for stroke and sudden death."[92] This escalates the importance of ensuring that surgical team members understand the pathophysiology of obesity and the impact of surgical positioning on cardiac and pulmonary functioning.[93]

- Skin Safety Plan: Routine skin assessment techniques may be ineffective due to patient size, chronic conditions, and lack of landmarks.[94] The skin safety plan must be individualized for each patient based on the patient's comorbid conditions and current medical history.

- Patient Positioning: The registered nurse is responsible to ensure appropriate positioning, body alignment, tissue perfusion, and skin integrity for the obese patient.[95] Padding and positioning (routine interventions and padding may be ineffective) should be sufficient to prevent respiratory, cardiac, and circulatory compromise.[96] "Retractors, equipment, or instruments resting on the patient and members of the perioperative team resting or leaning on the patient add to the risk of pressure injuries that cause nerve or tissue damage."[97] AORN has published "Recommended Practices for Positioning the Patient in the Perioperative Practice Setting."[98]

- Operative Skin Preparation: Surgical site preparation requires special attention to skin folds. Numerous studies have reported that obese patients are at a higher risk for surgical site infections.[99] "Obesity increases the risk of perioperative complications of the skin and underlying tissue, including wound infection, dehiscence, pressure ulcers, and deep tissue injury."[100] Surgical site infections are reported in the literature to involve between 15 and 25 percent of all bariatric patients.[101] "When prep solutions pool beneath a patient, there is increased risk for skin maceration."[102] A strategy to mitigate these risks is to develop a multidisciplinary evidence-based protocol for operative skin preparation and prophylactic antibiotic dosing. AORN has also published "Recommended Practices for Preoperative Patient Skin Antisepsis."[103]

- Surgical Counts: A retained instrument or sponge can have significant patient and legal implications. Retained surgical items are most often identified after a significant medical change in condition, infection (nearly 50 percent), fistula, perforation of an organ, or a bowel obstruction.[104] Patient size places the obese patient at a much higher risk for retained instruments and sponges.[105] A strategy to mitigate this risk is to have a surgical count policy, as well as procedures based on professional standards and recommendations that are endorsed and implemented by all members of the surgical team.

- Equipment and Mobility Safety: An individualized patient handling plan is an important safety element for obese patients and their assigned clinical care team. The plan should address a safe method for transferring the patient from the bed or gurney to the OR table and repositioning the patient (including the use of lateral transfer devices and patient lifts); safe transfer to the recovery area; and clinically safe transfer to the critical care unit or surgical care area.[106]

A Prepared OR Suite Every perioperative department should have appropriate equipment and supplies available to accommodate obese patients.

- Surgical Procedure Bed: All perioperative departments should have at least one automated extrawide operating table with appropriate weight capacity to accommodate the width and weight of the morbidly obese patient.[107,108] A bariatric surgical program would include additional specialty surgical beds supportive of the patient population served. "Many procedure beds are designed to safely support a 500-pound patient, but maximum weight for special functioning capabilities is an important consideration. Heavy-duty procedure beds are available that lift, articulate, and support patients weighing 800 to 1,000 pounds."[109]

- Surgical Instruments and Supplies: Design surgical trays for the obese patient, including longer forceps, retractors, scalpels, needles, needle holders, and extralong abdominal instrument sets,[110] and so forth. Ensure the surgical suite contains appropriately sized drains, tubes, catheters, packing materials, and sponges, etc.[111]

- Anesthesia Equipment and Supplies: Ensure anesthesia equipment includes a difficult intubation cart, long endotracheal tubes, appropriate cardiac and respiratory monitoring equipment, and anesthesia protocols for sedation and monitoring for obese patients.[112]

Radiology Department

Equipment associated with diagnostic tests often has manufacturer weight and size limitations that should not be exceeded to ensure staff and patient safety.[113] Organizational liability may include suboptimal quality of images and delay in treatment when patient weight exceeds diagnostic capability and plans have not been defined for safe and timely transfer.[114] The National Guideline Clearinghouse has published guidelines for radiology equipment for weight loss surgery programs. Recommendations include the following:

- Computerized tomography (CT) scanners with 400-pound weight capacity
- Magnetic resonance imaging (MRI) magnet with 400-pound weight capacity
- Fluoroscopic equipment with 300-pound capacity that can study patients in a standing position using high beam voltages
- Interventional facilities available twenty-four hours a day, seven days a week.[115]

SAFE PATIENT HANDLING

A safe patient handling program requires an organization-wide commitment across the continuum of care, including the provision of adequate resources for necessary equipment and staff training. A well-designed program protects both patients and staff. The U.S. Bureau of Labor statistics reports that in 2007 nursing aides, orderlies, attendants, emergency medical technicians, and paramedics had the two highest incidence rates per ten thousand workers for musculoskeletal injuries.[116] "When both caregiver and patient are obese the threat to safe patient handling is considerably greater."[117]

Equipment selection should be based on safety research, frontline staff evaluation of ease of set-up and use, the ease with which equipment moves in patient care areas (for example, on carpet and inclines), patient comfort, and staff and patient safety.[118] The old approach to ergonomic training as a one-day safety fair has not been effective in reducing musculoskeletal injuries.[119] A new paradigm for injury prevention involves an on-unit mentor to assist with the development of a safe patient handling care plan, provide training on appropriate equipment usage, and support a minimal lift philosophy.[120]

BARIATRIC SURGICAL PROCEDURES

In 1998, slightly more than 13,000 bariatric procedures were performed in the United States; 2008 estimates exceeded 200,000 cases.[121] Common bariatric procedures include the Roux-en-Y gastric bypass (the most common weight loss procedure performed in the United States), laparoscopic adjustable gastric banding, vertical banded gastroplasty, biliopancreatic diversion, and vertical sleeve gastrectomy.[122] A study conducted by LABS (Longitudinal Assessment of Bariatric Surgery), involving over 4,700 first-time bariatric patients admitted between 2005 and 2007 at ten facilities, reported a thirty-day mortality rate of 0.3 percent among patients who underwent a Roux-en-Y gastric bypass or laparoscopic adjustable gastric banding procedure.[123] "Within 30 days of surgery, 4.1 percent of patients had at least one major adverse outcome, defined as death, development of blood clots in the deep veins of the legs or in the pulmonary artery of the lungs, repeat surgeries, or failure to be discharged from the hospital within 30 days of surgery."[124] The LABS authors noted, "Owing to Center of Excellence programs and formal training programs, we anticipate that the low rates of perioperative death and adverse outcomes seen in LABS centers will be achievable elsewhere."[125] According to HealthGrades, patients at five-star hospitals were 67.23 percent less likely to experience a complication than patients at a one-star facility.[126]

Several professional organizations and societies have developed evidenced-based guidelines and protocols for weight loss surgery and bariatric care. Facilities providing bariatric and weight loss services should establish multidisciplinary committees for the "development of uniform minimum standards of multidisciplinary care for WLS [weight loss surgery] patients."[127] Many professional organizations have recognized the importance of multidisciplinary expertise (for example, nutrition services, nursing, pharmacy, physical therapy, and respiratory therapy) to provide optimal care for the obese and weight loss surgical patient.[128] A partial list of organizations providing professional and evidence-based recommendations includes the following:

- Society of American Gastrointestinal and Endoscopic Surgeons (SAGES)[129]
- American Society for Metabolic and Bariatric Surgery (ASMBS)[130]
- Betsy Lehman Center for Patient Safety and Medical Error Reduction[131]
- American College of Surgeons[132]

The ASMBS Bariatric Center of Excellence designation may be obtained by hospitals and surgeons through a comprehensive review process that evaluates the bariatric program for compliance with the program requirements, safe care, and short-term and long-term outcomes.[133] Specific requirements include the following:

- Ongoing education in bariatric surgery
- Minimum number of surgeries performed for the hospital (at least 125 bariatric surgical cases per year), with a minimum for each surgeon in the program of at least 125 total bariatric cases during his or her lifetime, of which at least 50 were performed in the preceding 12-month period
- A full complement of support staff, including staff certified in Advanced Cardiac Life Support
- A full line of equipment and instruments for the care of bariatric surgical patients
- Ongoing involvement in the field of bariatric surgery by the program's surgeons
- Use of clinical pathways and orders
- Use of nurses dedicated to serving bariatric surgical patients
- Organized and supervised support groups
- Provision for long-term patient follow-up[134]

· · · · · · · · ·

PROFESSIONAL LIABILITY RISKS

Bariatric surgery often involves high-risk patients with multiple comorbid conditions, thus increasing the potential for higher frequency and severity of complications and adverse outcomes. According to the 2009 HealthGrades report, the top five in-hospital bariatric complications include "respiratory complications (lungs failing to function adequately during and after surgery), followed by hemorrhages (excessive or uncontrolled bleeding), operative lacerations (arteries, nerves and/or other structures inadvertently cut or damaged during surgery), and gastrointestinal complications."[135] Strategies to mitigate professional liability risks include the following:

- Appropriate patient selection and preoperative evaluation, including medical, anesthesia, and psychological screening for possible risk factors and complications and evaluating the patient's ability to maintain a life-long commitment to lifestyle changes and medical follow-up[136]

- Appropriate provider education, training, credentialing, and procedure-specific privileging, for example, completing an accredited general surgery program and becoming board-certified, having documented training in weight loss surgery, completing a proctoring program with an experienced surgeon, and participating in criteria-based peer review process for a predetermined number of cases[137]

- Procedure-specific outcome criteria and volume-based criteria for reappointment, for example, a minimum number of twenty-five cases, with outcomes within accepted practice standards, performed at an accredited institution, and requirements to complete a minimum number of continuing medical education credits related to privileges and clinical care[138]

- Provision of adequate resources for preprocedure patient education and informed consent, which should include, but not be limited to, the following: risks and benefits, possible long-term and short-term complications, consequences of not having the procedure, potential benefits of weight loss, required behavioral and dietary changes, and nonsurgical treatment options[139]

- Bariatric program accreditation through such sources as the American College of Surgeons, Bariatric Surgery Center Network Accreditation program[140]

- Informed decision making and analysis of professional liability coverage, because not all insurance companies provide coverage for weight loss surgical procedures.

- Compliance with Emergency Treatment and Labor Act (EMTALA) requirements when providing care for the obese patient, including appropriate emergency response, triage, medical screening examinations, and transfer protocols.

· · · · · · · · ·

CONCLUSION

Even though obese patients may present unique challenges throughout the continuum of care, these risks can be appropriately managed. Recognizing and understanding the unique challenges that are specific to obese patients will better prepare the healthcare facility and clinical staff to care for obese patients and help mitigate risk. A prepared patient, a prepared facility, and a prepared healthcare team will facilitate a safe patient care experience.

Endnotes

1. World Health Organization (WHO). "Obesity and Overweight." Available at: www.who
   .int/dietphysicalactivity/publications/facts/obesity/en/print.html. (Accessed September
   2009.)

2. *Ibid.*

3. Khan, L. K., Sobush, K., Keener, D. et al. "Recommended Community Strategies and
   Measurements to Prevent Obesity in the United States." *Morbidity and Mortality
   Weekly Report*, 2009, 58(RR07):1–26. Available at: www.cdc.gov/mmwr/preview/
   mmwrhtml/rr5807a1.htm. (Accessed September 2009.)

4. Centers for Disease Control and Prevention (CDC). "U.S. Obesity Trends." Available
   at: www.cdc.gov/obesity/data/trends.html. (Accessed September 2009.)

5. American Obesity Association (AOA). "AOA Facts Sheets–Obesity in the U.S." Available
   at: http://obesity1.tempdomainname.com/subs/fastfacts/obesity_US.shtml. (Accessed
   September 2009.)

6. Khan, L. K., *op. cit.*

7. Centers for Disease Control and Prevention (CDC). "U.S. Obesity Trends," *op. cit.*

8. Khan, L. K., *op. cit.*

9. MayoClinic.com. "Obesity–Definition." Available at: www.mayoclinic.com/health/
   obesity/DS00314. (Accessed September 2009.)

10. American Obesity Association (AOA). "AOA Facts Sheets–Health Effects of Obesity."
    Available at: http://obesity1.tempdomainname.com/subs/fastfacts/Health_Effects.shtml.
    (Accessed September 2009.)

11. Finkelstein, E. A., Trogdon, J.G., Cohen, J. W., and Dietz, W. "Annual Medical
    Spending Attributable to Obesity: Payer- and Service-Specific Estimates." *Health
    Affairs*, July 29, 2009. Available at: www.deborahburnett.com/images/uploads/
    RisingHealthcarecostsandobesity.pdf. (Accessed September 2009.)

12. Commins, J. "Obesity Costs U.S. $147 Billion Annually." *HealthLeaders Media*, July
    28, 2009. Available at: www.healthleadersmedia.com/content/236558/page/1/topic/
    WS_HLM2_PHY/Obesity-Costs-US-147-billion-Annually.html. (Accessed September
    2009.)

13. Finkelstein, E. A., *op. cit.*

14. Fauntleroy, G. "Obesity Leads to More Hospital Admissions, Longer Stays." *Medical
    News Today*. Available at: www.medicalnewstoday.com/articles/91472.php. (Accessed
    September 2009.)

15. Centers for Medicare & Medicaid Services (CMS), "Hospital Acquired Conditions."
    Available at: www.cms.hhs.gov/HospitalAcqCond/06_Hospital-Acquired_Conditions
    .asp. (Accessed September 2009.)

16. ECRI Institute. "Managing Extremely Obese Patients in the Healthcare Setting."
    Healthcare Risk Control Risk Analysis, Vol. 1, Self-Assessment Questionnaires 33,
    July 2005.

17. Muir, M. "Space Planning for the Bariatric Patient." *Bariatric Times*, March 2009.
    Available at: www.bariatrictimes.com/2009/03/31/space-planning-for-the-bariatric-
    patient/. (Accessed September 2009.)

18. *Ibid.*

19. *Ibid.*

20. ECRI Institute, "Managing Extremely Obese Patients in the Healthcare Setting," *op. cit.*

21. *Ibid.*

22. *Ibid.*

23. *Ibid.*

24. ECRI Institute. "Facility Design and Bariatric Patient Safety." Available at: http://members2.ecri.org/Components/HRC/Pages/SpecClinPol3.aspx. (Accessed September 2009.)

25. ECRI Institute. "Managing Extremely Obese Patients in the Healthcare Setting," *op. cit.*

26. ECRI Institute. "Facility Design and Bariatric Patient Safety," *op. cit.*

27. Special Report. Commonwealth of Massachusetts, Betsy Lehman Center for Patient Safety and Medical Error Reduction. "Expert Panel on Weight Loss Surgery." Executive Report. December 12, 2007. Available at: www.mass.gov/Eeohhs2/docs/dph/patient_safety/weight_loss_executive_report_dec07.pdf. (Accessed April 13, 2010.)

28. *Ibid.*

29. *Ibid.*

30. *Ibid.*

31. ECRI Institute. "Managing Extremely Obese Patients in the Healthcare Setting," *op. cit.*

32. *Ibid.*

33. Arzouman, J., Lacovara, J. E., Blackett, A. et al. "Developing a Comprehensive Bariatric Protocol: A Template for Improving Patient Care." *MedSurg Nursing*, 2006, 15(1):21–26.

34. ECRI Institute. "Extremely Obese Patients in the Healthcare Setting: Patient and Staff Safety." *Healthcare Risk Control Risk Analysis*, Suppl. A, Special Clinical Services 13, July 2005.

35. Puhl, R. M. and Wharton, C. M. "Weight Bias: A Primer for the Fitness Industry." *ACSM's Health and Fitness Journal*, 2007, 11(3):7–11.

36. Rudd Center for Food Policy and Obesity. Yale University. "Weight Bias–The Need for Public Policy." 2008. Available at: www.naafaonline.com/dev2/about/Brochures/WeightBiasPolicyRuddReport.pdf. (Accessed September 2009.)

37. Puhl, R. "Understanding the Negative Stigma of Obesity and its Consequences." www.obesityaction.org/magazine/oacnews3/healthqanda2.php. (Accessed September 2009.)

38. Puhl, R. "Bias in Health Care–A Significant Struggle for Obese Patients." *WLS Lifestyles*, 2008. www.wlslifestyles.com/cached/_downloads/2729/Weight%20Bias%20In%20Health%20Care%20MAIN.pdf. (Accessed September 2009.)

39. Puhl, R. M. and Wharton, C. M., *op. cit.*

40. Rudd Center for Food Policy and Obesity, *op. cit.*

41. Schwartz, M. B., Chambliss, H. O., Brownell, K. D., et al. "Weight Bias Among Health Professionals Specializing in Obesity." *Obesity Research*, 2003, 11(9):1033–1039.

42. *Ibid.*

43. Rudd Center for Food Policy and Obesity, *op. cit.*

44. The Obesity Society. "Obesity, Bias, and Stigmatization." Available at: www.obesityusa. org/information/weight_bias.asp. (Accessed September 2009.)

45. Puhl, R. "Understanding the Negative Stigma of Obesity and its Consequences," *op. cit.*

46. American Society for Metabolic and Bariatric Surgery, "Obesity in America." Available at: www.asbs.org/Newsite07/media/asmbs_fs_obesity.pdf. (Accessed September 2009.)

47. Camden, S. "Obesity: An Emerging Concern for Patients and Nurses." *OJIN: The Online Journal of Issues in Nursing*, 2009, 14(1).

48. *Ibid.*, citing Okoro, C. A., Hootman, J. M., Strine, T. W. et al. "Disability, Arthritis, and Body Weight Among Adults 45 Years and Older." *Obesity Research*, 2004, 12:854–861.

49. The Risk Management and Patient Safety Institute (The RM&PSI). "Challenges Related to Care of the Obese Patient." Regional Program, 2009.

50. Wellness.com. "Obesity." Available at: www.wellness.com/reference/conditions/ obesity/symptoms-and-causes. (Accessed September 2009.)

51. Harris, H. "Nursing Care of the Morbidly Obese Patient." *Nursing Made Incredibly Easy!*, May/June 2008.6(3):34–43.

52. Camden, S. "Obesity: An Emerging Concern for Patients and Nurses," *op. cit.*

53. *Ibid.*

54. Harris, H., *op. cit.*

55. Camden, S. "Obesity: An Emerging Concern for Patients and Nurses," *op. cit.*

56. ECRI Institute. "Managing Extremely Obese Patients in the Healthcare Setting," *op. cit.*

57. Camden, S. "Obesity: An Emerging Concern for Patients and Nurses," *op. cit.*

58. Camden, S. G. "Shedding Health Risks with Bariatric Weight Loss Surgery." *Nursing* 2009, 39(1):34–42.

59. Davidson, J. E., Kruse, M. W., Cox, D. H., and Duncan, R. "Critical Care of the Morbidly Obese." *Critical Care Nursing Quarterly*, 2003, 26(2):105–116.

60. The American Society for Metabolic and Bariatric Surgery Clinical Issues Committee. "ASMBS Position Statement on Prophylactic Measures to Reduce the Risk of Venous Thromboembolism in Bariatric Surgery Patients." Approved by the ASMBS Executive Council, June 2007. Available at: www.asbs.org/Newsite07/resources/vte_statement. pdf. (Accessed September 2009.)

61. Anderson, Jr., F. A., and Audit, A. "Best Practices–Preventing Deep Vein Thrombosis and Pulmonary Embolism." Available at: www.outcomes-umassmed.org/dvt/best_ practice/. (Accessed September 2009.)

62. American Association of Clinical Endocrinologists, The Obesity Society, and American Society for Metabolic and Bariatric Surgery. *Medical Guidelines for Clinical Practice for the Perioperative Nutritional, Metabolic, and Nonsurgical Support of the Bariatric Surgery Patient.* Available at: www.guideline.gov/summary/summary .aspx?doc_id=13022&nbr=006716&string=gastric+AND+bypass. (Accessed September 2009.)

63. Camden, S. "Obesity: An Emerging Concern for Patients and Nurses," *op. cit.*

64. ECRI Institute. "Managing Extremely Obese Patients in the Healthcare Setting," *op. cit.*; Davidson, J. E., *op. cit.*

65. Bell, E. A. "Predicting Drug Dosing in Obese Patients Can Be a Challenge." Available at: www.endocrinetoday.com/view.aspx?rid=29906. (Accessed September 2009.)

66. Davidson, J. E., *op. cit.*

67. *Ibid.*

68. Camden, S. "Obesity: An Emerging Concern for Patients and Nurses," *op. cit.*

69. Brunette, D. B., "Hidden Mystery." *AHRQ Web M&M–Case & Commentary*, March 2005. Available at: www.webmm.ahrq.gov/case.aspx?caseID=88. (Accessed September 2009.)

70. Harris, H., *op. cit.*

71. Camden, S. "Obesity: An Emerging Concern for Patients and Nurses," *op. cit.*

72. Harris, H., *op. cit.*

73. Camden, S. "Obesity: An Emerging Concern for Patients and Nurses," *op. cit.*

74. Baldwin-Rodriquez, B. "Care of the Critically Ill Bariatric Patient." Available at: www.dynamicnursingeducation.com/class.php?class_id=134&pid=18. (Accessed September 2009.)

75. Camden, S. "Obesity: An Emerging Concern for Patients and Nurses," *op. cit.*

76. National Trauma Institute. "Trauma Statistics." Available at: www. nationaltraumainstitute.org/home/trauma_statistics.html. (Accessed September 2009.)

77. American College of Emergency Physicians (ACEP). "Obese and Super Obese Patients Challenge Emergency Care Providers." ACEP Press Release, September 21, 2007. Available at: www.acep.org/pressroom.aspx?id=30722. (Accessed September 2009.)

78. Zoler, M. L. "Obese Patients Are at Increased Risk for Trauma Complications." *Clinical Psychiatry News*, 2007, 35(3):45.

79. ECRI Institute. "Managing Extremely Obese Patients in the Healthcare Setting," *op. cit.*

80. *Ibid.*

81. American College of Emergency Physicians (ACEP), *op. cit.*

82. Camden, S. "Obesity: An Emerging Concern for Patients and Nurses," *op. cit.*

83. Abke, A. "Strategies for Risks Presented by Obese Patients in the ED." *ASHRM Journal* 2005; 25(4):33–35.

84. Lavery, J. P. The Risk Management and Patient Safety Institute (The RM&PSI). *Obstetric Obesity Suggested Management Guidelines*, January 28, 2009.

85. American College of Obstetricians and Gynecologists (ACOG), Committee on Obstetric Practice. "Obesity in Pregnancy." ACOG Committee Opinion, Number 315, September 2005.

86. Barclay, L. "ACOG Issues Guidelines on Managing Obesity in Pregnancy." *Obstetrics and Gynecology*, 2009, 113:1405–1413.

87. American College of Obstetricians and Gynecologists (ACOG), *op. cit.*

88. Lavery, J. P., *op. cit.*

89. *Ibid.*

90. American College of Obstetricians and Gynecologists (ACOG), *op. cit.*

91. The Risk Management and Patient Safety Institute (The RM&PSI). "Obesity and Bariatric Services." *Clinical Services Risk Management Manual.* For ordering information visit www.rmpsi.com/requestinginfoform.html. (Accessed April 12, 2010.)

92. AORN. "Recommended Practices for Positioning the Patient in the Perioperative Practice Setting." *AORN Perioperative Standards and Recommended Practices.* Ramona Conner, Clinical Editor, Deb Reno, Senior Editor. Denver, Colo.: AORN Inc., 2008, pp. 497–520.

93. *Ibid.*, p. 511, citing Brodsky, J. B. "Positioning the Morbidly Obese Patient for Anesthesia." *Obesity Surgery*, 2002, 12:751–758.

94. AORN, *op cit.* p. 500, citing Bushard, S. "Trauma in Patients Who Are Morbidly Obese." *AORN Journal*, 2002, 76:585–589.

95. AORN, *op. cit.*

96. *Ibid.*

97. AORN, *op. cit.* p. 513, citing O'Connell, M. P. "Positioning Impact on the Surgical Patient." *Nursing Clinics of North America*, 2006, 41:173–192; and Irwin, W., W. Andersen, P. Taylor, and L. Rice. "Minimizing the Risk of Neurologic Injury in Gynecologic Surgery." *Ostetrics and Gynecology*, 2004, 103:374–382.

98. AORN, *op. cit.*

99. Gupta, A., M. A. Schweitzer, K. E. Steele, A. O. Lidor, and J. Lyn-Sue "Surgical Site Infection in the Morbidly Obese Patient: A Review." *Bariatric Times*, June 2008. Available at: www.bariatrictimes.com/2008/06/11/surgical-site-infection-in-the-morbidly-obese-patient-a-review/. (Accessed September 2009.)

100. *Ibid.,* citing Baugh N., Zuelzer, H., Meador, J. et al. "Wounds in Surgical Patient [sic] Who Are Obese," *American Journal of Nursing*, 2007, 107(6):40–50; Derzie A. J., et al. "Wound Closure Technique and Acute Wound Complications in Gastric Surgery for Morbid Obesity: A Prospective Randomized Trial." *Journal of the American College of Surgeons*, 2000, 191(3):238–243.

101. Gupta, A., *op. cit.*

102. AORN, *op cit.,* p. 514, citing Armstrong, D. and Bortz, P. "An Integrative Review of Pressure Relief in Surgical Patients." *AORN Journal*, 2001, 73:645, 647–648, 650–653.

103. AORN, *op. cit.*

104. Iyer, P. "Retained Objects after Surgery." Available at: www.medleague.com/blog/tag/retained-sponges/. (Accessed September 2009.)

105. *Ibid.*

106. ECRI Institute. "Managing Extremely Obese Patients in the Healthcare Setting," *op. cit.*

107. *Ibid.*

108. Betsy Lehman Center for Patient Safety and Medical Error Reduction, *op. cit.*

109. AORN, *op cit.*, p. 499.

110. Betsy Lehman Center for Patient Safety and Medical Error Reduction, *op. cit.*

111. ECRI Institute. "Managing Extremely Obese Patients in the Healthcare Setting," *op. cit.*

112. *Ibid.*

113. ECRI Institute. "Managing Extremely Obese Patient in the Radiology Department." *Risk Management Reporter*, August 2005.

114. *Ibid.*

115. Betsy Lehman Center for Patient Safety and Medical Error Reduction, *op. cit.*

116. U.S. Department of Labor Statistics. "2007 Nonfatal Occupational Injuries and Illnesses–Case and Demographics." See Chart 21. Available at: www.bls.gov/iif/oshwc/osh/case/osch0038.pdf. (Accessed September 2009.)

117. Camden, S. G. "Recognizing Trends in Preventing Caregiver Injury, Promoting Patient Safety, and Caring for the Larger, Heavier Patient." *Bariatric Times*, March 2009. To access the article go to *Bariatric Times* homepage at http://bariatrictimes.com/. select the month and year from the Issues Archives on the left side of the Web page, then look for the article by title. (Accessed April 13, 2010.)

118. *Ibid.*

119. *Ibid.*

120. *Ibid.*

121. Bariatric Learning Center. "The Rising Popularity of Weight Loss Surgery." Available at: www.bariatriclearningcenter.com/the-rising-popularity-of-weight-loss-surgery/. (Accessed September 2009.)

122. Camden, S. G. "Shedding Health Risks with Bariatric Weight Loss Surgery," *op. cit.*

123. The Longitudinal Assessment of Bariatric Surgery (LABS) Consortium. "Perioperative Safety in the Longitudinal Assessment of Bariatric Surgery." *The New England Journal of Medicine*, 2009, 361(5):445–454.

124. "IH Study Finds Low Short-Term Risks After Bariatric Surgery for Extreme Obesity." *NewsRX Health & Science*, August 23, 2009. Available at: http://hcfpn.advisen.com/?resource_id=10023170520623218944#top. (Accessed September 2009.)

125. The Longitudinal Assessment of Bariatric Surgery (LABS) Consortium, *op. cit.*, p. 452.

126. HealthGrades. "The Fourth Annual HealthGrades Bariatric Surgery Trends in American Hospitals Study." July 2009. Available at: www.healthgrades.com/media/DMS/pdf/HealthGradesBariatricSurgeryTrendsStudy2009.pdf. (Accessed on September 2009.)

127. Betsy Lehman Center for Patient Safety and Medical Error Reduction, *op. cit.*

128. *Ibid.*

129. Society of American Gastrointestinal and Endoscopic Surgeons (SAGES). Available at: www.sages.org/publications/guidelines/. (Accessed September 2009.)

130. American Society for Metabolic and Bariatric Surgery (ASMBS). Available at: www .asmbs.org/Newsite07/resources/asmbs_items.htm. (Accessed September 2009.)

131. Massachusetts Department of Health and Human Services. "Betsy Lehman Center for Patient Safety and Medical Error Reduction." Available at: www.mass.gov/dph/ betsylehman. (Accessed April 13, 2010.)

132. American College of Surgeons. "Recommendations for Facilities Performing Bariatric Surgery." Available at: www.facs.org/fellows_info/statements/st-34.html. (Accessed September 2009.)

133. HealthGrades, *op. cit.*

134. *Ibid.*

135. *Ibid.*, p. 12.

136. ECRI Institute. "Bariatric Surgery." *Healthcare Risk Control Risk Analysis*, Suppl. A, Surgery and Anesthesia 29, March 2009.

137. Betsy Lehman Center for Patient Safety and Medical Error Reduction, *op. cit.*

138. *Ibid.*

139. *Ibid.*

140. American College of Surgeons. Bariatric Surgery Center Network (ACS BSCN) Accreditation Program. Available at: www.acsbscn.org/Public/index.aspx. (Accessed September 2009.)

19

Risk Management and Patient Safety in Oncology

Sylvia M. Brown

I t comes as no surprise to the risk management professional that circumstances triggering failure to diagnose cancer–related malpractice cases generally arise before the patient reaches an oncologist. Nevertheless, there is professional liability risk in oncology settings. For example, oncology care providers may be sued for failure to diagnose second malignancies in cancer survivors; chemotherapy-related errors, which can be catastrophic; and, in the last few years, inadequate pain management.[1]

Oncology care environments also generate unique employee health risks, such as chemotherapy exposure. In fact, these complex risk-prone settings require creative, comprehensive risk management and patient safety strategies. Following is an overview of oncology that identifies key exposures and suggests solutions for the risk management professional.

ORIGINS OF ONCOLOGY

The ancient Egyptians were the first to attempt treatment of cancer. They documented survival characteristics of women with breast and axillary masses and developed the first known tumor registry in approximately 1500 B.C. Also of tremendous significance, the Greek physician Hippocrates (460–370 B.C.) was the first to use classification systems to predict outcomes, including differentiation between benign and malignant tumors. He used the term *karkinos*, which is Greek for "crab," to describe malignant tumors because their vasculature reminded him of crab claws. Translated to early English, *karkinos* is "carcinos," the first English form of the term *cancer*.[2]

Since those early days, humans have attempted to address cancer with one innovative clinical solution after another, and theories have become increasingly optimistic. For example, John Hunter, MD (1728–1793), hypothesized in the eighteenth century that localized cancer might be amenable to surgical cure. Although validation of his ideas would need to wait for the arrival of general anesthesia in the nineteenth century, he laid the groundwork for the process of staging cancer. Another important milestone came in 1896 with the first radiographs, a diagnostic cornerstone of oncology and the beginning of radiation therapy. In the twentieth century, the development of chemotherapy (based initially on a study of the effects of mustard gas during war) and followed by hormone-related therapies made the oncology treatment choices even more powerful. However, as is illustrated throughout this chapter, risk accompanies such potent innovation.[3]

· · · · · · · · ·
THE ONCOLOGICAL CONTINUUM OF CARE

The oncological continuum of care can be extremely complex, depending on the diagnosis, which is framed in the context of a staging process.

Staging is a method of classifying a malignancy by the extent of its spread within the body. It is determined both clinically and histologically. The majority of staging classifications are based on the anatomical extent of disease. The most important goal of staging is to provide data for proper treatment planning, but it also assists with prognosis, treatment evaluation, and exchange of information between different treatment centers.

The TNM committee of the International Union Against Cancer (UICC) and the American Joint Committee on Cancer (AJCC) devised the *TNM staging system* as an internationally consistent staging scheme for solid-tumor malignancies. The three categories are quantified and graded to represent progressive size or involvement. The extent of the primary tumor (T) may be measured on the basis of combinations of depth of invasion, surface spread, and tumor size. The presence and extent of lymph node metastases (N) is assessed in terms of sizes and locations of involved nodes. Finally, the presence of distant metastases is determined. One should distinguish between a cTNM, based on clinical exam, and a pTNM, which relies on surgical findings. Once the TNM numerical values are assigned, the patient is placed into one of four stages (I, II, III, IV), with increasing stage indicating more advanced disease.

Nonsolid malignancies (leukemia, for example) do not conform to this staging scheme because of their inherently disseminated nature. Leukemias are often grouped according to their predominant cell types, whereas myeloma patients follow a three-stage prognostic system relating M proteins to myeloma cell mass.[4]

Depending on what type of cancer is involved, numerous healthcare settings touch the patient during the staging process. These may include radiology (magnetic resonance imaging, computed tomography, and/or positron emission tomography scans), pathology, laboratory, and in- or outpatient surgery. As the result of the staging process, the treatment plan may add numerous other care environments, including radiation therapy and inpatient or outpatient chemotherapy. Follow-up care, at minimum, is likely to include clinical monitoring such as blood tests and/or office visits. It may also include home visits and long-term adjuvant medication regimes such as tamoxifen for breast cancer patients.

· · · · · · · · ·
REDUCING RISK AND ENHANCING SAFETY IN ONCOLOGY
Communication with the Patient

Communication with patients and among providers is an important safety principle in all clinical settings, but the complex path followed by many oncology patients makes it absolutely essential. Providers must take extra pains to communicate clearly with a patient who is hearing complex, and possibly frightening, information. Both informed consent, where appropriate for a surgical procedure or investigational therapy, and education about a patient's treatment regime must be managed in an individualized and substantive way. (Please see Chapter 4 on informed consent and Chapter 5 on institutional review boards in this series for more information on those subjects.)

Communication among Oncology Providers

Providers must also ensure that the clinicians in the numerous disciplines involved in a patient's care communicate effectively to further individual patient care and quality of oncological care in general. The infrastructure to support true multidisciplinary care communication is challenging enough to establish and maintain when all providers are under one organizational roof. When they are based in multiple, distinct organizations, it may be weakened or nonexistent.

One care model that, theoretically, encourages real-time collaboration is vertical integration. As noted in a recent issue of the *Radiology Business Journal*, "Those who make a serious commitment to vertical integration are able to bring together distinct services that all play roles in comprehensive oncological care . . . everything is easier when experts are under the same roof, or at least nearby . . . When the radiation oncologists and medical oncologists are in the same practice and down the hall from each other, it fosters consistent access and open discussions."[5] However, this discussion focuses primarily on radiology services in the outpatient environment.

A more comprehensive approach was taken by physicians at the Medical College of Virginia, when they identified the following essential characteristics of an excellent oncology program:

- The program is easily accessed by patients and referring doctors.

- All specialties are available as the patient needs them.

- The separate and distinct divisions of care, such as radiation oncology, medical oncology, surgical oncology, would be transparent to the patient.

- There is an accountable physician at any given time.
- An internal communications structure is present that emphasizes the treatment plan based on best evidence.
- Outcomes and processes are tracked and reported through quality assurance, and there is visible accountability.
- Patients can call send e-mails and get answers to routine and complicated questions in short order. Patients do not have to decide who to call for what; one phone number is sufficient.
- The cost of care is worked out to the point that case rates for broad episodes of care are acceptable.
- Patients routinely report high satisfaction rates.
- Patients and professionals have access to information in the office and via the Internet.
- The physical setting for cancer care is appropriate.
- A written treatment plan or pathway is available at all times for patient and physician review.
- Follow-up strategies are well worked out to reduce travel and hassles for patients following treatment.
- There is a consistent and compassionate approach to end-of-life care.
- Advanced directives are raised early in the course of the illness and reviewed on a regular basis.
- Clinical trials are offered to all patients.[6]

In response to the questions, What would a model of excellence look like, and how would it be evaluable?, the physicians at the Medical College of Virginia also established the following to describe a care plan:

> . . . a comprehensive cancer care plan systematically evaluates the access, processes, and outcomes of care delivery; corrects problems; and evaluates results.[7]

In 1993, these physicians concluded that no organization had yet achieved the parameters they laid out. Indeed, many of these goals are still being sought after today. One resource that is potentially helpful to hospitals and free-standing centers seeking a cohesive, communicative approach for oncology is the accreditation process of the American College of Surgeons' Commission on Cancer (CoC). The CoC first began accrediting oncology programs in 1930 and is now endorsed by many oncology-associated professional organizations, including the American College of Radiology (ACR), the American Academy of Pediatrics (AAP), and the American Cancer Society (ACS). The 2009 CoC standards have the potential to promote effective oncology team communication. As is pointed out in CoC's standard 2.1, "Leadership is the key element in an effective cancer program, and program success depends on an effective cancer committee or other leadership body."[8] Elaborating on this statement, standard 2.1 requires that "the membership of the . . . leadership body is multidisciplinary, representing physicians from the diagnostic and treatment specialties and nonphysicians from administrative and support services."[9]

Resources in addition to accreditation that may strengthen oncology team communication include traditional team training tools, such as SBAR (situation, background, assessment and recommendations)[10] and other patient safety strategies discussed elsewhere in this series. Also important is a mechanism to keep oncology providers current with constantly changing care parameters such as the National Comprehensive Cancer Network Guidelines.[11] The electronic record is yet another resource that is likely to play a key role in facilitating safer care, connecting providers with one another and with patients, as patients begin to manage their own medical information.

Even though the previously discussed strategies can play an important role in lowering oncology setting risk, chemotherapy and radiation therapy require particular attention on the part of the risk management professional.

· · · · · · · · ·

CHEMOTHERAPY

Chemotherapy is a form of medication, and the reader is referred to the chapter elsewhere in this series on medication safety for general principles. However, there are four exposures that must be discussed here: chemotherapy administration–specific concerns, the use of oral chemotherapy, pediatric chemotherapy-related issues; and worker safety–related chemotherapy issues.

Chemotherapy-Specific Concerns

Much of the available literature on chemotherapy comments on its "narrow therapeutic index."[12] In other words, dosage must be precise. An underdose may be ineffective, and an overdose may be lethal. The death of a thirty-nine-year-old *Boston Globe Reporter* following a massive overdose of cyclophosphamide and heart damage to another patient from an overdose of the same chemotherapeutic agent, turned world-renowned Dana Farber Cancer Institute upside down. Among many steps taken to increase safety of chemotherapy administration were the following:

- New rules were adopted mandating close supervision of physicians in fellowship training.
- Nurses were required to double-check high-dose chemotherapy orders and to complete specialized training in new treatment protocols.
- Interdisciplinary clinical teams reviewed new protocols and reported adverse events and drug toxicities.
- A trustee-level quality committee was reorganized and strengthened.
- Discussions were begun regarding the transfer of inpatient beds to nearby Brigham and Women's Hospital.[13]

Many of the same steps were taken in many organizations across the country, and, in 2009, the American Society of Clinical Oncology and Oncology Nursing Society joined forces to create new Chemotherapy Administration Safety Standards that apply similar safety principles in the outpatient setting.[14] For example, standard 12 requires that

> a second person (a practitioner or other personnel approved by the practice to prepare or administer chemotherapy) independently verifies each order for chemotherapy before preparation, including confirming
>
> A. two patient identifiers,
> B. drug names,
> C. drug dose,
> D. drug volume,
> E. rate of administration,
> F. route of administration,
> G. the calculation for dosing (including the variables used in this calculation).[15]

The standards also require chemotherapy-specific training for all staff who administer chemotherapy and routine monitoring of competence.[16] Risk management professionals should note that, because these standards were generated by professional organizations rather than regulatory bodies, they are not required of all outpatient environments administering chemotherapy. Nevertheless, these standards arguably establish the standard of care and would most certainly be asserted by the plaintiff in a related negligence case.

Another safety-promoting resource that may be particularly valuable in the oncology setting is a medication ordering system equipped with computerized provider order entry (CPOE). For example, one sobering recent study of medication errors among cancer patients in four clinic settings identified 112 errors among 1,262 adult and 117 pediatric patient visits. Of the 112 total errors, 64 had potential to cause harm. However, the one site that had CPOE for chemotherapy reported only 1 error in 500 administrations.[17]

Still other strategies aimed at reducing chemotherapy-related medication errors include these, which were in a recent journal article:[18]

- Consistently use a reliable method to verify patient identity prior to chemotherapy administration to minimize errors associated with language barriers, close proximity of patients to one another, an overreliance on wrist bands or patient photographs, which can change significantly over time.

- If possible, measure height and weight in centimeters and kilograms, rather than feet and inches. To illustrate the problem, consider the following: When converting the height of 6 feet 3 inches to inches, it is often misunderstood to be 63 inches rather than the correct calculation of 75 inches.

- Have good lighting, employ magnification, and use high-visibility tools such as calculators with large number buttons and large lighted display areas. Errors have occurred when the wrong number is pushed on a calculator and the calculation is not confirmed.

- Organize the workspace and keep it free of clutter.

- If chemotherapy orders are transmitted by fax, use an original order sheet (as opposed to a copy) printed with a font larger than 12 points.

- Eliminate abbreviations and acronyms in all clinical documentation.

- Provide and use up-to-date, easily accessible chemotherapy drug information at the point of care.

- Follow the 80/20 rule because only a small percentage of medications are deemed high-alert, yet they are responsible for the greatest number of patient injuries. Parenteral chemotherapy is a small percentage of drugs administered, yet it is a high-alert medication and deserves full attention.

- Reduce potential for error by reducing the clinician's distractions, stress, and fatigue.

- Include the patient in chemotherapy error prevention efforts. The patient has the most to lose if an error occurs. Chemotherapy errors have been caught when the patient picked up on something different, for example, a larger than normal infusion bag. Visually reinforce chemotherapy education with cards that the patient can read immediately before each treatment. For those with limited ability to read, audiovisual resources such as head phones or videos may be used to convey information.

Oral Chemotherapy

In March of 2008, the National Comprehensive Cancer Network issued a task force report evaluating the impact of the increasing use of oral chemotherapy.[19] The group noted that routine administration of oral chemotherapy may be preferable to high-dose parenteral administration in some situations; however, they cautioned that there are significant patient safety issues. For example, although the convenience of self-administration is attractive to patients, the fact that they are taking a simple pill may result in the false assumption that daily compliance is not essential and underdosage may result in treatment failure. Equally or more concerning are situations in which highly motivated patients ingest tragic overdoses because they do not understand their regime. For example, a related article discussed the case of a patient who should have received temozolomide 320 mg for five days, yet died of leucopenia-related sepsis after erroneously taking the medication for twenty-two days. In yet another situation, a patient who was supposed to take lomustine 160 mg once every six weeks died after taking it every day for three weeks.[20] A broader perspective on these concerns was revealed by data from 356 follow-up telephone conversations between oncology nurses and patients receiving oral chemotherapy. Sixty-four of these interactions, or 18 percent of the sample, identified circumstances in which the patient needed further counseling and/or corrective action had to be taken. The authors of the article in which this survey was reported recommended that physicians write nonrefillable prescriptions for oral chemotherapy for only the amount of medication necessary for one cycle of treatment. They also recommended that the pharmaceutical industry take steps to ensure that chemotherapy is provided in a way that supports dispensing of safe and appropriate amounts and that there be further study of the impact of education on compliance.[21]

The task force also emphasized the critical role of education. As is noted in the report, "Some oncologists offer written material, video material, or group educational sessions, but the bottom line is that the extensive and ongoing patient education required to ensure safe and effective oral chemotherapy is uncompensated and perhaps underappreciated."[22]

They also discussed the potential role of technological solutions to facilitate monitoring of patient compliance.

> The ability to monitor symptoms in real time would help identify toxicities that may resolve by the next physician visit and consequently not be adequately recalled by the patient. Internet systems may improve communication for all patients. For example, patient-friendly Web-based programs have been developed that allow patients to communicate chemotherapy toxicities in real time, either from home or in the oncologist's office. One such program is called the STAR program, which has been investigated in patients with lung cancer and gynecologic malignancies. Patients were encouraged to log in and report symptoms at each follow up or to access the system from home. In one study involving 80 patients with gynecologic cancer, 42 severe toxicities (grade 3–4) entered from home prompted 7 clinician interventions. Additionally, online self reporting of toxicity symptoms was shown to be feasible in 107 patients with lung cancer. Patients reported high satisfaction with the program, and the nurses who received the symptom reports felt that the information was useful for clinical decisions, documentation, and discussions.[23]

Although oral chemotherapy may ultimately be more desirable from a clinical and patient satisfaction standpoint, the risk management professional should stay alert to development of specific guidelines that may improve safety. Please also see the discussion that follows regarding chemotherapy-related employee health issues. In addition to understanding their treatment regime, patients must be educated about how to protect themselves and their families through safe management of antineoplastic medication in the home setting.

Pediatric Chemotherapy

Pediatric medication-related safety issues already discussed in the pediatrics and medication management chapters of this series take on more significance in the context of chemotherapy administration. For example, much of the literature reviewed discussed the importance of standardizing a pediatric approach to chemotherapy to simplify dosage and administration and thus make it safer.[24]

Of particular note is the work of staff at the Children's Hospital of Philadelphia, who reduced their organization's medication error rate by 84 percent through participation in an intensive Breakthroughs Initiative project led by the Institute for Healthcare Improvement (IHI). Throughout the presentation of their results, they stress the importance of safety culture. For example, they describe the dramatic increase in reporting of intercepted adverse events, accompanied by a decline in actual adverse events, that occurred once they had reduced fear of incident reporting.[25] Other lessons learned that may be helpful to other operations include the following:

- Simplify and Standardize: Once they began to analyze their improved error and potential error reporting data, many issues related to the complexity of the chemotherapy ordering process were discovered. They then looked more closely at that complexity and found, for example, twenty-three different cyclophosphamide regimens in only fourteen protocols. One solution was a chemotherapy standards committee consisting of physicians, pharmacists, nurse practitioners, nurses, and a clinical research associate, who were charged with developing standard methods of chemotherapy administration. These standards apply to all uses of the drugs in oncology, except when a different protocol-directed method is central to the objectives of a clinical trial. Ultimately, the authors noted that "these changes have proven the most difficult and controversial of all that we have made, but (they are) also the most powerful."[26]

- Reduce Handoffs: Chemotherapy was sometimes given in more than one setting. Handoffs from the outpatient to inpatient setting, and among various shifts, unnecessarily complicated communication and impaired safety. They limited administration to one setting per cycle. Many settings only administer chemotherapy, whether pediatric or adult, in one place, but the principle of limiting handoffs is an important one.

- Pay Attention to Human Factors: The distractions in the various settings were very detrimental to safety. This was addressed in part by providing quieter places for order writing and equipped clinicians with reference materials.[27]

Two messages of particular importance for risk management professionals are the value of error reporting in understanding issues and the necessity of recognizing differences in children's ability to metabolize drugs (especially drugs such as chemotherapy) and the importance of standardizing related pediatric approaches.

Chemotherapy-Related Employee Health

In 2004, an Alert from the National Institute for Occupational Safety and Health (NIOSH) entitled "Preventing Occupational Exposure to Antineoplastic and Other Hazardous Drugs in Health Care Settings" was issued. The NIOSH Alert cites representative examples of employee health issues associated with chemotherapy, including allergies and cancer.[28] Corroborating the importance of the Alert is a recent study in which 7,094 pregnancies of 2,976 pharmacy and nursing staff were evaluated. Researchers determined that exposure of the mother to or the handling of antineoplastic agents during pregnancy was associated with significantly increased risk of spontaneous abortion.[29]

In the NIOSH Alert is a comprehensive guide to the procedures that must be followed in handling any antineoplastic medication, for instance, "use two pairs of powder-free, disposable chemotherapy gloves, with the outer one covering the gown cuff whenever there is risk of exposure to hazardous drugs."[30] It must also be emphasized that those who administer the medications are not the only ones at risk. Antineoplastic medication may enter the body when contaminated surfaces are touched, for example, by housekeepers, and when eating and drinking after having touched such surfaces. Exposure also occurs through aerosolization.

Surveillance for presence of antineoplastic agents should routinely be conducted by those skilled in this process, because these agents may occur in unexpected places. For example, in a study done to evaluate the presence of cytotoxic agents in the workplace, administration and pharmacy samples were swiped. Researchers identified measurable amounts of antineoplastic agents in 75 percent of the pharmacy samples, for example, the floor in the prep room, and 65 percent of the administration areas, for example, the floor around the bed or chair. Most important, every oncology setting should maintain a copy of the CDC Alert on the premises where it is accessible to staff, and those who may come in contact with these medications should be educated about potential dangers and how to protect themselves.

· · · · · · · · ·
RADIATION THERAPY

Radiation therapy has been in use as a cancer treatment for more than 100 years, and its earliest roots trace back to the discovery of X-rays in 1895 by Wilhelm Roentgen. However, the field of radiation therapy began to grow in the early 1900s largely due to the groundbreaking work of Nobel Prize–winning scientist Marie Curie, who discovered the radioactive elements polonium and radium.[31]

Radiation treatments are usually delivered by a linear accelerator, and dosage of radiation is generally fractionated; that is, the dose is divided and given at intervals to allow normal tissue to recover between treatments. It is also thought that radiation given in fractions is able to reach the tumor cells during different stages of cell growth, possibly causing more damage to those cells.[32]

The goal of radiation therapy is to deliver a prescribed dose of radiation to the patient's tumor site, while restricting the dose to all surrounding healthy tissue and organs to that less than or equal to normal tissue tolerance. Deviations of dosage of more than 5 percent may affect outcomes, so the stakes are high for oncology patients receiving radiation therapy. Also, the work of the radiation therapy team is complex, and involves many steps. The radiation oncologist, medical physicist, dosimetrist, and radiation therapy technician must communicate clearly and collaborate effectively to prescribe, plan, and deliver radiation therapy.[33]

As noted by the Pennsylvania Patient Safety Authority, errors in delivery of radiation therapy are relatively rare, at least in part because the Nuclear Regulatory Commission tightly controls the use of radioactive materials. Also, radiation therapy errors can usually be compensated for by reducing or increasing a later fractionated dose. However, "the real danger is if an error in administration goes undetected. This may result in healthy tissue being exposed to unnecessary levels of radiation or the tumor site not receiving a full effect of therapy. When radiation misadministrations are caught early, subsequent treatment doses can be adjusted so that the patient avoids receiving an underdose or overdose. However, a severe misadministration may result in radiation necrosis to vital organs and structures and can be fatal."[34]

A highly publicized case of radiation misadministration resulting in a fatality occurred in Glasgow, Scotland, in 2005, in which a young patient, Lisa Norris, received a 58 percent higher dose than ordered to her craniospinal area. An autopsy revealed that her tumor was still present despite radiation therapy. Another example of radiation misadministration involved the Therac-25 incidents, which occurred between 1985 and 1987. Two different computer software errors in a computerized linear accelerator resulted in massive radiation overdoses that injured six patients and caused two fatalities."[35]

Resources that can help reduce risk and promote safety in radiation therapy include use of ROSIS, a voluntary Radiation Oncology Safety Information System that houses data on radiation therapy–related events.[36] It was established in 2001 and, as of 2009, held seven hundred reports. Two hundred ninety-four of 600 events involved an element of data transfer. Significantly, of these 294 events, 130 of them involved a patient getting an incorrect treatment. Overall, the most common radiation misadministrations have resulted in patients receiving a wrong dose of radiation therapy, delivery of radiation therapy to the wrong site, or patients receiving radiation based on the wrong treatment plan.

Specific strategies to improve and maintain safety and effectiveness in radiation therapy include the following:

- Stay Current with Technology: Have a mechanism for staying current with new technology, and ensure that team member competencies are continually updated and monitored.

  The increasingly complex equipment in this area is leapfrogging current knowledge. For example, methods of performing quality assurance recommended by groups such as the American Association of Physicists in Medicine (AAPM) predate advances such as image-guided radiation therapy. Task Group 100 of the AAPM) is developing a framework for designing quality assurance activities with emphasis on failure mode and effects analysis. Still another down side of new technology may be corrupt computer files.[37]

  Against this backdrop, organizations performing higher volumes of new procedures must ensure that staff are proficient, that they feel comfortable in saying they need help with a new process, and that they question any apparently wrong computer-generated information. Beware of overreliance on technology. Most linear accelerators use a computerized record and verify (RV) system. The RV system's role is to verify that the treatment parameters entered at the time of administration are the same as those intended for the patient. Although the RV system is a safety mechanism that should be in effect in each linear accelerator, it is not foolproof. For example, in a study performed over one year at the University of Utah, of 22,542 external beam radiation therapy treatments administered, 38 errors were identified. Of these, 9 related to RV system use and included: overriding of the system by staff to allow use of an incorrect data file; an incorrect site was treated; and a wrong patient was treated.

  Similar issues were identified among 25 errors reported to the Pennsylvania Patient Safety Advisory between June 2004 and January 2009. The majority of events involved a patient receiving the wrong dose of radiation (40 percent). Other events included the wrong patient receiving the therapy (16 percent), wrong location (12 percent), wrong side (12 percent), and wrong set up (8 percent).[38] Examples from these data illustrating the impact of human error are as follows:

- The dosimetrist transcribed the radiation oncologist's prescription incorrectly to the planning system, and then to the recording system, causing the patient to receive 2.5 times the recommended dose.
- The patient was given one treatment of another patient's treatment plan. She wrongly responded to a similar sounding patient name when it was called in the waiting room. A picture of the patient and other identifiers on the computer screen that might have helped avoid the error were not picked up by staff.

   Despite volume-driven time constraints and the pressure of using complex technology precisely, staff should audit themselves to ensure that they are enforcing human-driven checks, such as patient identification checks.

- Check and Double-Check Dosage: In another study, more than half of all significant deviations (more than 5 percent discrepancy with ordered dose) resulted from errors made during manual input of data.

The American College of Radiology recommends that the treatment plan for each patient undergo an independent double-check and be signed by a radiation oncologist within one week of planned treatment. In a time of increasing volume with novel technology, processes to safeguard accuracy must be effective and used by all staff.

· · · · · · · · ·
FALL PREVENTION

Falls are more concerning in oncology than many other settings because of the frailty of much of the patient population. Because clinical characteristics associated with the disease and/or treatment include osteoporosis and low platelet count, fall-related harm may be significant in the oncological patient population. Although standard inpatient fall prevention measures may suffice for hospitalized patients, The Seattle Care Alliance, which includes Fred Hutchinson Cancer Center, was concerned by the fall rate they saw in their outpatient environment. Steps they took to address this issue included close monitoring of call lights and commonsense measures such as keeping family members and patients off rolling stools that sometimes exist in these settings. Given the move of oncology to the outpatient setting, the risk management professional should ensure that any infusion center or other oncology setting has implemented fall prevention strategies.[39]

· · · · · · · · ·
CONCLUSION

Higher volumes of oncology patients are receiving care from multiple providers who may or may not communicate with one another. Among the treatments they may receive in increasingly autonomous outpatient settings are complex and powerful radiation and chemotherapy treatments. The risk management professional is encouraged to use an enterprise risk management (ERM) analysis to prioritize exposures and help clinicians address them in this high-risk clinical environment.

Endnotes

1. Legant, P. "Oncologists and Medical Malpractice." *Journal of Oncology Practice*, Vol 2, No 4 (July), 2006: 164–169.

2. American Cancer Society. *The History of Cancer*. Available at: www.cancer.org/ docroot/cri/content/cri_2_6x_the_history_of_cancer_72.asp. (Accessed April 13, 2010.)

3. Sabel, M. S., K. M. Diehl, and A. E. Chang. "Principles of Surgical Therapy in Oncology," Chapter 4. *Oncology: An Evidence–Based Approach*. New York: Springer, 2006, p. 58.

4. Vapiwala, N.M.D. "MD2B — Introduction to Oncology — Diagnostic Evaluation, Classification, and Staging." *OncoLink*, Abramson Cancer Center of the University of Pennsylvania. Available at: www.oncolink.org/resources/article. cfm?c=9&s=19&ss=34&id=5. Last modified: December 22, 2001. (Accessed December 25, 2009.)

5. Thompson, G. "Vertical Integration of Outpatient Cancer Care." *Radiology Business Journal*. Available at: www.imagingbiz.com/articles/rbj_view/vertical-integration-of-outpatient-cancer-care/. (Accessed September 9, 2009.)

6. Smith, T. J., C. E. Desch, and B. E. Hillner. "The Quality of Cancer Care: Models of Excellence." Proposal submitted to the National Cancer Policy Board; August 31, 1998. Available at: www.iom.edu/~/media/Files/Activity%20Files/Disease/NCPF/modelfnl.ashx. (Accessed December 26, 2009.)

7. *Ibid*.

8. 2009 Commission on Cancer Revised Standards, page 17. Available from: www.facs. org/cancer/coc/programstandards.html.

9. *Ibid*., page 19.

10. "Communication Tool Empowers Nurses; Boosts Patient Safety." *Oncology NEWS International*, Vol 16, No 5 (May 1), 2007. Available at: www.cancernetwork. com/display/article/10165/61553?pageNumber=2. (Accessed December 26, 2009.)

11. National Comprehensive Cancer Network (NCCN) Guidelines. Available at: www.nccn. org/professionals/physician_gls/recently_updated.asp. (Accessed December 27, 2009.)

12. *op. cit.,* Legant, page 2.

13. "Organizational Change in the Face of Highly Public Errors: The Dana-Farber Cancer Institute Experience." Available at: www.webmm.ahrq.gov/perspective. aspx?perspectiveID=3. (Accessed December 26, 2009.)

14. Jacobson, J. O., M. Polovich, and K. K. McNiff. "The American Society of Clinical Oncology/Oncology Nursing Society Chemotherapy Administration Safety Standards." Available at: http://jco.ascopubs.org/cgi/content/short/JCO.2009.25.1264v1. (Accessed December 26, 2009.)

15. *Ibid.,* page 5.

16. *Ibid*., Standard 1, page 4.

17. Walsh, K. E., K. S. Dodd, K. Seetharaman et al. "Medication Errors Among Adults and Children With Cancer in the Outpatient Setting." *Journal of Clinical Oncology*, Vol 27, No 6 (February 20), 2009: 891–896.

18. Schulmeister, L. "Ten Simple Strategies to Prevent Chemotherapy Errors." *Clinical Journal of Oncology Nursing*, Vol 9, No 2, 2009: 201–205.

19. NCCN. "Report on Oral Chemotherapy." *Journal of the National Comprehensive Cancer Network*, Vol 6 Suppl 3, (March) 2008.

20. Birner, A. M., M. K. Bedell, J. T. Avery et al. "Program to Support Safe Oral Chemotherapy." *Journal of Oncology Practice*, Vol 2, No 1 (January) 2006: 5–6.

21. *op cit.,* NCCN.

22. *Ibid.*

23. *op. cit.,* NCCN Task Force at S-7.

24. David A. M., Rodriguez, A., Marks, S.W. "Risk Reduction and Systematic Error Management: Standardization of the Pediatric Chemotherapy Process." As published in Henriksen K., J.B. Battles, M.A. Keyes, and M.L. Grady, editors, *Advances in Patient Safety: New Directions and Alternative Approaches. Vol. 2. Culture and Redesign.* AHRQ Publication No. 08–0034–2. Rockville, Md. Agency for Healthcare Research and Quality, August 2008. Available at www.ahrq.gov/downloads/pub/advances2/vol2/Advances-David_13.pdf. (Accessed April 13, 2010.)

25. Womer, R. B., E. Tracy, S-H. Johnson et al. "Multidisciplinary Systems Approach to Chemotherapy Safety: Rebuilding Processes and Holding the Gains." *Journal of Clinical Oncology*, Vol 20, No 24 (December), 2002, 4705–4712.

26. *Ibid.*

27. *Ibid.*

28. NIOSH Alert "Preventing Occupational Exposure to Antineoplastic and Other Hazardous Drugs in Health Care Settings." September 2004. Available at: www.cdc.gov/niosh/docs/2004–165/pdfs/2004–165.pdf. (Accessed April 13, 2010.)

29. Valanis, B., W.M. Vollmer, and P. Steele. "Occupational Exposure to Antineoplastic Agents: Self-Reported Miscarriages and Stillbirths Among Nurses and Pharmacist." *Journal of Occupational & Environmental Medicine*, Vol 41, No. 8, 1999, 632–638.

30. *op cit.,* NIOSH Alert.

31. University of California San Diego Radiation Oncology "History of Radiation Therapy." Available at: http://radonc.ucsd.edu/patientinformation/history.asp. (Accessed April 13, 2010.)

32. "Intensity-Modulated Radiation Therapy." Available at: www.irsa.org/imrt.html. (Accessed April 13, 2010.)

33. "Errors in Radiation Therapy." *Pennsylvania Patient Safety Advisory*, Vol 6, No 3, (Sept) 2009, 87–92. Available at: www.patientsafetyauthority.org/ADVISORIES/AdvisoryLibrary/2009/Sep6(3)/Pages/87.aspx. (Accessed April 13, 2010.)

34. *Ibid.*

35. *Ibid.*

36. "Radiation Oncology Safety Information System." Available at: www.clin.radfys.lu.se/default.asp. (Accessed December 30, 2009.)

37. Amois, H.I. "New Technologies in Radiation Therapy: Ensuring Patient Safety, Radiation Safety and Regulatory Issues in Radiation Oncology." *Health Physics*, Vol 95, No. 5, (Nov) 2008, 658–665. Abstract available at: http://journals.lww.com/health-physics/Abstract/2008/11000/New_Technologies_in_Radiation_Therapy__Ensuring.24.aspx. (Accessed April 13, 2010.)

38. *op. cit.,* "Errors in Radiation Therapy."

39. Seattle Cancer Care Alliance Outpatient Fall Prevention Program. Available at: www.4elders.org/docs/20071024_Seattle_Cancer_Care_Alliance.pdf. (Accessed December 30, 2009.)

20

Seniors Housing and Long-Term Care

Kathryn Hyer
Mary Lynn Curran

T he U.S. population, estimated at over 304 million in 2008, is growing older at a rapid pace. The number of Americans aged sixty-five and older, estimated at 38 million in 2008, is expected to grow to 72 million by 2030 and to 88 million by 2050, according to the Bureau of the Census projections.[1] The bureau also projects that the fastest growing segment in the older population will be individuals aged eighty-five years and older. Because older persons have a much greater incidence of disability and chronic illness than do younger populations, health, medical, and social services are evolving rapidly to meet these needs. One health services market being transformed by elder needs is seniors housing, which now offers a wide array of medical and personal services options and in so doing creates numerous challenges for the risk management professional.

This chapter will describe three major types of seniors housing: independent living, assisted living, and skilled nursing facilities, including their regulatory environments. It will also identify key operational risk management issues and present solutions.

INDEPENDENT LIVING

The term *independent living* (IL) is used to describe housing for the elderly that offers apartment living, meals, transportation services, activities, housekeeping, and other personal services. Healthcare is not typically included in the program, but easy access to healthcare may be provided. IL arrangements for seniors may be found in a wide array of sizes, characteristics, and prices. The estimated number of such senior housing residences in the United States is approximately twenty-one thousand.[2] The IL residence may be an apartment building, a small group-home arrangement, or a large campus containing a combination of apartment buildings, stand-alone homes, duplexes, and, possibly, healthcare facilities. The IL community is not regulated by the state nor is it subject to state surveyor inspections. Each resident has a written agreement that should provide detail on all services provided by a particular community. Resident agreements run the gamut from a simple apartment lease agreement to a complex and sophisticated contract spelling out all associated services. A specific type of IL residence found in some communities is the *age-qualifying home*; these communities require residents to be a minimum age, such as fifty-five, sixty-five, or older.

IL for seniors is not a new concept; for many years, religious and cultural groups have set up residences where elders can receive living services they no longer are able to, or wish to, provide for themselves.[3] In the last decade, the seniors living market has tried to define itself as an independent setting, to set its operations apart from the nursing home environment that many seniors are trying to avoid. Marketing strategies endeavor to attract prospective residents and their families by suggesting that IL environments will relieve seniors of the worry of taking care of their own home and the work associated with meal preparation, as well as other tasks they must otherwise do for themselves. IL also appeals to those attempting to avoid isolation of the senior, with its associated social and safety ramifications. At the same time, this living arrangement may appear to create a safety net for elderly couples, because entering IL before a major medical event affects one or both spouses may reassure residents and their families that the couple is better prepared to manage such events.

IL for seniors is available in various forms:

- Entrance fee-based continuing care retirement center (CCRC). There are approximately 2,240 licensed CCRCs in the country with 745,000 residents.[4] In the CCRC setting, the resident(s), often a married couple, "buy in" to the IL side of the community. The CCRC offers healthcare services on the campus or healthcare is arranged. The healthcare component may include a skilled nursing facility, an assisted living facility, a memory support unit, home care, and/or rehabilitation services. Larger CCRCs may also offer physicians' services on the campus. The arrangement is much like a health insurance contract under which part of the entrance fee may be used to pay for healthcare services if they are needed at some future time. Another component of the fee paid at the inception of the arrangement usually covers purchase of the apartment or villa, usually treated as a condominium, and the senior or senior couple pay operational assessment fees each month. The property-related aspect of this arrangement generally constitutes an asset that is owned by the senior or seniors. However, the disposition of this asset on the death or move of the occupants is dealt with differently by each organization. Prospective residents should be encouraged to carefully review the resident contract with an attorney.

- Rental CCRC. This arrangement is similar to the one described above. However, the resident is a lessee, rather than a property owner. Healthcare services provided under this type of CCRC are typically fee for service or are covered partly or in whole by health insurance.

- Combined IL and assisted living (AL) community. In these communities, IL apartments may be separated from the AL area or located in the same facility. Often, the exact arrangement relates to how the community evolved. For instance, the building may have started out as IL apartments. However, as the residents of those apartments aged, the community acquired AL license(s) so that residents desiring to "age in place" could access a higher level of services.

- Free-standing IL. These communities are typically made up of apartment buildings that may or may not have been designed for seniors. Services may include housekeeping, one to three meals a day, full-amenity apartments, activities, transportation, and secure buildings. IL residents in these settings often have their own cars and may have their own personal care givers. The apartments may have emergency response systems or residents may be encouraged to wear pendants or bracelets to signal that they need assistance from local emergency medical services.

Any of the above arrangements may also be high-end communities, also known as luxury retirement communities. Living situations may include spacious IL apartments and/or AL facilities. Amenities may include swimming pools, spas, access to golf clubs, and numerous restaurants. Residents may be allowed to upgrade their apartments as desired.

Lower-end independent communities, also known as affordable housing, may be partly or wholly funded by states or municipalities. States increasingly view IL and AL operations as a better value than nursing homes, which must fulfill such expensive Centers for Medicare & Medicaid Services (CMS) mandates as providing 24-hour nursing care. Of note, most states require residents to be "nursing home eligible" to qualify for Medicaid benefits in an environment such as affordable housing.[5] To do so, they must meet a two-pronged test, showing that they are financially and medically in need of services. This clearly increases the risk in the population, which must be balanced against the need for independence, and the associated risk–benefit analysis must be clear to patients and families. As recommended in the 2008 report of an academic center–based task force evaluating the various ways in which states use Medicaid funds for the aging population,

> [p]ersons of all ages with disabilities have the right to choose and/direct a care plan involving "managed risk," in exchange for the advantages of personal freedom. Such risk taking presumes access to good information about the benefits and risk implications of alternatives.[6]

· · · · · · · · ·

OPERATIONAL RISKS AND EXPOSURES

Large numbers of people living in one building or on one campus increase risk and liability exposure, and such exposures are further exacerbated when the resident population is elderly and at risk for declining health and cognitive function. The median age of a new resident in a seniors housing residence is 82.8 years of age.[7]

ILs are expected to offer a warm, homelike, and secure environment where the resident can be self-sufficient. In an effort to reduce exposure to risk, some IL communities do not provide personal or healthcare services and screen out potential residents based on healthcare conditions, cognitive impairment, or disability that would jeopardize the resident's safety and create potential risk to the IL. (See the discussion of Fair Housing.) However, other ILs recognize that the market is increasingly willing to support residents with on-site resources such as home care and physical therapy. As residents age and functions decline or infirmities increase, IL managers and operators arrange additional services as needed.

Risk management concerns flow from the divergence in these approaches because they arguably create different standards of care with respect to long-term care. It is also important for the risk management professional to note that seniors housing–related exposures are partly driven by the marketing strategies employed by long-term care settings. Two potentially dangerous phrases commonly found in the marketing materials of these organizations are *aging in place* and *safe and secure.*

Aging in Place

Seniors' housing marketers use *aging in place* to attract seniors who are seeking their last home, where presumably all their needs will be provided as they age. The term also recognizes that the elder will have changing needs. If these needs are not met, and an injury occurs, there is potential for liability. The senior living community needs to specify what services can and cannot be provided and what actions may be taken if the resident needs a higher level of care or supplementary services. The resident agreement should address this, and so should the residents' handbook. An assessment process should be used to monitor changes in condition; in fact, this is required in government-licensed settings. Many IL communities have created a monitoring and tracking system whereby multiple departments in the community (dining services, concierge services, housekeeping, and so forth) meet and relate their observations and any events that have occurred. The purpose is to head-off any drastic change in the resident's status and provide a proactive basis for staff to judge when it is appropriate to bring in services that preserve independence, for instance physical therapy, companion services, and so on. From a liability reduction perspective, the community should have mechanisms in place so that residents' needs are properly met in the right setting and the organization does not increase risk to individual residents or become vulnerable to accusations of operating nursing homes without licenses.

The residents in IL and AL should also understand, through the residency agreement, handbook, and open discussions, that the community calls emergency services (9–1–1) following an incident such as a fall, not only to assist the resident to get up, but also to evaluate the resident for injury because nurses are not in the building 24 hours a day.

Safe and Secure   *Safe and secure* is another term commonly found in marketing materials. To prospective residents, the phrase may suggest that the setting offers a controlled environment that will address seniors' safety and security concerns. However, liability may later be incurred when events such break-ins, failure to respond to calls for help, and/or lack of a planned response to natural or human-caused disaster prove that the organization's claims of security were false.

Life Safety   Fire and/or smoke in a facility are critical risks with potential to affect many lives. In the United States, some senior housing settings have no fire suppression systems, creating a significant exposure. There are also many communities that allow smoking in the building. Even with fire suppression systems in place, residents may not hear alarms, understand how to shelter in place, or be clear on how to evacuate. Also, fire suppression systems have been known to fail in an emergency or to cause floods due to faulty signals.

One obvious strategy is an evacuation plan. However, such plans are challenging to implement in any occupied building, especially one that houses elders. An IL community of any size should have an active safety committee that is responsible for developing and overseeing the implementation of a comprehensive fire response and evacuation plan, as well as other life safety issues that pertain to both residents and staff. This plan, and other such processes, should be reviewed for accuracy at specified intervals and whenever the building is modified in any way. The fire response and evacuation plan should also be rehearsed on a regular basis by all potential participants. The community should maintain documentation of regular fire drills and evacuation plans.

The following risk control techniques are common strategies that can mitigate injury and property damage from fire:

- Work with the local fire department on response methods to a fire. Be certain the local fire department knows the building is for seniors and not nursing care.

- Test all fire alarms, smoke alarms, fire extinguishers, and sprinkler systems per state and manufacturers' guidelines.

- Drill, rehearse, and walk through disasters such as fire, sprinkler set-off, power outage, and other disasters.

- If smoking is allowed, have fire blankets stationed in the building.

- Have fire blankets and fire extinguishers visibly available near designated smoking areas.

- Control oxygen tank storage from access.

Please see Chapter 19 on emergency management in Volume 1 for more information. Recent natural disasters that have affected seniors housing help identify still more issues that must be addressed in life safety planning. These include hurricanes; brush fires; extreme heat, cold or snow; flooding and infrastructure failures, such as malfunctioning sewers; and infestations of vermin and insects. All of these perils, common in any residence, become more concerning in a setting in which they may affect many elderly people.

Falls   In IL settings, as in all seniors housing environments, the most frequent reason for a claim and/or lawsuit are falls and injuries from falls.[8] Falls occur in all venues of long-term care, including independent, assisted, skilled, and memory unit facilities, and they are a significant exposure, potentially leading to life-long disability and hastened death. (Please see the data specific to falls in other seniors living settings presented later in this chapter.) Numerous studies on causes of falls, prevention of falls, and the overall cost of falls to society have prompted many seniors housing organizations to mount aggressive campaigns aimed at preventing falls and/or reducing associated injuries. All seniors housing organizations should implement fall assessment and intervention processes. They should also continually refine such processes by evaluating effectiveness in light of data such as that yielded by tracking and trending of fall-related occurrences.

Third-Party Services   IL and AL facilities often allow third-party providers to augment services and care. These services may be personnel services, companion services, hospice, physical therapy, occupational therapy, dentistry, and so on. Care providers brought in to help the resident remain as independent as possible may come from other aspects of the organization, for example, an IL-based home care service; however, any introduction of third-party resources unrelated to the IL triggers a range of associated exposures. At minimum, the organization should require evidence of appropriate licensure or certification and current professional, general liability, and workers' compensation insurance. There should also be a criminal background history check performed, as well as a motor vehicle records check, as appropriate.

Another common third-party arrangement is illustrated by IL communities providing office space to physicians to make it more convenient for residents to see their doctor(s). A related example involves IL communities who set up clinics offering ophthalmology, dental, podiatric, as well as geriatric medicine resources. It is essential that the organization credential and privilege these professionals, just as a hospital would, to ensure their qualifications and promote defensibility of a corporate negligence case alleging that the organization did not properly oversee all activities within its walls. It is also critical that signage, name tags, and other strategies, such as provisions in the resident agreement, make clear to residents that these third-party caregivers are not employees of the IL organization. This is because a court may imply an employment relationship under the doctrine of apparent agency if it can be shown that the resident relied on his or her perception that the caregiver was an employee.

It is recommended that all third parties providing clinical services be subject to an agreement that outlines specific responsibilities between the physician(s) or other care provider(s) and the organization. In addition, as previously noted, the office or clinic area should post adequate signage and/or the IL should incorporate in the resident agreement a statement clarifying that physicians on the property and their staff are not employees of the senior community, but rather are independent contractors who will bill independently. Third-party physicians' office personnel should not wear any lab coats or name tags with the senior community's name and should not have business cards with the community name.

The risk management principles applicable to the resources discussed above also apply to contractors providing services anywhere on the campus, for example, plumbing, carpentry, roofing, electric, landscaping, and so forth. All such individuals should provide evidence of appropriate insurance. In addition to avoidance of corporate liability and other theories that might be alleged if a resident were injured as a result of these individuals' activities, any injury to an independently contracted worker might result in liability for the injured contractor's healthcare expenses unless that individual has his or her own coverage for on-the-job injury.

Occupancy-Related Issues   Seniors housing occupancy has recently been reduced by double digits in some areas of the country, in large part due to the real estate and economic crisis that began in 2008. This decreased occupancy is probably due in large part to the economic paralysis of prospective residents who were relying on the equity in their homes to pay for their move to seniors housing. Risk management issues that result from reduced occupancy are, in turn, tied to reduced financial capability of the IL. With less income, the organization will likely tighten budgets, delay maintenance, and may lay off employees. All of these issues add up to reduced services, which could result in increased resident and employee injuries. There may also be a relationship between low occupancy and increased claims due to economic incapacity and related anxiety of residents, residents, families, and employees.

Fair Housing Act   The Fair Housing Act prohibits discrimination against prospects based on race, religion, age, disability, marital status, and/or sexual orientation.[9] Physical and mental impairments; debilitating conditions such as heart disease, arthritis, blindness, Alzheimer's disease; and nonambulatory status are all examples of covered disabilities in the law. Clinically recognized mental and addictive conditions such as depression and alcoholism are also within the definition. Current use of illegal drugs is excluded from coverage of the law, but a recovering user is likely to be protected and therefore eligible to move into the community. To avoid potential allegations of Fair Housing Act violations,[10] which are associated with large fines (generally not covered by insurance) and negative publicity, it is wise for seniors housing organizations to review their marketing materials and the scripts that sales and marketing personnel follow to attract prospects. For instance, any perceived attempt of the senior housing community to dissuade a prospective resident who relies on a scooter or wheelchair from joining the community in an effort to attract more mobile residents may result in a violation.

· · · · · · · · ·

ASSISTED LIVING

For frail elders who want to avoid nursing home placement, yet require more support than can be provided in the community or ILs, assisted living facilities (ALFs) offer a broad array of resources in community-based residential models, including more health and social services than are generally available at home, although not as many as are provided in skilled nursing facilities. Similar to IL, the interest of prospective residents in ALFs is often based on the premise that autonomy, privacy, and other personal and healthcare needs can be met outside the institutionalized setting of the nursing home.

There are roughly 39,500 ALFs in the United States, housing over one million residents.[11] The number of residents residing in such facilities may range from several people to 300, but the most common occupancy is between 25 and 120. Depending on the state in which they are located, ALFs may also be known as personal care homes, sheltered homes, supportive living, domiciliary or residential care facilities, community residences, and/or custodial care. Although the distinction between AL and skilled nursing may be clear to the professional working in this area, the public and consumers of this service continue to confuse AL with skill nursing. See Table 20.1 for differences between these two elder care services.

TABLE 20.1   Differences Between Assisted Living and Skilled Nursing

Assisted Living	*Reimbursement*	*Regulation*	*Demographic Differences*	*Services*
Also known as residential care, personal care, supportive living, nursing home light, and other terms. One or more activities of daily living (ADLs) are provided, e.g., bathing, dressing, toileting, eating, grooming, ambulation, medication assistance. Extensive medical care not provided. Emphasis on privacy and autonomy. Residents typically bring their own furniture. A medical director is not required.	Private pay or Medicaid waiver or combined. Long-term care insurance may reimburse for the healthcare services rendered, but not room and board.	Every state has rules and regulations that come under the state's public health, healthcare, and/or social services department. State may have AL survey team; some states use the nursing home survey team. Visits may occur annually or biannually or on complaint only, depending on the state.	39,500 facilities in United States. Average size 25–120. Population estimated at one million.	3 meals a day 24-hour supervision Personal care Housekeeping Laundry Transportation Assistance with medication Security and emergency call system Health and exercise programs Social, cultural, and educational activities
Skilled Nursing/ Long-Term Care	**Reimbursement**	**Regulation**	**Demographic Differences**	**Services**
Skilled nursing and long-term care provides all ADLs plus nursing and medical care.	Medicare for skilled and rehabilitation services generally for short-stay (less than 100 days) and then private pay, secondary insurance, or Medicaid, if qualified.	Federal regulations, CMS rules.	15,000 facilities. Average size 108. Estimated population at 1.4 million.	Same as above, with emphasis on nursing and custodial care. Requirements include nursing care available 24 hours a day, 7 days a week, medical director, and licensed nursing home administrator.

Many elders and their families may not understand that states vary considerably in the regulation of AL services and settings. In some states, AL is viewed as an extension of social services. Oversight comes from the departments of social welfare rather than healthcare, because the states are intent on reducing the facilities' similarity to a medical model. The social model ALFs prefer to be associated with less medical management, less medication management oversight, and less assistance to immobile residents. Thus, they want to attract more independent, healthy, and mobile residents. Other states view ALs as an extension of the healthcare system, sometimes with oversight by the departments of public health or healthcare. Operations in these states tend to have more regulations on medication management, medical management, and resident care. Families may view ALFs as "light nursing homes," and do not have realistic expectations. For instance, they may assume there is 24-hour nursing care when that is actually rare in AL. In order to avoid misunderstandings, the wise AL organization takes time to understand the differences in the venues and then spends time and effort educating the consumer: residents and their families. From a risk management perspective, setting realistic expectations for the consumer of AL services is critical. Sales and marketing staff and those responsible for evaluating and assessing must understand these dynamics so that they can properly inform prospective residents and their families.

The care of residents with dementia-related diseases such as Alzheimer's often takes place in ALFs specifically designed to address the range of needs exhibited by those affected with dementia. Residents with dementia vary in their perception of their own safety. However, they are often ambulatory in the initial and intermediate phases of their disease process and may not require assistance with activities of daily living, such as ambulating, eating, dressing, and grooming. Skilled care settings may be too confining for residents with dementia because they often need to walk around, a characteristic of dementia-related diseases. Consequently, many states permit AL operations to provide a level of care designed to accommodate dementia-related conditions. One significant difference between a traditional AL setting and the dementia unit that may be adjacent is that the dementia operation is generally housed on a locked unit to prevent residents from wandering. Also, this unit may provide a formal program of activities to meet the needs of persons with memory impairment.

Operational Risks and Exposures in Assisted Living

Liability exposures in the AL setting are similar to those in independent and skilled environments. Although AL residents are assumed to have a greater level of self-sufficiency than skilled nursing residents, and are more capable of partnering with the organization in their care, the AL setting is just as likely as the skilled nursing environment to be found responsible for resident injuries.

This potential culpability emphasizes the need for the risk management professional to maintain awareness of and promote compliance with the requirements of each state in which their organization has locations. Specifically, the risk management professional should be familiar with key requirements such as those that pertain to admission criteria, caregiver-to-resident staffing ratios, medication management allowances, assessment requirements, and what is defined as *reasonable care*. Aside from each state's Web site addressing AL regulations, there is an annual compilation made available by the National Center for Assisted Living, *State Regulatory Review*, March 2009, at www.NCAL.org.

Assessments   In the AL sector, each state requires the needs of residents to be identified, and the degree to which ongoing needs are met must be assessed.[12] The assessment tools used in AL organizations range from handwritten tools to sophisticated computer programs that capture a detailed assessment, including service fees associated with a particular task. The frequency with which these assessments must be performed varies from monthly to annually, and depth of the required assessment is also variable. The most commonly seen requirement is that assessments be performed quarterly, but it is clearly important to be familiar with individual state requirements and assess the resident more often if there is a change in physical and/or mental condition.

It is also common practice to perform a mini-mental examination (MME) when the resident moves in, and periodically thereafter, to determine cognitive status. Other assessments commonly seen in AL environments include fall risk assessment, elopement risk assessment, and the self-administration medication management (SAMM) assessment.[13] From a risk perspective, these assessments, when completed, followed up, and well documented, can be critical to defending against an allegation of negligence, such as failure to monitor. For this reason, documentation in the narrative notes supporting these assessments is critically important to a defense. States require narrative notes to capture assessments and upon change in condition, and frequent notes are extremely helpful in promoting continuity of care and can be invaluable if there is a need to defend allegations of negligence involving the care of the resident. When the care of a resident becomes more complex, yet he or she is stable, it is common to see documentation of assessments and follow up on a monthly basis.

Medication Assistance or Administration   Requirements pertaining to medication-related activities, including qualifications of care providers who render this specialized aspect of care, vary widely from state to state, and the risk management professional should be familiar with pertinent regulations. The AL industry reports that 80 percent of seniors in AL facilities need help with managing their medications.[14] However, medication administration is a challenge in the AL setting because (1) AL residents on the average take seven to fourteen medications per day; (2) ALFs do not have a designated medical director, as is the case in skilled facilities in which the medical director oversees and standardizes medication regimes; and (3) state regulations pertaining to AL communities do not require a 24-hour nursing staff to administer medications. AL organizations, depending on state regulations, may employ nurses, nursing assistants who have taken courses and passed a competency test for administering medications, or medication technicians who administer medications. The medications themselves may include high-risk products such as warfarin, controlled substances such as morphine derivatives, and insulin. All such medications, if not given in a timely fashion or if overdosed or underdosed, may result in serious injuries.

If the resident is self-administering medication, he or she should be assessed for ability to self-administer. There are many such assessment tools available.[15] Some states require that this capability be assessed when the resident first enters an AL setting or when the resident determines that he or she wants to self-administer.

If a resident is no longer capable of managing his or her own medications, and the AL facility will take over responsibility for administration, it is essential that all medication risk-reduction mechanisms applicable in an acute care setting be employed. For example, unit dose should be used for all medications whenever possible, and those who administer medication should be taught to keep the medication in the unit dose packaging until it is actually given to the patient. Pouring medications from commercial pharmacy containers creates significant risk of error.

Another safety precaution for patients coming into the AL environment is a medication reconciliation process, in which the medications that patients bring with them to the AL are assessed against those for which orders are written. The same process should take place when the patient is transferred to or from the hospital, home, another unit, etc. Even though not all AL settings are accredited by The Joint Commission (TJC), the fact that TJC has required that medication reconciliation processes be in place in AL settings since 2005 arguably makes this practice the standard of care.[16] Recognizing the difficulty in reconciling medications for all transitions in care, TJC is not addressing medication reconciliation in the accreditation report and is not issuing any Requirements For Improvements (RFIs) for failure to comply.

Medication administration is one of the highest risk and most detailed care activities in the AL environment.[17] Therefore, it is essential that staff administering medication complete a comprehensive training program, including demonstration of related skills and periodic observation of their techniques by a nurse, physician, or pharmacist. Any medication error, or potential error, for example, a near miss, must be reported as an aspect of the facility's occurrence reporting system, the resultant data trended for issues, and any identified issues immediately addressed. Also, although having a medical director oversee medication administration is desirable, it may be as effective and more cost effective to involve a consulting pharmacist. Any pharmacy services should be contracted with adherence to the risk management principles previously discussed in the previous section of this chapter on regarding third-party services.

Another valuable component of medication administration–related quality improvement is periodic auditing of the medication administration record (MAR) against a current set of the resident's orders. This approach, closely related to medication reconciliation, can identify transcription or ordering issues. Any discrepancies should be documented on occurrence reports and followed up through the organization's quality improvement processes.

One mechanism used to prevent medication errors is to have residents and their families bring a list of current medications to every physician visit. Some facilities have a physician visit form that captures all medication changes during such visits (such as additional medications, deletions, or changes in dose). Other facilities attach the current medication administration record (MAR) to a physician visit form to enable the physician to review medications and dosages that are currently ordered.

Falls As previously noted, falls are the most frequent basis for a claim or lawsuit against an AL community. Falls are also the leading cause of fatal and nonfatal injuries for adults 65 and older. [18] The most serious injury is hip fracture; one-half of older adults hospitalized for hip fracture never regain their former level of function. Causes of hip fractures include age-related conditions, muscle weakness, environmental factors, several types of medications, and a history of falls. Also, lack of physical activity, osteoporosis, low body mass index, and a previous hip fracture are precursors to hip fracture. The highest average total paid, including indemnity and expense, in ALFs for falls is $191,438 and $186,635 in continuing care retirement communities (CCRCs). [19] Still other injuries that may be sustained from falls include deadly head injuries and fractures to the legs, arms, and wrist fractures. In AL as well as skilled care environments, every resident should be assessed for potential falls, and the service or care plan should address the interventions to prevent falls. Among many preventive strategies are the following:

- Check to see that shoes fit properly.
- Evaluate for ability to walk with and without physical devices, for example, a cane or walker.
- Evaluate environment for clear pathways, no loose rugs, ample grab bars, appropriate lighting, and access to chairs for rest periods.
- Evaluate the medication regime. In particular, consider the effects of polypharmacy (multiple medications) and use of antipsychotic drugs as well as other medications that alter sensory perception.

AL communities are advised to track the number of falls on a monthly basis, with particular attention to those who fall more than once. Prioritizing strategies to address issues identified in fall-related occurrences and orienting all staff to principles associated with fall prevention efforts are essential components of the organization's safety program.

Of particular importance with regard to loss mitigation strategies are the actions taken following a fall to check for fractures or head injuries. Because nurses are not usually present twenty-four hours a day in an AL community, it is essential that staff on duty be familiar with emergency procedures, including calling emergency medical services to evaluate the resident and determine if the resident requires a higher level of care (transfer to the emergency department). Residents and their families may sometimes resist going to the emergency department due to the cost or the inconvenience of an emergency department visit. However, if a resident is thought to have a head injury, or a fracture cannot be ruled out, staff is obligated to call for emergency assistance. Staff should be trained on how to persuade residents and their families when there is resistance to an emergency department visit. (As previously discussed, preparing residents and families for such contingencies in advance through education, including the resident handbook, is wise.) When an emergency department visit is not indicated, because there are no apparent injuries at all and the resident is able to assist himself or herself, it is extremely important to document the facts surrounding the situation, including the resident's resistance, notification to the family, and any interventions applied to prevent another fall. Also, the status (vital signs, observations, pain threshold) of the resident should be documented routinely, per protocol, for forty-eight to seventy-two hours following a fall. Additionally, all residents who fall should be evaluated for potential to fall again, with assessment for fall risk associated with multiple medications, underlying medical conditions, and potential environmental issues such as scatter rugs, and so forth. Another resource sometimes present in the AL environment that should be leveraged in fall reduction strategies is the physical therapist, who may provide an initial evaluation of the resident's gait and the environmental situation. AL residents may also benefit from gait-training and muscle-strengthening programs, which can help them to maximize their mobility and or transfer techniques, thereby reducing their risk of a fall.

Elopement Elopement is defined as an event in which the resident leaves a community on an unscheduled, unsupervised, and uncontrolled basis. Elopement is not just a concern for residents in dementia units. In any IL and AL setting, residents' cognitive status can change quickly, and disorientation clearly increases the resident's risk. Residents in all seniors living venues may be at particular risk when residents are new. In an unfamiliar environment, they may flee without any consideration of foul weather or other dangers, such as street traffic.

The injuries of residents who have been hurt due to the community's failure to provide a promised "safe and secure environment" may result in the organization being held accountable for significant damages. This is of particular concern now that some states' elder abuse laws provide for the award of punitive damages.

There are many important strategies for preventing elopement:

- Assessment of the resident for cognitive understanding and presence of agitation (the mini-mental examination is one tool that can facilitate this process)
- Controlled access and egress with key pad access, locks, alarms, and camera monitoring
- Internal control, with locked doors of areas not intended for residents, for example, storage, kitchen areas, model apartments, and so on.
- Accounting for all residents during all shifts
- Rehearsals or drills done routinely during the year, to refresh staff on how to respond to a missing resident, including how to conduct an orderly and expedient search

The expense of claims for elopement involving injury that have been brought against seniors living organizations varies, depending on the circumstances and the injury. In 2009, CNA HealthPro reported an average payout, including expenses, of $337,344 of cases involving elopement from AL facilities. However, there have been news media reports of cases settling for $1 million dollars or more for elopement cases that resulted in serious injuries or death.[20]

Behavioral Issues According to recent studies, at least half of assisted living residents age sixty-five or older have Alzheimer's disease, another disease or condition that causes dementia, or cognitive impairment that is probably caused by these diseases and conditions.[21] Of particular note, Alzheimer's and other dementia-related diseases may result in personality changes that involve residents' acting out aggressively, for example, shouting, yelling, pushing, shoving, hitting, and kicking. Residents, family members, and employees are all potential victims of this behavior. If this behavior is identified and not addressed, the organization may be liable for resultant injuries. Staff working with dementia patients should be trained in de-escalation techniques and incident response. By protocol, every new resident should also be assessed initially and then closely monitored for aggressive behavior while they acclimate to the community.

The organization's incident response plan should incorporate all resources that can and should be tapped when there is an out of control resident, for instance, a geriatric psychiatrist. Medications and behavioral management strategies are frequent remedies for such behavior. However, in some cases, transfer of the resident to a psychiatric facility may be necessary to protect the resident, other residents, family, and staff.

Abuse   *Elder abuse* is an all-inclusive term that incorporates all types of abusive behavior against the elderly.[22] It is also used to refer to specific acts of physical violence. Most experts agree that elder abuse can be an act of commission (abuse) or omission (neglect), intentional or unintentional, and that it can take one or more forms: physical, psychological (emotional and/or verbal aggression), and financial. In all these cases, such abuse and neglect results in unnecessary suffering, injury, pain, loss, and/or violation of human rights and decreased quality of life.

Allegations of abuse in AL are taken as seriously as in the skilled setting. All employees must be trained on what abuse is and their responsibility to report to the supervisor any activities or observations suggestive of abuse. This training is best done by an expert and then at least annually, when allegations occur, and when the community has challenging residents. Organizations should follow a zero tolerance policy for abuse, and it is particularly important that staff training include specific examples of what physical acts or voice tones might be construed as abuse.[23]

. . . .
NEGOTIATED RISK AGREEMENTS

AL residents (and their families) want to maintain independence for as long as possible and want to preserve their right to self-determine the role of the service provider in their need for continuing care. The judicious use of negotiated risk agreements (NRAs) (which are contracts) is one way to support resident independence while protecting the facility from liability. NRAs negotiated between the resident and facility identify activities that the residents will engage in and the autonomy that they will exercise over their own care. In many cases, these activities might be outside the scope of what would normally be permitted or tolerated in the absence of such an agreement. In other words, the resident has negotiated an accommodation or an exception to facility policy for a trade-off. This trade-off may be the forfeiture of residents' right to sue the facility, and the facility is, under the NRA, held harmless should residents become injured due to their negotiated activities. For example, smoking, walking unassisted, or other activities may be deemed risky by the facility and to mitigate that risk request the resident or family to sign a NRA. Additional information on contract review may be found elsewhere in this series.

NRAs have had some negative reviews because they have been used liberally and casually in some areas of the country. In some states, judges are quick to discount the agreement. Organizations are wise to view this agreement as an opportunity to have an informed consent discussion with the family and also to use the form as a temporary step until a more acceptable arrangement can be made, for instance, transfer to a higher level of care, the hire of a private caregiver, and so forth. In some large AL organizations, the completion of a NRA triggers a required consultation with a regional nurse or operations director to sort out all options and interventions.

Arbitration Agreements

This may be a separate document or wording that is incorporated into a residency agreement. There is debate on how this type of agreement is best articulated: a separate document referred to in the residency agreement or a provision embedded in the residency agreement. And some have argued that the best time to execute an arbitration agreement is at move-in, possibly as a condition of move-in, because it may be too late to negotiate such an arrangement when a serious incident occurs. In any case, signing an arbitration agreement obligates the resident or family to resolve any legal conflicts with the organization through arbitration or mediation processes, not in a court of law. Cases brought to mediators save significant trial-associated costs, including defense expenses, and time of the organization as well as of the parties bringing the case forward.

Congress stepped into the debate in late 2008 with the Fairness in Nursing Home Arbitration Act, which would essentially invalidate all preadmission arbitration agreements. The act did not clear the U.S. Senate Judiciary Committee, but the bill was reintroduced in early 2009. The essence of the proposed ban is that arbitration would be used only when a dispute arises and both parties agree to arbitrate.

· · · · · · · · ·
SKILLED NURSING FACILITIES

Approximately 15,000 nursing homes with 1.5 million beds in the United States participate in Medicare or Medicaid, and they served more than 1.4 million Americans in 2008.[24] The number of nursing home beds has increased slightly, but occupancy on average has fallen to 84 percent.[25] Nursing homes serve two distinct populations. Nearly half of all admissions are short-stay Medicare residents who return home within one month.[26] Medicare reimburses beneficiaries for up to one hundred days of nursing home care as long as the elder has a three-day hospital stay and qualifies for skilled services. Nursing homes seek to admit patients from the hospital for short-stay care because Medicare reimbursement is high for complex nursing and rehabilitative services. The other 50 percent of admissions are for residents with chronic care management needs and for cognitive impairments; generally, these residents stay more than one hundred days. Many long-stay residents eventually qualify for Medicaid after "spending down" as private payers. The risk management professional should be aware of the numerous federal requirements that pertain to quality of care and residents' rights in nursing homes.

Operational Risks and Exposures in Skilled Nursing Facilities

The issues discussed in regard to IL and AL are also important in the skilled nursing facility (SNF) environment, for instance, falls. Key differences are driven by the increased dependency of the SNF population on the seniors housing organization. For example, decubitus ulcers are much less of a concern in the more active IL and AL settings than they are in the SNF. Most important, public concern about the degree to which SNFs fulfill their care obligations to these much more dependent residents is largely responsible for two key senior housing phenomena. One is the fear of nursing homes that drives elders to avoid SNF care if they can, and the other is regulatory scrutiny of nursing homes that is more intense than that applied to any other healthcare setting. Finally, risk management professionals should be familiar with the information that CMS provides to the public at the CMS Web site "Nursing Home Compare" at www.Medicare.gov. There, data are available on every nursing home participating in Medicare or Medicaid. The information compares each home against the average for homes within the state and against other homes within the nation. The Web site features key information on each nursing home, including the results of the three most recent quality-of-care inspections; average minutes of nurse staffing by nursing level provided to each resident daily; and other important information data for consumers, families, and friends. It also contains the results of nineteen different quality-of-care measures for each nursing home, such as the percentage of residents who have pressure ulcers or are subject to physical restraints. An overall ranking by CMS provides every home with a summary score on quality. Scores for homes range from one to five stars, with five stars signifying the highest quality rating. In addition, CMS maintains a list of Special Focus Facilities, which are facilities identified as demonstrating poor quality care. Risk management professionals should frequently review these public records to determine if CMS has identified quality issues in their nursing homes.

Survey and Surveyors Issues

CMS defines the federal requirements of participation that nursing homes must meet to participate in the Medicare and Medicaid programs. The requirements establish specific care standards that affect residents' functional health status, including quality of care, quality of life, and the facility's management practices.[27] However, unlike other healthcare settings, the federal government does not accept nursing home accreditation by TJC or other certification agencies as *deemed status* (evidence that a Medicare SNF or a Medicaid nursing facility complies with program participation standards). Consequently, all nursing homes are inspected on average every twelve months by state surveyors. CMS contracts with the individual states to certify that homes meet these federal standards, and the state inspects to determine if state requirements that exceed federal regulations are met.[28] Any violation of the standards is cited as a deficiency, with a range of sanctions attached to the violation. To avoid predictability of an annual inspection, the window for the annual survey is from nine to fifteen months after the previous survey. In a further effort to ensure that facilities provide adequate care during nights and weekends, CMS requires at least 10 percent of all surveys occur during off-hours (before 8:00 A.M. or after 6:00 P.M.) or on weekends.

Citations for violations of federal regulations are determined through the annual survey process. Life and safety regulations, known as K-tags, fall under the federal regulations and are also addressed in the annual inspection. Surveyors are required to follow procedures and protocols established by CMS to determine if facilities are in compliance.[29] Two types of annual inspection, traditional survey and quality indicator survey (QIS), are currently used to evaluate nursing homes' compliance.[30] Federal law details regulations related to quality of residents' care and rights; these are F-tags. For each deficient practice identified in relation to any of these regulations, the severity and scope of the violation is determined; deficiencies varied in severity from A (least serious) to L (most serious). Severity has four levels of harm: Level 1, no actual harm with potential for minimal harm; Level 2, no actual harm with potential for more than minimal harm that is not immediate jeopardy; Level 3, actual harm that is not immediate jeopardy; Level 4, immediate jeopardy to resident health or safety.[31]

Scope is determined by how many residents of the facility were (or could have been) affected and is classified as isolated, a pattern of violation, or widespread.

When a deficiency is found, the state may recommend and CMS can impose sanctions, including monetary penalties, increased state monitoring, a ban on payment for Medicare or Medicaid admissions, or in rare cases for serious violations, closure of the facility.

The CMS Web site www.cms.hhs.gov/CertificationandCompliance provides information on nursing home survey processes, regulations, and studies or reports assessing quality of care.

Examples of Key Regulations

Whereas IL and AL operations are still defining clinical approaches to meet the standard of care, regulations define such approaches for the SNF.

For example, The Nursing Home Reform Act of 1987 specifies that a facility "must provide services and activities to attain or maintain the highest practicable physical, mental, and psychological well-being of each resident in accordance with a written plan of care."

CMS regulations further provide that "residents have the right to be free from verbal, sexual, physical, or mental abuse; corporal punishment; and involuntary seclusion, and to be free from any physical or chemical restraints imposed for purposes of discipline or convenience." Under federal regulations, facilities must do the following:

- Develop and implement written policies and procedures that prohibit mistreatment, neglect, abuse, and misappropriation of resident property.

- Report to the state's nurse's aide registry or licensing authorities any knowledge of actions by a court of law against an employee that would indicate unfitness for services.

- Ensure that all alleged violations involving mistreatment, neglect, or abuse including injuries from unknown sources, are reported immediately to the facility administrator, to the state survey or certification agency, and other officials as required by law.

- Be able to provide evidence that all alleged violations are thoroughly investigated and that further potential abuse is prevented.

- Report findings of the facility's investigation to the administrator, to the state survey and certification agencies, and to other officials in accordance with state law within five working days of the occurrence; if the violation is verified, corrective action must be taken.[32]

Complaint Survey

State surveyors may conduct a complaint investigation in response to a reported risk event or as part of a regularly scheduled inspection. Generally, complaint surveys require a review of clinical records and surveyor interviews with the resident, employee, and family. These interviews are conducted to determine whether an event constitutes a deficiency. It is best to advise staff to provide documentation and evidence that frames a particular event or complaint as dissatisfaction, not as a deficiency.

When investigating a potential risk event, managers should refer to all applicable standards, regulations, and survey protocols to assess whether a potential violation might have occurred. Consideration of the following requirements may facilitate investigation of a risk event.

- Quality of care. Prevention of pressure ulcers, pain management, facility responses to a resident's change(s) in condition, management of nutrition or hydration problems, and medication errors.

- Resident rights and facility practices. Prevention of abuse, neglect, and mistreatment; use of physical and chemical restraints, especially use of antipsychotic drugs; resident freedom of choice; advance directives; and informed consent.

- Administration. Injury investigation and reporting requirements, provision of physician services, supervision of medical care, and quality assurance committee.

- Quality of life. Activities or programs to promote the resident's highest practicable level of physical, mental, and psychosocial well-being.

- Resident assessment. Functional assessments, establishment of the interdisciplinary plan of care, and timing and management of changes in condition.

- Investigation and reporting obligations. A facility must investigate any injury to a resident and make a report to the facility administrator within five days. Findings of these investigations must also be forwarded to the state survey agency. State law may also establish separate reporting obligations under a vulnerable adult statute.

Facility Maintenance and Safety Issues

Regular assessment of the safety and environmental aspects of the facility will assist in risk identification and acknowledgment of the current policies and procedures.

The Safe Medical Devices Act (SMDA) of 1990 identifies nursing homes as device users and therefore subject to the medical device reporting (MDR) requirement. A medical device is any item that is used for the diagnosis, treatment, or prevention of a disease, injury, illness, or other condition, and that is not a drug. In nursing homes, this includes pressure manometers, thermometers, oxygen administering apparatus, infusion pumps, cardiac monitors, and the more recognizable long-term care staples such as walkers, canes, wheelchairs, crutches, hospital beds, and physical therapy equipment. A medical device also includes bandages, heating blankets, tongue depressors, and cotton swabs.

Nursing homes must have written procedures for internal MDR systems and documentation and recordkeeping. Adverse event files must also be kept. Reportable adverse events include only those incidents or reports of serious injury or death that the nursing home received or becomes aware of by other means that suggest the adverse event may be attributed to a medical device.

Personnel Issues in Skilled Nursing Facilities

Background Checking   Participation in Medicare and Medicaid programs requires long-term care facilities to query state nurse's aide registries for criminal history, specifically felonies, because this history puts residents at high risk. Facilities must check for findings of abuse, mistreatment, negligence, or misappropriation of property before allowing staff to work with residents. Also, facilities' administration should verify employees' driver's licenses and review their driving records before allowing anyone to use a facility vehicle to transport residents. Be familiar with the state's specific requirements for the transportation of residents. Depending on state-specific laws, type of vehicle being used to transport residents and the number of passengers being transported will determine the class of license that will be required. On at least an annual basis, the driving record of all known drivers should be accessed and reviewed.

Staffing Ratios   Over the past twenty-five years, numerous research studies have documented the important relationship between nurse staffing levels, particularly registered nurse (RN) staffing and the outcomes of care.[33] The average number of RN hours per resident day declined by 25 percent between 1998 and 2003 (from 0.8 to 0.6 hours) and then remained about the same between 2003 and 2008. The number of licensed practical nurses (LPNs/LVNs) with about one year of training, increased by 14 percent, and total nurse staffing increased by 5 percent between 2003 and 2008.[34] Studies have shown facilities with more RN staffing have higher quality of care on average. The average staffing levels are far below the level recommended by experts, which is 0.75 RN hours per resident day and 4.1 total hours of nurse staffing per resident day. The benefits of higher staffing levels, especially RN staffing, can include lower mortality rates; improved physical functioning; less antibiotic use; fewer pressure ulcers, catheterized residents, and urinary tract infections; lower hospitalization rates; and less weight loss and dehydration.[35]

Increasingly, states are mandating staffing levels required to care for nursing home residents. Facilities that care for chronically ill residents are staffed primarily by paraprofessional nursing aides who are responsible for providing the majority of personal care for residents. The aides are supervised by the licensed nursing staff, and the level of nursing supervision varies by state law. In some states, nursing aides can be supervised by LPNs. The majority of nurses in long-term care facilities are LPNs who are frequently charged with medication management. Unless a waiver is received, CMS requires that the long-term care facility designate a licensed nurse (RN, LPN, LVN) to serve as a charge nurse each shift and that the long-term care facility use the services of a RN for at least eight consecutive hours a day, seven days a week.[36,37] Usually, the director of nursing and assistant director of nursing are RNs; however, the director of nursing may serve as a charge nurse only when the facility has an average daily occupancy of sixty or fewer residents.[38] Increasingly, the level of RN staffing is of concern, because studies suggest that the skill level of nursing staff affects the quality of patient care. There remain, however, many open issues related to the suitability and level of staffing that is appropriate for nursing home care.

Medical Director   The required medical director is usually a part-time staff member and reports to the administrator. Medical directors vary considerably in their responsibility for oversight of the medical care of residents; however, regulations require this oversight, and surveyors can cite a facility for inadequate medical supervision.

Credentialing and Recredentialing Staff   All clinical staff, including medical, rehabilitation, and nursing staff, should be credentialed. When credentialing their practitioners, long-term care facilities often struggle with obtaining the needed documents from the primary or secondary sources. The correct method entails calling the state board, finding out whether the applicant holds an active license, and requesting written verification while cross-referencing the information to check for license restrictions. The purpose of primary sourcing is to reduce the possibility of forged credentials. Accepting photocopies of licenses does not meet the standard. Secondary source verification is confirmation of a healthcare practitioner's credentials based upon information from a credentialing verification organization or from another recognized and approved authority.

A secondary source should be a recognized independent authority. Do not rely on a hospital's process of privileges and verification of sources. When recredentialing, look at additional training that practitioners might have received since the original verification. Organizations must credential all staff and contract employees who come into contact with residents. Organizations have the right to limit a practitioner's provision of care, regardless of what state law allows. The delineation of specific clinical tasks that a practitioner may carry out is called *privileging*.

Credentialing also includes the checking of third-party providers' insurance coverage for current and adequate amounts.

The facility is wise to have an organized approach to credentialing that includes frequent reminders for third parties to comply or face suspension of their privileges.

Ergonomics and Workers' Compensation   According to the Bureau of Labor Statistics, through its statistical reporting and comparison with other industries, long-term care is a high risk setting from a workers' compensation standpoint. AL facilities are included within the same grouping as long-term care facilities in this information. Of note, the 2008 *Nonfatal Workplace Injuries and Illnesses Report* indicated an incidence rate of 3.9 cases per 100 equivalent full-time private industry workers, and nursing and residential care facilities reported a rate of 8.4 cases, the highest injury rates within healthcare.[39] The high rates of injury specifically involved injuries sustained from working with, transferring, and lifting residents. These injuries are typically serious and take time and medical intervention to treat, thus extending days away from work. It is essential for the organization to comply with the Occupational Safety and Health Association (OSHA) requirements and guidelines that have been developed to protect employees.[40] Several factors lead to workers' compensation claims in the long-term care setting:

- The nature of the job is conducive to losses. Lifting, transferring, bending, stooping, pushing, pulling, and so on, all may cause injury if not done properly.
- The industry turnover rate is high. This makes training difficult. Untrained or improperly trained employees injure themselves, which can lead to lost time or modified duty and add to staffing shortages.
- The workforce is aging, and many who are unskilled and uneducated seek positions in seniors housing, even though they may have underlying chronic conditions that make them vulnerable to injury.
- The commitment of time, staff, and resources to reduce losses might not be a priority.

Employees must be made aware of their responsibility to work safely by following policies and procedures and attending safety in-service education, which includes how to complete the accident form and what the expectation is if there is lost time or they are on modified duty. Studies have shown that supervisors' oversight can be very effective in reducing or avoiding injury by working with the new staff on proper body mechanics and teamwork.

Modified duty is a physician-approved temporary duty assignment that gets the employee back to work as soon as medically possible. A modified duty program should include

- communication with the physician and employee about the modified duty program and what the expectation is with regard to the employee returning to work and
- temporary job duties based on the restrictions, which should be reviewed with the employee.

OSHA standards that usually apply to nursing homes or AL include the following:[41]

1. Record Keeping: OSHA requires nursing homes and ALFs with more than ten workers to keep records of workplace injuries and illnesses.

2. Hazard Communication Standard: This standard is designed to ensure that employers and employees know about hazardous chemicals in the workplace and how to protect themselves. Employers with employees who may be exposed to hazardous chemicals in the workplace must prepare and implement a written hazard communication program and comply with other requirements of the standard.

3. Bloodborne Pathogens Standard: The standard is designed to protect employees from the health hazards of exposure to bloodborne pathogens. Employers are subject to OSHA's Bloodborne Pathogens standard if they have employees whose jobs put them at reasonable risk of coming into contact with blood or other potentially infectious materials. Employers subject to this standard must develop a written exposure control plan, provide training to exposed employees, and comply with other requirements of the standard.

4. Exit Routes Standard: All employers must comply with OSHA's requirements for exit routes in the workplace.

5. Electrical Standard. Electrical hazards, such as wiring deficiencies, are one of the hazards most frequently cited by OSHA. OSHA's electrical standards include design requirements for electrical systems and safety-related work practices. If flammable gases are used, special wiring and equipment installation may be required:

6. Emergency Action Plan Standard: OSHA recommends that all employers have an emergency action plan. A plan is mandatory when required by an OSHA standard. An emergency action plan describes the actions employees should take to ensure their safety in a fire or other emergency situation.

7. Fire Safety Standard: OSHA recommends that all employers have a fire prevention plan. A plan is mandatory when required by an OSHA standard.

8. Personal Protective Equipment (PPE): Employers must perform an assessment of each operation in their workplace to determine if their employees are required to wear PPE.

Exhibit 20.1 is a procedure suggested for seniors housing and long-term care organizations to address an OSHA inspection.

· · · · · · · · ·
PUBLIC AND MEDIA RELATIONS AND LONG-TERM CARE'S NEGATIVE IMAGE

To foster a positive perception by the public of the quality of care provided in long-term care facilities, each organization should consider developing public relations and media relations plans. Personnel designated to design a public relations program should work closely with the risk management professional to ensure that wording of any related press releases or advertisements is objective and realistic.

EXHIBIT 20.1   Responding to a Visit from an OSHA Inspector

1. The receptionist should notify the administrator or executive director or resident care director that an OSHA inspector is in the building. Also notify the maintenance director, safety committee officer, and human resource manager. These people should be available for an opening meeting.

2. The inspector may remain in the lobby until the group convenes. Make the inspector comfortable.

3. In the meantime, request the inspector's credentials and make a copy for the community.

4. The opening meeting will be conducted to discuss the reason for the inspection (target data specific, employee complaint, or referral from another agency such as state regulator).

5. Locate your 300 log, 300A log, and sharps injury log, which the inspector may wish to review.

6. Ask the inspector for a list of what will be reviewed. Have this ready for the inspector's review but wait until the inspector requests specific items.

7. Locate your safety manual, training materials, and training logs should the inspector wish to view.

8. Have housekeeping, maintenance, and clinical care conduct a quick walk-around to prepare the building while the opening meeting is underway.

9. The inspector may wish to tour immediately or may review records first. A director-level person should accompany the inspector at all times to answer questions.

10. If the inspector takes photos or video, a community director should take the same photos or video to use later when a report is received.

11. Following the tour and review of documents, a closing conference will be held. Violations will be discussed, along with any fines involved, the appeal process, and abatement deadlines.

12. On the tour and during document review, those involved in the meetings and tours should take notes that will be used in discussions with risk management.

13. The risk management department should be notified immediately following the inspection. Personnel involved in the inspection and any notes taken should be available for this call.

14. Any written correspondence from OSHA should be immediately faxed to the legal department prior to any further contact with OSHA.

15. Important points on the OSHA appeals process
    - If violations are cited, always request an informal conference, this is where fines and violation abatement issues are dismissed completely.
    - The next step is the notice to contest if issues are not resolved at the informal conference. Procedures on this are www.osha.gov/ and must be completed quickly because there are time limits.
    - Always involve the home office and the risk management department prior to making any appeals process decisions.

Media relations are particularly important in a time of emergencies, disasters, public trials, exposé of the industry, workplace violence issues, and so forth. As media coverage can affect the organization and its residents and employees, the organization and each of its facilities should follow a plan for managing the media during the aftermath of a clinical crisis.

The media relations plan should designate someone to speak to the press for the facility. The respective roles of public relations, legal counsel, risk management, administration, board representatives, and medical staff involvement should also be delineated.

Additionally, a media relations consultant might be helpful if the facility or organization has a serious risk management incident. The professional liability carrier, if pertinent, should be involved in such circumstances, and it must be remembered that HIPAA/HITECH requires the patient or resident to give consent for release of any protected health information (PHI). Of particular importance, any employee may be individually responsible for fines of up to $1.5 million dollars a year for HIPAA/HITECH violations. Please see Chapter 16 on HIPAA/HITECH in Volume 3 of this series for more information.

. . . .

INSURANCE FOR SENIORS HOUSING AND LONG-TERM CARE

Risk exposures associated with seniors housing are as varied and as significant to an organization's bottom line as a hospital's exposures. Pertinent insurance coverage for the long-term care organization to consider include property, general and professional liability, workers compensation, automobile/vehicular, employee benefits, employer liability, cyber liability, dram shop (liquor for social events) coverage, and directors and officers liability. Many long-term care organizations also have multiple settings and states to consider. These organizations purchase insurance for the whole organization, as opposed to buying separate coverage for each location, so that they may benefit from the group price associated with economies of scale. In some multisetting operations, however, location-specific issues may arise. For example, an organization may have private financial investors or lenders whose funding supports specific communities, locations, or portfolios of facilities. If these local investors or lending agencies have specific insurance requirements, the organization may find itself with multiple carriers for the same line of coverage, albeit these carriers operate in different locations.

Liability Claim Trends

Since the insurance crisis of the late 1990s, three organizations have published comparative data on liability claims associated with long-term care organizations. Each of these has access to large databases. However, to appreciate the significance of each organization's data, it is important to recognize that each organization's client base represents different types and volumes of long-term care organizations.

Aon Risk Services has published several benchmarking studies on the U.S. long-term care industry, including trends in general and professional liability claims. Their database includes 20,000 individual claims from twenty-four organizations operating 220,000 long-term care beds. These beds represent approximately 15 percent of the nursing home beds in the country and also includes AL, IL, rehabilitation and home care operations.[42]

CNA HealthPro has also examined the frequency and severity of general and professional liability claims in the long-term care environment in six reports published since 2001. The most recent study was published in 2009 and represents 1,644 open and closed claims from 2004 to 2008. These claims were valued at $5,000 or more. CNA's data represent claims against continuing care retirement centers, stand-alone AL facilities, and SNFs. CNA also looks at the differences between frequency and severity of claims of for-profit and non-profit organizations. Finally, CNA's report includes an analysis of injuries and their average costs to those insured, as well as risk reduction recommendations.[43]

The third organization that has evaluated professional liability/general liability claims is the American Seniors Housing Association (ASHA) in their report prepared in 2009 by the Willis Group (previously Thilman, Filippini, Hilb, Rogal, and Hobbs). Eight reports have been published since early 2000 detailing insurance rates, frequency and severity of professional and general liability, workers compensation, and employee benefit costs. The ASHA report also specifically analyzes insurance rates for the IL, AL, and CCRCs, as well as skilled facilities that are affiliated with the three types of seniors facilities. The ASHA 2008 survey report represents approximately 230,000 units of seniors housing owners or managers. IL units compose the majority of the sample (60 percent), followed by AL (30 percent) and skilled nursing (10 percent).[44]

All three of these organizations monitor and report the average claim dollar amount; frequency and severity of injuries resulting in claims; and per unit prices for general, professional liability, and workers compensation insurance coverage, as well as the types and amounts of insurance that seniors housing organizations are purchasing. This information is critical to long-term care organization's short-term planning process as they budget and allocate insurance costs across their companies. The organizations also need this information for medium and long-term strategic planning because this business segment engages frequently in transactions of locations, properties, and facilities via sales, mergers, and acquisitions.

Figures 20.1 to 20.4 are from the 2008 Aon General Liability/Professional Liability Long-Term Care Benchmarking Study and show loss cost per occupied bed for 2008 by state, loss cost per occupied bed–all states, claims frequency per occupied bed–all states, claim severity per occupied bed–all states.

Median and mean insurance costs for IL, AL, and skilled nursing are seen in Table 20.2.

Table 20.3 provides information on causes of severity and frequency.

The CNA study also tracks frequency and severity by type of facility (skilled, assisted, and continuing care) and whether the facility is for profit or not for profit.

Of closed claims with a total paid of $250,000 or more,

- 31.2 percent were not for profit and 68.8 percent for profit;
- 77.3 percent occurred in skilled facilities;
- 32.5 percent involved improper care as an allegation; and
- 65.6 percent involved a resident's death as the injury.

There were forty-four, or 7 percent of claims in this study representing total payment of $500,000 or more:

- 25 percent were not for profit.
- 75 percent were for profit.

FIGURE 20.1   2008 Loss Cost per Occupied Bed—Limited to $1M

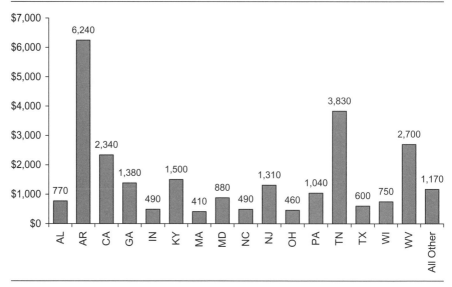

Source: Aon Risk Consultants, Inc. Actuarial and Analytics Practice.
Reprinted with Permission.

**FIGURE 20.2   Long-Term Care Benchmark General and Professional Liability
Loss Cost per Occupied Bed—Limited to $1M All States**

Overall Loss Cost Trends

The following graph shows the loss cost per occupied long-term care bed. The annual loss
cost decreased significantly in the period between 2001 and 2005. Overall loss costs have
stabilized since 2005.

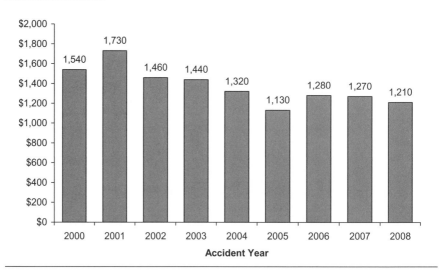

Source: Aon Risk Consultants, Inc. Actuarial and Analytics Practice.
Reprinted with Permission.

FIGURE 20.3   Long-Term Care Benchmark General and Professional Liability Claim Frequency per Occupied Bed All States

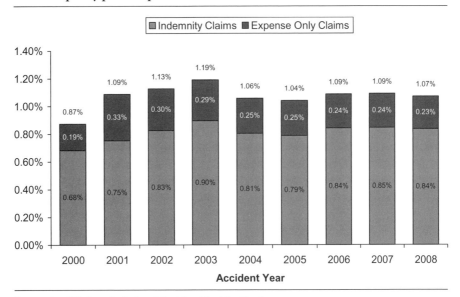

Source: Aon Risk Consultants, Inc. Actuarial and Analytics Practice.
Reprinted with Permission.

FIGURE 20.4   Long-Term Care Benchmark General and Professional Liability Claim Severity—Limited to $1M All States

Overall Severity Trends

The following graph shows the average size per long-term care claim (severity). The average severity decreased significantly over the period between 2000 and 2005. Since 2005 the average severity is stable.

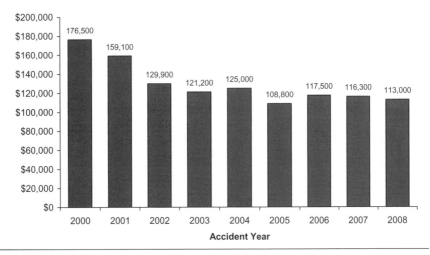

Source: Aon Risk Consultants, Inc. Actuarial and Analytics Practice.
Reprinted with Permission.

TABLE 20.2   Median and Mean Insurance Costs for Independent Living, Assisted Living and Skilled Nursing

Per Bed GL/PL Cost	Median / Mean
Independent living	$167 / $195
Assisted living	$343 / $405
Skilled and dementia unit	$491 / $441

GL, general liability; PL, professional liability.
Source: Data from ASHA Study 2008.

TABLE 20.3   CNA Study of Closed Claims

Most Frequent Allegations	Most Frequent Injuries
Resident fall	Death
Improper care	Fracture(s)
Pressure ulcers	Pressure ulcer
Failure to monitor	Unavailable information
	Amputation

Source: CNA HealthPro 2009 Study of Closed Claims occurring in 2004–2008, all venues of IL, AL, SNF.

- 90 percent occurred in the skilled setting.
- 9.1 percent occurred in AL.
- 34.1 percent of the allegations involved improper care.
- 61.4 percent involved death as the injury.

RISK MANAGEMENT PROGRAM

With multiple complex exposures in various kinds of settings, it is clear that a risk management program is essential to every seniors housing organization. For a multiple facility organization, risk management stems from the corporate offices where insurance decisions are made and filters down to the clinical areas of the facilities in day-to-day patient care.

An effective risk management program begins with a senior officer's statement of support and includes, or refers to, a comprehensive outline of how the organization addresses risk identification, risk control, and risk financing.

The program should be aimed at conserving the financial assets of the facility by seeking ways to reduce costs related to risk and reduce accident and injury claims while monitoring areas of high litigation risk. The top litigation targets in long-term care remain pressure ulcers, malnutrition, dehydration, falls, elopement, adverse drug events, burns, delay in diagnosis or treatment, and improper discharge. Claims also may allege several violations of residents' rights.

The following components are essential to include in any effective risk management program:

- Goals and objectives, which should include governing body approval of the program
- Designated individual responsible for developing, implementing, and monitoring all aspects of the risk management program
- Governance and committee structure, which include the integration of risk management information into the management of the organization through activities such as credentialing, contracting, performance reviews, quality improvement, resident satisfaction, standards of care, and investigations of legal allegations
- Resources for managing data from the incident reporting system
- Risk identification and tracking methodologies
- Documentation of findings and actions
- Annual program review with the governing body's input
- Loss control techniques identified and implemented
- Data analysis to identify trends
- Claims management
- Coordination of facility insurance and risk financing

Risk management should be a major goal of the administration, physicians, nurses, consultants, and all those who work in the setting. With the industry's increase in regulations and the public's concern about patient safety, it is essential that adverse outcomes be followed up quickly and thoroughly. The first step that follows notice of any such event should be an initial risk management investigation. Any related documentation should be labeled "Privileged and Confidential/Attorney Work Product/Completed in Anticipation of Litigation," and any specific statutory protection provisions should be cited if they are available.

Information documented should include the resident's name, date of occurrence, location, a brief description of the incident, witness identification, and location. Specific areas that are commonly investigated in following up an adverse event include environment of care; equipment management; communication between provider, patient, and family; medical record documentation; staffing; policies and procedures; and any identified barriers in the organization.

The information gathered through such adverse event reporting should also be tracked and trended so that priorities may be identified and addressed with the oversight of a multidisciplinary committee responsible for safety and quality improvement.

· · · · · · · · ·

CONCLUSION

As the U.S. population ages, the role and number of long-term care options for services and care will continue to grow. As the variety of these services proliferates, risk management professionals will be charged with more sophisticated loss prevention and patient safety measures in addition to reducing cost and loss for the organizations.

Endnotes

1. U.S. Census Bureau. U.S Population Projections (2008). *Projections of the Population and Components of Change for the United States: 2010 to 2050.* Available at: www.census.gov/population/www/projections/summarytables.html. (Accessed on October 27, 2009.)

2. American Seniors Housing Association (ASHA). Available at: www.seniorshousing.org. (Accessed April 5, 2010.)

3. Wylde, M. "The Independent Living Report." American Seniors Housing Association, 2009. Report can be purchased at: www.seniorshousing.org. (Accessed April 5, 2010.)

4. ASHA, *op. cit.*

5. Hendrickson, L. and Kyzr-Sheeley, G. *"Determining Medicaid Nursing Home Eligibility: A Survey of State Level of Care Assessment."* Rutgers Center for State Health Policy and National Academy for State Health Policy March 2008. Available at: www.adrc-tae.org/tiki-download_file.php?fileId=27272. (Accessed April 5, 2010) A state-specific example is available at: http://dhss.delaware.gov/dsaapd/medwaiver.html. (Accessed December 17, 2009.)

6. Kane, R.A., Kane R.L., Priester, R. & Homyak, P. "Research on State Management Practices for the Rebalancing of State Long-term Care Systems: Final Report." 2008, p. x. Available at: www.hpm.umn.edu/ltcresourcecenter/research/rebalancing/attachments/final_report.pdf. (Accessed on December 17, 2009.)

7. "The Independent Living Report," *op. cit.*

8. CNA HealthPro Transforming Aging Services, Long Term Care Study, 2001–2006. To read the study go to: www.cna.com/portal/site/cna. Once on the CNA site, search for WHAT'S NEW ARCHIVE in the search box. Then scroll down to the study issued December 12, 2007. (Accessed April 5, 2010.)

9. 42 U.S.C. 3601 Housing and Civil Enforcement Section discussion of law available at: www.justice.gov/crt/housing/housing_coverage.php. (Accessed December 4, 2009.)

10. Homes & Communities. U.S. Department of Housing and Urban Development. Fair Housing and Equal Opportunity. Available at: www.nls.gov/offices/fheo/seniors/index.cfm. (Accessed April 5, 2010.)

11. Assisted Living Federation of America, (ALFA) "2009 Overview of Assisted Living." Available for purchase from the AFLA Store at: www.alfa.org/Mall/StoreHome.asp?MODE=VIEW&STID=1&LID=0&PRODID=16&SNID=587473769. (Accessed April 5, 2010.)

12. National Center for Assisted Living. "Assisted Living State Regulatory Review," March 2009. Available at: www.ahcancal.org/ncal/resources/Documents/2009_reg_review.pdf. (Accessed April 5, 2010.)

13. Massachusetts Assisted Living Facilities Association. "Assisted Living: Including Options for People with Memory Loss and Dementia." Description of SAMM is on page 3. Available at: www.massalfa.org/docs/consumer_guide_text_only.pdf . (Accessed December 17, 2009.)

14. Assisted Living Federation of America, *op cit.*

15. Farris, K. B. "Instruments Assessing Capacity to Manage Medications." *The Annals of Pharmacotherapy* 2008; 42(7):1026–1036. Available at: www.theannals.com.

16. More information available at: www.ismp.org/newsletters/acutecare/articles/20050421. asp.

17. The Center for Excellence in Assisted Living has studies and resources for mediation assistance in assisted living under the CEAL Clearinghouse tab at www.theceal.org/. (Accessed April 5, 2010.) Information on training and protocols is available from the American Society of Consultant Pharmacists. "Medication Management in Assisted Living: Assuring Accuracy of Medication Administration." Issue paper available at: www.seniorcarepharmacy.org/advocacy/briefing/upload/accuracy.pdf. (Accessed April 5, 2010.)

18. Centers for Disease Control and Prevention. "Self-Reported Falls and Fall-Related Injuries Among Persons Aged ≥ 65 Years—United States, 2006." *MMWR Weekly* 2008; 57(9):225–229. Data and research information available at: www.cdc.gov/ mmwr/preview/mmwrhtml/mm5709a1.htm. (Accessed April 5, 2010.)

19. CNA HealthPro. *Reducing Risk in a Changing Industry, Aging Services Claims Analysis* 2004–2008. This study, as well as other CNA HealthPro client risk management resources, can be accessed at www.cna.com. Click Risk Control, then look for the study under What's New. (Accessed April 5, 2010.)

20. *Ibid.*, p. 20.

21. "People with Alzheimer's Disease and Dementia in Assisted Living." Alzheimer's Association Advocacy and Public Policy Division, October 2004, Available at: www.alz. org/national/documents/prevalence_Alz_assist.pdf. (Accessed April 5, 2010.)

22. Administration on Aging, National Center on Elder Abuse Web site provides laws and resource information. Available at: www.ncea.aoa.gov/ncearoot/Main_Site/index.aspx. (Accessed April 5, 2010.).

23. *Ibid.*

24. Harrington, C., Carrillo, H. & Blank, B.W. "Nursing Facilities, Staffing, Residents and Facility Deficiencies, 2003 through 2008." November 2009. Available at: www.nccnhr. org. (Accessed December 4, 2009.)

25. *Ibid.*

26. American Health Care Association. "2009 Annual Quality Report." Available at: www. ahcancal.org/research_data/quality/Documents/2009AnnualQualityReport.pdf. This report provides an overview of quality in U.S. nursing homes. (Accessed April 5, 2010.)

27. CMS State Operations Manual Chapter 7—Survey and Enforcement Process for Skilled Nursing Facilities and Nursing Facilities Available at: www.cms.gov/manuals/downloads/ som107c07.pdf. (Accessed April 5, 2010.)

28. NHRegsPlus serves as a one-stop location to examine and compare the content of state regulations related to nursing homes. It contains federal nursing home regulations and nursing home regulations for all states and the District of Columbia, updated as of July 2007. Available at: www.sph.umn.edu/hpm/NHRegsPlus/. (Accessed April 5, 2010.)

29. CMS Web site for more information on nursing home survey. Available at: www.cms. hhs.gov/CertificationandComplianc/12_NHs.asp#TopOfPage. (Accessed April 5, 2010.)

30. The Quality Indicator Survey (QIS) is in operation in five states, and CMS will replace the traditional survey as new states are trained and implemented. QIS survey involves

interviews with forty residents per survey. The interview includes questions on the residents' rights to individualized care. The Executive Summary from the Final Report on the Evaluation of the Quality Indicator Survey December 2007 is available at: www. cms.gov/CertificationandComplianc/Downloads/QISExecSummary.pdf. (Accessed April 5, 2010.)

31. CMS *State Operations Manual*, Appendix P–Survey Protocol for Long Term Care Facilities. Part I. Section IV Deficiency Categorization. B. Guidance on Severity Levels. p. 91. Available at: www.cms.gov/manuals/Downloads/som107ap_p_ltcf.pdf. (Accessed April 5, 2010.)

32. CMS released a protocol to examine policies on abuse and neglect during all nursing home inspections. *State Operations Manual*, Task 5G, p. P-62. Available at: www.cms. hhs.gov/Manuals/Downloads/som107ap_p_ltcf.pdf. (Accessed April 16, 2010.)

33. AHCA. Report Provides Objective, Independent Analyses of Quality Improvements in America's Nursing and Rehabilitation Facilities. News Release. September 28, 2009. www.ahcancal.org/News/news_releases/Pages/QualityReportNursingRehabilitation.aspx. (Accessed April 16, 2010.)

34. Harrington, C. et al., *op. cit.*

35. *Ibid.*

36. CMS. State Operations Manual Appendix PP–Guidance to Surveyors for Long Term Care Facilities §483.30(a)(2), p. 380. Available at: www.cms.gov/CFCsAndCoPs/Downloads/som107ap_pp_guidelines_ltcf.pdf. (Accessed April 5, 2010.)

37. CMS, State Operations Manual Appendix PP, *op. cit.*, §483.30(b)(1), p. 380.

38. CMS, State Operations Manual Appendix PP, *op. cit.*, §483.30(b)(3), p. 380.

39. U.S. Department of Labor, Bureau of Labor Statistics. "Workplace Injuries and Illnesses — 2008." News release, October 29, 2009.

40. Occupational Safety and Health Administration (OSHA) issued an ergonomics guideline for the nursing home industry on March 13, 2003. Guidelines, best practice examples, and other information are available at: www.osha.gov/ergonomics/guidelines/nursinghome/index.html.

41. U.S. Department of Labor, OSHA, "Compliance Assistance Quick Start: Health Care Industry." Available at: www.osha.gov/dcsp/compliance_assistance/quickstarts/health_care/index_hc.html. (Accessed April 5, 2010.)

42. For an overview of Aon's "Long Term Care 2008 General Liability and Professional Liability Actuarial Study" read the Q&R Strategist for July 2009 available at: http://ke.aon.com/communities/healthcare/us/publications/qr_strategist.jsp.

43. CNA HealthPro, *op cit.*

44. HRH. "Seniors Housing Liability Insurance, Health Benefit and Worker's Compensation Report, 2008." Available for purchase online in the bookstore at American Seniors Housing Association at: www.seniorshousing.org/default.aspx?id=32. (Accessed April 5, 2010.)

Glossary

637

Abuse	The willful infliction of injury, unreasonable confinement, intimidation, or punishment with resulting harm, pain, or mental anguish. "Fraud and abuse" describes practices that result in unnecessary costs to the Medicare or Medicaid program and other payer sources. "Patient abuse" is deliberate, nonaccidental contact or interaction that results in significant psychological harm, pain, or physical injury.
Academic medical center	Generally, a large inpatient teaching hospital with residency programs, faculty members, and research facilities and programs (see *Teaching hospitals*).
Access problem	Issues relating to impediments that restrict or limit persons in need of specific healthcare services from receiving them, such as lack of health insurance.
Accident (medical)	An unintended occurrence resulting in injury or death that is not the result of willful action. Generally, an accident means that it resulted in some degree of injury or harm to the person or persons involved. In the medical field, the term "*accident*" is generally not used to describe an event associated with clinical care but refers to other types of events, such as one that involves damage to a defined system that disrupts the ongoing or future output of the system.
Accidental loss	A loss that occurs by chance and is unexpected, unintended, and fortuitous.
ACEP	American College of Emergency Physicians.
ACGME	Accreditation Council for Graduate Medical Education.
ACHE	American College of Healthcare Executives.
ACLS	Advanced cardiac life support.
ACO	Ambulatory care organization.
ACOG	American College of Obstetricians and Gynecologists.
ACP	American College of Physicians: a national organization of internists, physicians who specialize in the prevention, detection, and treatment of illnesses in adults. ACP is the largest medical-specialty organization and second-largest physician group in the United States.
Acquired immune deficiency syndrome (AIDS)	A fatal, incurable disease caused by a virus (the human immunodeficiency virus) that can destroy the body's ability to fight off illness, resulting in recurrent opportunistic infections or secondary diseases afflicting multiple body systems.
Acquisition	A business transaction in which one corporation or entity purchases or otherwise acquires all of the assets or stock of another entity or organization.
ACR	American College of Radiology.
ACS	American Cancer Society.
ACS	American College of Surgeons.

Active error	An error that occurs at the level of the frontline operator, the effects of which are felt almost immediately and are readily apparent. This is sometimes called the "sharp end"; also called "active failure."
Active failure (3, 7)	A failure that results from an active error. Unsafe acts and deviation from expected and desired outcomes. Also called "active error" or "sharp end."
Actuarial analysis	A study performed by a professional known as an actuary aimed at predicting the frequency and severity of claims for a specific line of insurance coverage for a future time period. Such an analysis includes both an estimation of the ultimate value of known claims and an estimation of the number and value of claims that have occurred but have not yet been reported.
Actuarial study	An analysis performed by an actuary that determines appropriate funding levels required for operation of a self-insurance trust.
Actuary	A person who uses statistics to compute loss probabilities to establish premiums for insurance companies and self-insurance trusts.
Actual cash value	Basis for insurance reimbursement: cost new minus depreciation.
ACU	Ambulatory care unit.
Acuity	Degree or severity of illness.
Acute care hospital	Typically, a community hospital that has services designed to meet the needs of patients who require care for a period of less than thirty days.
ACV	Actual cash value.
ADA	American Dental Association; American Diabetes Association; Americans With Disabilities Act.
Additional insured	A person or entity added to an insurance policy by endorsement at the request of the named insured, often after the inception of the policy. Frequently required by contracts to give one contracting party the benefit of insurance coverage maintained by the other.
ADE	Adverse drug event.
ADEA	Age Discrimination in Employment Act.
Administrative agencies	Agencies within the executive branch of government. At the federal level, they generally fall under a cabinet official, such as, in the case of OSHA, the secretary of labor.
Administrative Procedure Act (18)	Law that governs the ways in which administrative agencies can promulgate and enforce regulations.
Admission	An out-of-court statement made by a person who is a party to an action. Admissions are normally admissible as evidence at trial.
Admitted insurer	An insurance company that has applied to be financially qualified in every state in which it wishes to conduct business. Once admitted, a carrier must obey all state laws regulating the operation of insurance companies, including filing forms and rates.

ADR	Alternative dispute resolution.
Advance directive	Written instructions recognized under law relating to the provision of healthcare when an individual is incapacitated. An advance directive may take either of two forms: living will and durable power of attorney for healthcare.
Adverse drug event (ADE)	An adverse event involving the use of medications; not necessarily related to error or poor quality of care. An adverse drug event may be the result of a medication error, but most are not.
Adverse drug reaction (ADR)	Adverse effect produced by the use of a medication in the recommended manner.
Adverse event	Any injury (undesirable clinical outcome) caused by medical care and not an underlying disease process.
Adverse outcome	A clinical outcome that, while neither desirable nor necessarily anticipated, may have been a known possibility associated with a particular treatment or procedure. This definition does not imply that any provider was negligent or that any error in process or that system factors contributed to the adverse outcome.
AED	Automatic external defibrillator.
AERS	Adverse event reporting system.
Affidavit	A written statement made under oath, without notice to the opposing party. A written or printed declaration or statement of facts, made voluntarily and confirmed by the oath or affirmation of the party making it, recorded before an officer having authority to administer such oath.
Age discrimination	Denial of privileges or other unfair treatment of employees because of their age. Age discrimination is prohibited by federal law under the Age Discrimination in Employment Act of 1978 to protect employees between the ages of forty and seventy years old.
Age Discrimination in Employment Act	The federal statute (29 USC 621 et seq.) prohibiting certain types of employment discrimination on the basis of age.
Agency by estoppel	See *Ostensible agency doctrine.*
Aggregate limit	The maximum amount the insurer will pay during the policy period, irrespective of the policy's limit of liability.
AHA	American Heart Association; American Hospital Association.
AHACC	American Hospital Association Certification Center.
AHCA	American Health Care Association.
AHERA	Asbestos Hazard Emergency Response Act.
AHIMA	American Health Information Management Association.
AHRQ	Agency for Healthcare Research and Quality: a component of the Public Health Services responsible for research on quality, appropriateness, effectiveness, and cost of healthcare.
AIC	Associate in claims.
AICPCU	American Institute for Chartered Property Casualty Underwriters.

AIDS	Acquired immune deficiency syndrome.
ALAE	Allocated loss adjustment expense.
ALF	Assisted-living facility.
Allegation	In a pleading, the assertion, declaration, or statement of a person setting out what the party to an action expects to prove.
Allied health professional	A specially trained nonphysician healthcare provider. Allied health professionals include paramedics, physician assistants, certified nurse midwives, phlebotomists, social workers, nurse practitioners, and other caregivers who perform tasks that supplement physician services.
Allocated loss adjustment expense	Money paid in the claims resolution process. Includes defense attorney fees, court costs, expert witness fees, and photocopy costs attributed directly to an individual claim.
All-risk coverage	Insurance that covers all losses that are not explicitly excluded.
ALS (4)	Advanced life support.
Alterations	To change the meaning or intent.
Alternative delivery systems	Health services provided in locations other than an inpatient, acute care hospital, such as skilled and nursing facilities, hospice programs, and home healthcare.
Alternative dispute resolution (ADR)	A process or system to resolve disputes outside the formal judicial process. It can include mediation, arbitration, or both, and can be voluntary or mandatory, depending on jurisdiction.
Alternative risk financing	Any of a number of mechanisms other than traditional insurance programs employed by individuals or organizations to pay for claims, including various types of captive insurance companies, risk retention groups, and self-insurance trust funds.
Alternative risk transfer	See *Alternative risk financing.*
Alternative treatment plan	Provision in managed care arrangements for treatment usually outside a hospital.
AMA	American Medical Association: the AMA helps physicians help patients by uniting them nationwide to work on the most important professional, public health, and advocacy issues in medicine.
AMAP	American Medical Accreditation Program.
Ambulatory	Not confined to a bed; capable of walking.
Ambulatory care	Medical care provided on an outpatient basis.
Ambulatory care organization (2)	A healthcare organization that includes multispecialty clinics, free-standing surgical centers, urgent care or walk-in medical clinics, and community health or public health facilities.
Americans With Disabilities Act	A federal statute (42 USC 12101 et seq.) aimed at prohibiting discrimination in employment and public accommodation against individuals with certain mental and physical disabilities.
ANA	American Nurses Association.

Ancillary	Describing services that relate to a patient's care, such as lab work, X-rays, and anesthesia.
Annual aggregate limit	The maximum amount the insurer will pay during the policy period (usually one year), irrespective of the policy's limit of liability.
Annuity	A fixed sum payable periodically, subject to the limitations imposed by the grantor.
ANP	Advanced nurse practitioner.
ANSI	American National Standards Institute.
Answer	A document filed with the court in response to a complaint or a petition. The answer must generally (1) admit that the plaintiff's allegations are true, (2) deny that the plaintiff's allegations are true, or (3) state that the defendant does not have information regarding the truth or falsity of the allegations.
Antikickback statutes	Medicare-Medicaid Antikickback Statute (42 USC 1320a-7b), outlawing "knowingly and willfully" seeking or receiving a bribe, rebate, or kickback for a referral (or the intent to induce a referral) for a program, reimbursable item, or service.
Antitrust laws	Laws designed to discourage or prohibit restraints of free trade, to unfairly reduce or eliminate competition, or to unfairly prevent entrance into a marketplace.
Any willing provider laws	Statutes in some jurisdictions prohibiting managed care organizations (MCOs) from discriminating among licensed providers of healthcare services and requiring that the MCO reimburse any licensed provider willing to accept the MCO's reimbursement schedule for the provision of covered services to a plan beneficiary.
AOA	American Osteopathic Association.
AONE	American Organizations of Nurse Executives.
AORN	Association of periOperative Registered Nurses.
APA	Administrative Procedure Act.
APC	Ambulatory patient classification.
Apparent agency	See *Ostensible agency doctrine*.
Appeal	An action that is taken after the trial of a matter or after a dispositive motion has been entered in a matter for the purpose of correcting an error made by the trial court or to obtain a new trial.
Appellate court	A court that is empowered to hear appeals. There are two tiers of appellate courts: an intermediate appellate court (such as the U.S. Circuit Courts of Appeal) and a supreme court (the U.S. Supreme Court, the New York Court of Appeals). Some states have only one appellate court tier.
APQC	American Productivity and Quality Center.
Arbiter	A neutral third party who issues a decision binding on the parties in a formal or informal hearing on a disagreement.

Arbitration	A method of dispute resolution used as an alternative to litigation where the hearing and determination of a case in controversy is by a person either chosen by the parties in opposition or appointed under statutory authority. May be binding (final) or nonbinding (aggrieved party may appeal or pursue conventional civil litigation).
Arbitration clause	A clause in a contract providing for arbitration of disputes arising under a contract. Arbitration clauses are treated as separable parts of the contract so that the illegality of another part of the contract does not nullify such agreements and a breach of repudiation of the contract does not preclude the right to arbitrate.
ARC	American Red Cross.
Archiving	Retaining and organizing expired insurance policies or revised policies and procedures to facilitate the determination of the provisions in place at a specific moment in the past.
ARES	Amateur Radio Emergency Services.
ARF	Alternative risk financing.
ARM	Associate in risk management.
ARM 54	Examination focusing on risk assessment; one of three required courses to obtain the designation as an associate in risk management (ARM) from the Insurance Institute of America.
ARM 55	Examination focusing on risk control; one of three required courses to obtain the designation as an associate in risk management (ARM) from the Insurance Institute of America.
ARM 56	Examination focusing on risk financing; one of three required courses to obtain the designation as an associate in risk management (ARM) from the Insurance Institute of America.
ARM-P	Associate in risk management for public entities.
ART	Accredited record technician.
ART	Alternative risk transfer.
ASA	American Society of Anesthesiologists.
ASC	Ambulatory surgery center.
ASCP	American Society of Clinical Pathologists.
ASHE	American Society for Healthcare Engineering.
ASHP	American Society of Health-System Pharmacists.
ASHRM	American Society for Healthcare Risk Management.
ASRS	Aviation Safety Reporting System.
Assault	An intentional act that is designed to make the victim fearful and produces reasonable apprehension of harm.
Assignment	The act of transferring to another party all or part of one's property, interest, or rights.

Assisted-living facility (4)
Facility that provides supervision, assistance, or both, with the activities of daily living (ADL), facilitates the delivery of services by outside providers, and ensures resident safety, health, and well-being by monitoring activities.

Associate in claims
A designation conferred by the Insurance Institute of America.

Association
An unincorporated group of persons assembled for a specific purpose or to complete a specific project. Unless the state has a specific statute governing the liabilities of the members, each member may be liable for the debts and obligations of the association.

Association or group captive
Jointly owned by a number of companies that are affiliated through a trade, industry, or service group.

Assumption of risk
Understanding the risks associated with a particular course of action and agreeing to accept those risks. Also, in a negligence case, an affirmative defense that alleges that the plaintiff knew of the danger involved in what he was doing, did nothing to prevent his own injury, and hence must bear the consequences of the action and cannot ask for the defendant to pay for his injury.

ASTM
American Society for Testing and Materials.

ATLS
Advanced trauma life support.

Attorney-client privilege
A legal doctrine recognized by both common and statutory law protecting certain confidential communications between an attorney and his or her client from discovery in a legal proceeding unless the privilege is waived by the client.

Attorney work product privilege
A legal doctrine recognized by both common and statutory law protecting the documents generated, theories devised, and legal strategies formulated by an attorney on behalf of a client from discovery in a legal proceeding unless the privilege is waived by the client.

Authentication (9)
Establishing or confirming that something is correct, accurate, or true.

Auto liability insurance
Insurance coverage for losses arising out of the ownership, maintenance, and use of automobiles and their equipment.

Automated dispensing cabinet
A cabinet that by its design has certain controls and documentation features that dispense medications pursuant to individualized patient drug profiles as ordered by a physician and confirmed by a pharmacist.

Autonomy (8)
The right to self-govern or self-manage; capacity to make an informed, uncoerced decision.

Aviation coverage
Insurance coverage for losses arising from the use of helipads by life-flight operators or other emergency helicopter landings.

AWHONN
Association of Women's Health, Obstetric, and Neonatal Nurses.

B

BAA	Business associate agreement.
Back pay	In employment practices liability claims, a demand for or award of damages asking the defendant to pay the employee's wages from the time of the alleged improper act (such as wrongful termination) to the time of the settlement or judgment by the court in the employee's favor. In cases in which it is alleged that the employee was improperly denied a promotion or salary increase, back pay represents the difference in the wages actually earned by the employee and those that would have been earned had the promotion or salary increase not have been denied.
Bad outcome	Failure to achieve a desired outcome of care.
Balancing measure	Measure used to ensure that changes to improve a system or process do not create or cause problems in other areas.
Bar coding technology	A computer identification system that uses bar-stripe codes to identify specific items, medications, or patients. Most often used with a scanning device to read or verify each unique code.
Battery	The touching of one person by another without permission. See *Medical battery*.
BBA	Balanced Budget Act of 1997.
BBI	Basic building information.
BBRA	Balanced Budget Relief Act of 1999.
BCAA	Blue Cross Association of America.
Belmont Report	Report describing the basic ethical principles on which all biomedical and behavioral research should be based.
Benchmarking	A process that identifies best practices and performance standards to establish normative or comparative standards (benchmarks) for use as a measurement tool. By comparing an organization against a national or regional benchmark, providers are able to establish measurable goals as part of the strategic planning and total quality management processes.
Beneficence	The concept of doing good.
Benevolent gesture	Action taken to communicate a sense of compassion or compensation arising from humane feelings when there is no implication (direct or implied) as to "fault" for having contributed to or caused the outcome.
BI	Business interruption insurance coverage.
Bioethics activities	Activities associated with issues such as end of life (advance directives, withdrawal or withholding treatment, do-not-resuscitate orders, and so on) and human subject research.
BIPA	Benefits Improvement and Protection Act of 2000.
BLS	Basic life support.

BLS	Bureau of Labor Statistics.
Blunt end	See *Latent failure*.
Board certified	Officially acknowledged as a specialist in the physician's particular area of practice. To achieve board certification, a physician must meet specific standards of knowledge and clinical skills within a specific field or specialty. Usually, this means completion of a supervised program of clinical residency and passing both oral and written examinations administered by a medical specialty group.
Board eligible	Status of a physician who has graduated from a board-approved medical school, completed an accredited training program, practiced for a specified length of time, and is eligible to take a specialty board examination within a specific amount of time.
BME	Board of Medical Examiners.
Boiler and machinery coverage	Insurance that protects against the explosion of boilers and other pressure vessels and accidental damage to equipment. Covers resulting damage to other property, including property in your care for which you are liable as well as the cost of temporary repairs and any additional cost incurred to expedite repairs. Coverage is written on a "cost to repair or replace" basis and is not subject to depreciation.
Borrowed servant	A common law legal doctrine that stipulates that the employer of a borrowed employee, rather than the employee's regular employer, is liable for the employee's actions that occur while the employee is under the control of the temporary employer despite the lack of a permanent employee-employer relationship between the temporary employer and borrowed employee.
BP	Blood pressure.
Brain death	Total irreversible cessation of cerebral function despite continued function of the respiratory and circulatory systems.
Breach of contract	Failure, without legal excuse, to perform any promise expressed in a contract. Also, hindrance by a party regarding the required performance of the rights and duties identified in the contract.
Breach of duty	One of the four elements necessary to prove negligence. The failure to fulfill (breach) an obligation or responsibility (duty).
Broker	A person who represents a buyer of insurance in negotiations with the underwriter and who serves as a consultant on various aspects of the buyer's insurance program.
BTLS	Basic trauma life support.
Builder's risk coverage	Insurance covering new construction.
BUN	Blood urea nitrogen.
Business interruption coverage	Insurance coverage typically provided as a part of a property insurance policy covering the lost revenues and extra operating expenses associated with a covered loss such as a fire.

C

CAA	Clean Air Act.
CAAS	Commission on Accreditation of Ambulance Services.
CABG	Coronary artery bypass graft.
CAH	Critical access hospital.
CAHPS	Consumer Assessment of Healthcare Providers and Systems. The CAHPS program is a public-private initiative to develop standardized surveys of patients' experiences with ambulatory and facility-level care.
CAMLTC	Comprehensive Accreditation Manual for Long-Term Care.
CAMTS	Commission on Accreditation of Medical Transport Systems.
CAP	College of American Pathologists.
Capitation	In managed care contracts, a payment method in which a provider is paid a set fee, often per member per month, to provide designated healthcare services to individuals covered by the managed care plan. The fee remains constant regardless of how much or how little healthcare service is actually provided.
"Captain of the ship" doctrine	A doctrine that imposes liability on a surgeon in charge of an operation for the negligence of his or her assistants during the period when those individuals are under the surgeon's control, even though they are also employees of the healthcare entity.
CAPTA	Child Abuse Prevention and Treatment Act.
Captive insurance company	An insurance company established to provide insurance coverage to a sponsoring entity as opposed to marketing and selling policies commercially to insureds. The sponsoring entity may be a parent corporation and its related subsidiaries, a professional association, or some other group.
CARF	Commission on Accreditation of Rehabilitation Facilities.
Cardiac catheterization	A procedure used to diagnose disorders of the heart, lungs, and great vessels.
CARME	Center for the Advancement of Risk Management Education.
Case management	A managed care technique in which a patient with a serious medical condition is assigned an individual who arranges for cost-effective treatment, often outside a hospital. See *Utilization management.*
CAT	Computerized axial tomography, a diagnostic technique that produces cross-sectional images of the head or body.
Catastrophic protection	Insurance that protects against the adverse effects of large losses from disasters of natural or human origin.
Cause of action	The facts that give the plaintiff the legal grounds to seek damages from another person. It is necessary to have a cause of action in order to bring and sustain a lawsuit.
CBC	Complete blood cell count.
CBRN	Chemical, biological, radiological, and nuclear (countermeasures).

CCAC	Continuing Care Accreditation Commission.
CCHSA	Canadian Council on Health Services Accreditation.
CCRC	Continuing care retirement community.
CCRN	Certification in critical care nursing.
CCU	Cardiac care unit.
CDC	Centers for Disease Control and Prevention.
CDRH	Center for Devices and Radiological Health, a division of the Food and Drug Administration.
Census	A count of the number of inpatients who receive hospital care each day, excluding newborns.
Centers for Disease Control and Prevention	An operating component of the Department of Health and Human Services whose mission is to promote health, prevent disease, injury, and disability and to prepare for new health threats.
Centers for Medicare and Medicaid Services	The federal agency responsible for administering Medicare, Medicaid, and the State Children's Health Insurance Program (SCHIP); formerly known as the Health Care Financing Administration (HCFA).
CEO	Chief executive officer.
CERCLA	Comprehensive Environmental Response, Compensation and Liability Act.
CERT	Centers for Education and Research in Therapeutics.
Certificate of insurance	A standardized form, usually produced by the insurance agent or broker who arranged for the coverage, evidencing specific insurance in place, the insurance carrier, policy period, policy number, and other particulars.
CfC	Conditions for coverage.
CFO	Chief financial officer.
CGL	Commercial general liability.
Chain of command	Communication route or hierarchy established by appropriate bodies (administration, medical staff and nursing) that allows staff members to air concerns and deal with difficult situations.
Chain of evidence	Procedure to ensure that the location and integrity of evidence (blood, clothing, weapons, and so on) collected from patients is accounted for, from the time it is collected until the time it is turned over to the police or court.
CHAP	Community Health Accreditation Program.
Charitable immunity doctrine	A doctrine that relieves a charity of liability in tort; most states have abrogated or restricted such immunity.
Chemotherapy	In the treatment of disease, the application of chemical reagents that have a specific and toxic effect on the disease-causing microorganism.
Chief executive officer	The corporate officer charged with responsibility for the financial and operational performance of the company. Often the CEO also carries the title of president.

Chief financial officer	The corporate officer charged with responsibility for overseeing the finance and accounting functions of the company, including reporting financial information to the public and to regulatory agencies, and interfacing with independent financial auditors.
Chief operating officer	The corporate officer charged with responsibility for the operations of the company.
Chief risk officer	The corporate officer charged with responsibility for identifying and managing a variety of financial, legal, strategic, and hazard risks faced by the organization. Distinguished from a traditional risk manager, whose role is generally confined to identifying and managing hazard risks.
Child Abuse Prevention and Treatment Act (CAPTA)	One of the key pieces of legislation that guides child protection.
Child Protective Service agencies	A governmental agency in many of the states of the United States that responds to reports of child abuse and neglect. Many states change the name to reflect a more family-centered practice, such as the Department of Children and Family Services (DCFS).
CICU	Cardiac intensive care unit.
CISM	Critical incident stress management.
Citation	A writ that orders a person to appear and do something, such as defend or answer a charge made by a governmental agency.
Civil false claim	A claim that is submitted by a person or a person who knowingly causes someone else to submit a claim to the federal government for payment that is false or fraudulent.
Civil law	The system of laws by which one person may bring an action against another person seeking compensatory or punitive damages or injunctive relief. Also refers to the predominant theory of laws established by the governments of most western European countries (with the exception of the United Kingdom).
Civil monetary penalties (CMP) (10)	Any penalty, fine, or other sanction that is for a specific amount, or has a maximum amount, as provided by federal law, and is assessed or enforced by an agency in an administrative proceeding or by a federal court pursuant to federal law.
Civil Rights Act of 1964	A broad federal statute (42 USC 2000 et seq) prohibiting discrimination on the basis of race, color, creed, or national origin in a variety of settings, including employment.
Claim	The amount of damage for which an insured seeks reimbursement from an insurance company. Once the amount has been determined, it becomes a loss.
Claimant	Someone who brings a claim for alleged injuries.
Claims investigation (11)	Process by which the necessary information to evaluate a claim is obtained. Information can be obtained through interviews, document review, visual inspection, and discovery requests.

Claims-made coverage	An insurance policy covering claims that are made during the policy period and that occurred since the policy retroactive date. Although policy definitions vary somewhat, most claims-made insurance policies consider a claim to be made when it is first reported to the insurance company, subject to certain terms and conditions. Claims-made policies are common for professional liability and directors' and officers' liability insurance.
Claims management	A systemized approach to reducing the financial loss and negative community image of a healthcare organization in situations where prevention fails and injury occurs.
Class action	A lawsuit, frequently a liability lawsuit, including a number of similarly situated plaintiffs whose cases are factually almost identical. Joining all of the plaintiffs into a single lawsuit expedites pretrial discovery and prevents multiple trials on the same issues and can provide a forum for plaintiffs whose individual damages may be quite small. Seen most frequently in product liability and employment practices litigation.
Clean Air Act	Law that defines EPA responsibilities for protecting and improving the nation's air quality and the stratospheric ozone layer.
CLIA	Clinical Laboratory Improvement Amendments: these are certification standards for laboratories established to consolidate the requirements for Medicare participation with rules for laboratories engaged in interstate testing; standards contain quality control and quality assurance, proficiency testing, and personnel requirements.
Clinical practice guidelines	See *Critical paths*.
Clinical research trials	Use of experimental drugs, devices, or protocols on human subjects in a clinical setting under a set of prescribed procedures as part of the FDA approval process.
CMP	Civil monetary penalties.
CMS	Centers for Medicare and Medicaid Services.
CNM	Certified nurse-midwife.
CNS	Central nervous system.
COB	Coordination of benefits, an antiduplication provision under group health insurance to limit benefits where there is multiple coverage in a particular case to 100 percent of the expenses covered and to designate the order in which the multiple carriers are to pay benefits.
COBRA	Consolidated Omnibus Budget Reconciliation Act of 1986.
Codefendant	A defendant who has been joined together with one or more other defendants in a single action.
Code blue	Designation indicating that an emergency situation has occurred and mobilizes staff to respond.
COI	Certificate of insurance.
COLA	Commission of Office Laboratory Accreditation.

Collateral-source benefits	Amounts that a plaintiff recovers from sources other than the defendant, such as the plaintiff's own insurance.
Collective bargaining	Negotiations between an employer and a group of employees to determine the conditions of employment, resulting in a collective agreement. Employees are often represented in bargaining by a union or other labor organization.
Combined ratio	The sum of two ratios, one calculated by dividing incurred losses plus loss adjustment expense (LAE) by earned premiums (the calendar year loss ratio), and the other calculated by dividing all other expenses by written premiums. A combined ratio below 100 percent is indicative of an underwriting profit.
Commercial auto coverage	Insurance that protects against loss arising out of the ownership, maintenance, and use of automobiles and their equipment, both those a person owns, hires, or borrows and those a person doesn't own but may be responsible for, such as the personal car of an employee used to run a company errand.
Commercial general liability coverage	Insurance that protects against financial loss resulting from liability to third parties arising out of the premises a person owns or occupies, acts of independent contractors a person has hired, products a person sells when they leave the seller's premises, and liability a person assumes under contract, subject to exclusions of the policy. Coverage applies to bodily injury, property damage, and personal injury.
Commercial insurance	A distinction in property and liability coverage that is written for business or entrepreneurial interests as opposed to personal lines.
Commission error	Incorrect action performed or an intended action that was improperly performed.
Common cause	Factor that results from variation inherent in a process or system.
Common law	A legal system in which the elements of the substantive law must be gleaned from decided cases, as opposed to statutory law.
Compensatory damages	Damages sought or awarded to a plaintiff in a liability action to compensate for losses, such as lost wages or medical expenses, and for pain and suffering.
Complaint	One of the initial filings with a court to begin a lawsuit. The complaint normally recites all of the allegations against the defendant and theories on which the plaintiff seeks to recover damages. May be called a *petition* in some jurisdictions.
Complementary medicine	Any of a number of therapies and treatment modalities used alone or in combination to treat or alleviate specific symptoms or disease that fall outside of those traditionally employed by physicians, surgeons, and dentists, including acupuncture, massage therapy, and herbal medicine. Sometimes referred to as alternative medicine. Complementary medicine treatments often take a holistic approach to care and treatment and may include an emphasis on the spiritual dimensions of healing.

Complication	Undesired and unintended but often known negative clinical symptoms or physical injury that resulted from medical treatment.
Comprehensive Environmental Response, Compensation and Liability Act (CERCLA)	This law created a tax on the chemical and petroleum industries and provided broad federal authority to respond directly to releases or threatened releases of hazardous substances that could endanger public health or the environment; established prohibitions and requirements concerning closed and abandoned hazardous waste sites; provided for liability of persons responsible for releases of hazardous waste at these sites; and established a trust fund to provide for cleanup when no responsible party could be identified. Also known as the "Superfund."
Computed tomography scan	Technique for gathering anatomical information from a cross-sectional plane of the body, presented as an image generated by a computer synthesis of X-ray transmission data obtained in many different directions through a given plane.
Computer-aided decision support system	A computerized system that provides scientifically based diagnostic and patient care information.
Computerized physician/ provider order entry (7, 14)	Computer system that allows direct entry of medical orders by the person with the licensure and privileges to do so.
CON	Certificate of need.
Conditions of participation	Requirements that hospitals must meet to participate in the Medicare and Medicaid programs; they are intended to protect patient health and safety and to ensure that high-quality care is provided to all patients.
Confidentiality	Parties to confidential communication cannot be compelled by law to disclose to any third party. Communication can be "confidential" in the sense that a person does not voluntarily disclose it to any other person. However, unless the law has defined a particular category of communications as confidential, anyone privy to that communication can be compelled to disclose it on penalty of law.
Confirmation bias	The human tendency to form a conclusion prematurely based on a preconceived expectation.
Consideration	In contract law, something of value exchanged for the promised performance of the other contracting party. Contracts frequently call for monetary consideration to be exchanged for the promise to provide specified goods or services.
Consolidated Omnibus Budget Reconciliation Act (COBRA)	Federal law that provides for the continuation of health coverage applicable to group health plans. Employers with more than twenty employees must extend group health insurance coverage for at least eighteen months after employees leave their jobs. Employees must pay 100 percent of the premium.
Constitution	A relatively short document enacted by a state or federal government that specifies the essential nature of governance by the elected legislature and generally restrains the actions of military or police forces and the power exercised by regulatory agencies.

Constructive termination	In employment law, a situation in which, even though an employee is not formally terminated from a job, the conditions of employment become so manifestly untenable that the employee had no choice but to quit and hence are treated by the court as a termination.
Contingency fee	A fee for service, collectable only if the outcome is favorable to the payee.
Contract	An agreement, either written or oral, involving an offer, the acceptance of the offer, and an exchange of consideration.
Contributory negligence	Conduct on the part of a plaintiff that falls below the standard to which he or she should conform for his or her own protection. If the claimant is negligent and this negligence combines with that of the healthcare provider in causing the injury, the claimant cannot recover damages.
COO	Chief operating officer.
CoP	Condition of participation.
Copayment	A specified flat fee per unit of service or unit of time charged to an enrollee for a service or supply. Many HMOs charge their members a nominal fee for all nonemergent ambulatory patient visits or for prescription medications.
COR	Cost of risk.
CORF	Comprehensive outpatient rehabilitation facility.
Corporate compliance	As relates to healthcare fraud and abuse, any of a number of programs and initiatives undertaken by providers to avoid civil and criminal investigations and charges related to improper billing procedures, inappropriate referrals, kickbacks, and other prohibited activities under federal statutes such as the Antikickback Act and the Stark I and Stark II amendments to the Medicare Act. Many healthcare providers have taken corporate compliance programs beyond these specific legislative and regulatory requirements to encompass broader corporate business ethics concerns.
Corporate liability	The liability of the healthcare entity for the failure of administrators and staff to properly supervise the delivery of healthcare in that entity, including negligence in hiring, training, supervising, or monitoring.
Corporation	A legal entity that may be created by one or more persons or entities to carry out a business purpose. Corporations are persons in the eyes of the law and may sue and be sued. Except in extraordinary circumstances, the owners of the corporation—shareholders or members (in nonprofit corporations)—are shielded from the liabilities of the corporation.
Cost-benefit analysis	A method comparing the costs of a project to the resulting benefits, usually expressed in monetary value.
Cost containment	Control or reduction of inefficiencies in the consumption, allocation, or production of healthcare services.

Counterclaim	A claim presented by the defendant in opposition to the claim of the plaintiff.
Countersignatures	A second signature confirming and endorsing a document already signed.
Coverage determination	A process that companies use to decide if coverage is applicable.
CPA	Certified public accountant.
CPCU	Chartered property casualty underwriter.
CPG	Clinical practice guidelines.
CPHQ	Certified professional in healthcare quality.
CPHRM	Certified professional in healthcare risk management.
CPI	Consumer price index, an inflationary measure encompassing the cost of a basket of consumer goods and services.
CPOE	Computerized provider order entry.
CPR	Cardiopulmonary resuscitation.
CPS	Child Protective Service.
CPT	Current procedural terminology.
CQI	Continuous quality improvement, an approach to organizational management that emphasizes meeting (and exceeding) consumer needs and expectations, use of scientific methods to continually improve work processes, and the empowerment of all employees to engage in continuous improvement of their work processes.
Credentialing	The process of verifying and reviewing the education, training, experience, work history, and other qualifications of an applicant for clinical privileges conducted by a healthcare facility or managed care organization. Typically performed for independent contractors such as physicians and allied health practitioners who frequently are not employed by the credentialing entity but who are granted specific clinical privileges to practice.
Credentialing and privileging	Process by which hospitals determine the scope of practice of practitioners providing services in the hospital; criteria are determined by the hospital and include personal character, competency, training, experience, and judgment.
Crew (cockpit) resource management (CRM)	A training concept originating at NASA, widely used in the aviation industry, and now adopted in healthcare to promote patient safety and enhance the efficiency of operations. Training elements include enhanced communications, situational awareness, problem solving, decision making, and teamwork.
Crime coverage	Insurance that provides coverage for losses arising out of employee or third-party theft or dishonesty.
Criminal false claim	Statute (18 USC 287) designed to "protect the government against those who would cheat or mislead it in the administration of its programs"; it has been employed to combat fraudulent claims filed under numerous federal programs, including Medicare and Medicaid.

Criminal law	The system of laws by which the state or federal government may bring suit against an individual, which suit may result in the loss of freedom or the person's life.
Critical access hospital	A small, limited-service, rural hospital that receives cost-based reimbursement for inpatient and outpatient care.
Critical paths	Any of a number of processes employed to define the generally accepted course of treatment for a specific medical condition or illness. Deviations from the prescribed critical paths must be explained by existing comorbidities, failure of prescribed treatments, and so on. Also known as *clinical practice guidelines* or care maps.
CRM	Crew resource management.
CRNA	Certified registered nurse-anesthetist.
CRO	Chief risk officer.
Cross-claim	A claim brought by a defendant against a plaintiff in the same action or against a codefendant concerning matters related to the original petition. Its purpose is to discover facts that will aid the defense.
C-section	Cesarean section, a procedure in which an incision is made through a mother's abdomen and uterus to deliver one or more infants.
CSO	Chief security officer.
CT	Cycle time, which records how responsive the process is. It is considered an efficiency measure.
CTS	Conformance to standard, which record how well the process is conforming to rules, regulations, standards, requirements, and specifications. These are quality measures.
CT scan	Computed tomography scan.
CVA	Cerebrovascular accident (stroke).
CWA	Clean Water Act.
Cycle time	The time it takes to complete a defined process—for example, the length of stay for a patient in the emergency department from triage to final disposition (transfer to unit; discharge or transfer out).
D	
D&C	Dilation and curettage.
D&O	Directors' and officers' (insurance coverage).
Damage cap	A legislatively imposed upper limit on the amount of a specific type of damages that may be awarded to a plaintiff in a specific type of lawsuit. State tort reform legislation frequently places a cap on the noneconomic damages that may be awarded to a plaintiff in a medical malpractice action.
Damages	Monetary compensation for an injury. The injuries for which the plaintiff (claimant) seeks compensation from the defendant (healthcare provider). May include economic losses, emotional distress, pain and suffering, and disability.

Dashboard	Dashboards are a management tool used to distill extensive data into succinct results often offering result comparison. They focus on performance, use key indicators or best practice, and show results graphically.
Date of occurrence	Date when an event or loss occurred.
Date of report	The date an event or loss was reported. Specific reporting requirements are generally outlined in coverage documents. The date of report is a "heading" on many loss runs.
DBA	"Doing business as," the legally required phrase preceding the designation of an alternative business name under which a company wishes to operate.
DDS	Doctor of dental surgery.
DEA	Drug Enforcement Administration.
Declaration	A statement made out of court; an unsworn statement or narration of facts made by a party involved in a transaction or by someone who has an interest in the existence of the facts recounted. Recounts of statements made by a deceased person are admissible as evidence in some cases.
Declaration of Helsinki	International declaration setting forth ethical standards for human subject research.
DED	Dedicated emergency department: as defined under the Emergency Medical Treatment and Labor Act, it means any department or facility of the hospital, regardless of whether it is located on or off the main hospital campus, that meets at least one of the following requirements: (1) It is licensed by the state in which it is located under applicable state law as an emergency room or emergency department; (2) it is held out to the public (by name, posted signs, advertising, or other means) as a place that provides care for emergency medical conditions on an urgent basis without requiring a previously scheduled appointment; or (3) during the calendar year immediately preceding the calendar year in which a determination under this section is being made, based on a representative sample of patient visits that occurred during that calendar year, it provides at least one-third of all of its outpatient visits for the treatment of emergency medical conditions on an urgent basis without requiring a previously scheduled appointment.
Deductible	In insurance, the amount of loss that must be paid by the insured before the insurer starts to pay. The use of deductibles allows insured parties to avoid paying for coverage for smaller claims they are capable of paying themselves.
Deemed status	Status conferred when a healthcare organization is certified as complying with the conditions of participation (standards) set forth in federal regulations, which is a prerequisite for participating in and receiving payment from Medicare or Medicaid programs.

Deep pocket	In claims, an informal term for the defendant having the most assets or available insurance coverage, which becomes the target of the plaintiff. The "deep pocket" may have less responsibility for the plaintiff's injuries than other codefendants but may be pursued more aggressively because of its financial resources.
Default judgment	A judgment entered by the court in a civil case in favor of the plaintiff and against the defendant when the defendant has failed to file some appearance in response to a summons. A defendant's failure to so file is deemed to be an admission that the demands of the plaintiff's complaint are valid.
Defendant	The party against whom relief or recovery is sought in an action or suit.
Defense	A denial, answer, or plea opposing the truth or validity of the plaintiff's case. This may be accomplished by cross-examination or demurrer. It is more often done by introduction of testimony of the plaintiff's case.
Demurrer	Admission of the truth of the allegations asserted by a plaintiff accompanied by a request for their dismissal due to legal insufficiency to state a cause of action. This has largely been replaced in the federal court system and in jurisdictions following the federal court rules of civil procedure by the motion to dismiss.
Deposition	Testimony (under oath) of a witness taken on interrogatories reduced to writing and used to support or substantiate testimony offered at trial. The deposition is an important phase of the discovery process. It consists of a question-and-answer session in which the witness is interrogated under oath, after which the testimony is transcribed.
DFASHRM	Distinguished Fellow of the American Society for Healthcare Risk Management.
Diagnosis-related group	Any one of the various categories in a resource classification system that serves as the basis for reimbursing hospitals under federal Medicare programs, based on the medical diagnosis for each patient. Hospitals receive a set payment amount determined in advance, based on the length of time patients with a given diagnosis are likely to stay in the hospital. Is also used as the basis of the Medicare inpatient prospective payment system and has been adapted for use by some managed care plans.
DIC (13)	Difference in conditions. Insurance coverage designed to close specific gaps in standard insurance policies; it allows coverage to be customized according to the insured's, needs extending coverage for exposures such as earthquake, landslide, flood, water damage, and collapse. Coverage may be provided by a separate insurance policy or it may be added by endorsement to the basic policy.
Diff.	Differential blood cell count.
Direct insurance	A contractual arrangement involving the purchase of insurance by an insured from an insurer.

Direct liability	Liability imposed on a party as a result of the party's acts or omissions.
Directors' and officers' insurance coverage	Policies covering liability in connection with any actual or alleged error, misstatement, or misleading statement or act or omission or breach of duty by directors and officers while acting in their individual or collective capacities or any matter claimed against them solely by reason of their being directors or officers of the company.
Disclosure	Communication of information regarding the results of a diagnostic test, medical treatment, or surgical intervention.
Discovery	The process in litigation by which each party to the action seeks to learn all relevant facts that either support the plaintiff's cause of action or support the defendant's asserted defenses or denials.
Dismissal with prejudice	Dismissal of a defendant in a suit that bars any future action against the defendant by the plaintiff.
Dismissal without prejudice	A dismissal that has no effect on the plaintiff's future actions with regard to the dismissed party.
DMAT	Disaster medical assistance team.
DME	Durable medical equipment.
DNR	Department of Natural Resources.
DNR	Do not resuscitate.
DO	Doctor of osteopathy.
DOC	Date of closure: the date a file or claim was closed.
Doctor of osteopathy	A doctor who employs the diagnostic and therapeutic measures of ordinary medicine in addition to manipulative measures. This approach is based on the idea that the normal body when in "correct adjustment" is a vital machine capable of making its own remedies against infections and other toxic conditions.
Documentation	The recording of pertinent facts and observations about an individual's health history, including past and present illnesses, tests, treatments, and outcomes. The legal evidence of professional accountability. See *Legal health record.*
DOD	U.S. Department of Defense.
DOE	U.S. Department of Education.
DOI	Date of incident.
DOJ	U.S. Department of Justice.
DOL	Date of loss; U.S. Department of Labor.
Do not resuscitate (8)	A physician's order that resuscitation efforts should not be performed on a person should the person have a cardiac or respiratory arrest. This order can be generated by an advance directive, living will, healthcare proxy, or other legally recognizable document in which the person's wishes were identified as desiring no life-sustaining measure.

DOR	Date of report.
DOT	Department of Transportation.
DPM	Doctor of podiatric medicine.
DPT	Diphtheria, pertussis, tetanus: three illnesses for which vaccines are often administered in a single injection.
DRG	Diagnosis-related group.
DRS	Designated record set: a group of records maintained by or for a covered entity that is the medical and billing records about individuals maintained by or for a covered healthcare provider; the enrollment, payment, claims adjudication, and case or medical management record systems maintained by or for a health plan; or information used in whole or in part by or for the covered entity to make decisions about individuals
DSM-IV	The fourth edition of the American Psychiatric Association's *Diagnostic and Statistical Manual of Mental Disorders,* published in 1994.
Dual capacity	In employer's liability, an individual or entity serving as both an injured party's employer in a workers' compensation claim and in some other role in which it is alleged to have caused injury, such as the manufacturer of a defective piece of equipment involved in the injury or as the provider of improper medical treatment for the injury.
Due diligence	The review of an entity targeted for acquisition by the acquiring party to ascertain pertinent information about its financial and operating history and current status. Corporate staff are generally held to the legal standard of having performed the review with due diligence before making a recommendation to the board of directors as to whether to proceed with the acquisition.
Due process	A procedural requirement that may be met by providing the affected party with (1) adequate notice of the proceeding, (2) the right to be represented by counsel, (3) the opportunity to be heard, (4) the right to call and cross-examine witnesses, and (5) the right to a written transcript of the proceeding.
Durable power of attorney for healthcare	Also called a "healthcare power of attorney," it is a directive prepared by a person in advance of becoming incapacitated that empowers the attorney-in-fact (proxy) to make healthcare decisions for the person, up to and including terminating care and disconnecting machines that are keeping a critically and terminally ill patient alive. Healthcare decisions include the power to consent, refuse consent, or withdraw consent to any type of medical care, treatment, service, or procedure.
Duty (4)	One person must be under a duty to another person (or to society) before negligence becomes an issue. In the context of professional liability, duty usually applies when the provider undertakes to care for a patient.

Duty of care (5)	The duty to act in good faith, with the care that an ordinarily prudent person in a similar position would use under those circumstances and in the reasonable belief that the actions taken are in the best interest of the corporation. Courts call this the "reasonable person standard" because the action or any failure to act by the board is judged by what a reasonable person would do.
Duty of loyalty (5)	The duty not to compete with the corporation, not to disclose confidential information obtained in the performance of one's duties as a board member, not to usurp corporate opportunity, and not to gain personal enrichment at the corporation's expense.
Duty to warn (4)	A psychotherapist treating a mentally ill patient has a duty to use reasonable care to give threatened persons such warnings as are essential to avert foreseeable danger arising from the patient's condition or treatment. The protective privilege between psychotherapist and patient ends where the public peril begins. In some jurisdictions, this duty extends to other healthcare practitioners.
DVM	Doctor of veterinary medicine.
Dx	Diagnosis.
E	
E&O	Errors and omissions (insurance).
EAP	Employee assistance program.
Early warning system (11)	A systemized method for the early detection of adverse events, medical error, or situations that can give rise to medical error to facilitate loss mitigation or implement prevention techniques.
ECF	Extended care facility.
Economic damages	Damages sought by or awarded to a plaintiff to compensate for out-of-pocket expenses, such as medical treatment or housekeeping services and lost wages resulting from an injury, as distinguished from noneconomic damages, such as pain and suffering and loss of consortium, for which a dollar value is more speculative.
ECRI	Current name of the former Emergency Care Research Institute.
ED	Emergency department.
EDP (13)	Electronic data processing.
EEG	Electroencephalogram.
EENT	Eye, ear, nose, and throat.
EEOC	Equal Employment Opportunity Commission.
HER (14)	Electronic health record.
EKG	Electrocardiogram.
Electronic data processing coverage (13)	Insurance that provides coverage for loss of information stored on cards, disks, drums, or tapes.

Electronic health record (14)	An electronic record of health-related information on an individual that conforms to nationally recognized interoperability standards and that can be created, managed, and consulted by authorized clinicians and staff across more than one healthcare organization.
Electronic incident reporting (6)	The reporting and entering of relevant incident data into a computer.
EMC	Emergency medical condition: an acute illness, injury, or condition requiring immediate attention.
Emergency Medical Treatment and Active Labor Act	Federal statute (42 USC 1395 et seq.) prohibiting the "dumping" of patients presenting to a hospital with an emergent medical condition or in active labor and limiting a hospital's ability to transfer them to other facilities. It also specifies when and how a patient may be refused treatment or transferred from one hospital to another when the patient is in an unstable medical condition.
EMF	Electromagnetic field.
EMG	Electromyogram.
Employee Polygraph Protection Act	Federal statute (29 USC 2001 et seq.) limiting most employers' ability to use polygraph testing in the applicant screening process.
Employer's liability	Any of a number of causes of action related to the employment relationship but falling outside of workers' compensation and employment practices liability insurance coverage, including dual capacity claims, spousal claims, and third-party-over claims.
Employment at will	Legal doctrine in most jurisdictions that an employer may discharge an employee for any reason, unless specifically prohibited by law.
Employment practices liability	Any of a number of violations by an employer, based on statute or common law, giving rise to damages outside of those covered by workers' compensation or similar statutes, including wrongful termination, discrimination, and sexual harassment.
Employment Retirement Income Security Act (ERISA)	Federal statute (42 USC 1002 et seq.) that regulates retirement plans and health insurance plans. If a lawsuit is brought under ERISA against a health insurance plan, it may be removed to federal court, and damages will include the value of services wrongfully withheld.
EMS	Emergency medical service.
EMT	Emergency medical technician.
EMTALA	Emergency Medical Treatment and Labor Act.
Enabling legislation (18)	A statute enacted by the legislature that permits an administrative agency to promulgate and enforce regulations.
Endorsement	A form attached to an insurance policy that either changes or adds to the provisions included in the policy. Endorsements may serve any number of functions, including broadening, limiting, or restricting the scope of coverage; clarifying coverage; adding other parties as insureds; or adding locations to the policy.
ENT	Ear, nose, and throat.

Enterprise liability	Liability to an organization or enterprise.
Enterprise risk management (ERM) (2)	An ongoing business decision-making *process* instituted and supported by a healthcare organization's board of directors, executive administration, and medical staff leadership. ERM recognizes the synergistic effect of risk across the continuum of care and aims to assist an organization to reduce uncertainty and process variability, promote patient safety, and maximize the return on investment through asset preservation and the recognition of actionable risk opportunities.
Environment of care (17)	The environment in which patient care is received and delivered. A category of standards promulgated by The Joint Commission.
Environmental impairment liability (13)	Negligent acts and/or omissions by individual(s) or organization(s) resulting in damage to The environment
Environmental Protection Agency (18)	The EPA leads the nation's environmental science, research, education, and assessment efforts. EPA's mission is to protect human health and the environment.
EOB	Explanation of benefits.
EOC (17)	Emergency operations center.
EOC	Environment of care.
EPA (18)	Environmental Protection Agency.
EPA (16)	Equal Pay Act.
EPL	Employment practices liability.
EPLI	Employment practices liability insurance.
EPO (4)	Exclusive provider organization.
Equal Employment Opportunity Commission	Federal agency charged with enforcing several federal statutes prohibiting various types of employment discrimination. Under some statutes, administrative hearing procedures before the EEOC must be exhausted before an employee has access to the court system.
Equal Pay Act	Federal statute (29 USC 206 et seq.) requiring equal pay for equal work without regard to the gender of the worker.
Equity	A system of justice that follows rules that differ and often override those of civil law and common law. In cases brought in equity, the court has the power, without a jury, to determine the facts of the matter and to make final determinations. Decisions are less affected by precedent than cases brought at law; they are generally based on principles of fairness to the parties. Examples of actions in equity include most domestic relations cases and cases for injunctive relief (restraining orders). Courts of equity have been merged with courts of law in the federal and most state systems.
Ergonomics (3)	The scientific discipline concerned with design according to human needs and the profession that applies theory, principles, data, and methods to design to optimize human well-being and overall system performance.

ERISA	Employee Retirement Income Security Act.
ERISA preemption	A provision of ERISA that preempts state law governing qualified pension and benefit plans and makes the remedies provided for by ERISA exclusive. Generally interpreted as preempting malpractice actions against managed care plans that are governed by the act.
ERM	Enterprise risk management.
ERP	Extended reporting period.
Error	Failure of a planned action to be completed as intended or use of a wrong plan to achieve an aim. The accumulation of errors results in accidents.
Errors and omissions insurance	An insurance policy providing coverage for negligent advice or business services provided by individuals or entities not eligible for professional liability insurance coverage, such as medical billing companies, insurance brokers, and managed care organizations.
Essential job functions	Under the Americans with Disabilities Act, the tasks associated with a particular job that an applicant must be able to perform, either with or without accommodation, to do the job.
Ethics (5)	A branch of philosophy, also called moral philosophy, that involves the systematizing, defending, and recommending of concepts of right and wrong behavior.
Ethics committee	A multidisciplinary group that convenes for the purpose of staff education and policy development in areas related to the use and limitation of aggressive medical technology and acts as a resource for patients, family, staff, physicians, and clergy regarding healthcare options surrounding terminal illness and assisting with living wills.
Event	An occurrence that is not part of the routine care of a particular patient or the routine operation of the healthcare entity.
Event reporting	A system in healthcare institutions by which employees use a standardized form to report any occurrence outside the routine so that the information can be used for loss prevention and claims management activities.
Evergreen clause	In contracts, a clause that makes the agreement perpetual unless terminated by one of the parties. Contracts with an evergreen clause have no set expiration date.
Evidence	Testimony, documents, objects, pictures, sound recordings, or other items that may prove that an occurrence did or did not occur. Such things may only be considered at trial if admitted into evidence by the court. Evidence may be excluded if it would unduly inflame the passions of the jury, if it is irrelevant, if it does not appear to be credible or probative, or for other reasons.
Evidence-based	Based on the best available scientific knowledge. Recommended evidence-based practices have generally gone through a rigorous review process by leading medical specialists.

Excess and surplus line carriers	Insurance companies that specialize in providing coverage above and beyond primary insurance policies or significant self-insured retentions. Under the insurance regulations of most states, such insurers may write coverage in the state according to certain specified conditions without going through the licensing provisions applicable to admitted insurance carriers.
Excess capacity	The difference between the number of hospital beds being used for patient care and the number of beds available.
Excess insurance policy	An insurance policy providing coverage above the limits provided by a primary insurer or a self-insurance program. Some insurance programs feature multiple layers of excess insurance policies.
Expense	Costs incurred associated with the generation of revenues.
Expenses within policy limits	A provision in some insurance policies that allocated- loss-adjusting expenses paid by the insurer are included when determining the applicable limits of coverage. For example, if $900,000 is paid to a claimant to settle a claim, expense costs come to $300,000, and the occurrence is covered by an insurance policy with a limit of $1 million that includes a provision for expenses within policy limits, the insurer will pay only $1 million. If the policy indicates that expenses are covered in addition to policy limits, the insurer will pay a total of $1.2 million. Expenses covered within policy limits are said to erode the limits.
Expert opinion (11)	An opinion rendered by a person who by virtue of education, training, skill, or experience is believed to have knowledge in a particular subject beyond that of the average person, sufficient that others may officially (and legally) rely on that person's specialized (scientific evidence [law], technical or other) opinion about an evidence or fact issue within the scope of the person's expertise.
Exposure	Risk: the chance of loss and potential liability that is covered by insurance. Also, a percentage, calculated by the attorneys and claims adjusters, that estimates the likelihood of losing a trial.
Extended reporting endorsement	An endorsement to a claims-made policy that extends the reporting period for claims.
Extended reporting period (13)	A designated period of time after a claims-made policy has expired during which a claim may be made and coverage triggered as if the claim had been made during the policy period.
Extra expense	Additional costs incurred in connection with to a covered loss.
F	
FAA	Federal Aviation Administration.
Face value	A perception that the level of validity of a concept is high, even when there is no scientific evidence to support that hypothesis.
FACHE	Fellow of the American College of Healthcare Executives.
Factitious disorder by proxy	See *Munchausen syndrome by proxy*.

Facultative	Describing a single transaction handled directly with a reinsurer.
Failure mode	Ways in which a process or subprocess can fail to provide the anticipated result.
Failure mode cause	Reasons why a process or subprocess would fail to provide the anticipated result.
Failure mode effects analysis or criticality analysis	A proactive, systematic assessment used to identify the steps of a process that may be subject to failure in order to design measures to either prevent or control such failures. If a criticality phase is used in this process, the perceived level of criticality of each type of potential failure is identified, to aid in setting priorities for establishing control mechanisms.
Fair hearing plan	A document, either freestanding or part of the bylaws of a medical staff, describing the procedures applicable to denial, revocation, and suspension of clinical privileges and other medical staff disciplinary issues. Such plans specify due process requirements such as the right to notice, hearings, representation by counsel, and appeals.
Fair Labor Standards Act	Federal statute (29 USC 201 et seq.) establishing the authority for the Department of Labor to promulgate wage and hour regulations and providing the framework for collective bargaining by employees.
False Claims Act	Two separate statutes defining false claims— 18 USC 287 and 31 USC 3729(a), 3730(a)–(b). See *Civil false claims* and *Criminal false claims.*
Family Education Rights and Privacy Act	Federal legislation (20 USC 1232G; 34 CFR 99) designed to protect the privacy of student education records. It is applicable to all schools that receive funds under designated U.S. Department of Education programs.
Family Medical Leave Act	Federal statute (29 USC 2611 et seq.) requiring certain employers to provide a period of unpaid leave to employees meeting specified criteria in order for them to receive medical treatment or to provide care to designated family members.
FASHRM	Fellow of the American Society for Healthcare Risk Management.
Fatigue factors	Manifestations of a person's physical or mental fatigue that may have contributed to an adverse event or outcome.
Fault tree analysis	A total quality management technique in which a complex process is broken down into a series of simpler steps and then particular areas of vulnerability for system breakdown are identified in an effort to anticipate and thereby avoid problems.
FDA	Food and Drug Administration.
Federal Emergency Management Agency (FEMA)	An independent response organization that reports directly to the president of the United States.
Federal Rules of Civil Procedure	Rules of practice and procedure and rules of evidence for cases in the U.S. district courts and courts of appeal.
Fee for service	A reimbursement mechanism that pays providers for each service or procedure they perform; opposite of *capitation.*

FEMA (17)	Federal Emergency Management Agency.
FERPA	Family Educational Rights and Privacy Act.
FFP (15)	Fitness for purpose, measures that record how well the process is satisfying stakeholders' interests, requirements, and desires. They define effectiveness measures.
Fiduciary duty	A duty to act for someone else's benefit while subordinating one's personal interests to those of the other person. It is the highest standard of duty implied by law (as in trustee and guardianship relationships).
Fiduciary liability (13)	Liability of trustees, employers, fiduciaries, professional administrators, and the plan itself with respect to errors and omissions in the administration of employee benefit programs as imposed by ERISA.
Financial guarantees	A form of financial security posted by the applicant to ensure timely and proper completion of a project, warranty materials, workmanship of improvements, and design. Financial guarantees include assignments of funds, cash deposits, surety bonds, or other financial securities.
FIRESCOPE (17)	Firefighting Resources of California Organized for Potential Emergencies, an interagency workgroup that developed the Incident Command System after several large wildfires in the early 1970s demonstrated the need for interagency cooperation.
First-dollar coverage	Commercial insurance providing protection against the entire loss covered by the policy, without requiring the insured to pay a deductible.
First-party coverage (13)	Insurance that provides coverage for the insured's own property and person so that the insured will be restored to the financial position that existed before the loss.
Float staff	Hospital staff, generally assigned to a specific patient care unit or not, made available to work on other units as required to yield appropriate staffing levels for a given patient volume and acuity.
FLV	Full liability value.
FMEA	Failure mode and effects analysis.
FMLA	Family Medical Leave Act.
FOIA	Freedom of Information Act.
Force majeure	Occurrences or situations over which one has no control, exempted from coverage in certain contracts. Clauses governing force majeure often declare the contracts, or specific provisions thereof, inapplicable in the event of natural disasters, such as earthquakes or hurricanes and sometimes other crises, such as war, riot, and civil commotion.
Forcing function	A technological design feature that forces the user to conform to a certain process, usually for a safety reason (for example, a car is designed not to permit ignition if the gearshift is in reverse).

Forensic examination (9)	The receiving, processing, documenting, analyzing, evaluating, and handling of evidence and work product for use in civil and criminal proceedings.
Formulary	A list of prescription medications that may be dispensed by participating pharmacies without health plan authorization. The formulary is based on effectiveness of the various drugs, as well as their cost. The physician is requested or required to use only formulary drugs unless there is a valid medical reason to use a nonformulary drug. Formularies may be open or closed. Closed formularies are restricted by the number and type of drugs included in the list.
Formulary system	A planned restriction on the inventory of medications stocked in a pharmacy, in order to limit the choice to essential drugs and promote safety by virtue of increasing staff familiarity with a more limited range of stocked medications.
For-profit hospital	A hospital operated for the purpose of making a profit for its owners. The initial source of funding is typically through the sale of stock, and profits are paid to stockholders in the form of dividends. Also referred to as a "proprietary hospital" or an "investor-owned hospital."
Forum non conveniens	A forum that is not convenient for the parties for some reason. Such a forum will normally have jurisdiction over the matter, and the venue of the action is appropriate, but hearing and deciding the matter there will work a hardship on the parties or the witnesses. Determining that a particular forum is not convenient is an exercise of the court's discretion.
FP	For profit.
FPO	Facility privacy official.
Fraud	Making false statements or representations of material facts in order to obtain some benefit or payment for which no entitlement would otherwise exist.
Fraud and abuse	Fraud is an intentional misrepresentation, deception, or act of deceit for the purpose of receiving greater reimbursement. Abuse is reckless disregard or conduct that goes against and is inconsistent with acceptable business, medical practices, or both, resulting in greater reimbursement. Terms are generally used together to refer to breach of federal statutes and regulations regarding inappropriate billing, kickbacks, referrals, related to the federal or state Medicare and Medicaid programs.
Free flow	The unrestricted flow of a fluid through an IV line.
Freestanding ambulatory surgery center	A medical facility that provides surgical treatment on an outpatient basis only.
Frequency (15)	The likelihood (probability) that a loss will occur; refers to a number of times a loss occurs.
FTC	Federal Trade Commission.

FTE	Full-time equivalent.
Full liability value	An estimate of the jury award if the plaintiff prevails on all issues.

G

Gag rule	A provision found in some managed care contracts with physicians prohibiting the physicians from discussing treatment alternatives, such as experimental procedures, with managed care plan patients when such treatments are not covered by the plan.
GAO (14)	Government Accountability Office.
Garage liability policy	Insurance that covers losses resulting from premises exposure of parking areas but excludes property in the care, custody, and control of the insured.
Gatekeeper	A primary care provider (PCP) who manages various components of a member's medical treatment, including all referrals for specialty care, ancillary services, durable medical equipment, and hospital services. The gatekeeper model is a popular cost-control component of many managed care plans because it requires a subscriber first to see the PCP and receive the PCP's approval before going to a specialist about a given medical condition (except for emergencies).
General liability (4)	A business organization's liability for claims for bodily injury and property damage arising out of premises, operations, products, and completed operations; advertising and personal injury liability.
General liability insurance	A standard insurance policy issued to business organizations to protect them against liability claims for bodily injury and property damage arising out of premises, operations, products, and completed operations; advertising and personal injury liability.
GI	Gastrointestinal.
GL	General liability.
GMP	Good manufacturing practice.
Government Accountability Office (14)	An independent, nonpartisan agency that works for Congress. Often called the "congressional watchdog," the GAO investigates how the federal government spends taxpayer dollars.
GP	General practitioner.
GU	Genitourinary.
Guarantee fund	A fund managed and controlled by the state to help pay the claims of financially impaired insurance companies. State laws specify the lines of insurance covered by these funds and the dollar limits payable. Coverage is usually for individual policyholders and their beneficiaries and not for values held in unallocated group contracts. Most states also restrict insurance agents and companies from advertising the funds' availability.

H

Hard insurance market	Insurance market conditions characterized by rising premiums and shrinking availability of coverage. Hard markets typically prompt insureds to accept larger deductibles or self-insured retentions, reduce coverage limits, or seek risk financing alternatives.
Hazard	A condition that increases the possibility of loss.
Hazard analysis	Collecting and evaluating information on hazards associated with a selected process so as to develop a list of hazards that are reasonably likely to cause injury or illness if not effectively controlled.
Hazard communication standard	To ensure chemical safety in the workplace, OSHA requires that standards are developed and information is disseminated about the identities and hazards of chemicals. Also known as the "employee right-to-know rule."
Hazardous condition	Any circumstance (beyond the disease or condition for which the patient is being treated) that significantly increases the likelihood of a serious adverse outcome.
Hazardous Waste Operations and Emergency Response standard	Applies to any person exposed or potentially exposed to hazardous substances, including hazardous waste, and who is engaged in one of five operations covered by HAZWOPER; certified by a qualified trainer.
HAZWOPER	Hazardous Waste Operations and Emergency Response.
HCCA	Health Care Compliance Association.
HCF (17)	Healthcare facility.
HCFA	Health Care Financing Administration; currently known as the Centers for Medicare and Medicaid Services.
HCO	Healthcare organization.
HCQIA	Health Care Quality Improvement Act.
Health Care Compliance Association	The professional society for healthcare corporate compliance officers.
Healthcare Facilities Accreditation Program	The AOA's Healthcare Facilities Accreditation Program (HFAP) has been providing medical facilities with an objective review of their services since 1945. The program is recognized nationally by the federal government, state governments, insurance carriers, and managed care organizations.
Healthcare Integrity and Protection Data Bank (HIPDB) (10)	A flagging system that may serve to alert users that a comprehensive review of a practitioner's, provider's, or supplier's past actions may be prudent. The HIPDB is intended to augment, not replace, traditional forms of review and investigation, serving as an important supplement to a careful review of a practitioner's, provider's, or supplier's past actions. The secretary of the DHHS, acting through the OIG, was directed by the Health Insurance Portability and Accountability Act of 1996 to create HIPDB to combat fraud and abuse in health insurance and healthcare delivery.
Healthcare organization	Entity that provides, coordinates, or ensures health and medical services for people.

Health Care Quality Improvement Act	Federal law (42 USC 11101 et seq.) that requires reports to the National Practitioner Data Bank and protects the confidentiality of peer review materials.
Health Insurance Portability and Accountability Act	Amendments to ERISA (42 USC 201 et seq.) addressing a variety of healthcare-related issues, including fraud and abuse and the portability of group health insurance benefits, and mandating specific patient privacy protections.
Health maintenance organization	A healthcare payment and delivery system involving networks of doctors and hospitals. Members must receive all their care from providers within the network. In a "staff model HMO," physicians are on the staff of the HMO and are usually paid a salary. In a "group model HMO," the HMO rents the services of the physicians in a separate group practice and pays the group a per-patient rate. In a "network model HMO," the HMO contracts with two or more independent physician group practices to provide services and pays a fixed monthly fee per patient.
Hearing (18)	A legal proceeding where an issue of law or fact is tried and evidence is presented to help determine the issue.
Hearsay	An out-of-court statement made by a person who is not a party to the action and is not available to testify that is offered to prove the truth of the matter asserted. Hearsay is normally not admissible as evidence.
HEDIS	Health Plan Employer Data and Information Set. A standard data reporting system developed in 1991 to measure the quality and performance of health plans. A main goal of HEDIS is to standardize health plan performance measures for consumers and payers. HEDIS concentrates on four aspects of healthcare: (1) quality, (2) access and patient satisfaction, (3) membership and utilization, and (4) finance. Within each focus area is a specific set of HEDIS data measures (for example, number of immunizations for pediatric enrollees). The National Committee for Quality Assurance (NCQA) is responsible for coordinating HEDIS and making changes each year.
HEICS	Hospital Emergency Incident Command System.
HFAP	Healthcare Facilities Accreditation Program.
HFE (3)	Human factors engineering.
HFMA	Healthcare Financial Management Association.
Hgb.	Hemoglobin.
HHC (6)	Home healthcare organization.
HHS	The U.S. Department of Health and Human Services.
HIAA	Health Insurance Association of America.
Hierarchy effect (steep hierarchy)	The effect that a perceived "pecking order" or relative differences in stature or status have on a lower person's level of willingness to question a higher person's actions or decisions.

High-alert medications (7)	Medications that have the highest risk of causing injury when misused.
High-low agreement	An agreement made between the plaintiff and defendant whereby the plaintiff will be entitled to at least the low amount but no more than the high amount and the defendant will be obligated to pay at least the low amount but no more than the high amount. If the jury returns a verdict between the low and high amounts, the case will settle for the amount of the verdict. A high-low agreement settles the case, and no appeal is permitted.
High-reliability organizations (7)	Organizations with systems in place that are exceptionally consistent in accomplishing their goals and avoiding potentially catastrophic errors.
High-risk patients (7)	Patients who are more susceptible to illness, injury, or disease or an exacerbation of an existing condition.
HIM	Health information management.
HIMSS (9)	Health Information Management Systems Society.
Hindsight bias	The tendency for a reviewer to focus most heavily on facts learned after an event or only the most obvious contributing factors, thereby failing to consider other, more subtle contributing factors.
HIPAA	Health Insurance Portability and Accountability Act.
HIPDB	Health Integrity and Protection Data Bank.
HIV	Human immunodeficiency virus.
HMO	Health maintenance organization.
Hold-harmless agreement	A contractual clause providing that one party agrees not to pursue a tort claim for vicarious liability against the other. Hold-harmless provisions are usually accompanied by indemnification provisions and are usually mutual.
Home healthcare	Healthcare services are provided in a patient's home instead of a hospital or other institutional setting; services provided may include nursing care, social services, and physical, speech, or occupational therapy.
Hospice	An organization that provides medical care and support services (such as pain and symptom management, counseling, and bereavement services) to terminally ill patients and their families; may be a freestanding facility, a unit of a hospital or other institution, or a separate program of a hospital, agency, or institution.
Hospital-acquired infection (1, 3)	An infection acquired in a hospital. Also known as a *nosocomial infection.*
Hospital Emergency Incident Command System (17)	A flexible, customizable plan developed to assist in the operation of a medical facility in time of crisis. HEICS was developed in 1991 by the Orange County Emergency Medical Services from the Incident Command System (ICS), a standard operating procedure for use by fire departments throughout the United States.

Hospitalist	A physician whose practice is caring for patients while in the hospital. A primary care physician (PCP) turns patients over to a hospitalist, who becomes the physician of record and provides and directs the care of the patient while the patient is hospitalized and returns the patient to the PCP at the time of hospital discharge.
HPL	Hospital professional liability (insurance).
HR	Human resources (department).
HRSA	Health Resources and Services Administration.
Human factors	The interrelationship between humans, the tools they use, and the environment in which they live and work.
Human factors engineering (3)	The discipline of applying what is known about human capabilities and limitations to the design of products, processes, systems, and work environments.
HVAC (17)	Heating, ventilation, and air conditioning (system).
I	
Iatrogenic	Adverse effects or complications caused by medical treatment or advice.
IBNR	Incurred but not reported.
IC (17)	Incident commander.
ICD-9-CM	The International Classification of Diseases, Ninth Revision, Clinical Modification (ICD-9-CM), is based on the World Health Organization's Ninth Revision, International Classification of Diseases (ICD-9). ICD-9-CM is the official system of assigning codes to diagnoses and procedures associated with hospital utilization in the United States.
ICF/MR	Intermediate care facility for the mentally retarded.
ICS	Incident Command System.
ICU	Intensive care unit.
ICUSRS (6)	Intensive Care Unit Safety Reporting System.
ID	Identification.
IDS	Integrated delivery system.
IHI (15)	Institute for Healthcare Improvement.
IHO (4)	Integrated health organization.
IIA	Insurance Institute of America.
IM (9)	Information management.
IM	Intramuscular.
IME	Independent medical examination.
Immediate jeopardy	A situation in which the provider's noncompliance with one or more requirements of participation has caused or is likely to cause serious injury, harm, impairment, or death to a patient or resident.
Immigration Reform and Control Act	Federal legislation (8 USC 1324 et seq.) requiring employers to verify the immigration status of prospective employees during the hiring process.

Impaired professional (4)	A professional who is unable to practice his or her profession with reasonable skill and safety to patients because of mental or physical illness, including deterioration through the aging process, loss of motor skills, or excessive use or abuse of drugs or alcohol.
Implementation (17)	Put into effect, carry out.
Improperly performed procedure or treatment	An appropriate procedure or treatment that is done incorrectly. Not to be confused with choosing the wrong procedure or treatment.
Inappropriate procedure or treatment	An incorrect procedure or treatment, usually as a result of poor medical judgment, skills, or techniques. Not to be confused with performing the correct procedure incorrectly.
Incident	Any occurrence not consistent with the routine operations of the facility or routine care of a particular patient; an unexpected event; an experience that leaves a patient, visitor, or other person feeling, rightly or wrongly, that he or she has been mistreated, neglected, or injured in some way.
Incident commander (IC) (17)	The individual responsible for the overall management of the response under HEICS.
Incident command system (ICS) 17	A standardized, on-scene, all-hazard incident management concept.
Incident report (6)	The documentation of an accident or an occurrence that is not consistent with normal operating routine or expected outcomes.
Incident reporting (1)	The filing of an incident report in an electronic, written, or verbal format.
Incident reporting system	Part of an early warning system intended to identify risk situations or adverse events in a timely manner to trigger prompt investigation from a claims management perspective as well as corrective action to prevent similar future events.
Incurred but not reported	Insurance and actuarial term applied to claims that have occurred but for which notification has not yet been received.
Indemnification (12)	A contractual agreement in which one party agrees to accept the tort liability and legal defense of another. Indemnification provisions are usually accompanied by hold-harmless provisions and are usually mutual.
Indemnification provision	A clause in a contract or agreement that identifies the terms of indemnification.
Indemnify	To secure against loss, damage, or expenses that may occur in the future which another may suffer.
Indemnity	An assurance or contract by one party to compensate for the damage caused by another; shifting an economic loss to the person responsible for the loss; the right that the person suffering the loss or damage is entitled to a claim; compensation given to make a person whole from a loss already received; a settlement or award made directly to a plaintiff as a result of the claims resolution process.

Independent medical examination	Medical examination of a claimant by a practitioner other than the claimant's treating practitioner at the request of a defendant to verify the claimant's diagnosis and prognosis.
Independent practice association	A group of independent physicians who have formed an- association as a separate legal entity for contracting purposes. IPA physician providers retain their individual practices, work in separate offices, continue to see their non–managed care patients, and have the option to contract directly with managed care plans. A key advantage of the IPA arrangement is that it helps its members achieve some of the negotiating leverage of a large physician group practice with some degree of flexibility for each provider. Also referred to as an "independent physician association."
Indicator	In quality improvement, a quantifiable objective standard against which performance is measured. Designed to be indicative of whether other care processes are also meeting established standards.
Information technology (14)	The study, design, development, implementation, support, or management of a computer-based information system, including software applications and computer hardware.
Informed consent	The legal doctrine that patients generally have a right to be informed regarding proposed medical and surgical treatments, including anticipated benefits, risks, and alternatives, and to accept or reject such proposed treatments.
Injunction	A court order prohibiting someone from doing some specified act or commanding someone to undo some wrong or injury.
INR (7)	International normalized ratio.
Insolvent	Lacking the available financial resources to pay covered claims.
Inspection (18)	A process in which an inspector (employed by an agency) comes onto the premises of an employer to interview employees, review documents, observe practices and conditions, take measurements or samples, and take photographs.
Institute for Safe Medication Practices (ISMP) (6)	The nation's only 501c (3) nonprofit organization devoted entirely to medication error prevention and safe medication use.
Institute of Medicine	A division of the National Academy of Sciences, a private nonprofit organization of scholars dedicated to research and publications related to engineering and the sciences. Noted for its 1999 publication *To Err Is Human: Building a Safer Health System*, which focused on medical errors.
Institutional review board	The body within a healthcare organization charged with establishing protocols for and overseeing clinical research trials and human experimentation.
Insurance	A contract to have internal losses paid for with funds external to the organization. A contractual relationship established when one party (the insurer), for consideration (the premium), agrees to reimburse another party (the insured) for loss to a specified subject (the risk) caused by designated contingencies (hazards or perils).

Insurance limits (13)	The total amount of losses to be paid expressed either on a per occurrence basis or on an aggregate basis, during an underwriting period. Limits vary by type of coverage, insurers, and insureds. Also referred to as "policy limits."
Insurance schedule	A document or graphic showing all of the insurance coverage in place for a given insured, usually including the names of insurers, policy limits, deductibles and retentions, policy numbers, and inception and expiration dates.
Insured versus insured exclusion	A provision common in insurance policies excluding coverage for claims in which one insured makes a claim against another.
Integrated care	A comprehensive spectrum of health services, from prevention through long-term care, provided via a single administrative entity and coordinated by a primary care "gatekeeper."
Integrated delivery system	A healthcare system made up of various types of providers, including hospitals, ambulatory care centers, surgery centers, home health agencies, and physician practices, and frequently a managed care organization, such as an HMO or a preferred provider organization (PPO).
Integrated health organization (4)	An organization that requires a separate legal entity, such as a parent organization, with at least two subsidiaries, such as a hospital and a management services organization, and often a third subsidiary such as an educational or research foundation.
Intentional acts	Purposeful actions by an insured that result in harm or loss, ordinarily excluded from coverage in most insurance contracts.
Interrogatories	A written set of questions that is served on the other party in litigation. All questions must be answered under oath and returned to the party that served them.
Intravenous	In or through the veins.
Investigation (11)	Detailed and careful examination to determine the facts surrounding an event, occurrence, or situation. The work of performing a thorough and systematic inquiry.
IOM	Institute of Medicine.
IP	Internet protocol.
IPA	Independent practice association.
IPPS (10)	Inpatient Prospective Payment System.
IRB	Institutional review board.
IRMI	International Risk Management Institute.
IRS	Internal Revenue Service.
ISMP	Institute for Safe Medication Practices.
ISO (16)	International Organization for Standardization.
IT (14)	Information technology.
IV	Intravenous, intravenously; also, an apparatus used for intravenous administration of a fluid.
IVP	Intravenous pyelogram (urogram).

J

JCR (16)	Joint Commission Resources.
JD	Juris doctor (doctor of law).
Joint and several liability	Liability in which each liable party is individually responsible for the entire obligation. Under joint and several liability, a plaintiff may choose to seek full damages from all, some, or any one of the parties alleged to have committed the injury. In most cases, a defendant who pays damages may seek reimbursement from nonpaying parties.
The Joint Commission	A voluntary nonprofit accreditation body that sets standards for hospitals and other healthcare organizations and conducts education programs and a survey process to assess-organizational compliance. Formerly known as the Joint Commission on Accreditation of Healthcare Organizations (JCAHO).
Joint Commission Resources	A not-for-profit affiliate of The Joint Commission that provides quality and safety innovations to healthcare organizations worldwide.
Joint defense	A defense of all defendants (for example, physician and hospital) in an integrated response.
Joint venture	An organization formed by two or more entities for a single purpose or undertaking that makes each member liable for all the organization's debts.
JUA	Joint underwriting association: Nonprofit risk-pooling associations established by state legislatures in response to availability crises concerning certain kinds of insurance coverage.
Judgment	The official decision of a court that determines the relative legal rights and obligations of parties to a legal proceeding.
Jurisdiction	The power of a court or other tribunal to hear and decide a legal matter. Also, the physical location in which a particular court is permitted to hear and decide cases.
Jury	A group of persons impaneled to hear a legal matter and to render a verdict. The jury typically finds the facts of the matter, and the court applies the law to the facts. The number of jurors necessary to form a jury varies by jurisdiction and sometimes by type of case.
Justice (8)	One of the three basic ethical concepts of the Belmont Report that refers to the fair distribution of the benefits and burdens of research.

L

LAE (11)	Loss adjustment expenses.
LAN (14)	Local area network.
Latent error	Errors removed from the direct control of the operator that include poor design, incorrect installation, faulty maintenance, bad management decisions, inadequate training, and poorly structured organizations whose effects typically lie dormant in the system for lengthy periods. Also called the *Blunt end.*

Latent failure (3, 7)	Weakness in an organization whose effects are usually delayed. Also called *blunt end* or *latent error.*
Law courts	Courts that have jurisdiction to hear most civil lawsuits (personal injury, breach of contract, and so on). For almost all practical purposes, law courts have been merged with courts of equity, but differences in actions based in law versus actions based in equity still remain.
LCF	Loss conversation factor: A factor that provides a charge to cover unallocated claims and the cost of an insurer's claim services. Used in formulas for retrospectively rated insurance programs.
LCL	Lower control limit.
LDF	Loss development factor, a common method of adjusting losses for the growth in claims and IBNR losses.
Leapfrog Group	A private business consortium for healthcare interests. A voluntary, member-supported program launched in 2000 aimed at mobilizing employer purchasing power to alert America's health industry that big leaps in healthcare safety, quality, and customer value will be recognized and rewarded.
Legal health record	Documentation of the healthcare services provided to an individual in any aspect of healthcare delivery by healthcare provider organizations. The legal health record is individually identifiable data, in any medium, collected and directly used in or documenting healthcare or health status. The term applies to records of care in any health-related setting used by healthcare professionals while providing patient care services, reviewing patient data, or documenting observations, actions, or instructions.
Legally cognizable injury	An injury for which the law can provide redress.
Legibility (9)	Understandable or readable based on appearance.
Length of stay	The period of hospitalization, measured in days billed; determined by discharge days divided by discharges.
LEP	Limited English proficiency.
LEPC (17)	Local emergency planning council.
Letter of intent	Formal notice to an organization that another organization is seeking to acquire or merge with it, setting due diligence in motion.
Libel	Defamatory language expressed in print, writing, pictures, or symbols intended to injure another's reputation, business. or means of livelihood.
Life Safety Code (10)	A code promulgated by the National Fire Protection Association (NFPA) and that addresses construction, protection, and occupancy features necessary to minimize danger to life from the effects of fire, including smoke, heat, and toxic gases created during a fire.
Limited liability company (LLC)	A company formed by one or more persons or entities to carry out a business purpose. The LLC shields its owners (members) from liability but enjoys certain tax advantages not available to corporations.

Limits (policy limits)	In insurance, the maximum the insurer will pay, typically expressed either per occurrence or as an annual aggregate (the maximum the insurer will pay during the year for all claims covered under the policy).
Living will	Document generated by a person for the purpose of providing guidance about healthcare and medical decisions to be provided if the person is unable to articulate those decisions. A living will does not designate another to speak in the patient's stead; it only offers written documentation of the person's wishes.
LLC	Limited liability company.
Long tail	Lines of insurance coverage for which there is frequently an extended period between the time an incident giving rise to a claim occurs and the time the claim is reported. Medical professional liability is generally considered long-tail insurance business.
Long-term care	A continuum of maintenance, custodial, and health services to the chronically ill, disabled, or mentally handicapped.
LOS	Length of stay.
Loss	The reduction in the value of an asset.
Loss adjustment expense (11)	All costs and expenses allocable to a specific claim that are incurred in the investigation, appraisal, adjustment, settlement, litigation, defense, or appeal of a specific claim, including court costs, costs of bonds, and postjudgment interest.
Loss control	Any of a number of programs and initiatives undertaken to prevent losses from occurring (loss prevention) or to decrease the severity of losses that do occur (loss reduction), including education and training, policy and procedure development, equipment maintenance, use of personal protective equipment, and installation of sprinkler systems.
Loss of consortium	Claim for damages relating to the loss of companionship, advice, and sexual relationship with an injured party, typically filed by the injured party's spouse.
Loss frequency	A measure of how many times a particular loss occurs or can be expected to occur in a given period of time.
Loss prevention	Reducing an organization's losses by lowering their frequency of occurrence.
Loss reduction	Actions taken to decrease the severity of a loss.
Loss reserve (12)	An estimate of the value of a claim or group of claims not yet paid.
Loss run	A listing, usually generated by computer, of claims brought against an insured for a specific line of insurance coverage; typically includes the name of the claimant, the date of occurrence, the date the claim was made, the status of claim (open or closed; suit, claim, or occurrence), amounts paid and reserved for both indemnity and loss adjustment expenses, and a description of the facts giving rise to the claim.

Loss severity	A measure of the size of an actual or expected loss; how much a loss will cost.
Lower control limit (LCL)	A formula that will calculate a lowermost limit for samples to evaluate to. Used in charts of statistical process control.
LSC (10)	Life Safety Code.
LPN	Licensed practical nurse.
LPT	Licensed physical therapist.
LTC	Long-term care.
LTD	Long-term disability.
LVN	Licensed vocational nurse.

M

M&A&D	Mergers, acquisitions, and divestitures.
M&M	Morbidity and mortality.
MA	Medical assistant.
Magnetic resonance imaging	Technology that uses radio and magnetic waves to create images of body tissue and monitor body chemistry.
Malfeasance	The wrongful or unjust doing of an act that the doer had no right to perform or had stipulated by contract not to do.
Malpractice	Improper professional actions or the failure to exercise proper professional skills by a professional adviser, such as a physician, dentist, or healthcare entity. Also, professional misconduct, improper discharge of professional duties, or failure to meet the standards of care of a professional, resulting in harm to another person.
Mammography Quality Standards Act (10)	A law focused primarily on issues related to improving the diagnostic and technical standards of mammography. The act also calls for the proper reporting of study results to referring physicians and their patients.
Managed care	The integration of healthcare delivery and financing that includes arrangements with providers to supply healthcare services to members, criteria for the selection of healthcare providers, significant financial incentives for members to use providers in the plan, and formal programs to monitor the amount of care and quality of services.
Managed care organization	Any of a number of organizations, such as HMOs and PPOs, that arrange for the provision of and payment for healthcare services with an eye toward reducing costs through managing access to specific providers.
Managed care E&O liability (13)	Insurance that covers allegations for wrongful acts in the design and administration of a managed care plan.
Management services organization (4)	An organization that provides management services to medical practices, large physician groups, and hospitals.

Mandatory settlement conference	A court-ordered meeting of the plaintiff and defendant held under the judge's direction with the goal of resolving a claim. This meeting is not voluntary, and the opposing parties are required to participate.
Manufacturers and User Facility Device Experience database (10)	A database of voluntary, user facility, distributor, and manufacturer reports of adverse events related to medical devices.
MAR	Medication administration record.
MAUDE (6, 10)	Manufacturers and User Facility Device Experience Database.
Maximum medical improvement (MMI)	In workers' compensation, the point at which the injured employee has recovered to the maximum extent medically expected (also called "permanent and stationary" or P & S improvement). When an employee reaches MMI, any residual disability, pain, or injury is expected to be permanent.
MBWA	Management by walking around.
MCO	Managed care organization.
MD	Medical doctor.
MDR	Medical device reporting.
MedPAC	Medicare Payment Advisory Commission.
Mediation	Intervention between parties in conflict to promote reconciliation, settlement, or compromise.
Medicaid	A federal public assistance program enacted into law in 1966 under Title XIX of the Social Security Act, to provide medical benefits to eligible low-income persons needing healthcare regardless of age. The program is administered and operated by the states, which receive federal matching funds to cover the costs of the program. States are required to include certain minimal services as mandated by the federal government but may include any additional services at their own expense.
Medical battery	Traditionally, a battery that occurs during the administration of medical care and procedures. May also include actions against medical care providers for prolonging the lives of patients who had previously requested that no "heroic measures" be undertaken when faced with a medical emergency.
Medical Injury Compensation Reform Act (MICRA) (10)	Legislation passed in California in 1975 to curb the high cost of medical professional liability insurance and "runaway" verdicts. Often promoted as the model for state and federal liability reform efforts.
Medical malpractice review panel	A panel consisting of two lawyers, two healthcare providers, and a circuit court judge that at the request of any party passes nonbinding judgments on claims of alleged medical malpractice. The panel may conclude that there was negligence, no negligence, or a question of fact that must be decided by a jury.
Medical professional liability (4, 13)	Insurance coverage for losses arising from the rendering or failure to render healthcare services.

Medical screening exam (10)	A screening examination to determine whether an emergency medical condition exists and to treat and stabilize any emergency condition. A requirement under EMTALA for all hospitals.
Medical services	The furnishing of professional healthcare services, including the provision of food, medications, or appliances; the postmortem handling of bodies; or service as a member of a formal accreditation review board.
Medical technology	Techniques, drugs, equipment, and procedures used by healthcare professionals in delivering medical care to individuals and the systems whereby such care is delivered.
Medicare	A federally administered health insurance program for persons aged sixty-five and older and certain disabled people under that age. Created in 1965 under Title XVIII of the Social Security Act, Medicare covers the cost of hospitalization, medical care, and some related services for eligible persons without regard to income. Medicare has two parts. Medicare Part A, the Hospital Insurance Program, is compulsory and covers inpatient hospitalization costs. Medicare Part B, the Supplementary Medical Insurance Program, is voluntary and covers medically necessary physicians' services, outpatient hospital services, and a number of other medical services and supplies not covered by Part A. Part A is funded by a mandatory payroll tax. Part B is supported by premiums paid by enrollees.
Medicare Modernization Act (10)	Short name for the Medicare Prescription Drug Improvement and Modernization Act of 2003.
Medication administration record	The record of all medications ordered and when each was administered, maintained by the nursing staff.
Medication error	Any preventable event that may cause or lead to inappropriate medication use or patient harm while the medication is in the control of the healthcare professional, patient, or consumer.
Medical Event Reporting System–Transfusion Medicine (MERS-TM)	Web-based medical event reporting system that documents, and allows for analysis of transfusion medicine-related events.
MedWatch (6)	The FDA's information and adverse event reporting program.
MER	Medication Errors Reporting (program).
Merger	The union of two or more organizations by the transfer of all assets to one organization that continues to exist while the others are dissolved.
MERS-TM	Medical Event Reporting System-Transfusion Medicine.
Metric (15)	Standard used to measure and assess performance or a process. Also, a system of measurement that includes the item being measured, the unit of measurement, and the value of the unit.
MGMA	Medical Group Management Association: The nation's principal voice for the medical group practice profession.

MHA	Master of health administration; master of hospital administration.
MHSA	Master of health services administration.
MI	Mental institution; mitral insufficiency; myocardial infarction.
MICRA (10)	Medical Injury Compensation Reform Act.
Microsystem	Organizational unit built around the definition of repeatable core service competencies. Elements of a microsystem include (1) a core team of healthcare professionals, (2) a defined population of patients, (3) carefully designed work processes, and 4) an environment capable of linking information on all aspects of work and patient or population outcomes to support ongoing evaluation of performance.
Misrepresentation	Any untrue or intentionally deceptive statement presented as fact.
MMA (10)	Medicare Modernization Act (official title: Medicare Prescription Drug Improvement and Modernization Act of 2003).
MOB	Medical office building.
Morbidity	Associated negative consequences relating to a clinical treatment or procedure; a complication. Also, the incidence and severity of illness and accidents in a well-defined class of individuals.
Mortality	Death rate; incidence of death in a well-defined class of individuals.
Motion	A filing with a court or other tribunal that requests that the court perform some function.
Motion for judgment notwithstanding the verdict	A filing that seeks to have a jury verdict set aside. In a trial process, the court normally enters judgment on a jury's verdict and thus gives effect to the verdict. This motion seeks to have the jury verdict set aside and judgment entered by the court that is not in accord with the verdict. Usually granted for the appearance of bias, prejudice, or possible jury misconduct.
Motion for new trial	A filing that seeks to invalidate the original trial and declare that the matter must be tried again. Usually granted when the verdict is contrary to the manifest weight of the evidence or when there is scant evidence to support the jury's verdict.
Motion for summary judgment	A filing that seeks to have a lawsuit decided because there are no genuine issues of material fact for the jury to decide.
Motion in limine	A filing to preclude the admission of certain facts, testimony, items, or proofs at trial. May be granted on the grounds that the evidence is not relevant, is redundant or duplicative of other evidence, will unduly arouse or inflame the jury, and so on.
Motion to dismiss	A filing that seeks to have a lawsuit rejected because the complaint or petition fails to state a cause of action on which relief may be granted. Such a filing often stays the period in which an answer must be filed.
Motion to strike	A filing to eliminate a cause of action in the complaint or petition or to preclude the defendant from mounting a defense based on a certain theory.
MPA	Master of public administration.

MPH	Master of public health.
MQSA	Mammography Quality Standards Act of 1992.
MQSRA (10)	Mammography Quality Standards Reauthorization Acts of 1998 and 2004.
MRI	Magnetic resonance imaging.
MSE (10)	Medical screening examination.
MSN	Master of science in nursing.
MSO	Management service organization.
MSW	Master of social work.
MT	Medical technologist.
Multihospital system	Two or more hospitals owned, leased, contract-managed, or sponsored by a central organization; they can be either not for profit or investor-owned.
Munchausen syndrome by proxy	A factitious disorder in which a person, usually a parent, exaggerates or feigns illness in a child or deliberately causes or exacerbates actual medical problems the patient is experiencing.
MVR (13)	Motor vehicle records.

N

Named peril coverage (13)	Insurance that covers only losses that fall under specific perils defined in the policy.
NASA	National Aeronautics and Space Administration.
National Center for Complementary and Alternative Medicine	An agency of the National Institutes of Health developed to study and provide information about complementary and alternative medicine treatments and therapies.
National Committee for Quality Assurance	A private nonprofit accrediting body for managed care organizations.
National Institute of Occupational Safety and Health	A research and education agency within the Department of Health and Human Services that has no enforcement powers.
National Labor Relations Act	The main body of law governing collective bargaining. It explicitly grants employees the right to bargain collectively and to join trade unions. Originally enacted by Congress in 1935 under its power to regulate interstate commerce.
National Organ Transplant Act (10)	Legislation passed by the Congress in 1984 to address the nation's critical organ donation shortage and improve the organ placement and matching process. The act established the Organ Procurement and Transplantation Network (OPTN) to maintain a national registry for organ matching.
National Patient Safety Goals (3, 9)	Goals developed by The Joint Commission to promote specific improvements in patient safety. They highlight problematic areas in healthcare and describe evidence and expert-based consensus to solutions to these problems and are updated yearly.

National Practitioner Data Bank	A data bank maintained by the federal government containing reports on certain individual practitioners. A report must be made by any entity that pays money on behalf of a practitioner to settle a legal claim asserted against the practitioner. Reports must also be made by any hospital that restricts, suspends, or terminates a practitioner's privileges to examine or treat patients at the hospital.
NB	Newborn.
NBC emergencies	Disaster scenarios involving nuclear, bioterrorism, or chemical warfare agents.
NCCH (16)	National Commission on Correctional Health Care.
NCC-MERP	National Coordinating Council for Medication Error Reporting and Prevention.
NCI	National Cancer Institute.
NCQA	National Committee for Quality Assurance.
NCVIA	National Childhood Vaccine Injury Act (42 USC 300); established the National Vaccine Injury Compensation Program.
NDS	National Disaster Medical System.
Near miss	Any variation in a procedure that did not affect the outcome but might have produced a serious adverse outcome. Also called a "good catch."
Neglect	Failure to provide goods and services necessary to avoid physical harm, mental anguish, or mental illness.
Negligence	A legal conclusion that is reached when it has been determined that (1) the defendant owed a duty of care to the plaintiff; (2) the defendant breached the duty of care; (3) the plaintiff was injured as a result of the breach of the duty of care; and (4) legally cognizable damages resulted from the injury. Less formally, carelessness: a failure to act as an ordinary prudent person would or action contrary to that of a reasonable party or the failure to use such care as a reasonably prudent and careful person would under similar circumstances.
Negligence per se (4)	A legal doctrine whereby an act is considered negligent because it violates a statute or regulation.
Neonatal	Referring to the first twenty-eight days of an infant's life. The infant is referred to as a newborn during this period.
NESHAP	National Emission Standard for Hazardous Air Pollutants.
Network	A self-contained, fully integrated system of providers.
Never events (7)	A list developed by the National Quality Forum of twenty-eight adverse events that are serious, largely preventable, and of concern to both the public and healthcare providers for the purpose of public accountability.
NF	Nursing facility.
NFP	Not for profit.

NFPA (17)	National Fire Protection Agency.
NICU	Neonatal intensive care unit.
NIH	National Institutes of Health.
NIMH	National Institute of Mental Health.
NIOSH	National Institute of Occupational Safety and Health.
NLRA	National Labor Relations Act.
NLRB	National Labor Relations Board.
NMHPA	Newborns' and Mothers' Health Protection Act.
No-fault system	A system of compensation for injured parties that is not based on the fault or negligence of the party causing the injury. Examples include the workers' compensation system and the personal injury protection automobile insurance mandated or available in some jurisdictions.
Nomenclature	A naming classification system, such as the FDA's system for choosing new medication names.
Nonadmitted insurer (13)	An insurance company that is exempt from rigorous state regulations. Because such companies do not file forms or rates and are not regulated by the state, they also do not participate in the state guaranty funds that protect insureds in case of insurance company failure.
Noneconomic damages (general damages)	Damages asserted by or awarded to a claimant for pain and suffering, loss of consortium, loss of enjoyment of life, and so on, for which no objective dollar value exists. The term technically includes punitive damages, but those are typically discussed separately.
Noninsurance transfer	The transfer of the financial obligations to pay for defense, expenses, verdicts, awards, and settlements. It reduces the transferor's loss exposure by contractually shifting legal responsibility for a loss through leases, contracts, and agreements (known as "exculpatory clauses").
Nonmaleficence (8)	Avoiding harm.
Nonsuit	A privilege granted to plaintiffs in Virginia that allows them to withdraw a civil lawsuit at any time before decision, without prejudice to their right or ability to bring it one more time.
NORA	National Occupational Research Agenda.
Nose coverage	Prior acts coverage.
Nosocomial infection	An infection acquired in a hospital.
NOTA (10)	National Organ Transplant Act.
Notice of claim	A letter from or on behalf of a claimant that puts a healthcare provider on notice that a claim of alleged medical negligence is being made and triggers certain rights of the parties to request a medical malpractice review panel.
NPDB	National Practitioner Data Bank.

NPSF	National Patient Safety Foundation.
NPSG	National Patient Safety Goals.
NQF	National Quality Foundation.
NRC	Nuclear Regulatory Commission.
NTSB	National Transportation Safety Board.
Nuclear medicine	The use of radioisotopes to study and treat disease, especially in the diagnostic area.
Nuremberg Code (8)	A ten-point statement delimiting permissible medical experimentation on human subjects. To some extent, the Nuremberg Code has been superseded by the Declaration of Helsinki as a guide for human experimentation.
Nurse practitioner	A licensed nurse who has completed a nurse practitioner program at the master's or certificate level and is trained in providing primary care services. NPs are qualified to conduct expanded healthcare evaluations and decision making regarding patient care, including diagnosis, treatment, and prescriptions, usually under a physician's supervision. NPs may also be trained in medical specialties, such as pediatrics, geriatrics, or midwifery. Legal regulations in some states prevent NPs from qualifying for direct Medicare and Medicaid reimbursement, writing prescriptions, and admitting patients to hospital. Also known as an "advanced practice nurse" (APN).

O

OASIS	Outcomes and assessment information set.
Oath of Hippocrates (8)	An oath, dating from the fourth century B.C.E. and widely attributed to Hippocrates, that pertains to the ethical practice of medicine. The oath has been revised to reflect modern medical practice.
OBA (8)	Office of Biotechnology Activities.
OBE	Occupied bed equivalent.
OB-GYN	(Specialist in) obstetrics and gynecology.
OBRA	Omnibus Budget Reconciliation Act.
OBS	Office-based surgery.
Obstetrics	The medical specialty concerned with the care of women during pregnancy and childbirth.
Occupational Safety and Health Act	Federal statute (29 USC 651 et seq.) that created the Occupational Safety and Health Administration.
Occupational Safety and Health Administration (OSHA)	Federal agency charged with responsibility for promulgating standards and enforcement mechanisms governing worker safety for most industries.
Occupational Safety and Health Review Commission (18)	An independent federal agency created to decide contests of citations or penalties resulting from OSHA inspections of American workplaces. The review commission functions as an administrative court with established procedures for conducting hearings, receiving evidence, and rendering decisions by its administrative law judges (ALJs).

Occurrence insurance	Insurance providing coverage for claims that arise during the policy period, regardless of when the claim is reported.
Occurrence screening	A systematic review of medical records and cases (conducted either retrospectively or concurrently) using predetermined screening criteria to identify cases that may warrant closer review—for example, unplanned returns to the ED within seventy-two hours of admission or prior treatment for a similar condition.
OCR	Office of Civil Rights.
OD	Doctor of optometry.
OD	Right eye.
Office for Human Research Protections (10)	Protects the rights, welfare, and well-being of subjects involved in research conducted or supported by HHS and helps ensure that such research is carried out in accordance with the regulations described at 45 CFR part 46.
Office for Civil Rights (10)	Promotes and ensures that people have equal access to and opportunity to participate in and receive services from all HHS programs without facing unlawful discrimination and that the privacy of their health information is protected while ensuring access to care.
Office of Inspector General (10)	Protects the integrity of HHS programs as well as the health and welfare of the beneficiaries of those programs.
Office of National Coordinator for Health Information Technology (14)	Provides counsel to the secretary of HHS and departmental leadership for the development and nationwide implementation of an interoperable health information technology infrastructure.
OHRP (8, 10)	Office for Human Research Protections.
OIG	Office of the Inspector General.
Older Workers' Benefit Protection Act	Legislation (29 USC 621 et seq.) amending the Age Discrimination in Employment Act restricting employers from making certain age-based distinctions in employee benefits plans.
OMB	Office of Management and Budget.
Omission error	Failure to carry out an intended action or to recognize that an action should have been carried out.
Omnibus Budget Reconciliation Act of 1987 (OBRA) (4)	OBRA 1987 or Federal Nursing Home Reform Act created a set of national minimum standards of care and rights for people living in certified nursing facilities.
ONC (14)	Office of the National Coordinator for Health Information Technology.
OPDRA	Office of Post-Marketing Drug Risk Assessment.
Operating margin	Net patient care revenues in excess of operating expenses.
Operating room	Locale where surgical interventions are performed.
OPO	Organ Procurement Organization.
OPPS (10)	Outpatient Prospective Payment System.

OPTN (10)	Organ Procurement Transplant Network.
OR	Operating room.
Ordinance	A law typically enacted by the elected legislative body of a city, town, county or other such minor political subdivision.
Organizational culture (3, 5)	A set of values, guiding beliefs, or ways of thinking that are shared among members of an organization.
Organ Procurement Transplant Network (10)	The unified transplant network established by the Congress under the National Organ Transplant Act of 1984.
ORYX	The Joint Commission's program for integrating performance measures into the accreditation process. A key component is the use of standardized core measures.
OS	Left eye.
OSCAR	Online Survey Certification and Reporting Database.
OSHA	Occupational Safety and Health Administration.
OSHA general duty clause	OSHA's general requirement that employers maintain a safe work environment. OSHA inspectors may cite the general duty clause whenever an unsafe workplace condition or work practice is identified, but no specific OSHA regulation applies.
OSHRC (18)	Occupational Safety and Health Review Commission.
Ostensible agency doctrine	The doctrine that permits a hospital to be held liable for the actions of an independent contractor. For example, in the absence of an employer-employee relationship, a managed care organization may still be held vicariously liable for the acts of provider physicians if the patient had a reasonable belief that the physician was the MCO's agent and that this belief was based on representations made by the MCO to that effect. The burden is on the plaintiff to prove that he or she relied on the fact that the MCO presented the physician as its agent.
OT	Occupational therapy.
OTC	Over the counter.
Outcome	The end result of medical care, as indicated by recovery, disability, functional status, mortality, morbidity, or patient satisfaction.
Outcomes measurement	The process of systematically tracking a patient's clinical treatment and responses to that treatment using generally accepted outcomes or quality indicators, such as mortality, morbidity, disability, functional status, recovery, and patient satisfaction. Such measures are considered by many healthcare researchers as the only valid way to determine the effectiveness of medical care.
Out-of-network (out-of-plan) services	In managed care, healthcare services required by a plan participant that are either not provided for by the plan (such as most experimental procedures) or must be provided for outside of the plan network (such as an emergency department visit for a participant who is traveling out of town).

Outpatient care	Treatment provided to a patient who is not confined in a healthcare facility. Includes services that do not require an overnight stay, such as emergency treatment, same-day surgery, outpatient diagnostic tests, and physician office visits. Also referred to as *Ambulatory care.*
Over-the-counter drugs	Medications that can be obtained without a written prescription from a physician.
Overuse	A healthcare quality problem involving the application or performance of unnecessary procedures or the provision of unnecessary services for patients.

P

P&P	Policy and procedure.
PA	Physician assistant; posterior-anterior.
PALS	Pediatric advanced life support.
Paradigm	A conceptual framework that aids in the explanation of a complex phenomenon or field of inquiry.
Parallel processes	Two or more processes being performed simultaneously.
Partnership	An entity formed by two or more persons to undertake a business purpose for profit. Each partner is liable for the obligations and liabilities of the partnership. Income to the partnership is considered income to the partners; there is no taxation at the level of the partnership.
Patient-controlled analgesia (7)	A means for a patient to self-administer analgesics (pain medications) intravenously by a computerized pump, which introduces specific doses into an intravenous line.
Patient safety	Freedom from accidental injury. Ensuring patient safety involves the establishment of operational systems and processes that minimize the likelihood of errors and maximize the likelihood of intercepting them when they occur.
Patient Safety and Quality Improvement Act of 2005 (6)	Legislation signed into law in 2005 to improve patient safety by encouraging voluntary and confidential reporting of events that adversely affect patients. It creates patient safety organizations to collect, aggregate, and analyze confidential information reported by healthcare providers.
Patient safety evaluation system (6)	The process of collecting, managing, or analyzing information the patient safety organization receives from healthcare providers.
Patient safety event taxonomy (6)	A voluntary system for classifying patient safety incidents to enable different patient safety reporting systems to communicate with each other.
Patient safety work product (6)	Data submitted by a healthcare provider to a listed patient safety organization; the data developed by the listed organization are privileged and confidential under the Patient Safety Act.

Patient Self-Determination Act of 1990	Federal statute (42 USC 1395 et seq.) requiring that certain healthcare organizations, including hospitals and HMOs, provide patients with information regarding advanced directives.
PC (15)	Process cost: the fixed or investment costs associated with the process.
PC	Professional corporation.
PCA	Patient-controlled analgesia.
PCE	Potentially compensable event: any event that in the opinion of a risk management professional could give rise to a formal demand for compensation or an event that could generate an indemnity payment.
PDCA (15)	The "plan, do, check, act" cycle offers healthcare systems a simple yet effective way to measure and modify change based on the effect on the quality outcome of the change they are attempting to achieve.
Peer review	A process whereby possible deviations from the standard of patient care are reviewed by an individual or committee from the same professional discipline to determine whether the standard of care was met and to make recommendations for improving patient care processes. Most jurisdictions provide at least a limited protection from discovery in civil actions for peer-review activities.
Per diem staff	Staff of a healthcare provider called in to work on an "as-needed" basis, depending on patient volume and acuity, as opposed to having their work schedules determined in advance.
Performance improvement (15)	Analyzing a particular process or procedure, then modifying the process or procedure to increase the output, efficiency (economics), or effectiveness of the process or procedure.
Peril	The cause of a loss.
Perinatal care	The care of a woman before conception, of the woman and her fetus throughout pregnancy, and of the mother and her neonate until twenty-eight days after childbirth.
Personal health record (14)	An electronic record of health-related information on an individual that conforms to nationally recognized interoperability standards and that can be drawn from multiple sources while being managed, shared, and controlled by the individual.
PET	Positron emission tomography.
Petition	See *Complaint*. Also used to denote the written instrument that initiates certain proceedings, such as bankruptcy.
Pharmacy patient profile	The specific record created for each patient in the pharmacy that typically notes the patient's name, diagnoses, weight, allergy history, and medications prescribed and dispensed.
PHI	Protected health information.
PHN	Public health nurse.
PHO	Physician-hospital organization.

PHR (14)	Personal health record.
PHRP	Program for Human Research Protection.
PHS	Public Health Service.
Physician assistant	A specially trained and licensed allied health professional who performs certain medical procedures previously reserved to the physician. PAs practice under the supervision of a physician.
Physician-hospital organization	An integrated delivery system that links hospitals and a group of physicians for the purpose of contracting directly with employers and managed care organizations. A PHO is a legal entity that allows physicians to continue to own their own practices and to see patients under the terms of a professional services agreement. This type of arrangement offers the opportunity to better market the services of both physicians and hospitals as a unified response to managed care.
PI	Performance improvement; process improvement.
PIAA	Physician Insurers Association of America.
PICU	Pediatric intensive care unit.
PIE (9)	Problem, interventions, and evaluations of interventions.
PIP	Personal injury protection.
PL	Professional liability.
Plaintiff	A person who brings a civil lawsuit.
Pleadings	The formal allegations by the parties involved in a lawsuit that delineate the claims and defenses of each party and request judgment by the court prior to resolution.
PM	Preventive maintenance.
PMA	Premarket approval application.
PoC (10)	Plan of correction.
Policy	A predetermined course of action established as a guide toward accepted business strategies and objectives.
POMR (9)	Problem-oriented medical record.
POS	Point of service.
Positron emission tomography	An imaging technique that tracks metabolism and responses to therapy. Used in cardiology, neurology, and oncology; particularly effective in evaluating brain and nervous system disorders.
Postloss damage control	Any of a number of initiatives taken after a potentially compensable event to build rapport with the patient and family and to decrease the likelihood or severity of a subsequent claim.
Potentially compensable event	An occurrence for which a claim can be reasonably anticipated but for which no claim has yet been asserted.
PPE	Personal protective equipment.
PPO	Preferred provider organization.
PPS	Prospective payment system.

Practice guidelines	Formal procedures and techniques for the treatment of specific medical conditions that help physicians achieve optimal results. Practice guidelines are developed by medical societies and medical research organization such as the AMA and the Agency for Health Care Policy and Research, as well as many HMOs, insurers, and business coalitions. Practice guidelines serve as educational support for physicians and as quality assurance and accountability measures for managed care plans.
Precedent	A previously decided case that turned on the same facts, circumstances, or legal theory as the case under consideration. Lower courts are bound to follow precedents set by higher courts in the jurisdiction in which the lower court is located. Cases decided by courts in other jurisdictions may be considered "persuasive authority" by the court rendering judgment in a given case. In this event, the court may follow the decision of the other court, although it is not legally required to do so. The doctrine requiring the binding effect of precedent is called *stare decisis.*
Preemption	Doctrine adopted by the U.S. Supreme Court holding that certain matters are of such a national, as opposed to local, character that federal laws take precedence over state laws.
Preexisting condition	A physical or mental condition that an insured has prior to the effective date of coverage. Policies may exclude coverage for such condition for a specified period of time.
Preferred provider organization	A plan that contracts with independent providers at a discount for services. Generally, a PPO's network of providers is limited in size. Patients usually have free choice to select other providers but are given strong financial incentives to select one of the designated preferred providers. Unlike an HMO, a PPO is not a prepaid plan but does use some utilization management techniques. PPO arrangements can be either insured or self-funded. An "insurer-sponsored PPO" combines a large network of providers and utilization management programs; an "administrative-sponsored PPO" combines a large network of providers, utilization management programs, administrative services, and healthcare insurance. A "self-funded PPO" generally excludes administrative and insurance services from the plan package. However, employers can purchase these services separately.
Preparation (17)	Readiness, to make ready.
Preventable adverse event	An adverse event that could have been avoided if actions were taken before the final step of the process.
Prevention (17)	Action to make sure something does not happen; a risk control technique that decreases the probability of an event occurring.
Primary care	Basic healthcare, including initial diagnosis and treatment, preventive services, maintenance of chronic conditions, and referral to specialists.

Prior acts coverage	Insurance coverage that extends a claims-made policy to claims that occurred before the inception date of the policy but subsequent to a specified retroactive date for which a claim is made during the policy period. Sometimes referred to as *Nose coverage.*
Privileged communication	The exchange of information in an environment of confidentiality. A breach in privileged communication can result in a civil suit or tort.
Privileging (delineation of clinical privileges)	The process of granting specific clinical privileges, based on training, experience, and competency, for individuals credentialed to provide healthcare services under medical staff bylaws.
Privity (4)	A derivative interest founded on a contract or a connection between two parties; a mutuality of interest.
PRN	*Pro re nata,* Latin for "on an as-needed basis."
Procedure	A method by which a policy can be accomplished; it provides instructions necessary to carry out a policy statement.
Professional corporation	A corporation formed by individuals to practice their profession (as by physicians to practice medicine). The PC is typically licensed to practice the profession of the owners. Only members of the profession can be owners (shareholders) of the PC.
Professional liability insurance	Coverage for liability arising from the rendering of or failure to render professional services.
Promulgation	The process for creating rules or regulations. It typically involves announcement of a proposed regulation, allowance of a reasonable period for public comment, consideration of the comments received, and announcement of the final regulation.
Property coverage	Insurance on buildings, their contents, attached equipment, and equipment used for cleaning and maintenance.
Prospective payment system	A payment method in which the payment a hospital will receive for patient treatment is set up in advance; hospitals keep the difference if they incur costs less than the fixed price in treating the patient, and they absorb any loss if their costs exceed the fixed price. Also called "prospective pricing."
Protected concerted activity	A group activity that seeks to modify wages or working conditions.
Protected health information	Medical record information and other individually identifiable information for which privacy protection is afforded under HIPAA.
Provider-sponsored organization	A public or private entity established or organized and operated by a healthcare provider or a group of affiliated healthcare providers that performs a substantial proportion of services under the Medicare+Choice contract and shares substantial financial risk.
Provider stop-loss coverage (13)	Reimbursement to healthcare providers, subject to daily limitations and coinsurance requirements, for losses in excess of a stipulated amount per member per year.
PSA	Prostate-specific antigen.
PSDA	Patient Self-Determination Act.

PSES (6)	Patient safety evaluation system.
PSET (6)	Patient Safety Event Taxonomy.
PSO	Provider-sponsored organization.
PSQIA (6)	Patient Safety and Quality Improvement Act of 2005.
PSRS (6)	Patient Safety Reporting System.
PSWP (6)	Patient safety work product.
PT	Physical therapy.
PTO	Paid time off.
Punitive damages	Damages sought or awarded to punish or deter a defendant or others from similar conduct rather than to compensate the injured party. The awarding of punitive damages generally requires a showing of gross negligence or willful and wanton misconduct. Such damages are not insurable in some jurisdictions and may be excluded by insurance policies. Also known as "exemplary damages."
Q	
QA	Quality assurance.
QAPI	Quality assessment and performance improvement.
QI	Quality improvement.
QIO	Quality improvement organization.
QS	Quality system regulation for medical devices (21 CFR 820).
Quality assurance	Attempts by managed care organizations to measure and monitor the quality of care delivered.
Quality improvement organizations	QIOs are private contractor organizations working under the auspices of CMS to improve the effectiveness, efficiency, economy, and quality of services delivered to Medicare beneficiaries QIOs are required under sections 1152–1154 of the Social Security Act. CMS contracts with one QIO in each state, the District of Columbia, Puerto Rico, and the U.S. Virgin Islands to serve as that state or jurisdiction's QIO contractor. QIO contracts are three years in duration, with each three-year cycle referenced as an ordinal statement of work (SOW).
Quality of care	The degree to which health services for individuals and populations increase the likelihood of desired health outcomes and are consistent with current professional knowledge.
Quid pro quo	Latin for "this for that": something received in exchange for something given.
Qui tam plaintiff	A plaintiff in an action under the False Claims Act that is brought on behalf of the federal government. The False Claims Act prohibits the presentation of false claims to the federal government. (*Qui tam* is the start of a Latin phrase meaning "Who sues on behalf of the king and himself.")
Qui tam relator	One who brings an action on behalf of the government (originally on behalf of the king).

R

RAC (8)	Recombinant DNA Advisory Committee.
RAC	Rent-a-captive.
Radio-frequency identification (14)	Technology that incorporates the use of electromagnetic or electrostatic coupling in the radio-frequency portion of the electromagnetic spectrum to uniquely identify an object, animal, or person.
RBC	Red blood cell count.
RCA	Root cause analysis.
RCRA	Resource Conservation and Recovery Act.
Realm of control (15)	An area over which one exercises control; span of control.
Reasonable accommodation	Under the Americans With Disabilities Act, actions required by an employer to allow an otherwise qualified individual with a disability to perform a specific job. Reasonable accommodations include modifications to work processes and schedules and to physical facilities that are not "unduly burdensome."
Reconstruction Civil Rights Acts	Post-Civil War federal legislation (42 USC 1981, 1983) prohibiting certain types of racial discrimination.
Recovery (17)	Postevent activities to restore an organization's operation to the same status as before an event.
Regulation	An enactment issued (promulgated) by a regulatory (nonelected) agency. Regulations must be promulgated pursuant to a statute that gives the agency the authority to do so and typically must go through a promulgation process.
Rehabilitation Act	Prohibits discrimination on the basis of disability in programs conducted by federal agencies, in programs receiving federal financial assistance, in federal employment, and in the employment practices of federal contractors.
Reimbursement (9)	Compensating a person or entity for an expense; to pay back, refund, or pay.
Reinsurance	A contractual arrangement involving the purchase of insurance by an "insurer" from "another insurer" to protect against extraordinary losses.
Release	A document executed by the plaintiff, usually in exchange for a monetary settlement, that releases the defendant from any further obligation or threat of suit.
Reliability (15)	Producing similar results with different users.
Rent-a-captive	A captive insurance company owned by investors rather than insureds and organized to insure or reinsure third-party risks.
Replacement cost (13)	Basis for insurance reimbursement that is defined by the cost to repair or replace without any deduction for depreciation.
Reporting of claims (11)	The process by which claims are reported to parties in an organization, such as the risk manager, and external to the organization, such as to the organization's insurance company.

Request for admission	A set of questions served on a party in litigation during discovery that asks that party to admit or deny the allegations presented.
Request for production	A written set of requests served on a party in litigation during discovery that asks the party to produce tangible things (records, photographs, equipment, and so on).
Request for proposal (6)	A structured process by which an organization will invite external parties (vendors) to respond to their request for services.
Reservation of rights (11)	An insurance carrier's attempt to preserve the rights to deny coverage at a later date even though the carrier may initially investigate and defend a claim.
Reserves	Money set aside, based on estimates of the amount that will ultimately be required to settle a claim or pay a judgment ("indemnity reserve") and to provide for a defense and pay other allocated expenses related to managing a claim ("expense reserve").
Res ipsa loquitur	Latin for "The thing speaks for itself"; a legal theory that applies in situations where the instrumentality was in the defendant's exclusive control and the accident was one that ordinarily could not happen in the absence of negligence.
Resource Conservation and Recovery Act (18)	Authorizes the EPA to regulate the dumping of solid and hazardous waste. It also provides the EPA with the authority to regulate underground storage tanks.
Respondeat superior	Latin for "Let the master answer"; a doctrine of law under which the employer is responsible for the legal consequences of the acts and omissions of the employees who are acting within the scope of employment. While the employee is also generally liable for his or her own negligence, the employer remains vicariously liable.
Response (17)	One of four categories in emergency management.
Responsiveness (15)	One of the characteristics of a good measure. The item being measured is responsive or sensitive to risk management activities.
Restraint	Restriction of a person's freedom of movement. A "chemical restraint" is a medication used to control behavior or to restrict the patient's freedom of movement that is not a standard treatment for the patient's medical or psychiatric condition. A "physical restraint" is any manual method or physical or mechanical device, material, or equipment attached or adjacent to the patient's body that restricts freedom of movement or normal access to the body.
Retrospective premium plan	An insurance policy for which an initial deposit premium is paid, with the ultimate premium determined based on the loss experience of the insured. Some plans adjust the premium based on losses incurred (which include reserves for claims not yet settled), while others make adjustments based on paid losses only. Common in workers' compensation insurance programs.
Reuse	Using a single-use device more than once, as after reconditioning.

Reviewable sentinel event	An event that resulted in an unanticipated death or major permanent loss of function not related to the natural course of the patient's illness or underlying condition.
RFID (14)	Radio-frequency identification.
RFP	Request for proposals.
Risk	The chance of loss. "Pure risk" is uncertainty as to whether loss will occur. "Speculative risk" is uncertainty about an event that could produce loss. Pure risk is insurable, but speculative risk usually is not.
Risk acceptance	The decision not to transfer an identified risk but instead to assume its financial consequences.
Risk-adjusted data	Data that have gone through the process of matching different groups in a manner that takes into account significant differences and equalizes them prior to performing comparisons. For example, prior to comparing mortality rates of different physicians, the patient population groups are "risk-adjusted" to equalize for age and other clinical status differences.
Risk analysis	The process used by the person or persons assigned risk management functions to determine the potential severity of the loss from an identified risk, the probability that the loss will happen, and alternatives for dealing with the risk.
Risk avoidance	The decision not to undertake a particular activity because the risk associated with the activity is unacceptably high. This is the only risk control technique that completely eliminates the possibility of loss from a given exposure.
Risk control techniques	Techniques designed to prevent the likelihood of an occurrence or reduce the frequency of occurrences that give rise to losses or to minimize at the least possible cost those losses that strike an organization.
Risk financing	Any of a number of programs implemented to pay for the costs associated with property and casualty claims and associated expenses, including insurance, self-insurance, and captive insurance companies.
Risk identification	The process of identifying problems or potential problems that can result in loss.
Risk management	The process of making and carrying out decisions that will help prevent adverse consequences and minimize the negative effects of accidental losses on an organization.
Risk management ethics (2)	An articulated code of conduct to which a risk management professional must adhere if he or she is a member of the American Society for Healthcare Risk Management.
Risk management information system (14)	Systems used to automate the gathering, reporting, storage, retrieval, analysis, evaluation, benchmarking, and display of risk information.

Risk purchasing group	Groups of policyholders with similar risks who may group together to purchase liability insurance authorized by the Federal Liability Risk Retention Act of 1986. Authorization under the federal statute allows a group to be incorporated in one state but to purchase insurance in all states, subject to specific restrictions.
Risk reduction	Reducing the severity of losses that other risk control techniques do not prevent.
Risk retention group	A liability-only domestic insurance captive for a group whose members are engaged in similar activities.
Risk transfer	The procedure of shifting risk of loss to another party who agrees to accept it.
RMIS	Risk management information system.
RN	Registered nurse.
Root-cause analysis	A multidisciplinary process of study or analysis that uses a detailed, structured process to examine factors contributing to a specific outcome (such as an adverse event).
RPG	Risk purchasing group.
RPLU	Registered professional liability underwriter.
RRG	Risk retention group.
Rx	Prescription. (Originally the symbol ℞, standing for the first letter of the Latin word *recipe*, "take.")

S

Safe Medical Devices Act	Federal statute (21 USC 360 et seq.) governing the tracking of certain implantable medical devices and requiring reporting of patient deaths and serious injuries involving the use of medical devices or equipment.
Safety	Freedom from accidental harm.
Sarbanes-Oxley Act	The Public Company Accounting Reform and Investor Protection Act of 2002, also known as the Sarbanes-Oxley Act of 2002, introduced major changes to the regulation of financial practice and corporate governance. The legislation established new or enhanced standards for all U.S. public company boards, management, and public accounting firms. Named after Senator Paul Sarbanes and Representative Michael Oxley, who were its main architects.
SBAR (3)	Situation, background, assessment, and recommendation.
SBS	Sick building syndrome.
SC	Subcutaneous.
SCCM	Society of Critical Care Medicine.
SCHIP	State Children's Health Insurance Program.

Scorecard (15)	An evaluation tool that specifies the criteria a healthcare facility's key stakeholders will use to rate performance in relationship to the requirements.
SE	Sentinel event.
SEC	Securities and Exchange Commission.
Segregation	The separation of exposure units to reduce the uncertainty of losses by increasing the predictability of both loss frequency and severity.
Self-governing medical staff	The Joint Commission requirement that the hospital medical staff elect its own officers and approve its own bylaws and rules and regulations.
Self-insurance trust fund	A mechanism for funding claims and related expenses under a program of self-insurance whereby the insured establishes a segregated fund administered by a trustee, that is replenished from time to time according to actuarially determined estimates of future loss costs.
Self-insured retention	The portion of a claim that the insured is required to pay before the insurer begins to pay. This is similar to a deductible but is frequently funded through a mechanism such as a self-insurance trust fund and is larger than a deductible. The insured generally manages claims falling entirely within the SIR (or contracts with a third party to do so) so that the insurer is involved only if the amount of the claim exceeds or is anticipated to exceed the amount of the retention. Common in hospital professional liability programs.
Sentinel event	An unexpected occurrence involving death or serious physical or psychological injury or the risk thereof, including loss of limb or function. The phrase "or risk thereof" includes any process variation for which a recurrence would carry a significant chance of a serious adverse outcome.
Sentinel event policy (6)	A policy developed by The Joint Commission to encourage the self-reporting of medical errors to learn about the relative frequencies and underlying causes of sentinel events and to share lesions learned with other healthcare organizations, thereby reducing the risk of future sentinel events occurring.
Sentinel event reporting (3)	The voluntary reporting of a sentinel event to The Joint Commission.
Settlement	An agreement between the parties in which consideration is paid and the matter is concluded with respect to those parties. Settlement may occur at any time.
Severance agreement	A contract between an employer and a terminated employee. Generally, severance agreements provide a lump sum payment or a period of salary continuation in return for the employee's agreement not to make certain claims against the employer.

Sexual harassment	Any of a number of statutorily prohibited kinds of unwanted sexual contact, remarks, or conditions of employment. In "quid pro quo sexual harassment," participation in sexual activity or performance of sexual favors is made an explicit or implicit condition of employment. A "hostile environment" exists when jokes, comments, cartoons, or touching of a sexual nature in the workplace interfere with an employee's ability to perform his or her job comfortably.
Sharp-end (7)	See *Active failure.*
SICU	Surgical intensive care unit.
SIDS	Sudden infant death syndrome.
Single-payer system	A financing system such as Canada's in which a single entity—usually the government—pays for all covered healthcare services.
Single-point weakness	A step in the process so critical that its failure would result in system failure or in an adverse event.
Single-use device (10)	Devices manufactured for single use only.
SIR	Self-insured retention.
Skilled nursing facility	A facility, either freestanding or part of a hospital, that accepts patients in need of rehabilitation and medical care. To qualify for Medicare coverage, SNFs must be certified by Medicare and meet specific qualifications, including round-the-clock nursing coverage and availability of physical, occupational, and speech therapies.
Slander	A false and defamatory statement about a person.
Slip	Human error, usually occurring during an activity that the person is proficient in and is performing "automatically and hence somewhat inattentively."
SMDA	Safe Medical Devices Act.
SNF	Skilled nursing facility.
S.O.A.P. (9)	Subjective, objective, assessment, plan: a popular problem-oriented model of documentation for use in progress notes.
S.O.A.P.I.E.R. (9)	Subjective, objective, assessment, plan, interventions and evaluation, revision: a model of documentation that includes revision to the original plan of care.
SOB	Shortness of breath.
Special cause	A factor that intermittently and unpredictably causes a variation in a system.
SOM (10)	State Operating Manual.
Specials	The elements of a plaintiff's damages that can be computed with relative precision, including lost wages, medical expenses, and future expenses.
SSA	Social Security Act.
SSI	Supplemental security income.

SSN	Social Security number.
Stair stepping (11)	Periodic increases in the reserve by set amounts absent any circumstances that would support such an increase.
Standard	A minimum level or target range of acceptable performance or results. The American Society for Testing and Materials defines six types: (1) standard test methods: a procedure for identifying, measuring, and evaluating a material, product, or system; (2) standard specifications: a set of requirements to be satisfied and the procedures for determining whether each is satisfied; (3) standard practice: a recommended procedure for performing one or more specific operations or functions; (4) standard terminology: acceptable terms, definitions, descriptions, explanations, abbreviations, or acronyms; (5) standard guide: a series of options or instructions that suggest but do not dictate a specific course of action; and (6) standard classification: a systematic arrangement or division of products, systems, or services into groups based on similar characteristics.
Standard of care	As a measure of the competency of a medical professional, the typical level of skilled care and diligence exercised by members of the same professional or specialized field in light of the present state of medical and surgical science. In a legal proceeding, the degree to which the defendant acted as an ordinary, prudent person with similar training and skill would have acted in a similar situation. If the defendant's conduct falls below this standard, the defendant may be determined to have acted negligently.
Standing	The right or authority by which a person may bring and sustain a legal proceeding. It is normally conferred on a person who has suffered an injury or that person's legal proxy.
Stat	Immediately.
Statement of fault	An acknowledgment of responsibility for a specific event or outcome.
Statute	A law enacted by the elected legislature of a state or the federal government.
Statute of limitations	The legal deadline by which a claimant must file a claim for damages or be barred from so doing. Most jurisdictions extend the deadline for individuals who are injured as minors, and many include a discovery rule extending the deadline for individuals whose injuries were not readily discoverable.
Statute of repose	A statute that sets a maximum period of time in which a suit may be brought. This statute is always longer than the statute of limitations and is generally subject to fewer, if any, exceptions or extension provisions.
STD	Sexually transmitted disease; short-term disability.

Stop loss	Insurance coverage for healthcare and managed care organizations that have agreed in advance to accept financial risk for the provision of healthcare services under capitated managed care contracts. Stop-loss policies limit the losses experienced by such entities when utilization of services exceeds estimates.
Subacute care	A level of care that is between acute care and long-term care.
Subpoena	A document issued by the court commanding a person to appear at a certain time and place to give testimony.
Subpoena duces tecum	A form of subpoena requiring not only the appearance of the subpoenaed party but also the production of books, papers, and other items.
Subrogation	The process of collecting from the person responsible for damages. It allows the insurer who is making a payment to the insured to assume the insured's right of recovery against the third party responsible for the loss.
SUD	Single-use device.
Summary judgment	A judgment rendered by the court before a verdict because no material issue of fact exists and one party or other is entitled to a judgment as a matter of law.
Summons	A brief (usually one-page) document commanding a defendant to appear and answer before a court.
Supreme court	The highest appellate court in most states and the federal government. Appeals entered after trial of a lawsuit are ultimately heard by this tribunal.
Surety (13)	A party that guarantees the performance of another.
Surety bond	A three-part contract in which two parties, the surety and the principal (or obligor), agree to be bound by a promise to a third party, the obligee. If the principal defaults on the promise, the surety, for a premium paid in advance by the principal, steps in and fulfills the obligation. Surety bonds typical in the healthcare setting include patient trust fund bonds (to ensure that patient funds and valuables held by hospitals and nursing homes are appropriately safeguarded), performance bonds (to ensure that construction projects are completed as agreed), and various license bonds (to ensure appropriate performance of the licensee's duties). A surety who fulfills the obligations to the obligee may seek reimbursement from the principal.
Surge capacity	Reserve capacity in terms of staff, space, equipment, and supplies built into a healthcare provider's operations to accommodate emergency situations in which the demand for services may exceed normal levels.
Surgicenter	A healthcare facility that is physically separate from a hospital and provides prescheduled surgical services on an outpatient basis, generally at a lower cost than inpatient hospital care. Also called a *Freestanding ambulatory surgery center.*

Swing beds	Acute care hospital beds that can also be used for long-term care, depending on the needs of the patient and the community; only hospitals with fewer than one hundred beds located in a rural community, where long-term care may be inaccessible, are eligible to have swing beds.
System	A set of interdependent elements interacting to achieve a common aim. These elements may be both human and nonhuman (equipment, technologies, and so on).
Systemic or system-related issue	An issue that arises due to some design, process, or other operational aspect of a complex, multiple-entity "system" or multistep process.

T

T&A	Tonsillectomy and adenoidectomy.
Tail	The delay between an actual incident of malpractice or alleged action and the filing of a claim. An insurance company underwriting occurrence policies will be covering claims for many years after the policy has expired due to this long tail. In contrast, a claims-made policy covers only claims that are actually made during validity of the policy. Therefore, if you cancel your claims-made policy and wish to have continued coverage, you must purchase an extended reporting endorsement or tail coverage.
Tail coverage	Extended reporting endorsement.
TB	Tuberculosis.
Teaching hospital	A hospital that has an accredited medical residency training program and, typically, is affiliated with a medical school.
Telehealth	See *Telemedicine*.
Telemedicine	The use of telecommunications to provide medical information and services.
Tertiary care	Highly technical services for a patient who is in imminent danger of major disability or death.
Therapeutic privilege	A doctor's right to bar a patient's access to certain parts of the patient's medical records, out of a concern that the patient will not be able to cope with the information contained therein.
Third party	A party other than the insurer or the insured.
Third-party administrator	An independent organization that contracts to provide claims management services to a self-insured entity. Unlike insurance carriers, TPAs do not underwrite the insurance risk.
Third-party coverage (13)	Insurance coverage for a party other than the insured to make that person whole for loss or injury caused by the insured.
Third-party overclaim	A claim by an injured employee against a party other than his or her employer, such as the manufacturer of a machine involved in the injury, in which the third party brings the employer in as an additional defendant, as for failure to properly maintain the machine. Third-party overclaims fall outside workers' compensation coverage and are generally covered by employers' liability policies.

Threat envelope	In disaster planning, analysis of the types of occurrences most likely to occur, as well as those less likely but having particularly serious consequences for a community or organization for which it determines it must prepare.
Tight coupling	Dependence of each step of a process so closely on the preceding step that a variation in or adverse consequence resulting from the prior step affects the ensuing step and hence the entire desired outcome.
Title VII of the Civil Rights Act of 1964 (4)	Antidiscrimination legislation prohibiting harassment and discrimination of an employee based on that employee's race, gender, and national origin. Also prohibits sexual harassment.
Tomography	A diagnostic technique using X-ray photographs that do not show the shadows of structures before and behind the section under scrutiny.
Tort	A private or civil wrong or injury for which the court will provide a remedy in the form of an action for damages.
Tortfeasor	Party deemed liable as a result of the party's acts or omissions.
Total cost of risk (15)	A report that captures a financial snapshot of the cost to an organization of a risk management program across all lines of coverage and operating units.
Total quality management	A systematic set of processes and tools designed to improve quality on an ongoing basis.
Toxic Substances Control Act (18)	Federal statute that gives the Environmental Protection Agency the authority to track and control the toxic or potentially toxic chemicals used by industry.
TPA	Third-party administrator.
TPO	Treatment, payment, and operations.
TQI	Total quality improvement.
TQM	Total quality management.
Transitional duty	Altered working conditions put in place for an injured employee during the employee's period of recovery. Also known as "alternative duty," "light duty," and "modified duty."
Transparency	Full disclosure to the consumer or patient, as opposed to providing limited information or a policy of secrecy.
Treaty	A contract specifying that a reinsurer agrees in advance to accept certain classes of exposures. The insurer assumes underwriting authority on behalf of the reinsurer.
Triage	When multiple patients present for treatment, evaluating the urgency and seriousness of each patient's condition and establishing a priority list for their care to ensure that medical and nursing staff and facilities are used most efficiently.
Trial court	Usually, the lowest-level court in a given jurisdiction and the court in which the actual trial of the matter will be conducted.

Trust (12)	A funding vehicle that, in its simplest terms, is a bank account administered by an independent third party (trustee); a common form of self-insurance for healthcare organizations.
Trustee (5)	An individual or organization appointed to hold or manage and invest assets for the benefit of another.
TSCA	Toxic Substances Control Act.
Tx	Treatment.

U

UCL	Upper control limit.
Ultrasonography	An imaging technology for outlining various tissues and organs in the body.
UM	Utilization management.
Umbrella coverage	An insurance policy providing limits above those of a primary policy, such as for professional and general liability and auto liability. Umbrella policies may also include some specific coverage not found in the underlying policies.
Unanticipated outcome	A result of a treatment or procedure that differs significantly from what was anticipated.
Underground storage tank (UST) (18)	A tank that has at least ten percent of its volume underground. Generally referred to in terms of an "underground storage tank system," which includes the tank and any piping attached to the tank. USTs often house petroleum and other hazardous materials.
Underuse	Failure to provide a healthcare service or procedure for persons for whom it was clinically indicated or needed.
Underwriter	An insurance company employee who makes determinations regarding the acceptability of a given risk for insurance coverage and for specific terms, conditions, and pricing of such coverage.
Underwriting	The process of identifying, evaluating, and classifying the potential level of risk represented by a group seeking insurance coverage in order to determine appropriate pricing and administrative feasibility. The chief purpose of underwriting is to make sure that the potential for loss is within the range for which the premiums were established. Underwriting can also refer to the acceptance of risk.
United Network for Organ Sharing (10)	A nonprofit scientific and educational organization that brings together medicine, technology, public policy, and science to facilitate every organ transplant performed in the United States. UNOS ensures that all organs are procured and distributed in a fair and timely manner.
United States Pharmacopeia	The U.S. Pharmacopeia is a nongovernmental, nonprofit public health organization whose independent volunteer experts work under strict conflict-of-interest rules to set scientific standards for all prescription and over-the-counter medicines and other healthcare products manufactured or sold in the United States. They also set widely recognized standards for food ingredients and dietary supplements and for the quality, purity, strength, and consistency of these products critical to the public health.

Universal coverage	Making healthcare services available to all citizens.
UNOS (10)	United Network for Organ Sharing.
Upper control limit	Used in quality control charts, it is a horizontal line representing the uppermost limit for samples to evaluate to. It is the upper limit of process capability in quality control for data points above the control (average) line. Opposite of LCL.
UR	Utilization review.
URAC	The former Utilization Review Accreditation Commission, also known as the American Accreditation HealthCare Commission.
Urgent care	Care for injury, illness, or another type of condition (usually not life-threatening) that should be treated within twenty-four hours. Also refers to after-hours care and to a health plan's classification of hospital admissions as urgent, semiurgent, or elective.
URL	Uniform resource locator, also known as a "Web address."
USA PATRIOT Act	Federal legislation (officially titled the Uniting and Strengthening America by Providing Appropriate Tools Required to Intercept and Obstruct Terrorism Act) that enhances the ability of law enforcement to deter and detect acts of terrorism, including cyberintelligence gathering, wiretapping, and other means of gathering information from designated private records.
USC	United States Code.
USERRA	Uniformed Services Employment and Reemployment Rights Act.
USP	United States Pharmacopeia.
USPHS	United States Public Health Service.
UST (18)	Underground storage tank.
Utilization	Pattern of usage for a particular medical service such as hospital care or physician visits.
Utilization management	The function of monitoring the utilization of healthcare resources by individual patients (to verify that surgery was indeed required or that the length of a hospital stay is justified, for example). Also referred to as *Case management*.
Utilization review	An evaluation of the care and services that patients receive, based on preestablished criteria and standards.
V	
VAERS (6)	Vaccine Adverse Event Reporting System: a program for vaccine safety of the CDC and the FDA. It collects, analyzes, and disseminates information about adverse events (possible side effects) that occur after the administration of U.S. licensed vaccines.
VAHRPAP	Veterans Administration Human Research Protection Accreditation Program.
Validity (15)	The degree to which a test measures what it is designed to measure; support for the intended conclusion drawn from the results; one of the characteristic of a good measure.

VBAC	Vaginal birth after C-section.
VDRL	Venereal Disease Research Laboratory. VDRL is a screening test for syphilis that measures antibodies that can be produced by *Treponema pallidum,* the bacteria that causes syphilis.
Venue	The physical location, or the tribunal in that location, in which a legal proceeding may be brought. This is usually the place where the injury is alleged to have occurred.
Verdict	The formal decision or definitive answer of a jury impaneled to hear and decide the facts of a legal proceeding, which is reported to the court.
VHA	Veterans Health Administration.
Vicarious liability	The imposition of liability on one person for the actionable conduct of another, based solely on a relationship between the two persons, such as the liability of an employer for the acts of an employee.
VIP	Very important person.
Voir dire	The process of questioning jurors, prior to seating them, to determine if any jurors have knowledge of the case, personally know or know of the parties, or may otherwise have preconceptions that would prevent them from hearing and deciding the case impartially.
Volume-outcome relationship	The basis of a theory that for certain procedures, higher volume (by either a specific provider or a hospital) is associated with better health outcomes.
Voluntary protection program (18)	A voluntary program created by OSHA in 1982 that recognizes businesses and work sites that show excellence in occupational safety and health and that are committed to effective employee protection beyond the requirements of OSHA standards.
Volunteer Protection Act of 1997 (5)	Signed into law by President Clinton in 1997, this law provides immunity from tort claims that might be filed against the volunteers of nonprofit organizations.
VPP (18)	Voluntary protection program.
Vulnerability analysis (17)	The process of identifying, quantifying, and prioritizing (or ranking) the vulnerabilities in a system.
W	
WAG (18)	Waste anesthetic gases.
Waiver of subrogation	A contractual provision in which one party agrees not to seek indemnification by the other in the event of a subsequent loss for which the second party may bear responsibility.
Warrant (18)	A type of writ that is a formal written order issued by a body with administrative or judicial jurisdiction that commands or authorizes a person to do a particular thing. In modern usage, this public body is normally a court.

War risk exclusion	An exclusion found in many types of insurance policies excluding losses caused by acts of war or military action.
Waste anesthetic gas (18)	Anesthetic gas and vapors that leak out into the surrounding room during medical and surgical procedures.
WC	Workers' compensation.
Whistleblower	An individual, frequently an employee or former employee, who reports unlawful activity, such as healthcare fraud and abuse or OSHA violations, to the government or an administrative agency. Some statutes provide for the whistleblower to receive a share of fines levied against the organization for making the report. Most statutes prohibit retaliatory discharge or other discriminatory actions against an employee who makes such a report.
WHO	World Health Organization.
WIC	Women and Infant Children Program.
Withholds	A provision in some managed care contracts withholding a portion of a healthcare provider's reimbursement until the end of a specific time period. If certain utilization targets are met for the period, the provider then receives the withheld reimbursement payments.
WBC	White blood cell count.
WMD	Weapons of mass destruction.
Workers' compensation	Statutory obligation requiring employers to provide compensation to employees for injuries arising out of and in the course of their employment.
Working memory	The concentrated short-term memory used by persons when learning any new task or process.
Worried well	Individuals who, in a disaster, contact healthcare providers for information or present at treatment sites for reassurance, even though they have no specific injuries or symptoms, inhibiting the provider's ability to assess and treat those truly in need of medical services.

Index

Page references followed by *fig* indicate illustrated figures; *t* indicate tables; *b* indicate boxes; *e* indicate exhibits.